Tracheostomy

Terence Pires de Farias
Editor

Tracheostomy

A Surgical Guide

Springer

Editor
Terence Pires de Farias, M.D., Ph.D., M.Sc., Researcher
National Cancer Institute
INCA, Rio de Janeiro, Brazil

ISBN 978-3-319-67866-5 ISBN 978-3-319-67867-2 (eBook)
https://doi.org/10.1007/978-3-319-67867-2

Library of Congress Control Number: 2017964088

Printed on acid-free paper

This Springer imprint is published by Springer Nature
The registered company is Springer International Publishing AG
The registered company address is: Gewerbestrasse 11, 6330 Cham, Switzerland

I dedicate this book to all patients suffering from head and neck cancer or any serious illness that causes an ICU hospitalization and requires a temporary or permanent tracheostomy. I especially dedicate it to my wife Izaura and our beloved Valentina, the most important part of our lives; to my parents, who have always boosted me in my career; and finally, to my preceptors, who taught me the art of head and neck surgery, allowing me to disseminate this information to the younger generations.

Terence Pires de Farias

Foreword

Surgical procedures range from safe and simple to extremely complex, technically demanding, and potentially life-threatening. In this realm, tracheostomy is often thought of as a mundane topic for discussion because it is a relatively safe, simple, and often lifesaving procedure. However, if embarked upon without foresight, proper planning, and an assessment of the clinical scenario (including the patient, problem, anatomy, and pathology), without adequate support, or in a suboptimal environment, tracheostomy can be a very hazardous and potentially life-threatening procedure. Dr. Terence Farias and his coauthors are to be commended for assembling this comprehensive and exhaustive treatise on the topic of tracheostomy. Their knowledge, wisdom, judgment, and experience are reflected in each chapter.

The book begins with an interesting chapter on history, in which the authors delve into the detailed anatomy of the trachea. Photographs of cadaver dissection are accompanied by beautiful artwork to illustrate the anatomy. An exhaustive listing of tracheostomy tubes and their specific indications follows. A series of chapters on surgical technique follows, describing conventional and percutaneous procedures in great detail. The advantages, disadvantages, pearls, and pitfalls of both approaches are discussed.

The next chapters address the specific scenarios and indications for tracheostomy, with detailed discussions on the specific issues pertaining to each condition. Throughout these chapters, photographs of case examples and artwork are included to illustrate the issues. The remaining chapters in the techniques section focus on tracheostomy and cricothyrotomy in trauma and orthognathic surgery, including the appropriate place to perform the procedure—either bedside, in the intensive care unit, or in the operating room. Furthermore, an important chapter on difficult endotracheal intubation addresses management of the difficult airway. The final chapters deal with complications, postoperative care, rehabilitation, and decannulation.

This comprehensive text on tracheostomy covers the depth and breadth of the topic. The book is a "must read" for the surgical trainee, while also being a superb reference for surgeons and anesthesiologists who are faced with a difficult airway or a challenging tracheostomy. Thus, this book should have a definite place in the libraries of medical schools, hospitals, departments of surgery and anesthesia, and even in the operating room, intensive care unit, and emergency rooms. The text is an invaluable resource on this common but occasionally difficult operation.

Jatin Shah, M.D., Ph.D. (Hon), D.Sc. (Hon)
Head and Neck Oncology
Memorial Sloan Kettering Cancer Center
New York, NY, USA

Contents

Contributors

Juliana Maria de Almeida Vital, M.D. Head and Neck Department, Irmandade Santa Casa de Sao Paulo, Sao Paulo, SP, Brazil

Head and Neck Surgeon, Private Practice, São Paulo, SP, Brazil

Lica Arakawa-Sugueno, Ph.D., Speech Therapist. School of Medicine, University of São Paulo-USP, São Paulo, SP, Brazil

Carlos Manoel Mendonça de Araujo, M.D. Department of Radiotherapy, Brazilian National Cancer Institute, Rio de Janeiro, RJ, Brazil

Marcelle Morgana Vieira de Assis, P.T. Physiotherapist, Department of Home Care, Waldemar de Alcantara General State Hospital, Fortaleza, Brazil

Carlos Eduardo Santa Ritta Barreira, M.D., Ph.D. Department of Head and Neck Surgery, Santa Luzia Hospital, Brasília, DF, Brazil

Antonio Augusto T. Bertelli, M.D. Departamento de Cirurgia da Irmandade da Santa Casa de Misericórdia de São Paulo, Faculdade de Ciências Médicas da Santa Casa de São Paulo, São Paulo, SP, Brazil

Antônio Albuquerque de Brito, D.D.S., M.D., M.Sc. Private Practice, Belo Horizonte, MG, Brazil

Marcelo de Camargo Millen, M.D. Head and Neck surgeon of Barra Mansa, RJ, Brazil

Monique Pierosan Cardoso, M.D. Hospital Universitário Evangélico de Curitiba – Paraná, Curitiba, PR, Brazil

André Leonardo de Castro Costa, M.D., M.Sc. Department of Stomatology, Federal University of Bahia, Salvador, BA, Brazil

Department of Head and Neck Surgery, Aristides Maltez Hospital, Salvador, BA, Brazil

Department of Head and Neck Surgery, Portuguese Hospital, Salvador, BA, Brazil

Paulo Jose de Cavalcanti Siebra, M.D. Department of Head and Neck Surgery, Brazilian National Cancer Institute (Instituto Nacional de Câncer - INCA/MS), Rio de Janeiro, RJ, Brazil

Ricardo Lopes da Cruz, M.D. Private Practice, Rio de Janeiro, RJ, Brazil

Department of Craniomaxillofacial Surgery, National Institute of Traumatology and Orthopedics, Rio de Janeiro, RJ, Brazil

Fernando Luiz Dias, Chairman, M.D., Ph.D., M.Sc., F.A.C.S. Head and Neck Surgery Department, Brazilian National Cancer Institute – INCA, Rio de Janeiro, RJ, Brazil

Head and Neck Department, Pontifical Catholic University of Rio de Janeiro, Rio de Janeiro, RJ, Brazil

Thiago Pereira Diniz, M.D. Department of General Surgery, University of the State of Piauí, Piauí, Brazil

Terence Pires de Farias, M.D., Ph.D., M.Sc., Researcher. Department of Head and Neck Surgery, Brazilian National Cancer Institute—INCA, Rio de Janeiro, RJ, Brazil

Department of Head and Neck Surgery, Pontifical Catholic University, Rio de Janeiro, RJ, Brazil

Luciana Paiva Farias, MSc., Speech Therapist. Sírio-Libanês Hospital, São Paulo, SP, Brazil

Department of Neurolinguistics, Faculty of Medicine, Hospital Das Clinicas, University of São Paulo, São Paulo, SP, Brazil

Federal Speech Therapist Council, Belo Horizonte, MG, Brazil

Gustavo Trindade Henriques-Filho, M.D. Intensive Care Specialist by the Brazilian Intensive Care Medicine Association (AMIB) and Brazilian Medical Association (AMB), Recife, Pernambuco, Brazil

Santa Joana Recife Hospital, Recife, Pernambuco, Brazil

Oswaldo Cruz University Hospital, Universidade de Pernambuco (HUOC/UPE), Recife, Pernambuco, Brazil

Jorge Pinho Filho, M.D., F.A.C.S. Memorial Hospital São José, Recife, PE, Brazil

Pedro Collares Maia Filho, M.D. Head and Neck Surgeon, Department of Home Care, Waldemar de Alcantara General State Hospital, Fortaleza, Brazil

Adilis Stepple da Fonte Neto, M.D. Department of Head and Neck Surgery, Integral Medicine Institute of Pernambuco (Instituto de Medicina Integral de Pernambuco-IMIP), Recife, PE, Brazil

Pernambuco Cancer Hospital (Hospital de Câncer de Pernambuco), Recife, PE, Brazil

Department of Head and Neck Surgery, Brazilian Head and Neck Surgery Society (Sociedade Brasileira de Cirurgia de Cabeça e Pescoço), São Paulo, SP, Brazil

Carlos Eduardo Ferraz Freitas, M.D. Intensive Care Specialist by the Brazilian Intensive Care Medicine Association (AMIB) and Brazilian Medical Association (AMB), Recife, Pernambuco, Brazil

Santa Joana Recife Hospital, Recife, Pernambuco, Brazil

Esperança Recife Hospital, Recife, Pernambuco, Brazil

Esperança Recife Hospital, Olinda, Pernambuco, Brazil

Marcos Antonio Cavalcanti Gallindo, M.D. Intensive Care Specialist by the Brazilian Intensive Care Medicine Association (AMIB) and Brazilian Medical Association (AMB), Recife, Pernambuco, Brazil

Santa Joana Recife Hospital, Recife, Pernambuco, Brazil

Agamenon Magalhães Hospital, Recife, Pernambuco, Brazil

Royal Portuguese Hospital, Recife, Pernambuco, Brazil

Rodrigo Gonçalves, D.D.S. Department of Bucco-Maxillo-Facial Surgery and Traumatology, Hospital Santa Casa de Piracicaba, Piracicaba, SP, Brazil

Antonio José Gonçalves, M.D. Departamento de Cirurgia da Irmandade da Santa Casa de Misericórdia de São Paulo, Faculdade de Ciências Médicas da Santa Casa de São Paulo, São Paulo, SP, Brazil

Norberto Kodi Kavabata, M.D. Departamento de Cirurgia da Irmandade da Santa Casa de Misericórdia de São Paulo, Faculdade de Ciências Médicas da Santa Casa de São Paulo, São Paulo, SP, Brazil

William Kikuchi, M.D. Departamento de Cirurgia da Irmandade da Santa Casa de Misericórdia de São Paulo, Faculdade de Ciências Médicas da Santa Casa de São Paulo, São Paulo, SP, Brazil

Rafael Vianna Locio, M.S., (Medical Student). Faculdade Pernambucana de Saúde/IMIP – Maternity Childhood Institute of Pernanbuco, Recife, PE, Brazil

Fernando Cesar A. Lima, D.D.S., M.D. Department of Oral and Maxillofacial Surgery, Hospital Federal dos Servidores, Rio de Janeiro, RJ, Brazil

Private Practice, Rio de Janeiro, RJ, Brazil

Ronald Lima, M.D., Ph.D. National Cancer Institute – INCA, Rio de Janeiro, RJ, Brazil

Catherine Lumley, M.D. Department of Otolaryngology–Head and Neck Surgery, Georgetown University, Washington, DC, USA

Gabriel Manfro, M.D., Ph.D. Department of Head and Neck Surgery, Santa Teresinha University Hospital, Universidade do Oeste de Santa Catarina, UNOESC, Joaçaba, Santa Catarina, Brazil

Marcus Antônio de Mello Borba, Ph.D. Faculty of Medicine, Department of Experimental Surgery and Surgical Specialties, Federal University of Bahia, Salvador, BA, Brazil

Department of Head and Neck Surgery, Portuguese Hospital, Salvador, BA, Brazil

Department of Head and Neck Surgery, Aristides Maltez Hospital, Salvador, BA, Brazil

Marcelo Benedito Menezes, M.D. Departamento de Cirurgia da Irmandade da Santa Casa de Misericórdia de São Paulo, Faculdade de Ciências Médicas da Santa Casa de São Paulo, São Paulo, SP, Brazil

Sissi Monteiro, M.D. Head and Neck Department of the Federal Hospital of Bonsucesso, Bonsucesso, RJ, Brazil

Brazilian National Cancer Institute—INCA, Rio de Janeiro, RJ, Brazil

Ruiter Diego de Moraes Botinelly, M.D. Department of Head and Neck Surgery, National Cancer Institute—INCA, Rio de Janeiro, RJ, Brazil

Diego Chaves Rezende Morais, M.D. Department of Radiotherapy, Brazilian National Cancer Institute, Rio de Janeiro, RJ, Brazil

Adriana Eliza Brasil Moreira, M.D. Department of Head and Neck Surgery, Hospital Santa Casa de Piracicaba, Piracicaba, SP, Brazil

Maria Eduarda Lima de Moura, M.S., (Medical Student). Faculdade de Medicina Nova Esperança (FAMENE), João Pessoa, PB, Brazil

Marianne Yumi Nakai, M.D. Departamento de Cirurgia da Irmandade da Santa Casa de Misericórdia de São Paulo, Faculdade de Ciências Médicas da Santa Casa de São Paulo, São Paulo, SP, Brazil

Lúcio Noleto, M.D., Ph.D. Department of Head and Neck Surgery, University of The State of Piaui, Teresina, Piaui, Brazil

Juliana Fernandes de Oliveira, M.D. Department of Head and Neck Surgery, Brazilian National Cancer Institute – INCA, Rio de Janeiro, RJ, Brazil

Alexandre Ferreira Oliveira, M.D., Ph.D. Department of Surgery, Federal University of Juiz de Fora, Juiz de Fora, MG, Brazil

Jose Gabriel Miranda da Paixão, M.D. Department of Head and Neck Surgery, Brazilian National Cancer Institute (Instituto Nacional de Câncer – INCA/MS), Rio de Janeiro, RJ, Brazil

Maria Beatriz Nogueira Pascoal, M.D., Ph.D. Department of Head and Neck Surgery, São Leopoldo Mandic Medical School, Campus of Campinas, Campinas, Brazil

Department of Head and Neck Surgery, Dr. Mário Gatti Municipal Hospital, Campinas, SP, Brazil

Department of Integrated Clinical Meeting, São Leopoldo Mandic Medical School, Campus of Campinas, Campinas, Brazil

Roberta Melo Calvoso Paulon, Ph.D., MSc. Speech Therapist. Sírio-Libanês Hospital, São Paulo, SP, Brazil

Department of Oncology, A.C. Camargo Cancer Center, São Paulo, SP, Brazil

Oswaldo Cruz Foundation, Rio de Janeiro, RJ, Brazil

Paola Andrea Galbiatti Pedruzzi, M.D., M.Sc. Hospital Erasto Gaertner de Curitiba –Paraná, Curitiba, PR, Brazil

Lucio Pereira, M.D. Department of Otolaryngology, Hofstra Northwell School of Medicine, Long Island Jewish Medical Center, New Hyde Park, NY, USA

Marina Azzi Quintanilha, M.D. Department of Head and Neck Surgery, Santa Luzia Hospital, Brasília, DF, Brazil

Ricardo Mai Rocha, M.D. Assistant Professor of Head and Neck Surgery, Universidade Federal do Espirito Santo, Vitoria, Brazil

Assistant Professor of Head and Neck Surgery, Faculdade Brasileira Multivix, Vitoria, Brazil

Pedro Rotava, M.D., M.Sc. National Cancer Institute – INCA, Rio de Janeiro, RJ, Brazil

José Francisco de Sales Chagas, M.D., Ph.D. Federal University, São Paulo, SP, Brazil

Department of Head and Neck Surgery, São Leopoldo Mandic Medical School, Campus of Campinas, Campinas, Brazil

São Leopoldo Mandic Medical School, Campus of Araras, Araras, Brazil

Leonardo Vianna Salomão, M.D. National Cancer Institute-INCA, Rio de Janeiro, RJ, Brazil

Daniela Silva Santos, M.D. Department of Head and Neck Surgery, Portuguese Hospital, Salvador, BA, Brazil

Dorio Jose Coelho Silva, M.D. Department of Head and Neck Surgery, Evangelic Hospital of Vila Velha, Vila Velha, Brazil

Ricardo Alexander Marinho da Silva, D.D.S. Department of Oral and Maxillofacial Surgery, Hospital Santa Casa de Piracicaba, Piracicaba, SP, Brazil

Paulo Soltoski, M.D., M.Sc. Assistant Professor of Surgery, Universidade Federal do Paraná, Curitiba, PR, Brazil

João Lisboa de Sousa Filho, D.D.S. Department of Bucco-Maxillo-Facial Surgery and Traumatology, Hospital Santa Casa de Piracicaba, Piracicaba, SP, Brazil

Alexandre Baba Suehara, M.D. Departamento de Cirurgia da Irmandade da Santa Casa de Misericórdia de São Paulo, Faculdade de Ciências Médicas da Santa Casa de São Paulo, São Paulo, SP, Brazil

Maria Alice Gurgel da Trindade Meira Henriques, M.S., (Medical Student). Centro Universitário Maurício de Nassau (UNINASSAU), Recife, PE, Brazil

Maria Eduarda Gurgel da Trindade Meira Henriques, M.S., (Medical Student). Faculdade Pernambucana de Saúde (FPS), Recife, PE, Brazil

Célia Maria Pais Viégas, M.D., Ph.D., M.Sc. Department of Radiotherapy, Brazilian National Cancer Institute, Rio de Janeiro, RJ, Brazil

Priscila Rodrigues Prado Prado Zagari, MSc., Speech Therapist. Hospital Sírio-Libanês, São Paulo, SP, Brazil

Pontifical Catholic University of São Paulo, São Paulo, SP, Brazil

Department of Oncology, A.C. Camargo Cancer Center, São Paulo, SP, Brazil

Check for updates

The History of Tracheostomy

Sissi Monteiro, Terence Pires de Farias,
Marcelo de Camargo Millen, and Rafael Vianna Locio

Introduction

The tracheostomy is one of the most ancient surgical procedures, which consists of opening the anterior wall of the trachea to allow a patient to breathe. In its first references the tracheostomy was used in cases of acute airway obstruction, such as trauma, inflammatory conditions, and foreign body aspiration. The history of tracheostomy can be divided into very specific periods, as discussed below.

The Period of Legend (3100 BC–AD 1546)

> *"The bountiful one who without ligature, can cause the windpipe to reunite when the cervical cartilages are cut across, provided that they are not entirely severed."* Rig Veda, Sacred Book of Hindu Medicine

The oldest recorded surgical procedure on the airway is in the Edwin Smith Papyrus, an ancient Egyptian medical text thought to date to around 1600 BC, which

S. Monteiro, M.D. (✉)
Head and Neck Department of the Federal Hospital of Bonsucesso, Bonsucesso, RJ, Brazil

Brazilian National Cancer Institute—INCA, Rio de Janeiro, RJ, Brazil
e-mail: sissi@rscap.com.br

T.P. de Farias, M.D., Ph.D., M.Sc., Researcher.
Department of Head and Neck Surgery, Brazilian National Cancer Institute—INCA, Rio de Janeiro, RJ, Brazil

Departament of Head and Neck Surgery, Pontifical Catholic University, Rio de Janeiro, RJ, Brazil

M. de Camargo Millen, M.D.
Head and Neck surgeon of Barra Mansa, Barra Mansa, RJ, Brazil

R. Vianna Locio, M.S., (Medical Student).
Faculdade Pernambucana de Saúde/IMIP — Maternity Childhood Institute of Pernanbuco, Recife, PE, Brazil

T.P. de Farias (ed.), *Tracheostomy*, https://doi.org/10.1007/978-3-319-67867-2_1

demonstrates a procedure thought to be a tracheostomy to provide an emergency airway in trauma [1]. It is impossible to know exactly when the first tracheostomy was attempted, but there is evidence from hieroglyph slabs belonging to King Djer in Abydos and King Aha in Saqqara that tracheostomy was performed in ancient Egypt in about 3100 BC. Hippocrates, in 400 BC, condemned the procedure, mentioning the risks of carotid artery lesions. In AD 131, Galeno described the larynx and tracheal anatomy and identified the site of laryngeal voice generation and larynx innervation. In the fourth century BC, Alexander the Great is said to have saved the life of a soldier who was choking from a bone lodged in his throat by "puncturing his trachea" with the point of his sword [2].

The first elective tracheostomy is credited to Asclepiades of Bithynia in 100 BC [3]. This procedure was described by the physician Claudius Galen in AD 131, who also contributed to the understanding of the tracheostomy by describing the anatomy of the head and neck [4]. In the same century, Aretaeus, in his book *The Therapeutics of Acute Diseases*, confirmed the work done by Asclepiades of Bithynia on the subject of tracheostomy, but he condemned it on the grounds that "cartilage wounds do not heal." Albucasis (936–1013) contributed to the history of tracheostomy by suturing a tracheal wound, and demonstrating its ability to heal, in a servant girl who had tried to commit suicide by cutting her throat.

Many authors of this period described tracheostomy in detail, but none of them claimed to have performed it themselves. References were made to tracheostomy, but the operation was considered both useless and dangerous due to the high risk of wound infection and a belief that cartilage rings could not heal.

The Period of Fear (AD 1546–1833)

> *"The terrified surgeons of our times have not dared to exercise this surgery and I also have never performed it; it is a scandal."* Fabricius Aquapendente

In this specific period the procedure was considered dangerous and brutal, and only 28 successful tracheostomies were recorded in the literature [5].

What is considered the first surgical description of a tracheostomy was given in 1546 by an Italian physician, Antonio Musa Brasavola, in a patient with an "abscess in the throat"; the patient was refused by barber surgeons before being treated by Brasavola [6]. In 1620 the French author Nicholas Habicot published a book of 108 pages totally dedicated to the procedure (Fig. 1).

In the early 1600s, tracheostomy was considered acceptable for acute upper airway obstruction caused by foreign body ingestion, aspiration, and infection [7]. In Fig. 2 we can see an illustration of the procedure from that period. Renaus Moreau suggested its use in mumps, recommending that the procedure be performed with the patient in the supine position, a recommendation that was ignored for nearly 200 years [8].

When George Washington (the first president of the USA) presented with airway obstruction secondary to a peritonsillar abscess, Dr. Elisha Dick suggested a

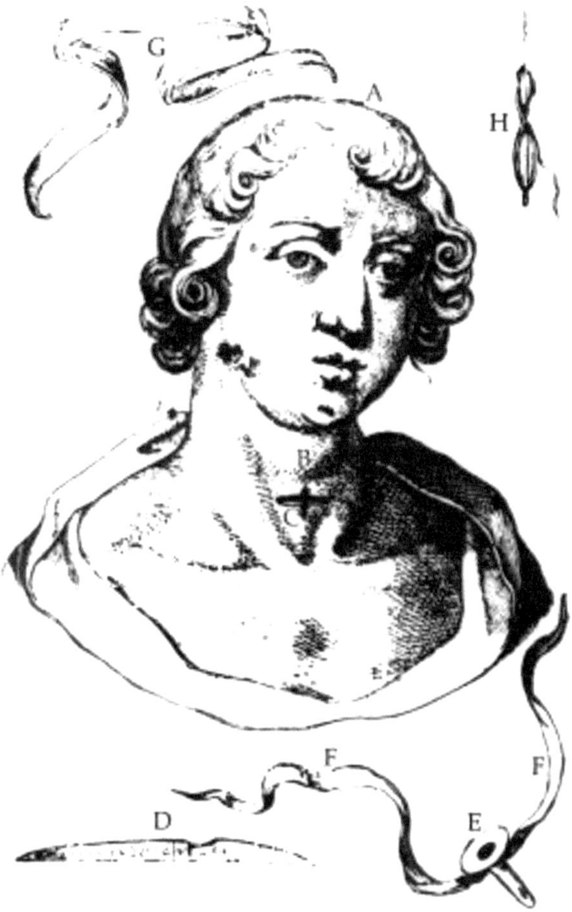

Fig. 1 Tracheostomy pictured by Nicolas Habicot in Question Chirurgicale. J. Corrozet, Paris, 1620. *A*, the patient. *B*, the larynx. *C*, the wound or bronchotomy. *D*, the instrument for bronchotomy. *E*, the hollow cannula. *F*, the straps for fastening it on the neck. *G*, the plain smooth band to apply over the cannula to scatter the air stream. *H*, the needle to suture the wound when one removes the dressing to make the wound heal

tracheostomy, but Dr. James Craig and Dr. Gustavus Brown did not concur; instead they treated him with bloodletting to release "evil humors." The patient presented worsening of symptoms within 36 hours after its onset and passed away on December 14, 1799 (Fig. 3).

Until 1707 the procedure was known as "laryngotomy." It was Pierre Dionis who started calling it "bronchotomy" [9]; in 1718, Lorenz Heister recommended that it should be called "tracheostomy" and that all other terms should be discarded [10]. In the illustration reproduced in Fig. 4, the procedure was reproduced and the two terms were used.

In 1730, the British surgeon George Martin introduced the double-lumen cannula with the advantage of an inner cannula that could be removed and cleaned, thus preventing tube obstruction with mucus. There is no record of whether he used it [11].

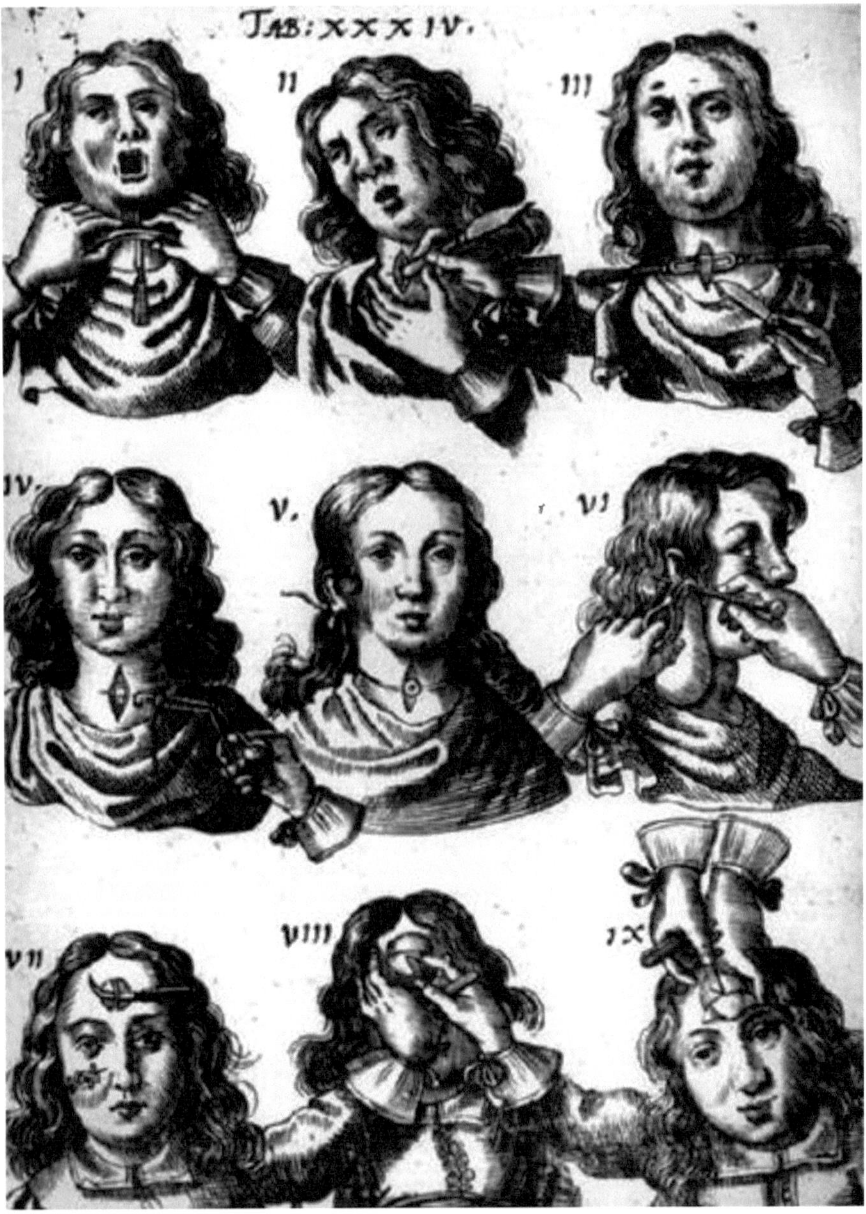

Fig. 2 Ancient engraving illustrating a tracheostomy procedure. From Armamentarium Chirurgicum Bipartitum, 1666

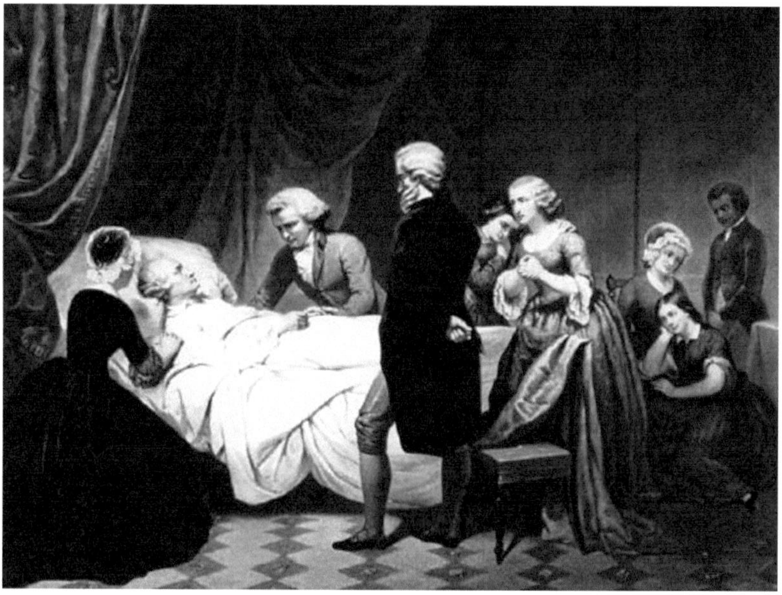

Fig. 3 George Washington, on his death bed, diagnosed with a peritonsillar abscess

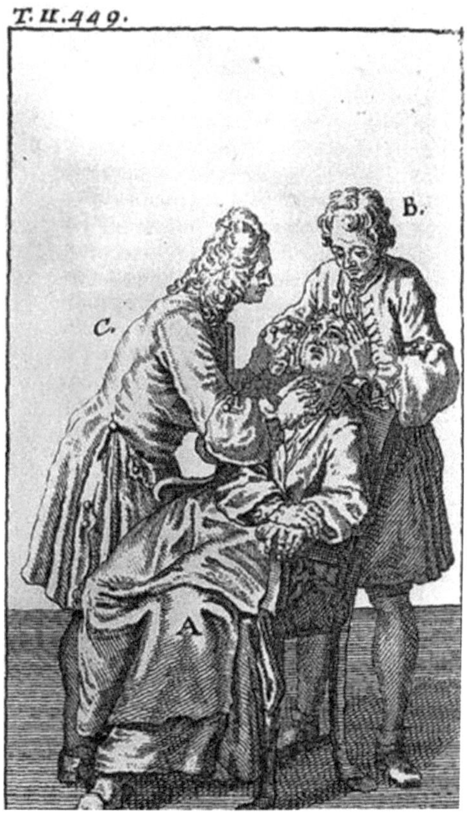

Fig. 4 Performing a bronchotomy (tracheostomy). Chirurgie Scènes de la vie médicale: Traité des opérations de chirurgie. Paris: G. Cavelier, 1731

The Period of Dramatization (AD 1833–1932)

> *"The question always arises in the mind of the young surgeon whether the symptoms are sufficiently urgent to render the operation necessary."*McKenzie [11]

This sentence by McKenzie helps us to understand the idea that physicians had of the procedure back then. Trousseau, in 1833, described 200 cases of tracheostomies performed in patients with diphtheria (also known as croup). Patients usually develop a membrane on one or both tonsils, with extension to the tonsillar pillars, uvula, soft palate, oropharynx, and nasopharynx. *Corynebacterium diphtheria* multiplies on the surface of the mucous membrane, resulting in formation of the pseudomembrane. He reported that 25% of these interventions were successful.

In 1869, Dr. Erichsen described four complications of tracheostomy: exposing of the air tube, hemorrhage, opening of the air passage, and misplacement of the tracheostomy tube. He further recommended that the tube be cleaned with a sponge and a solution of silver nitrate [12].

With time, tracheostomy became an accepted technique to bypass upper airway obstruction. In 1909, Chevalier Jackson defined factors that predisposed to complications, such as a high incision, use of an improper cannula, poor postoperative care, and splitting of the cricoid cartilage. He designed a metal double-lumen tube of proper length and curvature with just the right fitting to avoid excessive pressure on the anterior or posterior wall of the trachea and to reduce the risks of ulceration and tracheal erosion (Fig. 5). Jackson favored a vertical

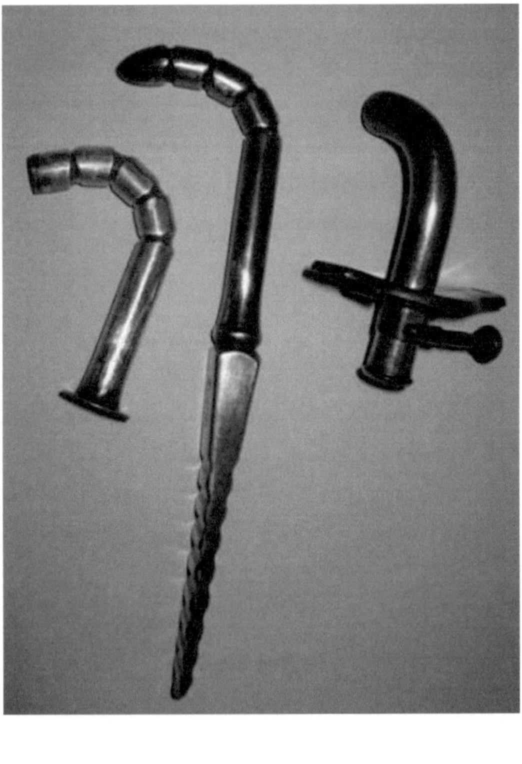

Fig. 5 Durham Flexible Pilot (introducer) Lobster tail. Tracheostomy tube, inner cannula, and introducer

incision from the thyroid notch to the suprasternal notch for best visibility of the surgical field. His teachings significantly reduced the complication rate and mortality rate of tracheostomy [13].

With the introduction of immunization for diphtheria and the discovery of sulfonamides to help reduce other upper respiratory infections, the need for emergency tracheostomy became less common. For a brief period, tracheostomy was the only means of securing airways through general anesthesia, but the increasing popularity of endotracheal intubation replaced the need for tracheostomy.

The Period of Enthusiasm (AD 1932–1965)

> *"If you think tracheostomy … do it!"* Unknown author

Almost in direct opposition to McKenzie's statement, this sentence became very popular during this period. The indications for tracheostomy were being actively pursued by the medical world. In 1932, with the outbreak of bulbar poliomyelitis, tracheostomy was used to prevent impending pulmonary infection, since the affected patients were unable to cough and raise secretions. For the first time, tracheostomy was considered as an elective procedure [14]. Polio remained an epidemic until the early 1950s, when the invention of positive pressure respiration, together with tracheostomy, greatly reduced its mortality.

Tracheostomy was openly advocated for tetanus; head, chest, and maxillofacial injuries; drug overdose; and following major surgery where airway patency was compromised [7]. During the Spanish Civil War (1936–1939), while soldiers with maxillofacial trauma were waiting for surgery, they underwent tracheostomy to prevent aspiration and respiratory distress. This practice decreased mortality rates for soldiers waiting for such surgeries [15]. Tracheostomy became more prevalent as intensive care and postanesthetic care units were established in the 1950s, with better care for tracheostomy patients [16].

With the control of many infectious diseases, the indications for tracheostomy were changing. In 1961, Meade, in a series of 212 cases, showed that 41% of tracheostomies were still carried out on patients with upper airway obstruction due to tumors, infectious disease, and trauma, and 55% were performed to assist in mechanical ventilation [17].

The Period of Rationalization (AD 1965–Present)

With improvements in the techniques of orotracheal and nasotracheal intubation, these have become safer and faster alternatives to tracheostomy. Improvements in tracheostomy tubes, aspiration equipment, and use of biocompatible materials have improved the safety of the procedure.

Goldenberg et al. showed that 76% of tracheostomies were prophylactically performed in patients requiring prolonged mechanical ventilation, while only 6% of patients were tracheostomized due to upper airway obstruction. Only 0.26% of tracheostomies were performed on an emergency basis [18].

Percutaneous dilational tracheostomy (PDT) is an alternative to open tracheostomy because it can be comfortably performed at the bedside (Fig. 6). In 1953, Seldinger introduced the technique of percutaneous guide wire needle placement for arterial catheterization. In 1985, the guide wire technique was adapted to percutaneous tracheostomy by Ciaglia et al. In 1969, Toy and Weinstein developed a tapered straight dilator for performing percutaneous tracheostomy over a guiding catheter [19], and in 1989 Schachner et al. developed dilating tracheostomy forceps over a guide wire.

The development of PDT using serial dilators over a guide wire made the procedure safer in elective situations and can be performed by various medical personnel at the beside [20]. We now have two possible techniques for performing tracheostomy in intensive care units for patients requiring prolonged mechanical ventilation.

Carried out in the operating room, intensive care, and intermediate care units—and even in locations with minimal medical support—tracheostomy remains one of the most important and commonly performed surgical procedures to this day. It may be dreaded, scorned, and carried out with extreme hesitancy, or in other instances, a noble and dramatic life-saving procedure.

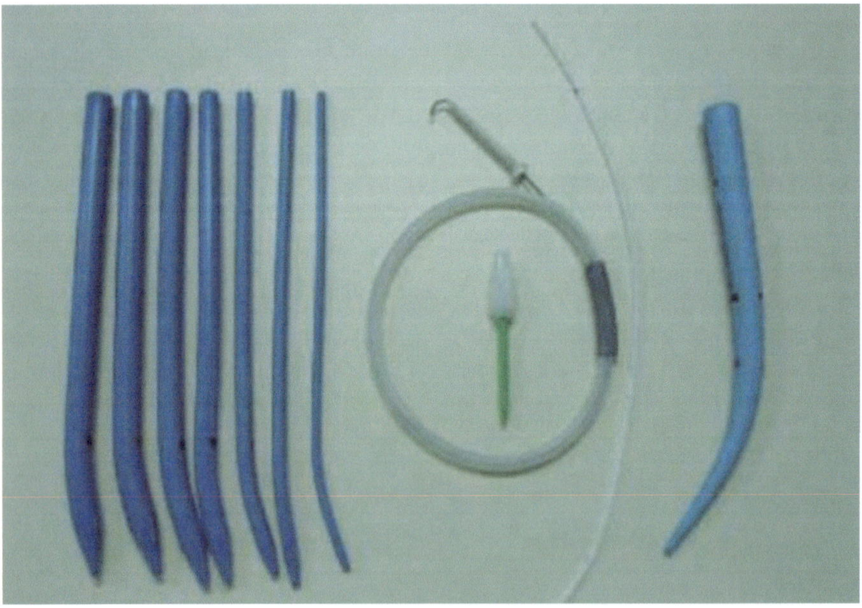

Fig. 6 Ciaglia dilators, guide wire, rigid dilator, guide catheter, and Blue Rhino dilator

References

1. Cooper JD. Surgery of the airway: historic notes. J Thorac Dis. 2016;8(Suppl 2):S113–20.
2. Gordon BL, FA Davis. The romance of medicine. 1947;461.
3. Wright JA. History of laryngology and rhinology. Philadelphia: Lea & Feiber; 1914. p. 65.
4. CG Kuhn. Galen. Introductio Seu Medicus. (Trans) Leipzig; 1856. P. 406. Adam F. Areataeus: the therapeutics of acute diseases. (Trans) London: Syndenham Society; 1856. P. 406.
5. Goodall EW. The story of tracheostomy. Br J Child Dis. 1934;31:167–76, 253–72. 618–24.
6. Stock CR. What is past is prologue: a short history of the development of tracheostomy. Ear Nose Throat J. 1987;66(4):166–9.
7. Frost EA. Tracing the tracheostomy. Ann Otol Rhinol Laryngol. 1976;85(5 Pt.1):618–24.
8. Borman J, Davidson JT. A history of tracheostomy. Si Spiritum Ducit Vivit Br J Anesthesiol. 1963;35:388–90.
9. Dionis P. Cours d'operatione de chirurgiris, ed. Paris: L dHoury; 1751.
10. Heister L. General system of surgery, vol. 2. 8th ed. London: Printed for W Innys, J Richardson, C Davis, and J Clark; 1768. p. 52.
11. McKenzie M. Diseases of the pharynx, larynx and trachea. New York: Wood and Co.; 1880. p. 397.
12. Erichsen JE. The science and art of surgery. Philadelphia: Henry C Lea; 1869. p. 919.
13. Jackson C. Tracheostomy. Laryngoscope. 1909;19:285.
14. Wilson JL. Acute anterior poliomyelitis treatment of bulbar and high spinal types. N Engl J Med. 1932;206:887.
15. Booth JB. Tracheostomy and tracheal intubation in military history. J R Soc Med. 2000;93:380–3.
16. Collins CG. Rationale and value of tracheostomy in severe preeclampsia and eclampsia. Postgrad Med. 1955;17:259–66.
17. Meade JW. Tracheostomy—its complications and their management. N Engl J Med. 1961;265:519–23.
18. Goldenberg D, Ari EG, Golz A, Danino J, Netzer A, Joachims HZ. Tracheostomy complications: a retrospective study of 1130 cases. Otolaryngol Head Neck Surg. 2000;123:495–500.
19. Toy FJ, Weinstein JD. A percutaneous tracheostomy device. Surgery. 1969;65(2):384–9.
20. Schachner A, Ovil Y, Sidi J, Rogev M, Heilbronn Y, Levy MJ. Percutaneous tracheostomy, a new method. Crit Care Med. 1989;17(10):1052–6.

Anatomy of the Trachea

Juliana Fernandes de Oliveira, Terence Pires de Farias, Juliana Maria de Almeida Vital, Maria Eduarda Gurgel da Trindade Meira Henriques, Maria Alice Gurgel da Trindade Meira Henriques, and Maria Eduarda Lima de Moura

For practice of any surgery, it is essential to know the anatomy of each structure involved in the technique, as well as the elements that surround it. The trachea is not just a tube that connects the larynx to the bronchi, as well as other organs of the respiratory tree; it has the function of cleaning and heating the air that transits in its lumen. Anatomical variations, whether congenital or acquired, are challenging and should never be overlooked. In this chapter, we will provide an explanation illustrated with a photographic and schematic collection, with emphasis on surgical details.

J.F. de Oliveira, M.D. (✉)
Head and Neck Surgery at Brazilian National Cancer Institute – INCA, Rio de Janeiro, RJ, Brazil
e-mail: ju.foliveira@yahoo.com.br

T.P. de Farias, M.D., Ph.D., M.Sc., Researcher.
Department of Head and Neck Surgery, Brazilian National Cancer Institute—INCA, Rio de Janeiro, RJ, Brazil

Department of Head and Neck Surgery, Pontifical Catholic University, Rio de Janeiro, RJ, Brazil

J.M. de Almeida Vital, M.D.
Head and Neck Department, Irmandade Santa Casa de de São Paulo, São Paulo, SP, Brazil

Head and Neck Surgeon, Private Practice, São Paulo, SP, Brazil
e-mail: jujuliana.a@gmail.com

M.E.G. da Trindade Meira Henriques, M.S., (Medical Student).
Faculdade Pernambucana de Saúde - FPS, Recife, PE, Brazil

M.A.G. da Trindade Meira Henriques, M.S., (Medical Student).
Centro Universitário Maurício de Nassau (UNINASSAU), Recife, PE, Brazil

M.E.L. de Moura, M.S., (Medical Student).
Faculdade de Medicina Nova Esperança - (FAMENE), João Pessoa, PB, Brazil

T.P. de Farias (ed.), *Tracheostomy*, https://doi.org/10.1007/978-3-319-67867-2_2

Macrostructure

The trachea is a tube located in the midline, connecting the cricoid cartilage in the neck to the main bronchi in the thorax. In its cervical portion, it begins at the height of the sixth or seventh vertebra, and is deep to the cervical fascia and infrahyoid muscles (Figs. 1 and 2). It is bordered by the thyroid gland on the anterior face, with lateral recurrent laryngeal nerves. As it progresses caudally, it remains anterior to the esophagus, between the common carotid arteries, internal jugular veins, and vagus nerve (Figs. 3, 4, 5, and 6). The brachiocephalic or innominate artery is the first blood vessel found in pretracheal dissection during airway

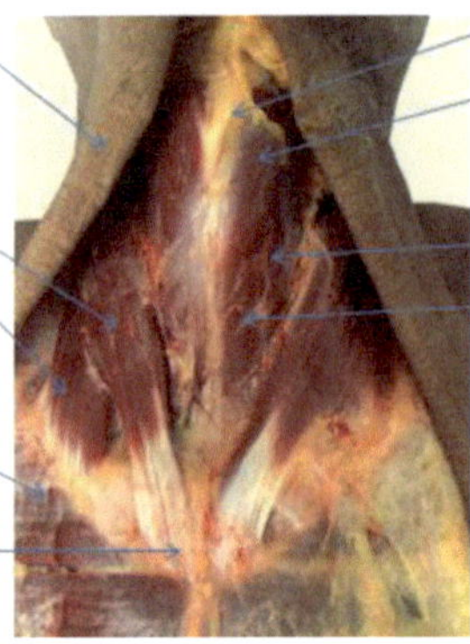

Fig. 1 Cervical region with the subplatysmal myocutaneous flap highlighted. Infrahyoid muscles arise medially and the sternocleidomastoid laterally

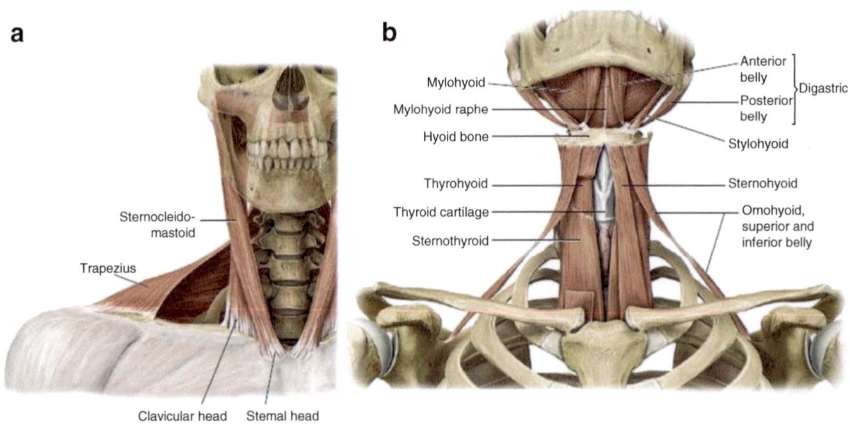

Fig. 2 Individualized neck muscles . (**a**) Anterior view. (**b**) Anterior view.The sternohyoid has been cut (right)

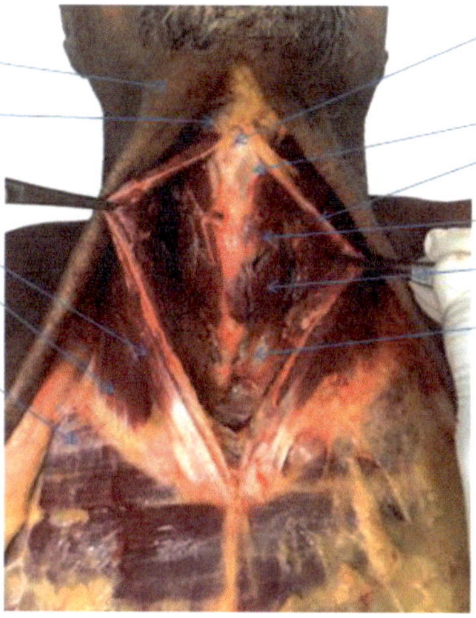

Fig. 3 Dissection through the pretracheal visceral fascia exposing the midline organs

mobilization, justifying the reason for trachea–innominate fistula occurrence. The brachiocephalic vein crosses the front of the innominate artery in a plane even more anterior to the trachea. The carina is in the lower border of the trachea, where the two primary bronchi originate, at the height of the fourth or fifth thoracic vertebra (Figs. 7 and 8) [1].

The trachea surfaces with cervical extension allowing half of it to be accessible by this route, facilitating most surgical procedures. Maximal flexion leads to cricoid cartilage at the level of the sternum, minimizing the tension of anastomoses after resection of the tracheal segment. With current anatomical knowledge and blood supply, good mobilization promotes greater safety for resection and reconstruction of half the length of the trachea [2].

The trachea has an incomplete cartilaginous ring structure, the posterior face filled by smooth muscle with longitudinal (external) and transverse fibers (internal tracheal muscle). The annular ligament is found between the tracheal rings and it is composed of two layers of fibrous membrane: an external layer, covering the surface of each ring; and another internal layer. In the intervals of the cartilage, these membranes meet, conferring both flexibility and fixation to the respiratory tract.

The external diameter of the trachea measures approximately 2.3 cm in the coronal cut, and 1.8 cm in the sagittal cut in men, forming a U-like structure. In females these dimensions are 2.0 cm and 1.4 cm, respectively, forming an elliptical framework in the axial section. The length in the adult phase is, on average, 11.8 cm and

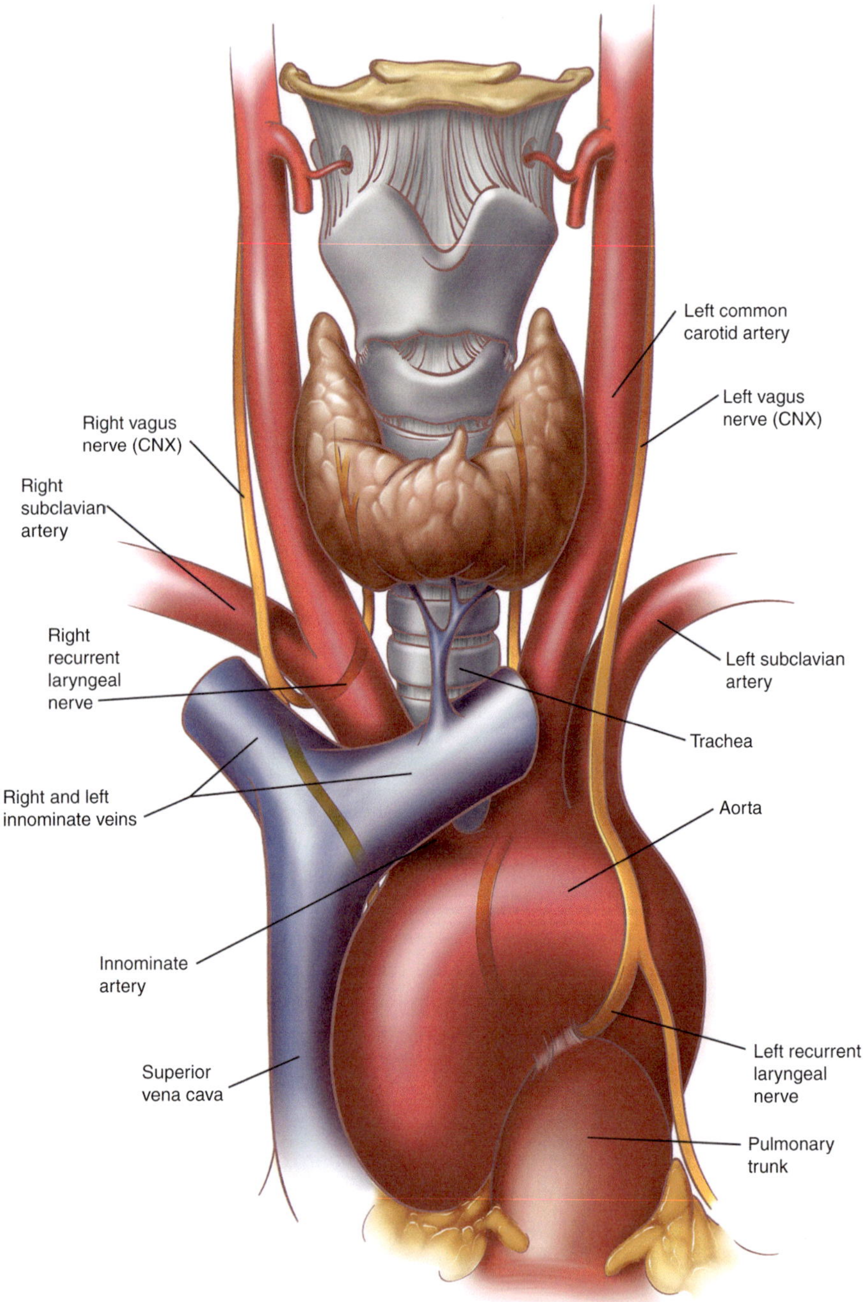

Fig. 4 Relationships of trachea to surrounding structures. Anterior view. Note the tight packing of major mediastinal vessels adjacent to the trachea

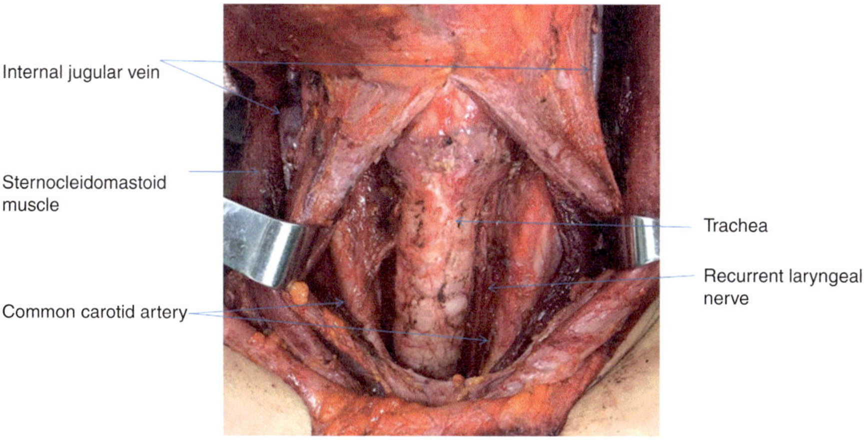

Fig. 5 Vessels and nerves lateral to the tracheal compartment

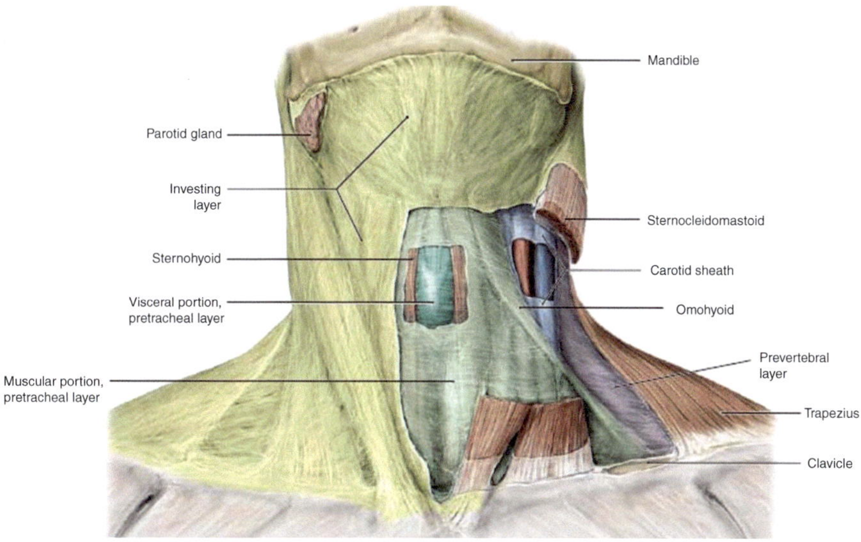

Fig. 6 Cervical fascia and neck muscles illustrating the planes until identification of the trachea

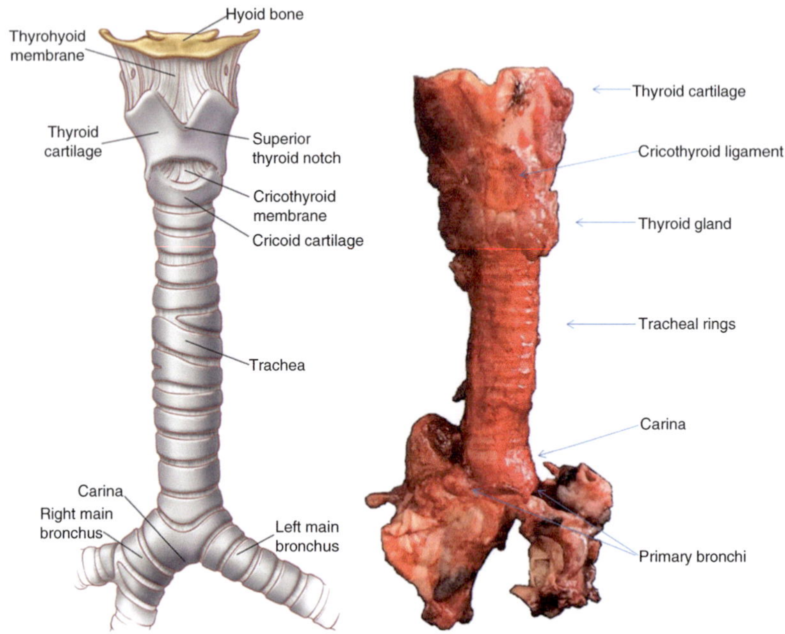

Fig. 7 Laryngeal case and inferior airway. Cricothyroid ligament where access is made for cricostomy. Trachea divided into cervical and thoracic portions. Conventional cervical tracheostomy allows easier and safer organ exposure

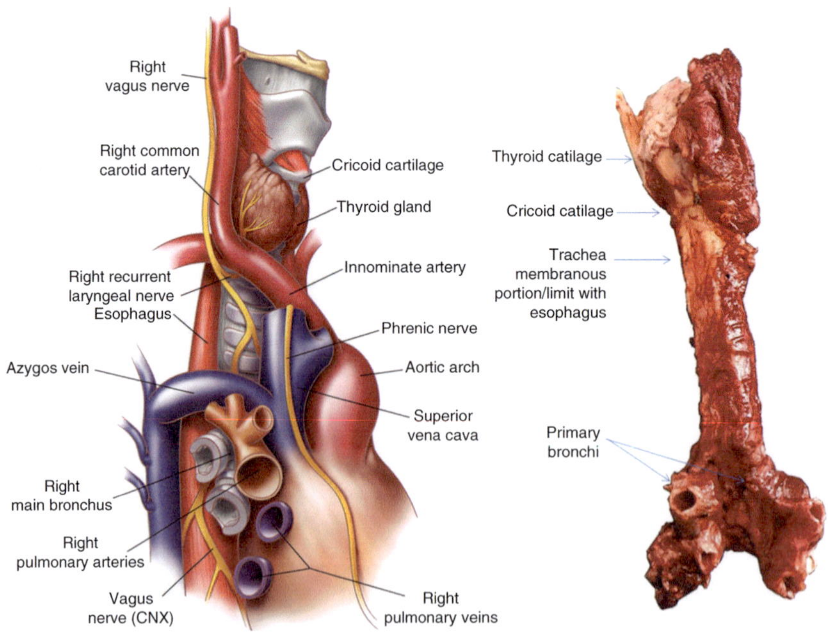

Fig. 8 Right oblique cut shows the posterior area membranous direct limit with the esophagus. In the emergence of the thoracic portion, the innominate artery crosses the trachea, which is accompanied by the vagus nerve until its bifurcation in the source bronchi

can vary, according to sex and height, between 10 and 13 cm, and its thickness is, on average, 3 mm. At each centimeter of extension, there are approximately two rings, and every organ has a total of 18–22 cartilaginous rings [3]. The first tracheal ring has a larger diameter and is connected to the cricoid cartilage cricothyroid ligament, while the last tracheal ring is thicker and broader in the midline, since its lower border extends in a triangular-shaped process, curved down and behind the two bronchi.

These rings prevent the collapse of the tracheal mucosa during inspiration. Airflow depends on the tracheal diameter. The resistance is inversely proportional to the radius to the fourth power. Thus thickening of the mucosa, constriction of muscles, masses/tumors that compress the respiratory tract, and even endotracheal tubes trigger reduction of the lumen and generate turbulent airflow [4].

Microstructure

The cartilaginous arch is covered externally by the adventitial tunica and internally lined by mucosa of ciliated cylindrical pseudostratified epithelium. This is composed of hair cells, goblet cells, basal cells, and neuroendocrine cells. In smokers or in individuals with a chronic irritation process, squamous metaplasia and loss of hair cells may occur. The submucosal layer is composed of a loose connective tissue network, which houses nerves, blood vessels, and mucus-producing glands (Figs. 9 and 10).

The air is heated to about 37 °C and humidified to 100% saturation during inspiration. In case of reduction of the airway—in tracheostomies or

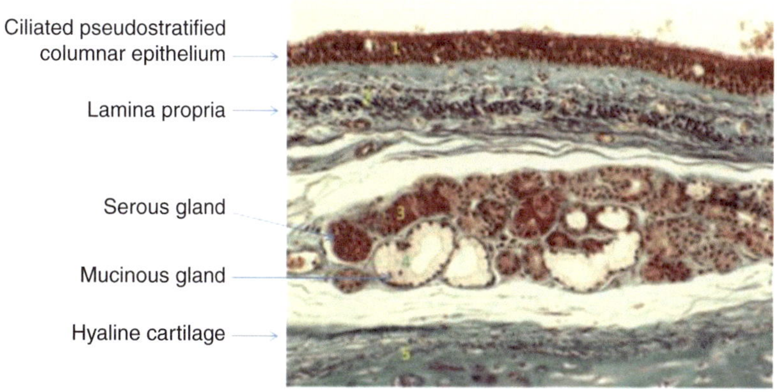

Fig. 9 Tissue layers constituting the tracheal wall: respiratory epithelium, the submucosa filled with glands, and the hyaline cartilage of the rings

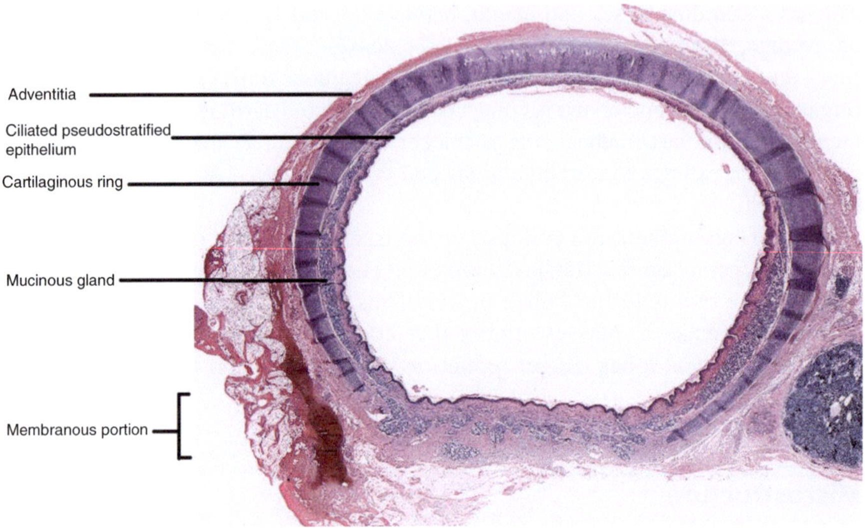

Fig. 10 Cross-section in the trachea evidencing the annular shape and structural difference conferred by the cartilage rings

intubations, for example—the air that will reach the lungs will be less hot and humid. This difference in heat loss raises energy consumption to reach temperature homeostasis [4].

Vascularization

The blood supply to the trachea occurs through lateral pedicles. This is important to rule out lateral dissection in tracheal resection, being limited to 1–2 cm to prevent devascularization or anastomosis dehiscence.

The cranial portion of the trachea is supplied by the lower thyroid arteries and their tracheoesophageal branches, while the bronchial arteries nourish the distal portion, carina, and bronchi (Figs. 11 and 12).

Between the rings a submucosal plexus of intercartilaginous arteries is present, filling the tissue and irrigating the cartilaginous portion, while the membranous trachea is nourished by branches from the esophageal arteries (Fig. 13).

The venous drainage converges to the brachiocephalic vein through the plexus of the inferior thyroid vein, while the lymphatic drainage converges to the paratracheal lymph node and deep cervical lymph nodes.

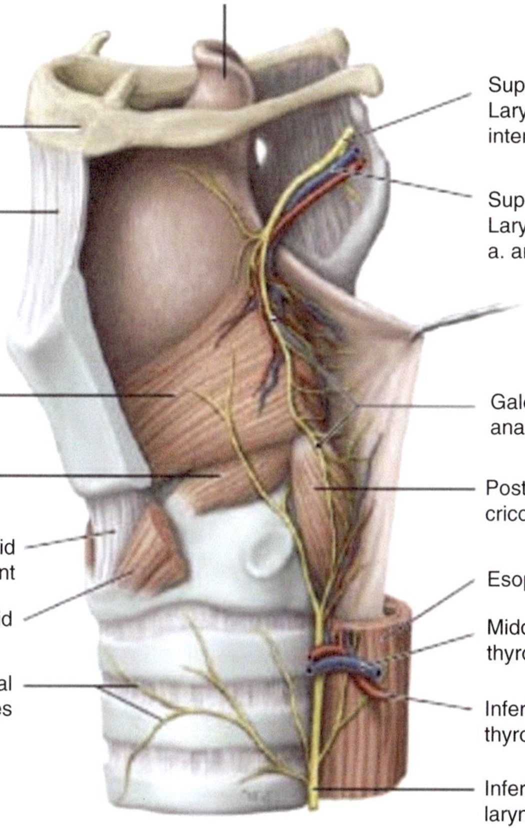

Fig. 11 The cervical portion of the trachea is supplied by the lower thyroid arteries

Innervation

The innervation of the trachea comes from tracheal branches originating from the thoracic sympathetic chain and the inferior ganglion of the vagus nerve (Fig. 14). The former is responsible for tracheobronchial muscle tone, allowing bronchodilation and bronchoconstriction, production of mucoid secretion, and vascular permeability. The vagal innervation in turn is responsible for the reflex of coughing and sternutation.

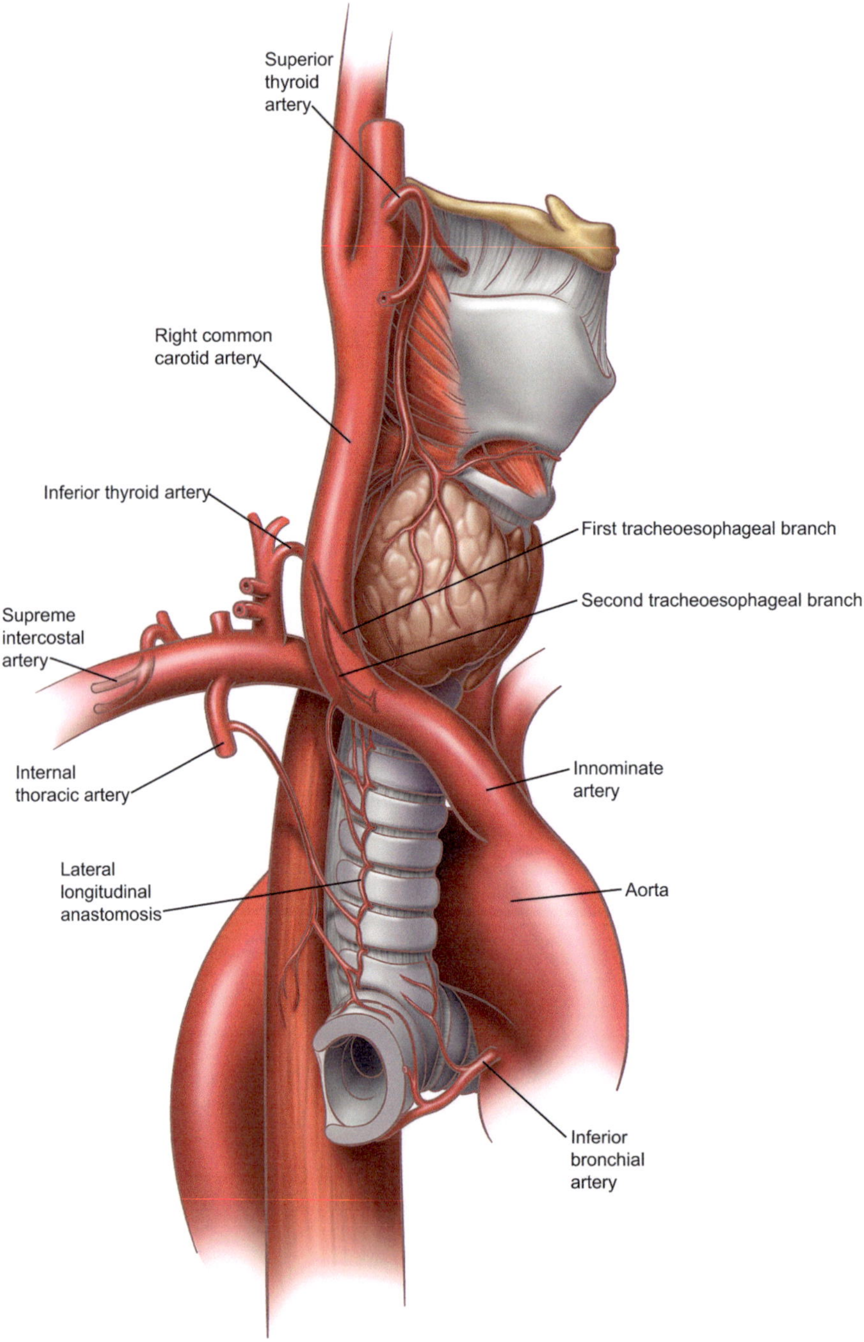

Fig. 12 The thyrocervical trunk, a direct branch of the aorta, emits the inferior thyroid artery, and this originates tracheoesophageal branches nourishing the cranial portion. The internal thoracic artery also gives branches to the caudal portion, which anastomoses to the bronchial arteries

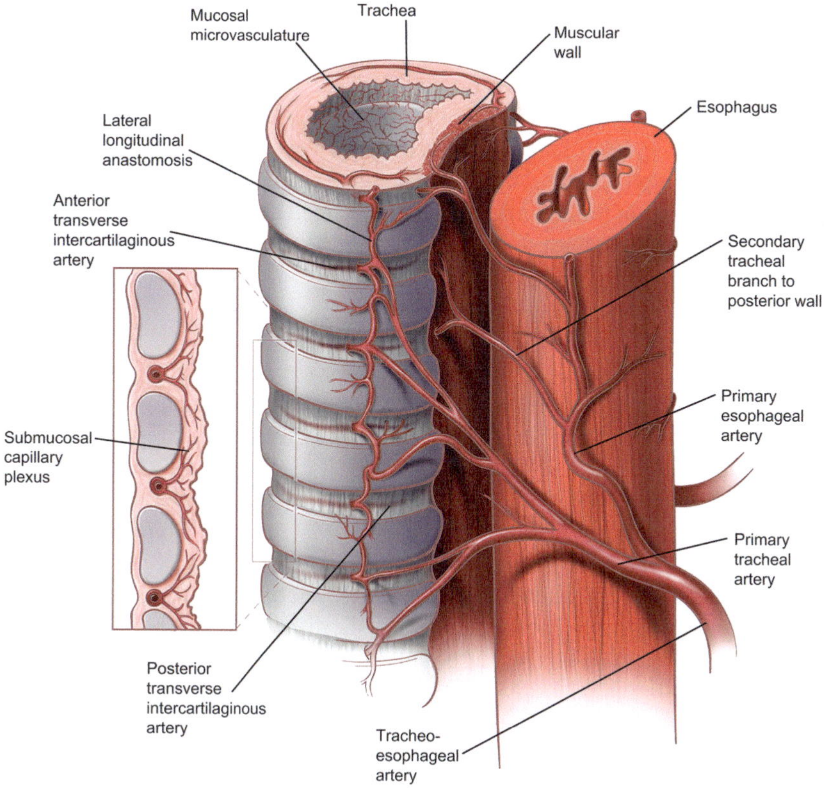

Fig. 13 Submucous capillary plexus formed by the tracheoesophageal branches inserted into the intercartilaginous membranes of the rings

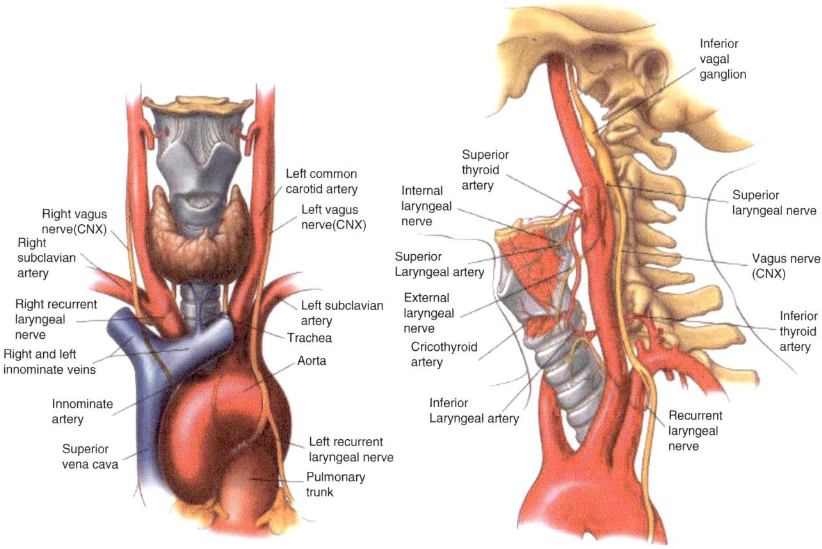

Fig. 14 Vague lateral nerve to the trachea emitting the recurrent laryngeal branch after circumventing the large intrathoracic vessels

Anatomy in Children

In children, the neck and trachea are smaller. The trachea is more elastic and extensible—properties that are reduced with the aging calcification process. It is also deeper and more mobile than in adults; pulmonary reserve is also reduced in cases of apnea, for example. In this way, accidental displacement of the cannula is a high-risk maneuver. Fixing the cannula to the skin through single stitches is an option to prevent this accidental removal.

Anatomical Variations

There is variety in the conformation of the tracheobronchial tree, which can reach an incidence of 1–12% and is usually asymptomatic. When variations are symptomatic, cough, hemoptysis, and recurrent episodes of respiratory infection may occur. The importance of recognition is evident when the patient undergoes procedures such as bronchoscopy, intubation, and pulmonary recruitment. Some variations are accessory bronchi, tracheal diverticulum, and a bronchial bridge [5]. It is suggested that these changes are justified by the theory of selection, in which the bronchial abnormalities result from local morphogenesis disorders. The bronchial mesenchyme itself is able to induce budding if grafted onto the tracheal epithelium [6].

References

1. Burdett E, Mitchell V. Anatomy of the larynx, trachea and bronchi. Anaesth Intensive Care Med. 2008;9:329–33.
2. Drevet G, Conti M, Deslauriers J. Surgical anatomy of the tracheobronchial tree. J Thorac Dis. 2016;8(Suppl 2):S121–9.
3. Minnich DJ, Mathisen DJ. Anatomy of the trachea, carina, and bronchi. Thorac Surg Clin. 2007;17(4):571–85.
4. Epstein SK. Anatomy and physiology of tracheostomy. Respir Care. 2005;50:476–82.
5. Wooten C, Patel S, Cassidy L, et al. Variations of the tracheobronchial tree: anatomical and clinical significance. Clin Anat. 2014;27:1223–33.
6. Alescio T, Cassini A. Induction in vitro of tracheal buds by pulmonary mesenchyme grafted on tracheal epithelium. J Exp Zool. 1962;150:83–94.

Tracheostomy Tube Types

Juliana Maria de Almeida Vital, Fernando Luiz Dias, Maria Eduarda Gurgel da Trindade Meira Henriques, Maria Alice Gurgel da Trindade Meira Henriques, Maria Eduarda Lima de Moura, and Terence Pires de Farias

Introduction

The word *tracheostomy* is derived from the Greek *trachea arteria* (hard artery) and *tome* (cut) [1]. The procedure consists of an incision in the trachea. It has been reported since ancient times [1, 2], but it was only at the beginning of the twentieth century that its technique and indications were defined and described by Chevalier Jackson [3].

A tracheostomy tube is used to secure the airway in this procedure, which can be performed in patients on prolonged invasive mechanical ventilation [4, 5], with upper airway obstruction, undergoing laryngectomy, or at high risk of recurrent aspiration [6].

J.M. de Almeida Vital, M.D. (✉)
Head and Neck Department, Irmandade Santa Casa de São Paulo, São Paulo, SP, Brazil

Head and Neck Surgeon, Private Practice, São Paulo, SP, Brazil
e-mail: jujuliana.a@gmail.com

F.L. Dias, M.D., Ph.D., M.Sc., F.A.C.S.
Head and Neck Surgery Department, Brazilian National Cancer Institute – INCA, Rio de Janeiro, RJ, Brazil

Head and Neck Department, Pontifical Catholic University of Rio de Janeiro, Rio de Janeiro, RJ, Brazil

M.E.G. da Trindade Meira Henriques, M.S., (Medical Student).
Faculdade Pernambucana de Saúde (FPS), Recife, PE, Brazil

M.A.G. da Trindade Meira Henriques, M.S., (Medical Student).
Centro Universitário Maurício de Nassau (UNINASSAU), Recife, PE, Brazil

M.E.L. de Moura, M.S., (Medical Student).
Faculdade de Medicina Nova Esperança (FAMENE), João Pessoa, PB, Brazil

T.P. de Farias, M.D., Ph.D., M.Sc., Researcher.
Department of Head and Neck Surgery, Brazilian National Cancer Institute—INCA, Rio de Janeiro, RJ, Brazil

Department of Head and Neck Surgery, Pontifical Catholic University, Rio de Janeiro, RJ, Brazil

T.P. de Farias (ed.), *Tracheostomy*, https://doi.org/10.1007/978-3-319-67867-2_3

Tracheostomy cannulae, when compared with endotracheal tubes, allow a reduction in respiratory work, less laryngeal injury, and easier oral hygiene, and may also enable oral feeding [1].

There is a wide range of tracheostomy tubes available, with different materials, sizes, and styles. On the tube's neckplate, its characteristics are marked, such as its inner and outer diameters and its length. Clinicians, intensive care professionals, and surgeons must know the differences between them in order to select suitable tubes for patients' needs [7–9].

Structure

Tracheostomy tubes have a main shaft (cannula) attached to a neckplate (or flange), and cuffed tubes have a pilot balloon, which shows whether the cuff is inflated. The neckplate has a slot where ties can be placed, and fenestrated tubes can have a cuff and/or inner cannula. Their insertion is aided with an obturator [10]. Figures 1 and 2 show the tracheostomy tube parts.

Materials

Tracheostomy tubes can be made from metal (silver or stainless steel) or, most commonly, from plastic (polyvinyl chloride, silicone, or polyurethane) [11, 12].

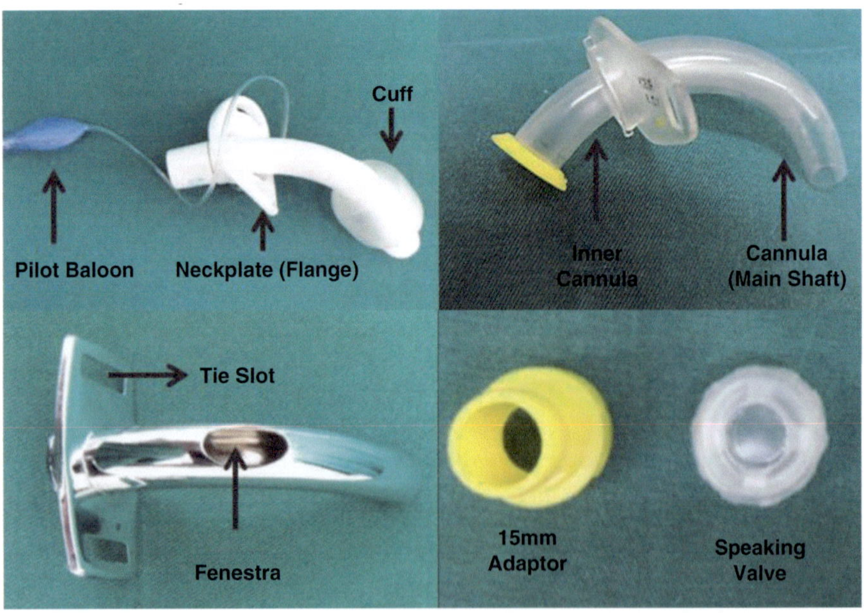

Fig. 1 Tracheostomy tube structure and parts

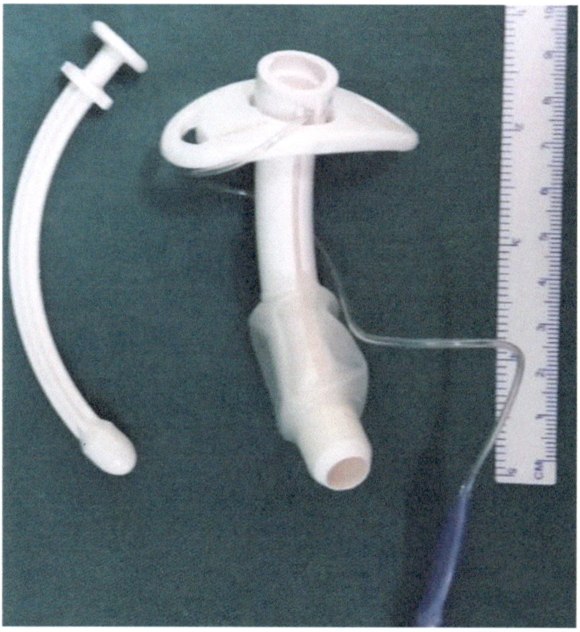

Fig. 2 Obturator and cuffed tracheostomy tube without an inner cannula

Metallic Tubes

The advantages of metal tubes are that they are endurable, inert, and resistant to biofilm formation; they limit bacterial growth; they are easily sanitized and can be sterilized [12]; and they are more cost effective for long-term use [10]. On the other hand, they are inelastic, do not have a cuff or a connector for mechanical ventilation, and can harm the trachea by heat or cold injury, hence they are not suitable for patients on radiation therapy whose radiation field is near the device [10, 12]. They are available from size 00 to size 12. Figure 3 shows standard metallic tubes and their inner cannulae from sizes 2 to 6.

The tube is inserted with the aid of a rounded-tip obturator through its lumen [12]; it has an inner cannula, and it can have fenestration and/or a speaking valve (Figs. 4, 5, and 6).

Plastic Tubes

Plastic tubes can be semiflexible or rigid. The first type adapts to the patient's anatomy, normally has a right angle, and has a longer cannula. The second type does not collapse or deflect, does not have a right angle, and is usually used for neck swelling, but it is not suitable for patients with thick necks, since its main shaft is short [10]. As with metal tubes, their insertion is aided by an obturator.

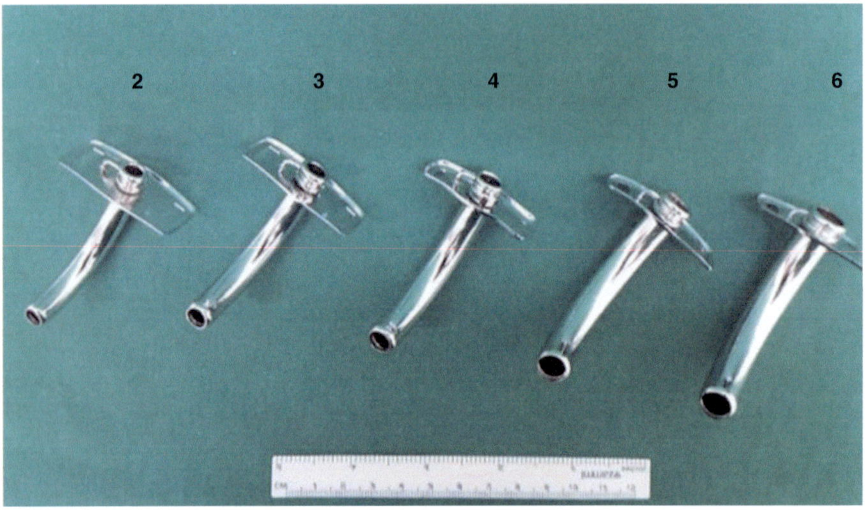

Fig. 3 Metallic conventional tracheostomy tube sizes 2, 3, 4, 5, and 6 with inner cannulae inserted

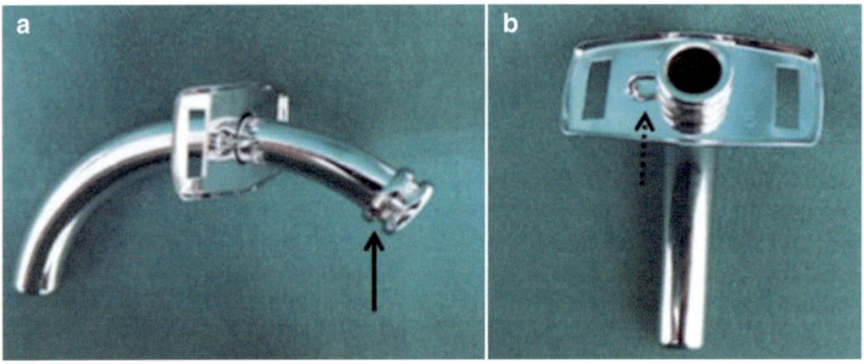

Fig. 4 (**a**) Metallic conventional tube and its inner cannula being inserted. The *arrow* points to the notch for the locking device (hook). (**b**) Front view of the same tube with the inner cannula already inserted. The inner cannula is turned (either clockwise or counterclockwise) after it is fitted to the hook (shown by the *dotted arrow*)

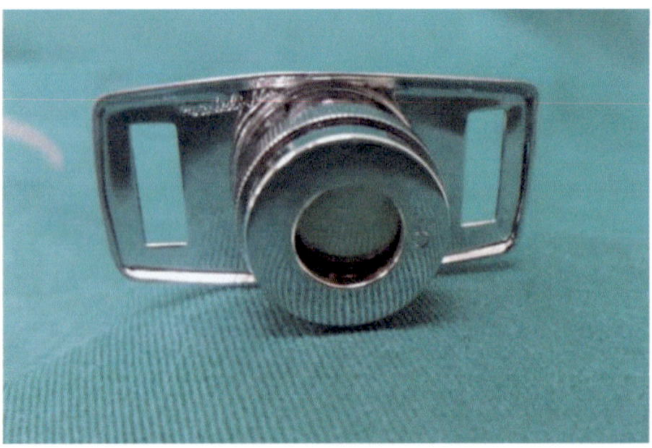

Fig. 5 The metallic speaking valve is a cap with a mobile plate; it is attached to the cannula and allows speech and breathing without manual occlusion or a cap

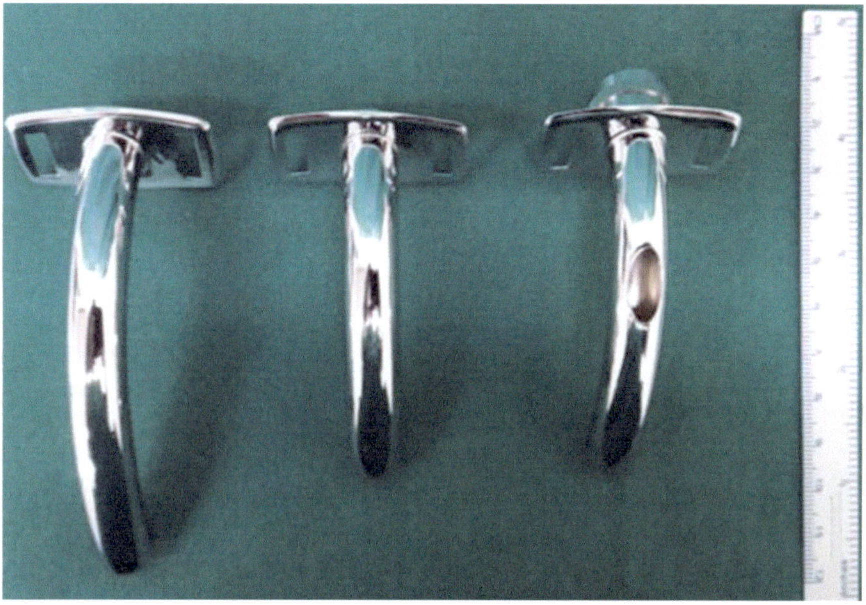

Fig. 6 Long conventional and fenestrated metallic tubes. The long tube is used for large necks or where there is a tumor in the stoma. The fenestrated tube is used to enable speech and can be used with or without a speaking valve

Polyvinyl chloride (PVC) adjusts to the patient's temperature and anatomy; silicone is soft, does not retain heat or cold, is resistant to colonization and biofilm, and can be sterilized [12] (Figs. 7, 11, 12, and 14).

Some authors recommend the use of plastic-cuffed tracheostomy tubes with an inner cannula, such as Bjork-Shiley tubes or Portex® tubes [1].

Cannula Types

Tracheostomy tubes may have an inner cannula or not. Those that do are dual-cannula tracheostomy tubes, and this feature allows periodic cleaning without removing the tube's main shaft or, when it occludes, ensures a patent airway [10–12]. Nonetheless, there is a lack of evidence that this helps to prevent pneumonia, and changing the inner cannula regularly in critical care units is not necessary [13]. Some inner cannulae may have an attachment for mechanical ventilation or fenestration [12]. Figure 8 shows capped, conventional, and 15 mm adapter inner cannulae.

On the other hand, an inner cannula decreases the inner diameter, resulting in additional work for breathing and paradoxical secretion adhesion [14, 15]. Carter et al. evaluated the effect of the inner tube of the Portex® Blueline Ultra® on the resistance and work of breathing through tracheostomy tubes. It was observed that the placement of the inner cannula significantly increased the work of breathing,

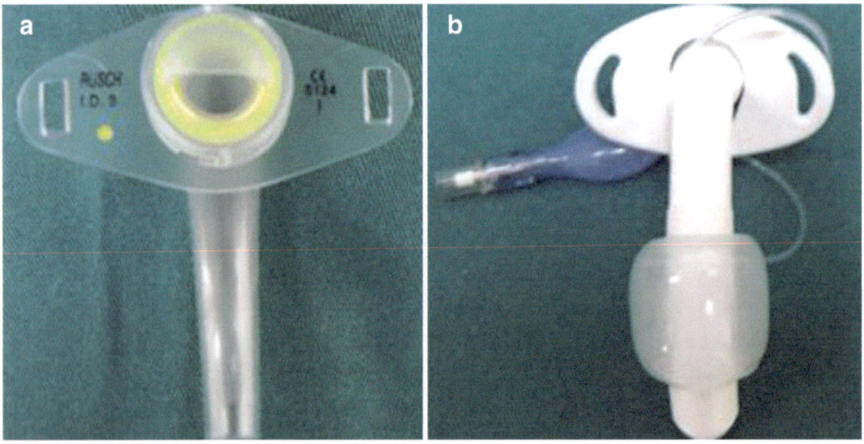

Fig. 7 **a** Rüsch® number 9 (inner diameter 9.0 mm) plastic uncuffed tube with an inner cannula and cough cap. **b** Shiley™ number 8 (inner diameter 7.6 mm) cuffed tube with an inner cannula

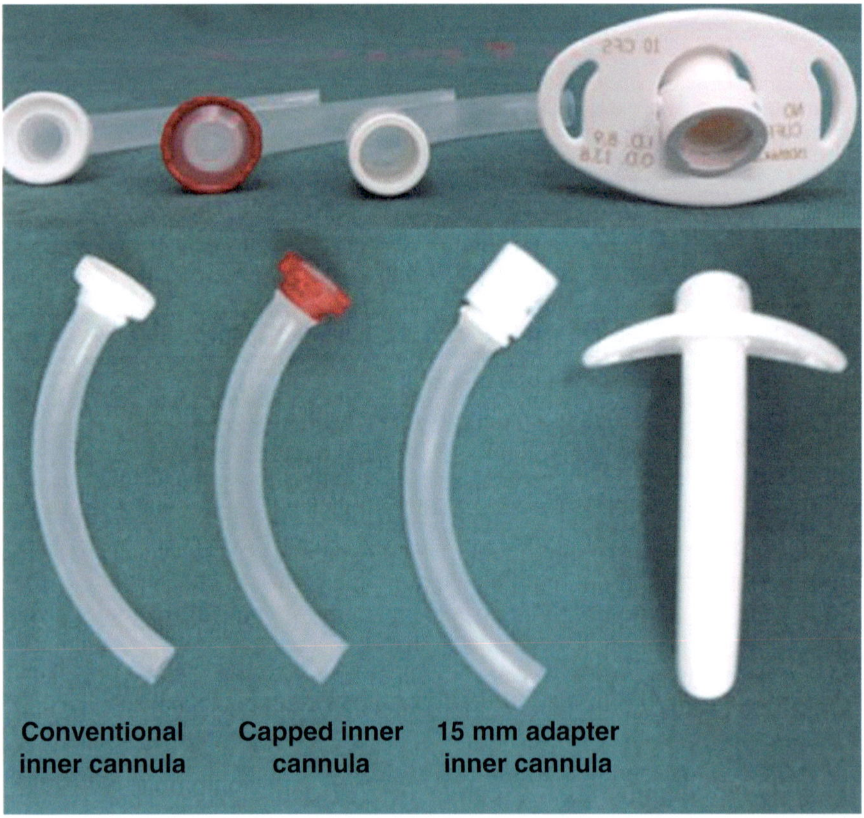

Fig. 8 Different inner cannulae. The capped inner cannula is used when the patient is being weaned, and it can be used with an uncuffed tube or a deflated cuffed tube. The 15 mm adapter connects to a mechanic ventilator, but a cuffed tube is needed in this scenario

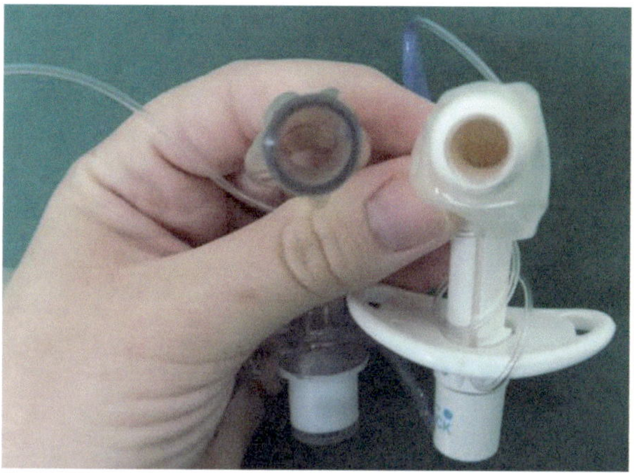

Fig. 9 Portex® number 9 tube without an inner cannula, and Shiley™ number 9 tube with an equivalent outer diameter; there is an important difference between their inner diameters

and this effect was greatest with a size 7.0 tube [16]. However, this disadvantage must be weighed against the benefits of cleaning, and encrusted secretions may also reduce the inner tube diameter [17]. Figure 9 shows the difference in the inner diameters of plastic cannulae with the same outer diameter size but with and without an inner cannula.

A single cannula prevents an increase in the work of breathing, but it is not suitable for patients with excessive secretions or poor clearing [10].

Dimensions

The specifications of tracheostomy tubes are related to the dimensions of their length, curvature, and inner and outer diameters. These dimensions are not standardized; different manufacturers' tube sizes are not equivalent to each other, and the size usually corresponds to neither the inner nor the outer diameter [10–12]. Hence, different tube brands with the same size numbers might actually be quite different [12]. The size and the inner and outer diameters are usually marked on the neckplate of the tracheostomy tube (see Fig. 10) [10].

The International Organization for Standardization (ISO) has determined a sizing method based on the inner diameter of the outer cannula at its smallest dimension. Dual-cannula sizing considers the inner cannula as the functional diameter and the outer diameter as its largest diameter [12] (Table 1).

I.D. inner diameter, *NA* not available, *O.D.* outer diameter

With regard to tube length, tubes may be angled, standard, extra-length, or adjustable flange. For patients with large necks, long-flange tubes are necessary [11], and adjustable-flange tubes enables changing the tube's lenght when necessary—for instance, when there is granulation tissue or a tumor within the airway or between the skin and the trachea [18]. Figures 11, 12, and 13 show the distinctions

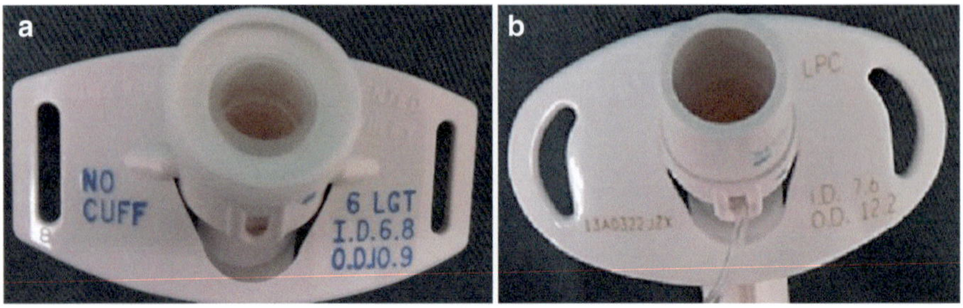

Fig. 10 Tracheostomy measurement specifications for a Shiley™ tube flange. **a** LGT (laryngectomy tube) number 6. **b** LPC (low-pressure cuff). Both have a nondisposable inner cannula. *I.D.* inner diameter, *O.D.* outer diameter

Table 1 Tracheostomy tube sizes

Size	Portex®		Shiley™		Jackson (metallic)	
	I.D. (mm)	O.D. (mm)	I.D. (mm)	O.D. (mm)	I.D. (mm)	O.D. (mm)
4	–	–	5.0	9.4	5.0	9.4
5	NA	NA	NA	NA	6.0	9.0
6	6.0	8.2	6.4	10.8	6.4	10.8
7	7.0	9.6	–	–	7.0	11.0
8	8.0	10.9	7.6	12.2	7.6	12.2
9	9.0	12.3	–	–	8.3	13.0
10	10.0	13.7	8.9	13.8	8.9	13.8

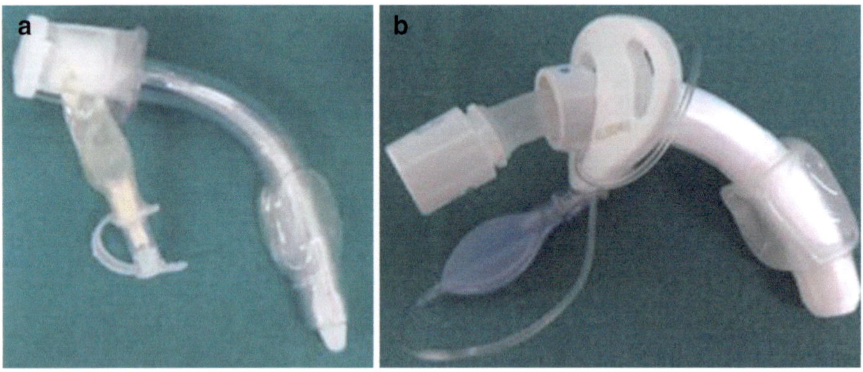

Fig. 11 (**a**) Plastic-cuffed angled tube without an inner cannula. (**b**) Plastic-cuffed curved tube with an inner cannula

in the curvature and length of tracheostomy tubes. The locking device must be secured so the tube will not be dislodged or move out of position [18]. In Fig. 14, an adjustable Portex® locking device mechanism is demonstrated.

When choosing the tracheostomy tube size, some factors must be considered, such as the size of the patient's neck, the stoma and trachea size, the presence of tumors or granulation tissue, the quality and quantity of secretions, and ventilator

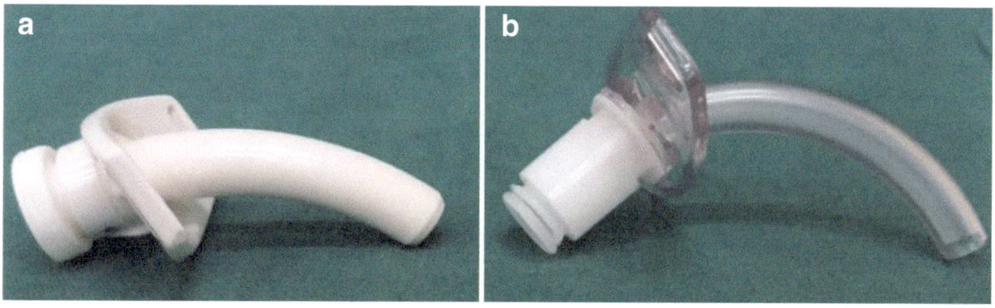

Fig. 12 (**a**) The Shiley™ LGT (laryngectomy tube) is shorter than the conventional Shiley™ DCFS (cuffless with disposable inner cannula) tube; the 6LGT length is 50 mm and the 6DCFS length is 76 mm. (**b**) The Portex® Blue Line size 6 is a standard cuffless tube with a disposable inner cannula tube, like the Shiley™ 6DCFS. Its length is 64.5 mm

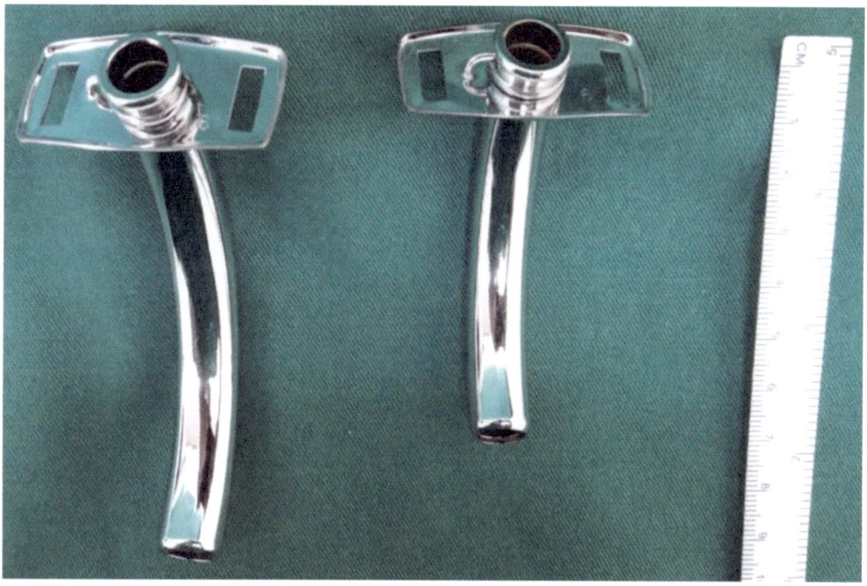

Fig. 13 Extra-length and standard metallic tubes

and weaning needs [10]. If the inner diameter is too small, the resistance through it and respiratory work will be increased, and the cuff pressure required to seal the tracheal lumen will be higher. A large outer diameter prevents the patient from speaking when the cuff is deflated [12]. Figure 15 shows a schematic drawing of the difference between inner and outer diameter sizes.

The trachea in adult females has a smaller inner diameter than that in males, and tubes with a 6.0–6.5 mm inner diameter (10 mm outer diameter) are usually adequate for females, while tubes with a 7.0–8.0 mm inner diameter (11 mm outer diameter) are suitable for males [10, 12, 18]. In children, the diameter of the fifth finger is similar to the trachea size [10].

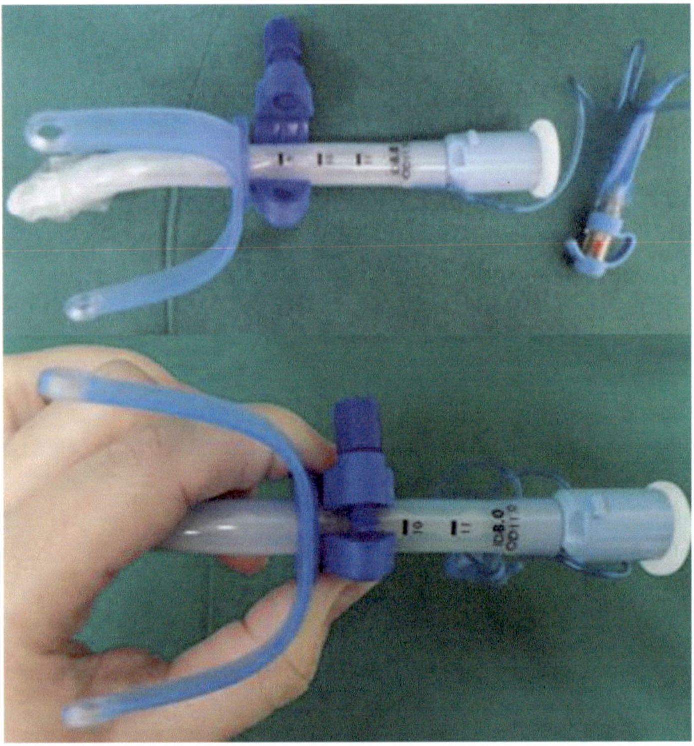

Fig. 14 Adjustable-flange tracheostomy tube. The flange size is set and then the locking device must be closed with the plastic screw

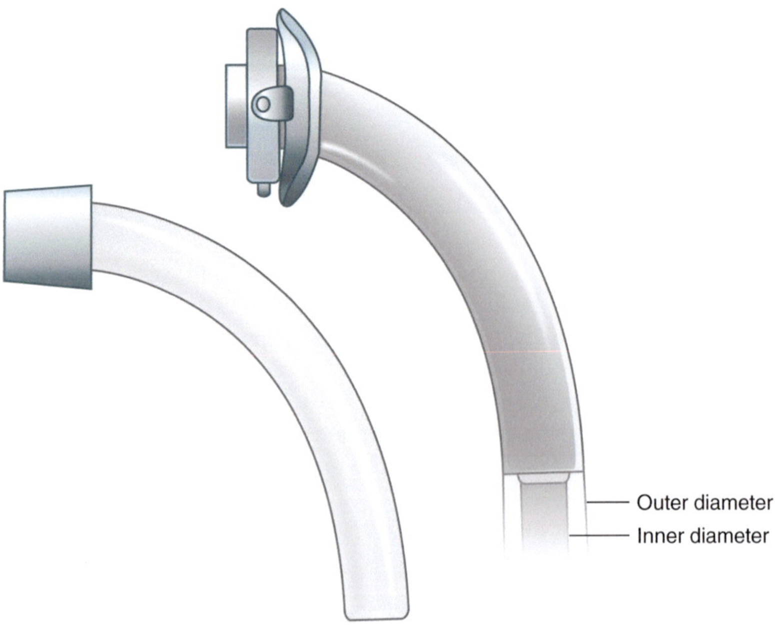

Fig. 15 Difference between inner and outer diameters

Fenestration

Fenestrated tubes have an opening on the posterior wall of the cannula, which allows the air to flow and be exhaled through it. This opening may consist of one large opening or several small ones [10–12]. A dual-cannula tube may or may not have a fenestrated inner cannula and may be cuffed or cuffless [10]. Figure 16 shows examples of metallic tube size 3, 4, 5, and 6 fenestrated cannulae.

This feature is important for preparing the patient for decannulation and phonation. When it is plugged and the cuff (if present) is deflated, the air flows to the upper airway through this opening and around the cannula. This makes it possible to assess the patient's ability to breathe using the upper airway, and allows phonation. When the patient is using a cuffed tube, it must be deflated before occluding the cannula [10–12]. A fenestrated tube model, showing its inner cannula and cap, is shown in Fig. 17.

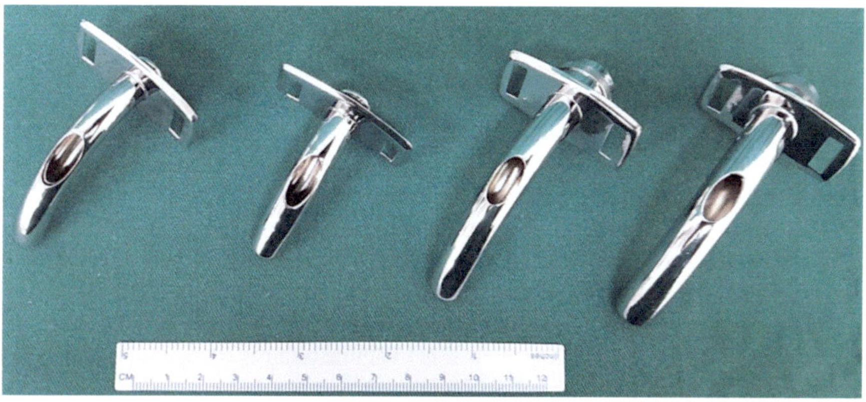

Fig. 16 Metallic fenestrated tubes with fenestrated inners

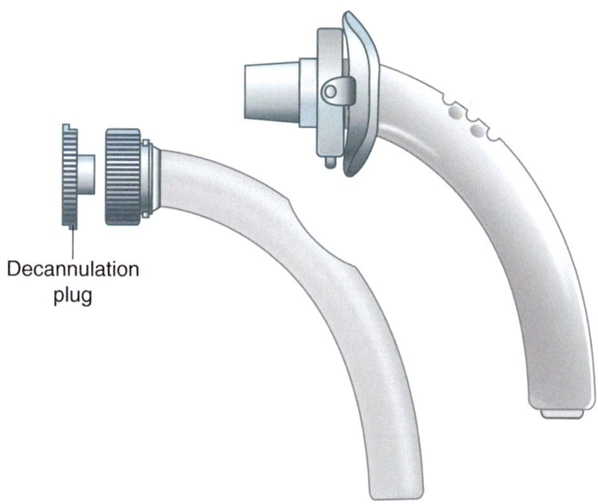

Fig. 17 Model of a fenestrated tube and inner cannula. The decannulation plug can be used while the patient is being weaned

These tubes may be difficult to fit, and the distance from the neckplate to the fenestration should be 1 cm longer than the stoma tract length for better adaptation [19]. Otherwise, the air will not pass to the upper airway and there will be an increase in flow resistance. Despite correct positioning, there may be other problems—such as granulation tissue induced by the fenestrations, resulting in impairment of the airway—and the position of the fenestrations should be checked periodically [20].

Cuffed and Cuffless Tracheostomy Tubes

Cuffed Tubes

Tracheostomy tubes may be cuffed or uncuffed (cuffless). The cuff is a rounded dilatation located in the distal part of the cannula, which seals the airway, providing a closed system for airway protection and ventilation [10–12, 21]. There are high-volume low-pressure, low-volume high-pressure, and foam cuffs [12].

High-volume low-pressure cuffs are the most commonly used type. They have a large diameter and a large residual volume, so the resting volume is larger than the patient's tracheal diameter, and the thin flexible material of the wall adapts easily to the tracheal wall when inflated [22]. Nonetheless, if excessive pressure is applied to the tracheal wall, there may be damage to its mucosa [23].

The cuff pressures used in current standard practice range from 20 to 30 cm H_20 (15–22 mmHg) to provide sealing of the airway and to prevent aspiration, preventing damage to the tracheal wall [12, 23]. Monitoring of the intracuff pressure should be performed at least once per shift and more often if necessary (e.g., if a leak occurs, if the position or the tube are changed, or if the volume of air is changed) [12]. Besides the risk of tracheal wall injury, higher cuff pressure impairs the swallowing reflex [24].

High pressure is commonly caused when the tube is small and the cuff must be overfilled in order to seal the trachea, or by tube malpositioning, low-pressure high-volume cuffs, and tracheal dilatation [12].

A low-volume high-pressure cuff is suitable for patients receiving intermittent cuff inflation, because it allows the air to flow around the tube while deflated, so speech and upper airway use are possible. It is a silicone cuff, which should be filled with sterile water, because if it is inflated with air, it will deflate due to gas permeability [12]. Figure 18 compares low-volume high-pressure cuffs and high-volume low-pressure cuffs, demonstrating how those cuffs interact with the tracheal wall.

Foam cuffs are not commonly used; they contain autoexpanding foam composed of polyurethane foam covered by a silicone sheath, which conforms to the patient's airway shape [12, 25]. These cuffs inflate passively at ambient atmospheric pressure and, if used properly, this pressure will not exceed 27 cm H_20 (20 mmHg). Their insertion and removal are harder, and the air should be removed with a syringe, which is disconnected when the tube is in place. The pilot tube is opened and the cuff keeps its pressure balanced with the atmospheric pressure (observe in Fig. 19 the Bivona® tube device for cuff inflation control). Nonetheless, they have to be

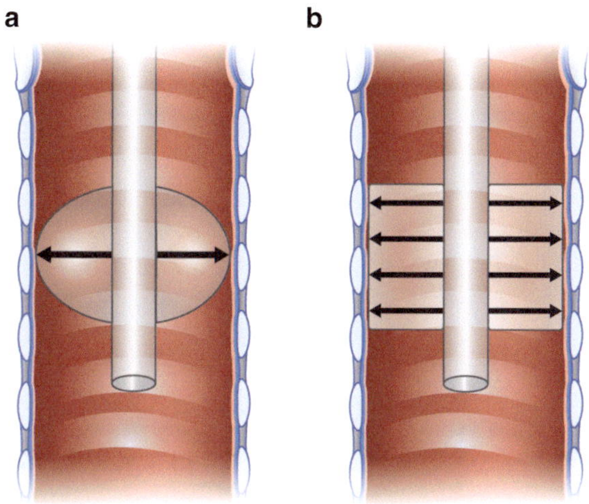

Fig. 18 Pressure is force per unit area. (**a**) Low-volume high-pressure cuffs are spherical and have a smaller area of contact with the tracheal wall, thus a higher pressure. (**b**) High-volume low-pressure cuffs are barrel-shaped and touch a bigger area, with lower pressure applied to the tracheal mucosa

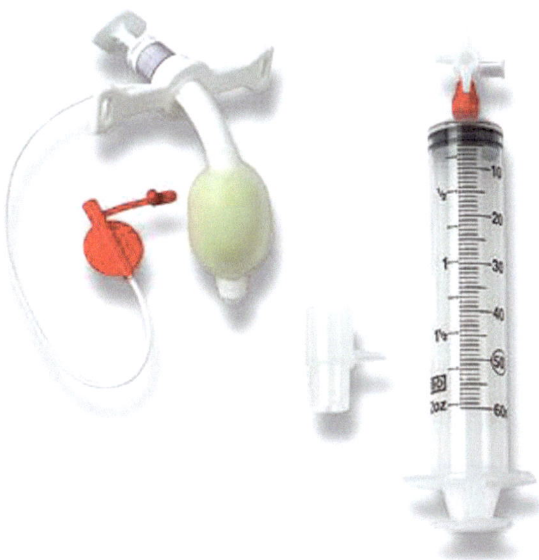

Fig. 19 The Bivona® Adult Fome-Cuff® has a foam cuff and comes with a 60 mL syringe, which helps in controlling the cuff's inflation while attached to a three-way stopcock, aiding insertion and measurement of the cuff volume. (Reproduced from Smiths Medical [34])

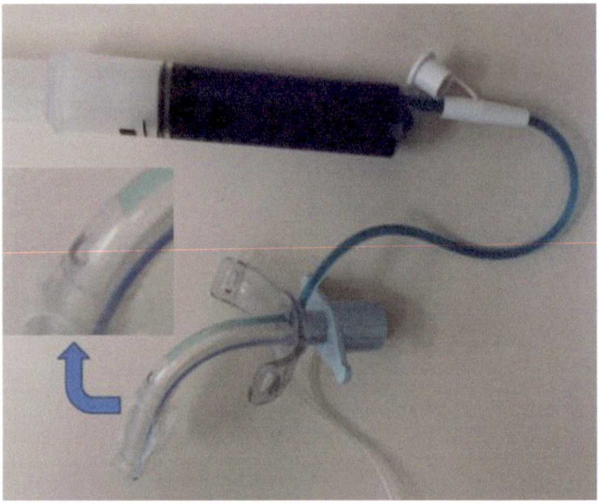

Fig. 20 Plastic tube with a supraglottic suction device. *Blue dye* highlights the suction port path in this picture

periodically deflated so that humidity is removed from the sponge and to keep the silicone sheath from adhering to the tracheal wall. They are not suitable for patients with one-way speaking valves, since they seal the lower airway, and so they are reserved for patients with tracheal injury caused by cuffed cannulae [12, 26].

Cuffs, either deflated or inflated, may increase the work of breathing, and they should be replaced with a cuffless tube while the patient is in the process of weaning [27].

Some cuffed tracheostomy tubes have a suction port above the cuff to remove subglottic secretions [18]. Their role in preventing ventilator-associated pneumonia (VAP) in patients with endotracheal tubes has been shown in meta-analyses, with a reduction in VAP of approximately 50% [28, 29]. Ledgerwood et al. also observed fewer cases of VAP and trends toward reductions in the intensive care unit stay and the time of mechanical ventilation in patients with a tracheostomy tube and a subglottic suction port [29]. Nonetheless, there have been no large clinical trials, nor meta-analyses, on subglottic suction devices in tracheostomy tubes. A tracheostomy tube with a suction port is shown in Fig. 20, with its path highlighted and distal port magnified.

Cuffless Tubes

Cuffless (uncuffed) tracheostomy tubes allow air to flow to the upper airway and allow stomal maintenance. They are used when mechanical ventilation is no longer required but the airways still need to be accessed. There are plastic and metal models available. Figure 21 shows plastic and metallic uncuffed tubes.

Some factors must be addressed before a cuffless tracheostomy tube is used. First the patient has to be able to breathe spontaneously and swallow without significant aspiration. Once the patient is fitted with the cuffless tube, its opening can

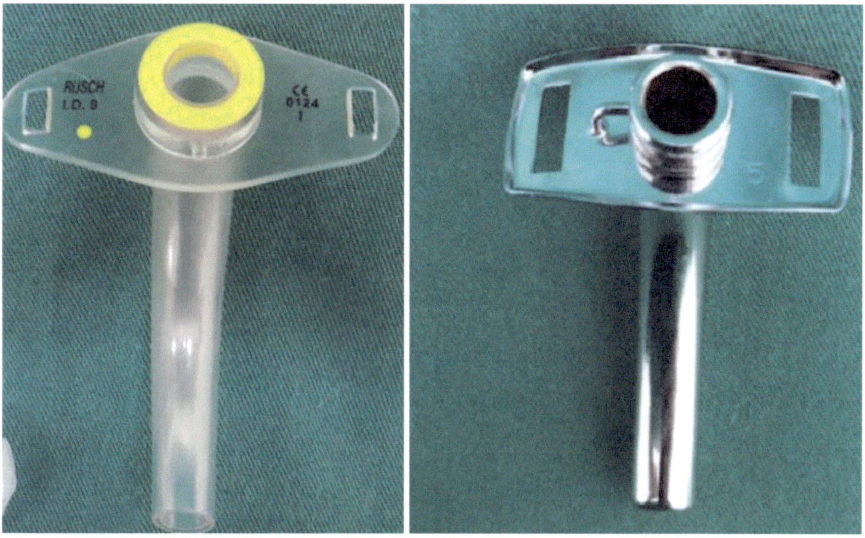

Fig. 21 Plastic and metallic cuffless tubes

Table 2 Sizing chart for Portex® cuffed tracheostomy tubes (Blue Line Ultra® with Suctionaid® and Blue Line Ultra®)

Size	I.D. (mm)	I.D. with inner cannula (mm)	O.D. (mm)	Length (mm)	Cuff O.D. (mm)
6	6.0	5.0	9.2	64.5	20.0
7	7.0	5.5	10.5	70.0	24.0
7.5	7.5	6.0	11.3	73.0	30.0
8	8.0	6.5	11.9	75.5	30.0
8.5	8.5	7.0	12.6	78.0	30.0
9	9.0	7.5	13.3	81.0	30.0
10	10.0	8.5	14.0	87.5	30.0

Adapted from the Austin Health Tracheostomy Review and Management Service [30]
I.D. inner diameter, *O.D.* outer diameter

be closed with the patient's (or caregiver's) finger, be capped, or a speaking valve can be used for speech.

Plastic uncuffed tubes are used in patients receiving head and neck radiotherapy to prevent stoma and tracheal wall burn [10, 12, 18, 26].

Tracheostomy Tube Sizes

The sizing charts shown in Tables 2, 3, 4, 5, 6, 7, 8, 9, and 10 are adapted from the Austin Health Tracheostomy Review and Management Service (TRAMS) tracheostomy sizing chart [30] (see also Figs. 22, 23, 24, 25, 26, 27, 28, 29, 30, 31, 32, and 33).

Table 3 Sizing chart for Portex® adjustable-flange tracheostomy tubes (Blue Line Ultra®)

Size	I.D. (mm)	O.D. (mm)	Length (mm)	Cuff O.D. (mm)
6	6.0	8.3	59–81	20.0
7	7.0	9.7	64–84	24.0
8	8.0	11	73–97	30.0
9	9.0	12.4	78–111	30.0
10	10.0	13.7	84–123	30.0

Adapted from the Austin Health Tracheostomy Review and Management Service [30]
I.D. inner diameter, *O.D.* outer diameter

Table 4 Sizing chart for Portex® Uniperc™ Adjustable Flange Tracheostomy Tubes

Size	I.D. (mm)	I.D. with inner cannula (mm)	O.D. (mm)	Length (mm)
7	9.3	7.0	11.6	62
8	10.3	8.0	12.6	68
9	11.3	9.0	13.6	74

Adapted from the Austin Health Tracheostomy Review and Management Service [30]
I.D. inner diameter, *O.D.* outer diameter

Table 5 Sizing chart for Bivona® foam cuff tracheostomy tubes (Bivona® Adult Fome-Cuff®)

Size	I.D. (mm)	O.D. (mm)	Length (mm)
5	5.0	7.3	60.0
6	6.0	8.7	70.0
7	7.0	10.0	80.0
8	8.0	11.0	88.9
9	9.0	12.3	98.0
9.5	9.5	13.3	98.0

Adapted from the Austin Health Tracheostomy Review and Management Service [30]
I.D. inner diameter, *O.D.* outer diameter

Table 6 Sizing chart for Shiley™ cuffed tracheostomy tubes: cuffed with an inner cannula (LPC) and fenestrated (FEN)

Size	I.D. (mm)	O.D. (mm)	Length (mm)
4	5.0	9.4	65
6	6.4	10.8	76
8	7.6	12.2	81
10	8.9	13.8	81

Adapted from the Austin Health Tracheostomy Review and Management Service [30]
I.D. inner diameter, *O.D.* outer diameter

Table 7 Sizing chart for Shiley™ tracheostomy tubes with a disposable inner cannula: cuffed (DCT), cuffed and fenestrated (DFEN), percutaneous (PERC), cuffless (DCFS), and cuffless and fenestrated (DCFN)

Size	I.D. (mm)	O.D. (mm)	Length (mm)
4	5.0	9.4	62
6	6.4	10.8	74
8	7.6	12.2	79
10	8.9	13.8	79

Adapted from the Austin Health Tracheostomy Review and Management Service [30]
I.D. inner diameter, *O.D.* outer diameter

Table 8 Sizing chart for Shiley™ flexible tracheostomy tubes: cuffed and uncuffed (CN/UN)

Size	I.D. (mm)	I.D. with inner cannula (mm)	O.D. (mm)	Length (mm)
4	6.5	5.5	9.4	62.0
5	7.0	6.0	10.1	68.0
6	7.5	6.5	10.8	74.0
7	8.0	7.0	11.4	77.0
8	8.5	7.5	12.2	79.0
9	9.0	8.0	12.7	79.0
10	10.0	9.0	13.8	79.0

Adapted from the Austin Health Tracheostomy Review and Management Service [30]
I.D. inner diameter, *O.D.* outer diameter

Table 9 Sizing chart for Shiley™ XLT tracheostomy tubes with extra length

Size	I.D. (mm)	O.D. (mm)	Proximal length (mm)	Distal length (mm)	Total length (mm)
5 distal	5.0	9.6	5.0	48.0	90
5 proximal	5.0	9.6	20.0	33.0	90
6 distal	6.0	11.0	8.0	49.0	95
6 proximal	6.0	11.0	23.0	34.0	95
7 distal	7.0	12.3	12.0	49.0	100
7 proximal	7.0	12.3	27.0	34.0	100
8	8.0	13.3	15.0	50	105
8	8.0	13.3	30.0	40.0	105

Adapted from the Austin Health Tracheostomy Review and Management Service [30]
I.D. inner diameter, *O.D.* outer diameter

Table 10 Sizing chart for Cook® Versa™ tracheostomy tubes

Size	I.D. (mm)	I.D. with inner cannula (mm)	O.D. (mm)	Length (mm)	Cuff O.D. (mm)	Angle (°)	Color
7	7.0	6.0	10.0	78.0	25.0	96	Green
8	8.0	7.0	11.0	86.0	28.0	96	White
9	9.0	8.0	12.0	98.0	30.0	98	Blue

Adapted from the Austin Health Tracheostomy Review and Management Service [30]
I.D. inner diameter, *O.D.* outer diameter

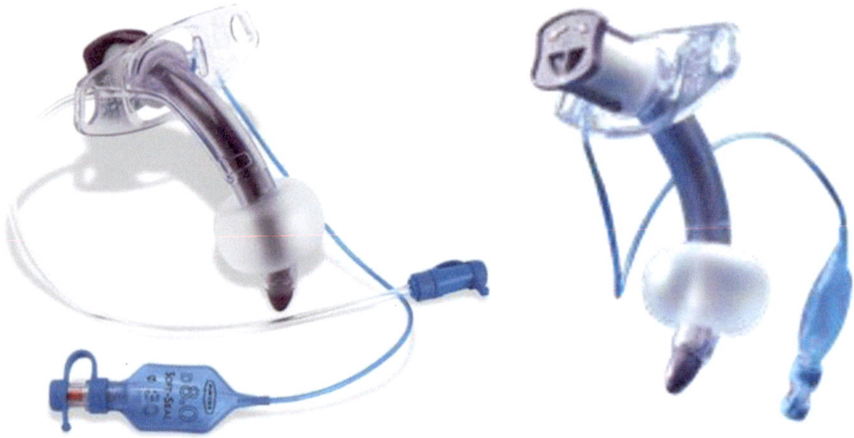

Fig. 22 Two tube models with inflated cuffs. The first is a model with a subglottic suction port and the second is without one. (Reproduced from Smiths Medical [34])

Fig. 23 Portex® Blue Line Ultra® adjustable-flange tube. (Reproduced from Smiths Medical [34])

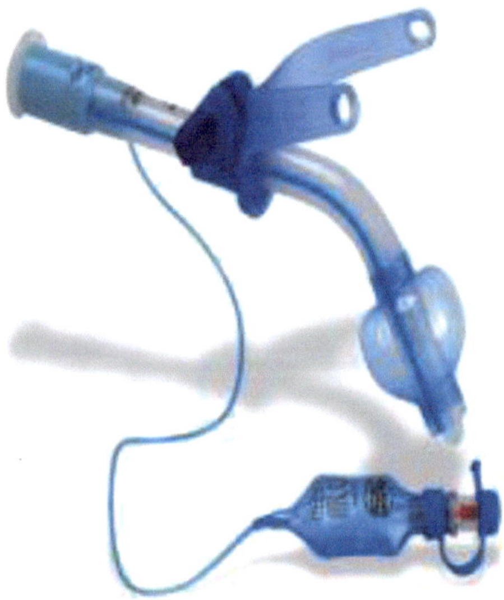

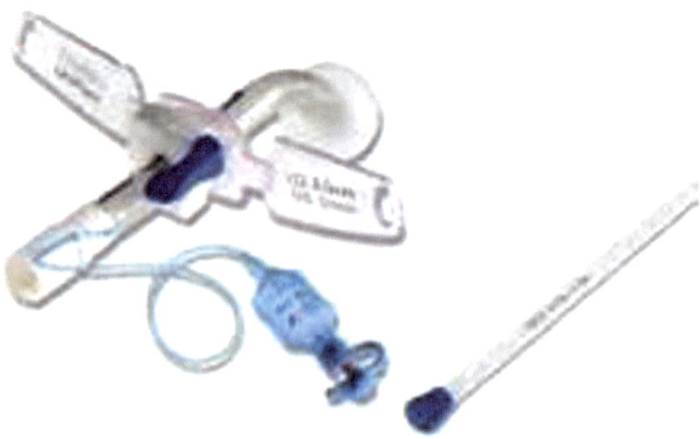

Fig. 24 The Portex® UniPerc® adjustable-flange tube is a percutaneous tube with a flexible polytetrafluoroethylene (PTFE) inner cannula with a nonstick surface. (Reproduced from Smiths Medical [34])

Fig. 25 Bivona® Fome-Cuff® and cuff maintenance device (CMD™). (Reproduced from Smiths Medical [34])

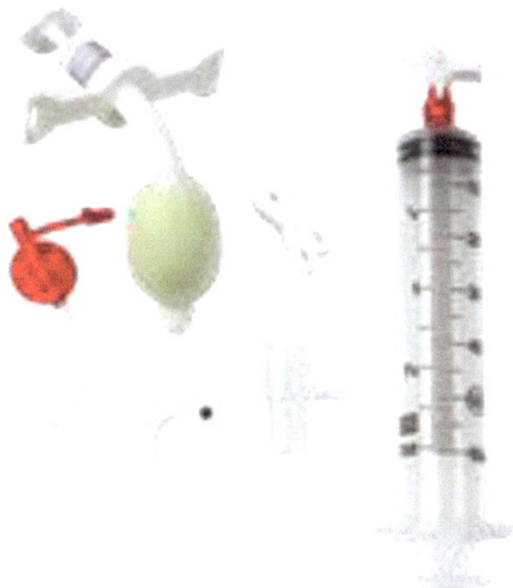

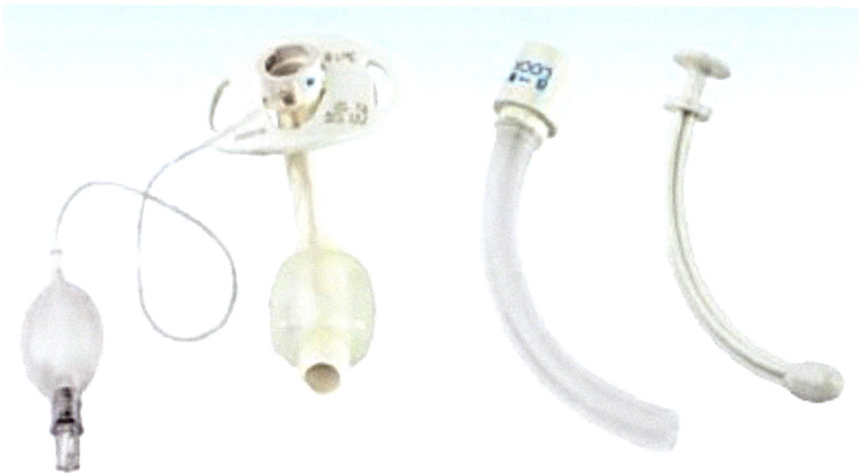

Fig. 26 Shiley™ LPC (low-pressure cuff). (Reproduced from Medtronic [31])

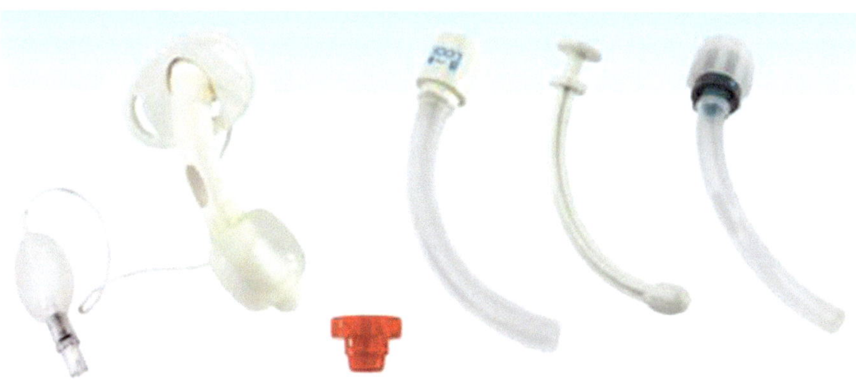

Fig. 27 Shiley™ FEN (fenestrated) tube with its cap (in *red*), inner cannula with a 15 mm adapter, obturator, and fenestrated inner cannula. (Reproduced from Medtronic [31])

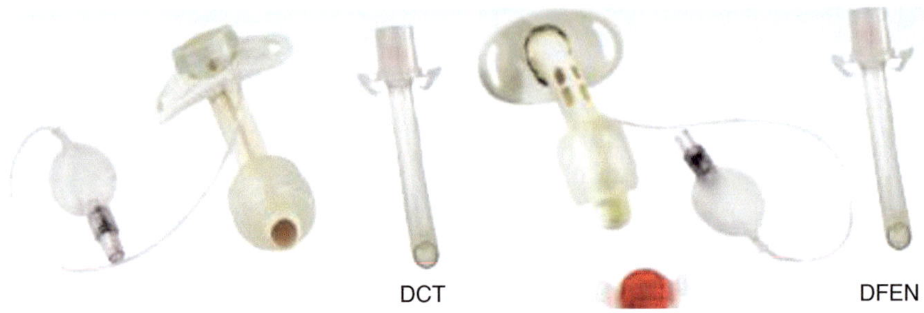

Fig. 28 Shiley™ DCT (disposable cuffed tube) and Shiley™ DFEN (cuffed and fenestrated tube). The *red plug* is the cap for tube occlusion. (Reproduced from Medtronic [31])

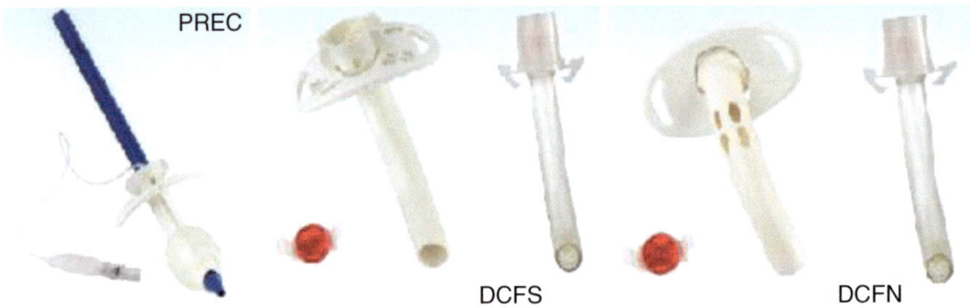

Fig. 29 Shiley™ PERC (percutaneous) tube with its introducer, Shiley™ DCFS (cuffless with disposable inner cannula) tube, and Shiley™ DCFN (cuffless and fenestrated) tube, each with its inner cannula and cap. (Reproduced from Medtronic [31])

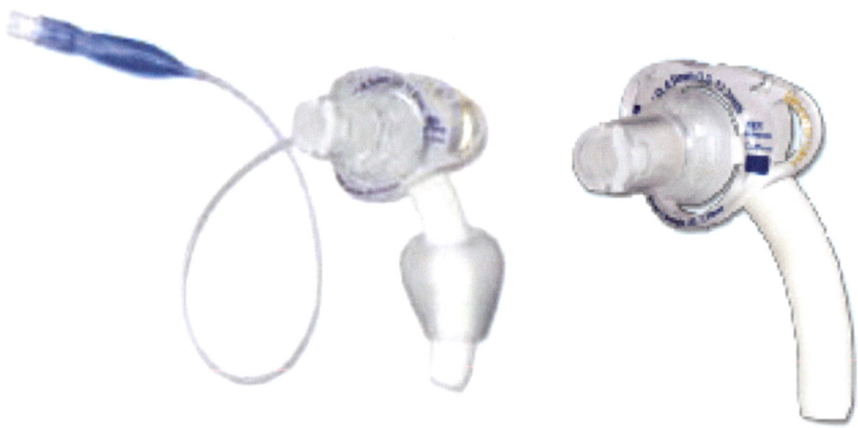

Fig. 30 Cuffed and uncuffed Shiley™ flexible tubes. (Reproduced from Medtronic [31])

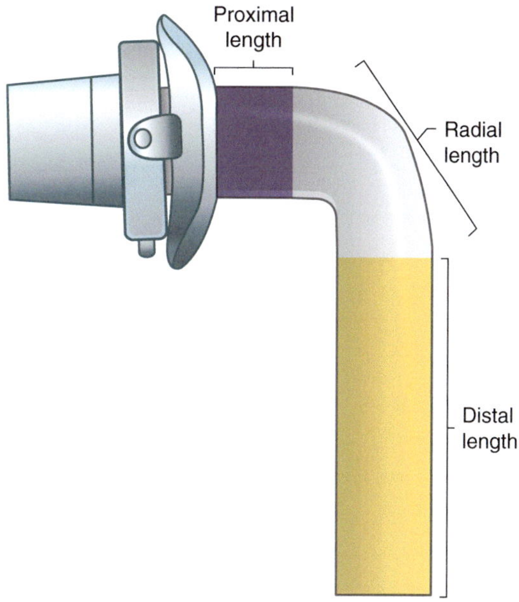

Fig. 31 Tracheostomy tube length measurements

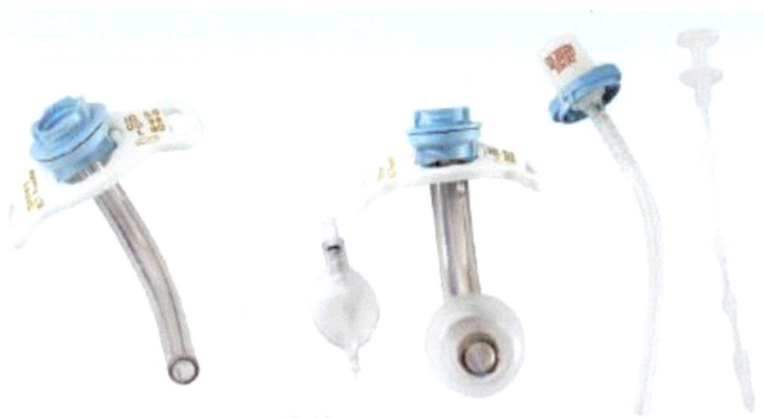

Fig. 32 Uncuffed and cuffed Shiley™ XLT tubes. (Reproduced from Medtronic [31])

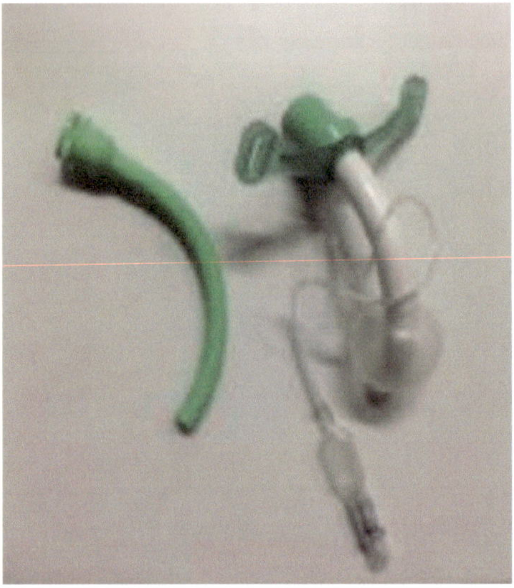

Fig. 33 Cook® Versa™ tracheostomy tube size 7. (Reproduced from Austin Health Tracheostomy Review and Management Service [30])

Conclusion

There is a wide range of tracheostomy tubes available for different clinical settings. The clinician must be familiar with them to choose a suitable tube for each patient and occasion.

References

1. De Leyn P, et al. Tracheotomy: clinical review and guidelines. European Journal of Cardiothoracic Surgery. 2007;32:412–21.
2. Pierson DJ. Tracheostomy from A to Z: historical context and current challenges. Respir Care. 2005;50(4):473–5.
3. Jackson C. High tracheotomy and other errors. The chief causes of chronic laryngeal stenosis. Surg Gynecol Obstet. 1923;32:392.
4. White AC, O'Connor HH, Kirby K, White AC, O'Connor HH, Kirby K. Prolonged mechanical ventilation: review of care settings and an update on professional reimbursement. Chest. 2008;133(2):539–45.
5. Esteban A, Anzueto A, Frutos F, Alia I, Brochard L, Stewart TE, et al. Characteristics and outcomes in adult patients receiving mechanical ventilation: a 28-day international study. JAMA. 2002;287(3):345–55.
6. Cox CE, Carson SS, Holmes GM, Howard A, Carey TS, Cox CE, et al. Increase in tracheostomy for prolonged mechanical ventilation in North Carolina, 1993–2002. Crit Care Med. 2004;32(11):2219–26.
7. Wilson DJ. Airway appliances and management. In: Kacmarek RM, Stoller JK, editors. Current respiratory care. Philadelphia: PC Decker; 1988.

8. Wilson DJ. Airway management of the ventilator-assisted individual. Prob Resp Care. 1988;1(2):192–203.
9. Godwin JE, Heffner JE. Special critical care considerations in tracheostomy management. Clin Chest Med. 1991;12(3):573–83.
10. Weilitz PB, Dettenmeier PA. Back to basics: test your knowledge of tracheostomy tubes. Am J Nurs. 1994;94(2):46–50.
11. Engels PT, et al. Tracheostomy: from insertion to decannulation. Can J Surg. 2009;52(5):427.
12. Hess DR, Altobelli. NP. Tracheostomy tubes discussion. Respir Care. 2014;59(6):956–73.
13. Burns SM, Spilman S, Wilmoth D, Carpender R, Turrentine B, Wiley B, Marshall M, Marten S, Burns JE, Truwit JD. Are frequent inner cannula changes necessary? A pilot study. Heart Lung. 1998;27(1):58–62.
14. Cowan T, Op't Holt TB, Gegenheimer C, Izenberg S, Kulkarni P. Effect of inner cannula removal on the work of breathing imposed by tracheostomy tubes: a bench study. Respir Care. 2001;46(5):460–5.
15. Loh KS, Irish JC. Traumatic complications of intubation and other airway management procedures. Anesthesiol Clin North Am. 2002;20:953–69.
16. Carter, et al. The work of breathing through tracheostomy inner tubes. Anaesthesia. 2013;68:276–82.
17. Wilson AM, Gray DM, Thomas JG. Increases in endotracheal tube resistance are unpredictable relative to duration of intubation. Chest. 2009;136:1006–13.
18. White AC, Kher S, O'Connor HH. When to change a tracheostomy tube. Respir Care. 2010;55(8):1069–75.
19. Dunn PF, Goulet RL. Endotracheal tubes and airway appliances. Int Anesthesiol Clin. 2000;38:65–94.
20. Siddharth P, Mazzarella L. Granuloma associated with fenestrated tracheostomy tubes. Am J Surg. 1985;150(2):279–80.
21. Morris LL, Whitmer A, McIntosh E. Tracheostomy care and complications in the intensive care unit. Crit Care Nurse. 2013;33(5):18–30.
22. Carroll RG, McGinnis GE, Grenvik A. Performance characteristics of tracheal cuffs. Int Anesthesiol Clin. 1974;12(3):111–41.
23. Maguire S, Haury F, Jew K. An in vitro comparison of tracheostomy tube cuffs. Med Devices (Auckl). 2015;8:185.
24. Amathieu R, Sauvat S, Reynaud P, Slavov V, Luis D, Dinca A, et al. Influence of the cuff pressure on the swallowing reflex in tracheostomized intensive care unit patients. Br J Anaesth. 2012;109(4):578–83.
25. Eber, Ernst, Oberwaldner B. Tracheostomy care in the hospital. Paediatr Respir Rev. 2006;7(3):175–84.
26. John RES, Malen JF. Contemporary issues in adult tracheostomy management. Crit Care Nurs Clin North Am. 2004;16(3):413–30.
27. Beard B, Monaco MJ. Tracheostomy discontinuation: impact of tube selection on resistance during tube occlusion. Respir Care. 1993;38(3):267–70.
28. Muscedere J, et al. Subglottic secretion drainage for the prevention of ventilator-associated pneumonia: a systematic review and meta-analysis. Crit Care Med. 2011;39(8):1985–91.
29. Leasure AR, Stirlen J, Shu Hua L. Prevention of ventilator-associated pneumonia through aspiration of subglottic secretions: a systematic review and meta-analysis. Dimens Crit Care Nurs. 2012;31(2):102–17.
30. Austin Health Tracheostomy Review and Management Service (TRAMS). Tracheostomy sizing chart. http://tracheostomyteam.org/data/uploads/pdf/sizing-chart.pdf. Accessed
31. Medtronic. Shiley™ tracheostomy products quick reference guide. http://www.medtronic.com/content/dam/covidien/library/us/en/product/tracheostomy/shiley-tracheostomy-products-quick-reference-guide-ous.pdf. Accessed
32. Szmuk P, Ezri T, Evron S, et al. A brief history of tracheostomy and tracheal intubation, from the Bronze Age to the Space Age. Intensive Care Med. 2008;34:222–8.

33. Ledgerwood LG, Salgado MD, Black H, Yoneda K, Sievers A, Belafsky PC. Tracheotomy tubes with suction above the cuff reduce the rate of ventilator-associated pneumonia in intensive care unit patients. Ann Otol Rhinol Laryngol. 2013;122(1):3–8.
34. Smiths Medical. Tracheostomy products. https://www.smiths-medical.com/products/tracheostomy. Accessed

Tracheostomy: Conventional Technique

Adilis Stepple da Fonte Neto, Terence Pires de Farias, Juliana Maria de Almeida Vital, Jose Gabriel Miranda da Paixão, Juliana Fernandes de Oliveira, and Paulo Jose de Cavalcanti Siebra

Introduction

Tracheostomy, a term derived from two Greek words meaning "to cut the trachea," is a procedure known for approximately 3500 years.

The literature concerning its early history is quite scarce and open to various subjective interpretations, which hinder understanding of the technique. Most articles reference the procedure alone or, at most, its indications [1].

A.S. da Fonte Neto, M.D. (✉)
Department of Head and Neck Surgery, Integral Medicine Institute of Pernambuco (Instituto de Medicina Integral de Pernambuco-IMIP), Recife, PE, Brazil

Pernambuco Cancer Hospital (Hospital de Câncer de Pernambuco), Recife, PE, Brazil

Department of Head and Neck Surgery, Brazilian Head and Neck Surgery Society (Sociedade Brasileira de Cirurgia de Cabeça e Pescoço), São Paulo, SP, Brazil
e-mail: adilisdafonte@gmail.com

T.P. de Farias, M.D., Ph.D., M.Sc., Researcher.
Department of Head and Neck Surgery, Brazilian National Cancer Institute—INCA, Rio de Janeiro, RJ, Brazil

Department of Head and Neck Surgery, Pontifical Catholic University, Rio de Janeiro, RJ, Brazil

J.M. de Almeida Vital, M.D.
Head and Neck Department, Irmandade Santa Casa de São Paulo, São Paulo, SP, Brazil

Head and Neck Surgeon, Private Practice, Sao Paulo, SP, Brazil
e-mail: jujuliana.a@gmail.com

J.G.M. da Paixão, M.D. • J.F. de Oliveira, M.D. • P.J. de Cavalcanti Siebra
Department of Head and Neck Surgery, Brazilian National Cancer Institute (Instituto Nacional de Câncer – INCA/MS), Rio de Janeiro, RJ, Brazil

T.P. de Farias (ed.), *Tracheostomy*, https://doi.org/10.1007/978-3-319-67867-2_4

Information about the procedure is included in two of the world's three oldest medical references. The sacred book of Hinduism, written between 2000 and 1000 BC, mentions the convergence of the tracheal rings without ligatures after tracheostomy as apparently not warranting great concern [2]. Since that time, surgical closure of the tracheostomy was considered unnecessary, a principle adopted in the current era. The Ebers Papyrus, an Egyptian text from 1550 BC, refers to caution in the approach to the neck and diligence concerning the blood vessels, which still guide the hemostatic precautions adopted with current techniques. In their third medical book, the Chinese did not reference the procedure because the body was considered sacred and surgery deemed unnecessary.

Circa 100 BC, Asclepiades of Bithynia, a surgeon from a Roman province in northern Asia Minor, was the first to perform the procedure electively, in an infectious disease case. The procedure was later condemned because it was believed that the cartilage would not close [3].

With the fall of the Roman Empire and the beginning of the Byzantine Empire, one of the most prominent surgeons of that era emerged, Paul of Aegina (AD 625–690). He was born on the island of Aegina and practiced medicine in Alexandria. He wrote a series of seven books titled *The Medical Compendium in Seven Books*, which merged information from the ancient Greek and Roman empires. The chapter referring to the head and neck was the first to describe the technique of tracheostomy, fundamentally unchanged since this time, and its indications might be accurate here. According to Paul of Aegina, the patient should be placed in the supine position with the head extended for better exposure of the trachea. Next, a transverse excision of the membrane between the tracheal rings would be performed with a subsequent forceful expulsion of air or an inability to vocalize. Later, the skin would be sutured but not the cartilage [4].

New reports of the procedure and technical developments were possible only after the end of the Barbarian invasions, at the start of the High Middle Ages. Initially, due to much fear and skepticism, the procedure was discouraged.

Major technical advances occurred during the sixteenth century. In 1546, Musa Brassarolo Ferrara described the surgical technique. Notwithstanding its additional indications, his technique resembled that described by Paul of Aegina. In 1590, Sanatorius introduced the concept of cannula changing and leaving a cannula in place for 3 days. At that time, the preparation of a tracheocutaneous fistula was already an emerging concern.

In the seventeenth century, experiments performed by Robert Hooke on an animal model and inspired by the studies of Vesalius (1543) demonstrated the possibility of mechanical ventilation using cannulae with endotracheal balloons. At the University of Padua, using a vertical incision in the trachea, Fabricius ab Aquapendente and his pupil Casserius developed straight cannulae with rings and curved cannulae that enabled the patient to remain tracheostomized for a long period [1, 4].

The procedure was established during the eighteenth century despite extensive discussion and contrary opinions, such as those regarding its safety and extended indications. An important milestone in the nineteenth century was the publication in 1830 of a book by McKenzie, titled *Diseases of the Pharynx, Larynx and Trachea*, which discussed the appropriate time for the surgical approach. A literature review by Dr. Max Schuller in 1880 showed that great disagreement persisted at that time about the technique—for example, regarding the level chosen for the incision and the optimal opening of the trachea, anesthesia, and technique in children and adults.

An important development at the end of the nineteenth century and the beginning of the twentieth century was the possibility of airway control by orotracheal intubation. This advance allowed reduced comorbidities resulting from complex types of respiratory failure and consequently contributed to surgical technique improvement [24].

A 1909 publication in *Laryngoscope* by the author Chevalier Jackson, followed by other publications in 1921, set forth the technical fundamentals used today. He proposed a long and low incision in the fourth/fifth ring, which avoided dissection of the cricoid and thyroid cartilages and aimed to reduce stenosis. Jackson also proposed the dissection and sectioning of the tracheal isthmus for better exposure along with the development of various instruments for laryngotomy, bronchoscopy, and tracheostomy [18].

Currently, the surgical technique remains similar to that developed over 3000 years of history. More objective indications; technically improved scalpels, suture materials, and hemostatics; and the development of specific cannulae have contributed to a noteworthy reduction in morbidity.

Legislation

In Brazil, several opinions, consultations, and resolutions guide the Regional and Federal Medical Councils, standardization of the procedure and its good practice, and expertise and responsibilities.

The most common guidelines for proper procedural performance are discussed subsequently.

Who Is Qualified to Perform the Procedure?

In principle, any physician may perform the procedure, whether a clinician or surgeon, as long as they judge themselves capable and are willing to assume responsibility. Prudence demands that such individuals be professionals whose residency programs are standardized by the Ministry of Health and specialty societies and have included adequate training.

General surgeons, head and neck surgeons, oncological surgeons, pediatric surgeons, thoracic surgeons, and intensivists are specialists qualified for this purpose [5–7].

In cases of emergency care for craniofacial trauma for which an oromaxillofacial surgeon is available, the on-duty clinician or surgeon is responsible for securing the airway, whether by tracheostomy or another method, before referring the patient to the specialist [8].

In emergencies, physicians must be prepared to perform cricothyroidotomy or perhaps tracheostomy if it is within their capability.

In cases of elective tracheostomy, it is prudent for the surgical team to perform the procedure [5].

What Is a Suitable Location for the Procedure?

Bedside tracheostomy should be discouraged and should be performed only when patient transport to the operating room generates greater risks than those of the intensive care setting. Nonetheless, adequate technical conditions such as lighting and surgical instruments and a multidisciplinary team cannot be disregarded [6].

Elective tracheostomy should be performed primarily in the operating room with the participation of a multidisciplinary team to provide adequate health care support [9].

Emergency tracheostomies may be performed outside the operating room and within the emergency care environment, respecting the need to support well-defined cases. These procedures should be performed in an isolated environment that provides the technical support required to ensure good practice.

Is Informed Consent Necessary?

In urgent cases, performing a tracheostomy without any prior authorization is acceptable because the objective of this procedure is to safeguard the patient's life and health. Thus, its immediate performance is indisputable and unavoidable, as is any other procedure performed without informed consent.

In elective cases, prior authorization from the patient or legal representative is necessary whereby the risks and benefits of this procedure are clearly explained.

In cases of patients with unknown identities for whom no legal guardian is identified, the legal department of the institution must request the procedure judicially. The technical/clinical director is not responsible to authorize any type of invasive procedure [10].

Surgical Technique

No major changes to the conventional surgical tracheostomy technique have ensued since it was proposed by Brassarolo in 1546 and later described and refined by Chevalier Jackson in 1909. The anatomical knowledge held by the Egyptians, Greeks, and Persians was expanded, described, and studied in the Renaissance era, which makes the technique a widespread and consolidated procedure.

In the early twentieth century, Chevalier Jackson summarized the tracheostomy technique according to the following important aspects [18]:

1. Preservation of the cough reflex
2. Careful tissue dissection with minimal bleeding
3. Posttracheostomy care

4. Technique following aseptic principles
5. Trendelenburg position to decrease airway infection and bleeding
6. Appropriate size and length of the cannulae

Substantial advances have clearly ensued in terms of indications, damage control, reduction of complications, and development of minimally invasive techniques.

However, some myths related to the procedure warrant examination. First, some medical professionals believe that tracheostomy is a low-risk secondary procedure without complications. Although mortality has decreased considerably, as recently as the early twentieth century it was 10–15% [18].

Thus, although the procedure is well established and has quite precise indications, the fact that some complications and sequelae exist that may be fatal for the patient must be clarified for the medical professional, patient, and patient's family members. The informed consent form must be completed properly and must not represent an institutional formality. Although this suggestion may appear innocuous, it may potentially confer heightened significance should court proceedings ensue.

The purpose of this chapter is not to discuss indications and contraindications for the procedure, which will be discussed and detailed in other chapters. Next, the conventional technique of tracheostomy will be addressed and the procedure clarified.

The following checklist must be followed before procedural execution.

Training of the Multidisciplinary Team

Less-informed professionals may believe that the simple presence of a surgeon, or one assisted by a nursing technician or other professional, makes the surgery achievable with risks inherent in the procedure. The assumption of impeccable surgical skills may represent the most critical error in such surgery.

The team should always be multidisciplinary [22, 23, 25]; its needs depend on the situation and are determined by the reason the procedure was indicated.

In elective tracheostomy on stable patients able to undergo the procedure under local anesthesia, the team will be composed of the surgeon, a qualified medical assistant, a scrub nurse, and a circulating nurse.

In hemodynamically unstable patients with an inadequate ventilation pattern or those from intensive care units (ICUs) or similar units, the presence of an anesthesiologist is necessary and prudent because simultaneous maintenance of vital functions and judicious performance of the procedure by the same person are not possible.

For patients undergoing tracheostomy in the ICU, the intensivist may sedate the patient to perform the procedure. In this situation, the presence of a respiratory physiotherapist is crucial to assist in the patient's full adaptation to the respirator.

In emergency tracheostomy, the team should be tailored according to the situation. The crucial consideration is to open the airway as rapidly as possible and with the least damage.

In all cases, nursing teams and technicians who are trained in the procedure are necessary, and they should be available at the exact time of the intervention. The success of the procedure depends on the ability of this team to respond appropriately and effectively.

Surgical Instruments

Because of high demand and low resources in Brazil's Unified Health System (Sistema Único de Saúde (SUS)), practitioners must perform the procedure without minimal conditions being met; they thereby assume unnecessary risks and, in the worst cases, cause harm to patients.

The following surgical instruments are required for tracheostomy in any situation: surgical mask, surgical cap, sterile surgical gowns and drapes, electrosurgical knife, cold scalpel, dissecting forceps with and without teeth, hemostatic curved forceps, straight and curved scissors, Farabeuf retractors, 10 cc and 20 cc syringes, lidocaine with and without a vasoconstrictor, suction catheter, gauze and bandages, field forceps, 2–0/3–0 surgical cotton yarn, 3–0/4–0 nylon thread, 3–0/4–0 Prolene, tracheostomy cannulae, and fixation tape. The choice of the cannula to be used depends on various factors and needs. Generally, for patients undergoing tracheostomy in the ICU and on mechanical ventilation regardless of the need for end-expiratory pressure, a polyethylene cannula with a balloon is required, which ensures full adaptation to the respirator. In cases in which the patient does not require ventilatory support, the best option is a simpler cannula, such as a metal cannula or a polyethylene cannula with or without a cuff (with or without risk of bronchial aspiration, respectively), with or without fenestration (with or without vocal potential, respectively) and with a subcannula. The availability of at least two cannulae that may be used and are chosen in advance is essential. Regarding size, the use of the largest possible cannula is always recommended because it guarantees the best ventilatory flow and allows better cleaning and less bronchoaspiration. For adults, metal cannulae sizes 5 and 6 and cuffed polyethylene cannulae sizes 7.5, 8, and 8.5 are commonly used (for the latter, the endotracheal tube that is used may provide guidance regarding the size of the tracheostomy tube). In special cases, the need for long cannulae due to unusual anatomical conditions should be considered initially and assessed in advance. This decision cannot be untimely, and the cannula must be accessible before the procedure begins (Fig. 1).

Location

Like any other surgical procedure, tracheostomy is associated with indications, contraindications, surgical techniques, and complications. It is not an inconsequential or second-tier procedure. Rather, unusual technical situations that may lead to early or late complications may exist and should not be overlooked.

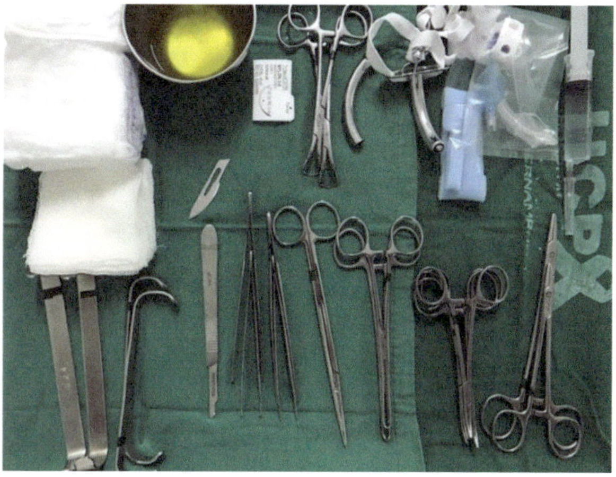

Fig. 1 Surgical instruments mounted on a Mayo table with instruments and cannulae

For these reasons, as defined in advance according to technical recommendations, the tracheostomy should be performed in a large room, wherein a multidisciplinary team may circulate. The procedure should follow all of the principles of asepsis, including those pertaining to the gas supplies (oxygen, nitrogen, and nitrous oxide), anesthesiology equipment, and technical arsenal for intravenous and inhaled general anesthesia. Also required are laryngoscopy, nasal endoscopy, and bronchoscopy equipment; an electrosurgical knife; appropriate tables and surgical lighting; a support table; and surgical aspirators. The room may be part of the operating center or adapted for operation in emergencies (Fig. 2).

Tracheostomy performance in the intensive care unit has always been subject to criticism [19]. The management of critically ill patients—including, among other factors, adequate transportation to the operating room for the procedure—has prompted many discussions about technical deterioration and the consequent percentage increase in complications. In their review, Futran et al. found no differences in the incidence of early and/or late complications between groups undergoing tracheostomy at the bedside or in the operating room. However, tracheostomy at the bedside was associated with lower cost and greater convenience in terms of the surgeon's time and was independent of the operating room schedule. Furthermore, less movement of critically ill patients was required, which avoided potential complications or less movement of critically ill patients, an activity associated with potential complications, was required—if either retains the intended meaning [20]. Regardless, the aforementioned minimum necessary conditions must be provided in that environment to avoid the risks associated with negligence or carelessness.

In extrahospital environments in which control of the appropriate parameters is typically not possible, providing a large site for the exclusive use of the rescue team is vital. An oxygen supply must always be considered. Correct patient mobilization must be followed to avoid exacerbation of the underlying pathology. The use of a preassembled kit is suggested. Finally, the most suitable technique for the specific condition should be chosen.

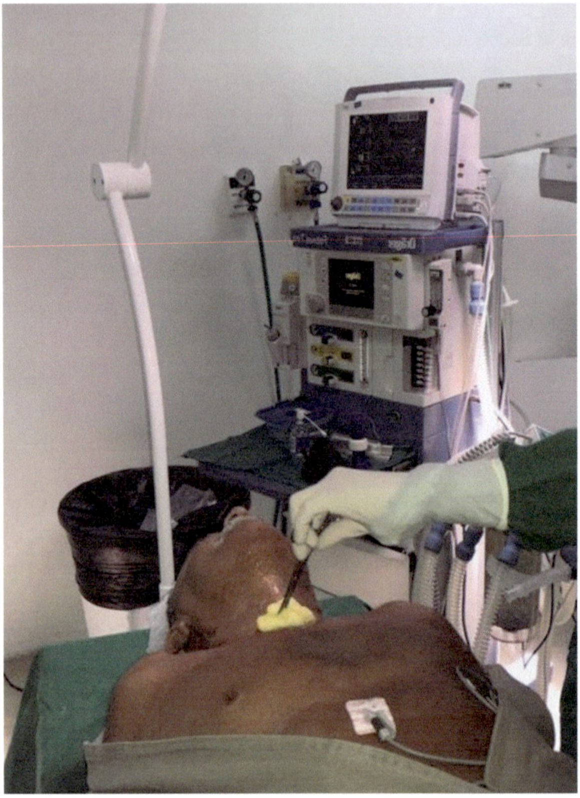

Fig. 2 Adequate monitoring is essential when performing the procedure in the operating room under an aseptic technique

General Conditions

Once tracheostomy is indicated (as discussed in specific chapters), the doctor responsible for performing the surgery must formulate an overview of the patient from a practical perspective, foreseeing difficulties and complications.

Although the procedure is widely practiced and has a low major complication rate, it may nonetheless lead to considerable morbidity in the short term, medium term, and long term; thus, tracheostomy encompasses great technical responsibility.

A careful analysis of each case is therefore needed from the outset. No type of pressure or inadvertent act may be permitted. The indication must be questioned whenever necessary. The patient's clinical condition must be meticulously evaluated (drug dependence, mechanical ventilation, oxygen therapy, degree of respiratory discomfort, associated comorbidities, prescription drugs, etc.). The conditions at the hospital where the procedure will be performed (location, instrumentation, and multidisciplinary team) must be evaluated. Adherence to these steps will allow the establishment of minimum safety measures and aid in minimizing mortality associated risks.

Positioning

The patient's positioning clearly dictates the success of the procedure. This step must not be considered a poor use of time nor assigned to the medical assistant or nursing staff. The purpose of this step is to ensure optimized accessibility to the laryngotracheal complex.

In most cases, the patient is placed supine on a rigid surface, properly monitored (physical pressure curves, electrocardiographic tracings, oximetry) with peripheral or central venous access, oxygen supplementation as necessary, and anesthesiology assistance. A bolster, which should also be hard, is then placed between the rigid surface and the shoulders, ensuring anteriorization of the laryngotracheal complex. The head is hyperextended and supported on a comfortable cushion [17, 19, 21, 26] (Figs. 3 and 4).

Frequently encountered or unexpected situations may occur. For ICU patients who require bedside tracheostomy, the following considerations must be addressed:

1. When the cushion used does not have sufficient rigidity to maintain the patient's position, one option is to increase the size of the bolster used below the shoulders or to support the entire chest/neck and head on a rigid surface.

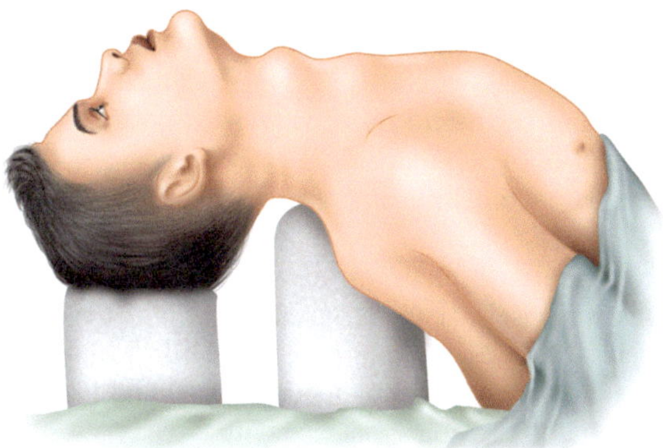

Fig. 3 Proper positioning with mild cervical hyperflexion, facilitating exposure with tracheal anteriorization

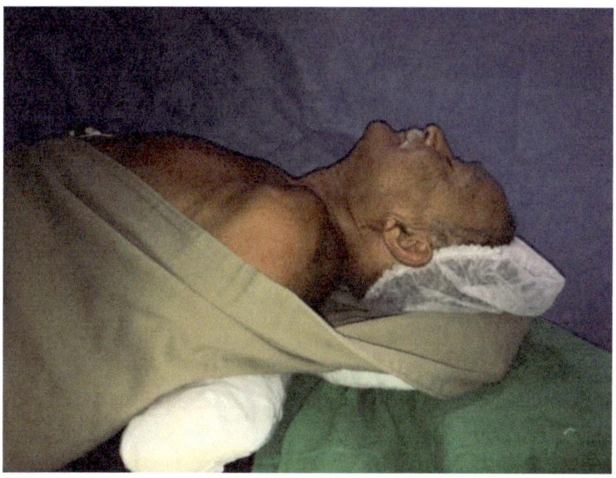

Fig. 4 Positioning in surgical practice. The bolster used under the shoulders should be sufficiently firm to maintain hyperflexion. Consent for Publication

2. The distance between the surgeon and the patient is much greater than when using a surgical table, which increases the difficulty of the procedure throughout its course. In such cases, this difficulty should be foreseen and a suitable table or patient transportation to the operating room should be requested.
3. Lighting must be adequate, preferably providing white light and front focus.
4. The multidisciplinary support team is crucial at this time; the patient will require sedation under the care of the ICU physician or anesthesiologist.

In other situations, the aforementioned positioning of the patient is not possible, whether due to breathing difficulties or due to facial or cervical trauma [17]. These patients should be placed in the best possible position to optimize the breathing pattern, typically in a seated or lateral decubitus position. At that juncture, full anatomical knowledge combined with rapid decision making will shape the outcome of the case.

After placing the patient in the optimal position and with the previous measures ensured, tracheostomy should be performed when necessary [21, 26]. Properly attired staff should perform antisepsis of the surgical field. For this purpose, a 10% polyvinylpyrrolidone iodine-based solution, 2% or 4% chlorhexidine gluconate antiseptic solution, or 0.5% alcohol solution should be used. The solution should be spread evenly, from the chin region to the nipple, and from one shoulder to the other (Fig. 5).

The excess is removed with a dry swab. Consensus has not been reached regarding the use of antibiotics [17, 21]. When an antibiotic is provided, the indication is prophylaxis for specific skin pathogens; it should be administered between 30 and 60 min prior to the procedure [26]. The placement of sterile fields is next, leaving an adequate opening for the procedure (Fig. 6).

This approach should be considered for most patients. In conscious patients, the placement of fields in the mouth and nose area may lead to greater respiratory distress and may cause psychomotor agitation. Placing a fenestrated drape in this area is advised; thus, in such cases, the fashioning of a sterile field with two openings is useful (Fig. 7).

Spatial access to the patient's bedside and bedside access for anesthesiologists are crucial to provide assistance with the oxygen supply, ventilation, aspiration, or perhaps positioning of the endotracheal tube when performing the tracheostomy.

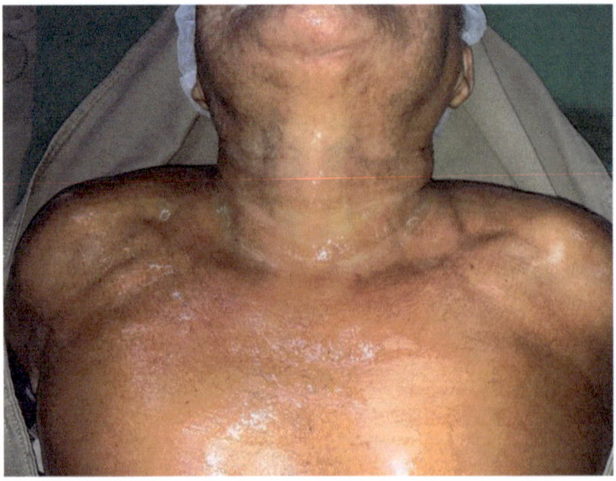

Fig. 5 Delimitation of the surgical field using chlorhexidine antiseptic solution. The upper limit is the chin area with lateral extent to the shoulders and the lower limit at nipple height

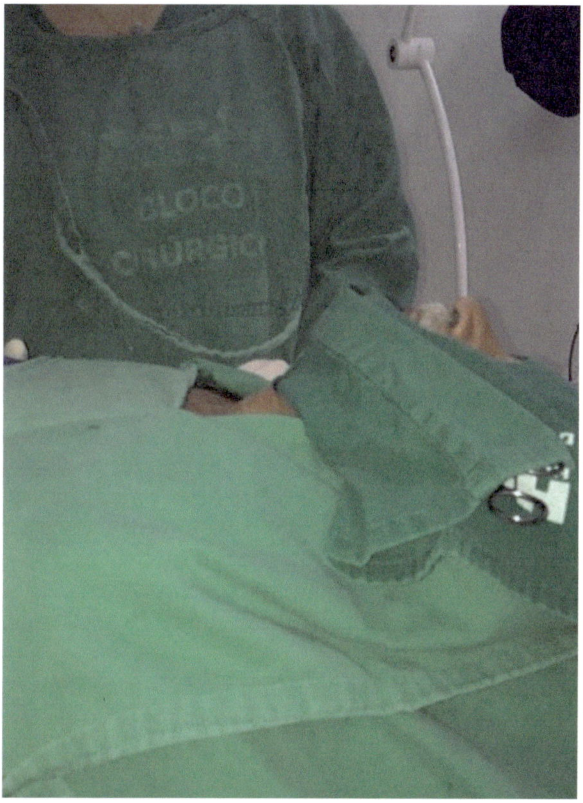

Fig. 6 Positioning of the sterile field. Note the positioning of the fenestrated field on the face, which in conscious patients decreases the perception of suffocation and facilitates patient collaboration

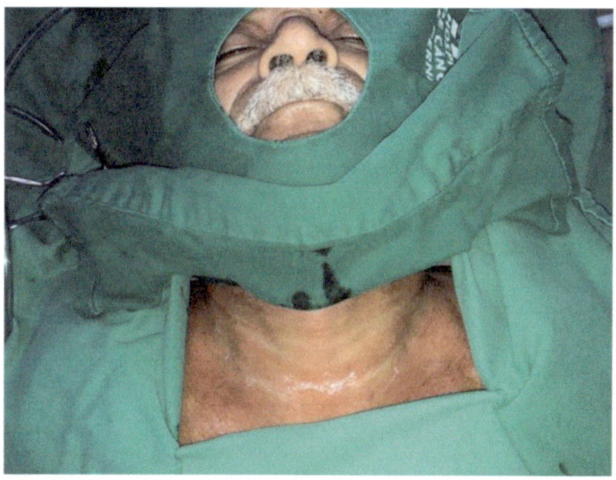

Fig. 7 Detail of a fenestrated drape on the face, which is separated from the surgical field. Consent for Publication

Notably, however, the technique previously described typically would not be followed during emergency tracheostomy because the primary goal would be to save the patient's life. An airway should be opened rapidly, whether by cricothyroidotomy or perhaps by establishing a tracheostomy, with the technique assuming secondary importance. Chevalier Jackson's observation in the early twentieth century in reference to execution of the emergency tracheostomy, which remains valid today, was that surgery should be performed using two incisions: the first in the skin and pretracheal soft tissues and the second in the trachea, into which an endotracheal cannula is inserted. This sequence ensures the opening of the airway, with blood loss evaluated subsequently [18].

Anesthesia

Intubated patients and those in an ICU should be sedated and eventually myorelaxed for mechanical ventilatory adaptation during the procedure [18, 20, 21].

Patients undergoing elective tracheostomy should be sedated judiciously, and local anesthesia with 2% lidocaine with or without a vasoconstrictor should be used. The use of an anesthetic with a vasoconstrictor may reduce bleeding during the surgery [21, 26]; epinephrine in a 1/100,000 dilution should be administered in such cases [20]. The local anesthetic must be introduced using a hypodermic needle throughout the incisional area, followed by exchange to a large-bore needle and subsequent anesthesia of the deep paratracheal planes (Figs. 8, 9, 10, and 11).

Because the introduction of intratracheal anesthesia may cause a choking sensation, cough, and dyspnea, its use is inadvisable [2, 3].

The procedure is similar in patients undergoing emergency tracheostomy, in whom positioning is the greatest difficulty. Invariably, anesthesia is performed in the usual manner.

In emergency tracheostomy, as previously discussed, procedural execution is possible only within the constraints of the patient's respiratory emergency.

Incision

The incision should be made between the following anatomical landmarks: the edge of the cricoid cartilage superiorly, the sternal notch inferiorly, and the sternocleidomastoid muscles laterally [17, 19, 21, 23]. In some cases, because the trachea may be displaced due to various causes, the space thus delineated by these anatomical landmarks may not in fact correspond to the actual location of the trachea. When

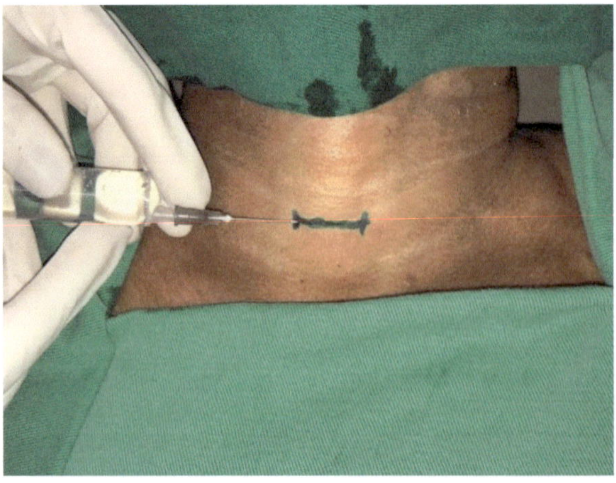

Fig. 8 Skin infiltration with local anesthetic throughout the incisional area at the level of the epidermis and dermis

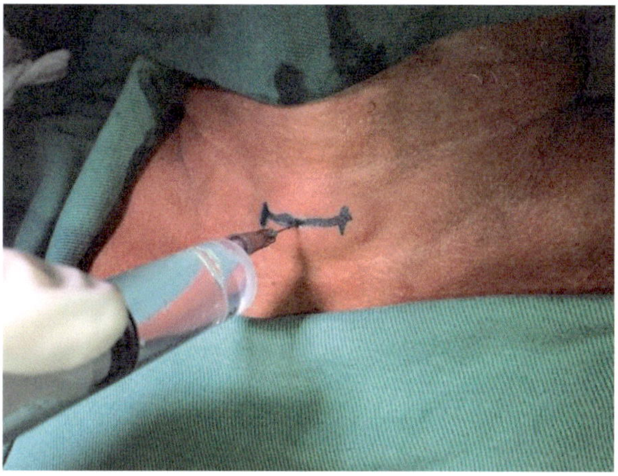

Fig. 9 Deep median infiltration with local anesthetic at the prelaryngeal musculature level

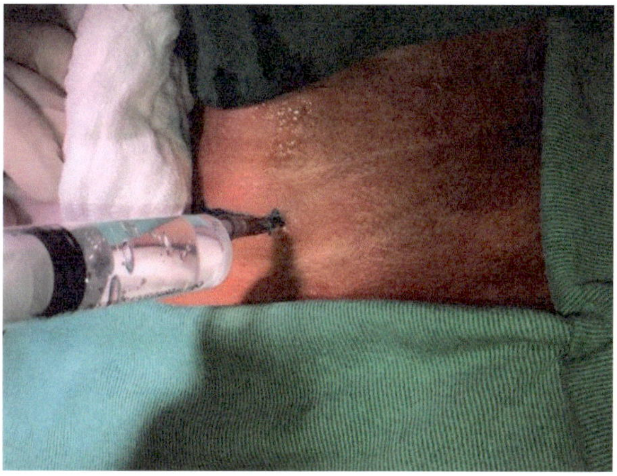

Fig. 10 Deep left paratracheal infiltration to aid analgesia related to lateral traction using retractors

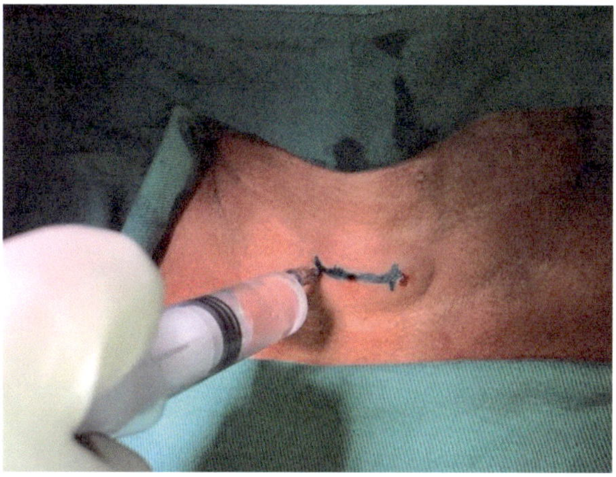

Fig. 11 Deep right paratracheal infiltration to aid analgesia related to lateral traction using retractors

possible, the tracheal location should be identified using imaging to allow the planning of precise access (Figs. 12 and 13).

In principle, the ideal skin incision should be tailored to a size sufficient for optimum tissue exposure during dissection and to ensure less intra- and postoperative morbidity. The incision may be performed with a cold knife or an electrosurgical knife (Figs. 14, 15, 16, and 17).

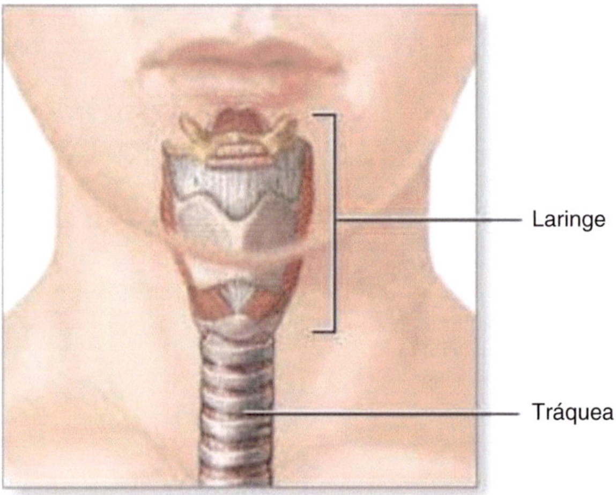

Fig. 12 Anatomical laryngotracheal relationships. *Laringe* larynx, *Tráquea* trachea

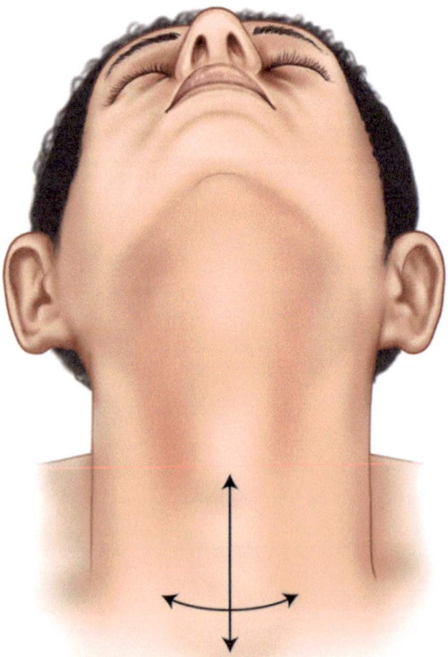

Fig. 13 Cervical incision options

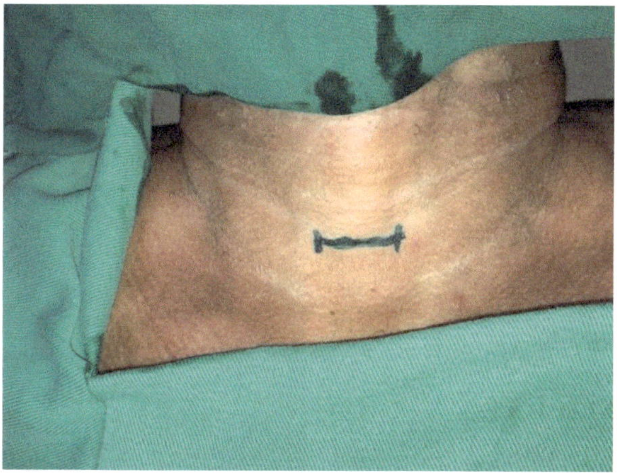

Fig. 14 Horizontal skin incision approximately 3–4 cm in diameter at a distance 1–2 cm from the sternal notch

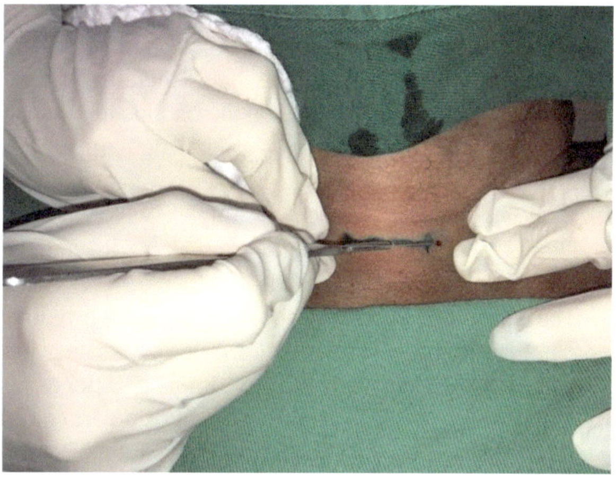

Fig. 15 The skin is opened using a cold scalpel along a previously marked line

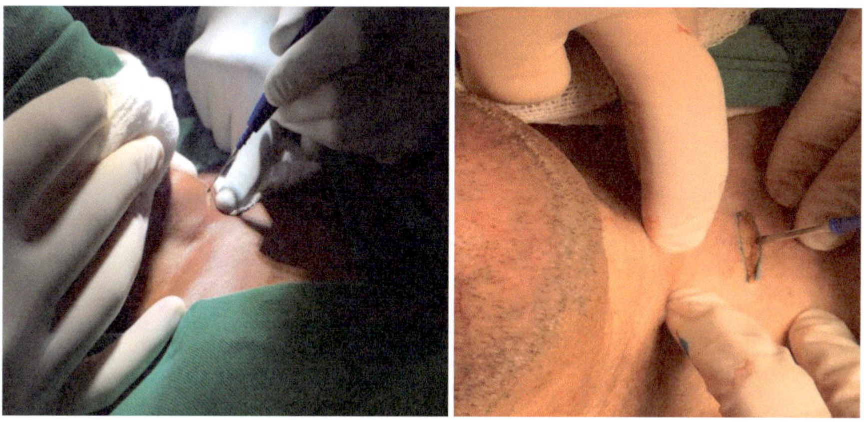

Fig. 16 Subcutaneous dissection using an electrosurgical knife along a previously marked line

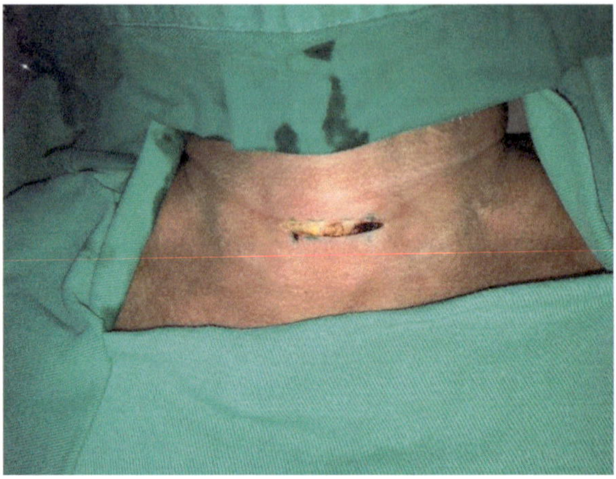

Fig. 17 Exposure of the panniculus adiposus and premuscular fascia deep planes

The skin incision may be vertical or horizontal, each of which has advantages and disadvantages. Ideally, the choice should therefore be based on the merits of each case.

The vertical incision is made on the midline in the space between the cricoid and the sternal notch. Approximately 3–4 cm in length, it permits tissue dissection on the midline with less risk of bleeding. Another advantage is that it allows vertical movement together with the laryngotracheal complex, which is more physiological. However, lateral limits to the tracheal planes exist, making dissection difficult, particularly with displacement of the trachea, or perhaps restricting access when inadvertent bleeding occurs.

The horizontal incision should be made approximately 2 cm above the sternal notch, between the sternocleidomastoid muscles, and should be approximately 3–4 cm in length. Because this incision is parallel to other neck skin cleavage lines, its aesthetic result is far superior to that of a vertical incision. This incision is indicated when surgery in this region is undertaken—for example, laryngectomy or thyroidectomy. As a more static incision, it may cause more discomfort, friction, and resulting granulomas [2, 3, 11, 12, 23, 26].

The aforementioned incisions have strengths and weaknesses, limitations, and inconveniences. Each incision type holds no technical superiority over the other. The final decision will depend on the constraints imposed by the patient, whether according to anatomical considerations or morbidities. The choice should be made based on the experience or training of a multidisciplinary team.

For patients with cervical hyperextension difficulties, whether due to spinal deformity, trauma, or a short neck, a vertical incision appears to offer a larger field of surgical exposure and reduced procedural morbidity. For patients who prioritize the aesthetic result, those with long necks, or those with previous cervical lesions that obstruct access, horizontal incisions appear to offer greater advantages and lower morbidity.

Because obtaining a patent airway is of paramount importance in an emergency tracheostomy, the incision factor has lower priority. Notably, however, in such cases, a need for combined incisions may exist—for example, cricothyroidotomy may be required prior to tracheostomy.

In our routine practice, we have performed horizontal incisions in all reported cases, elective and emergency. Generally, this incision type may be performed quickly and offers low morbidity, a low complication rate, and early decannulation without the need for any intervention to close the incision.

Dissection

After the skin incision, the dissection of the pretracheal tissue begins. The salient factor at this stage is knowledge of the deep anatomy and its variations.

Initially, the top and bottom or lateral flaps are pulled back, depending on whether the incision is horizontal or vertical, respectively. This is accomplished using an electrosurgical knife. Care should be taken to interrupt this step to cauterize or connect vessels when bleeding is encountered (Figs. 18 and 19).

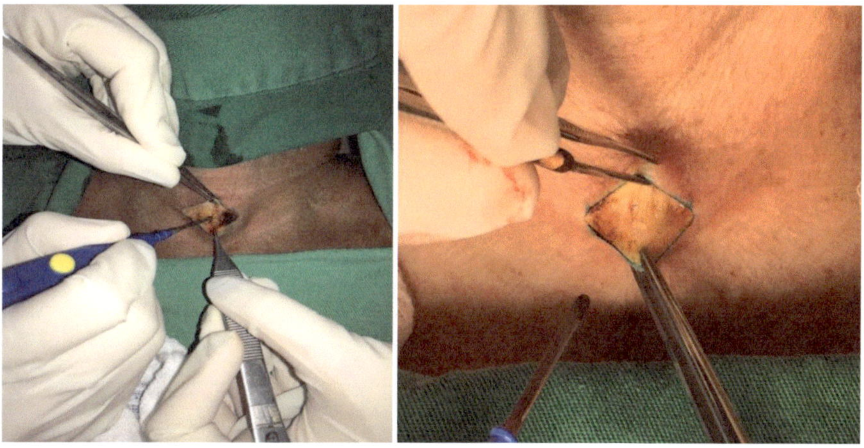

Fig. 18 Dissection of planes on the midline through the premuscular fascia

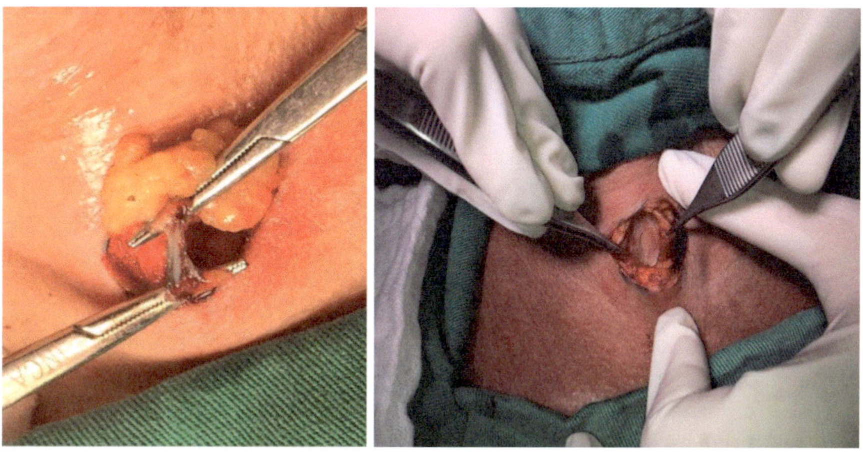

Fig. 19 Ligation of the prefascial vessels; fascial opening and cervical musculature on the midline

The midline is then sought, due to the lower risk of bleeding. The opening is made using the electrosurgical knife or Metzenbaum scissors. Then, with the aid of curved dissecting and hemostatic forceps, inferior–lateral–superior movements are performed to dissect the sternohyoid and sternothyroid muscles, displacing them laterally using Farabeuf retractors [17, 19, 20, 21, 26] (Figs. 20, 21, and 22).

At this stage, the thyroid gland is exposed, particularly its isthmus. The thyroid gland is fixed loosely to the laryngotracheal complex via its vascular communications, Berry's ligament, and the pretracheal fascia. Thus, it is possible to carefully dissect the inferior poles with curved hemostatic forceps and to suspend the gland cranially, maintaining the field using Farabeuf retractors [20, 26, 27] (Fig. 23).

In some cases, whether due to a short neck, an enlarged thyroid gland, or an ectopic gland, ligation of the isthmus may be necessary to gain wide access to the trachea. This step follows next and demands caution to obtain adequate hemostasis

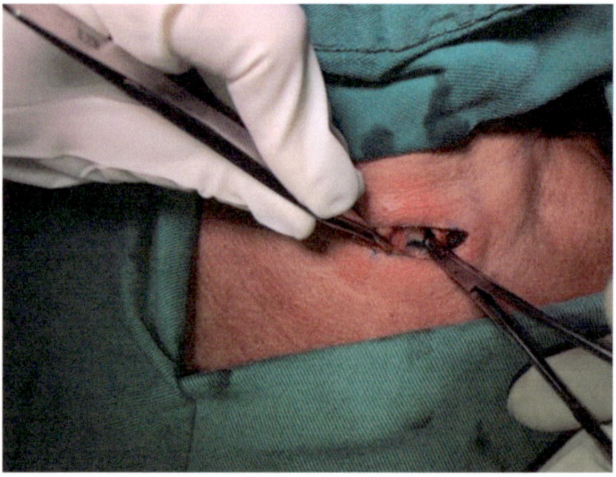

Fig. 20 Blunt dissection using hemostatic forceps from the midline with inferior–superior–lateral movements

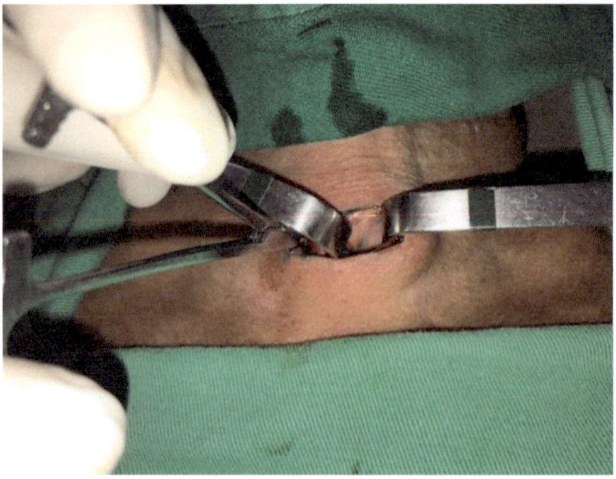

Fig. 21 Separation of cervical structures on the midline after sequential opening and placement of retractors

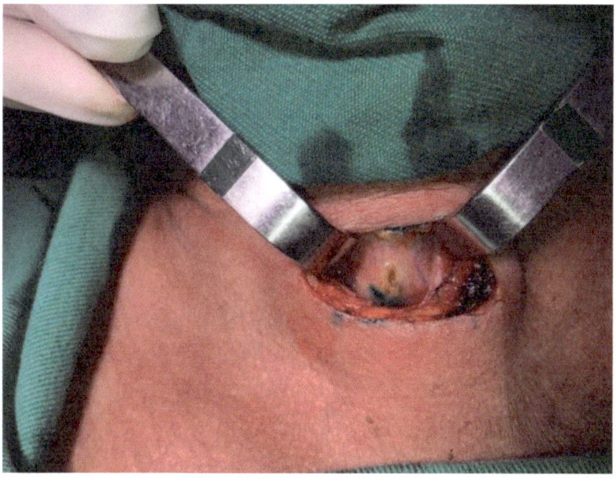

Fig. 22 Prethyroid fascial dissection and lateral separation, exposing the thyroid

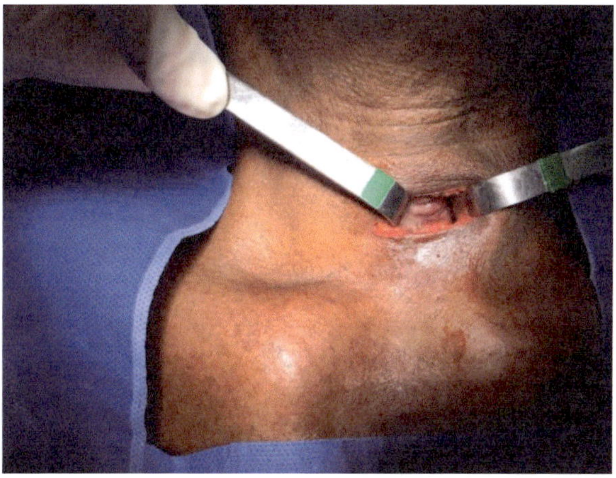

Fig. 23 Superolateral thyroid displacement, which completely exposes the trachea and avoids bleeding

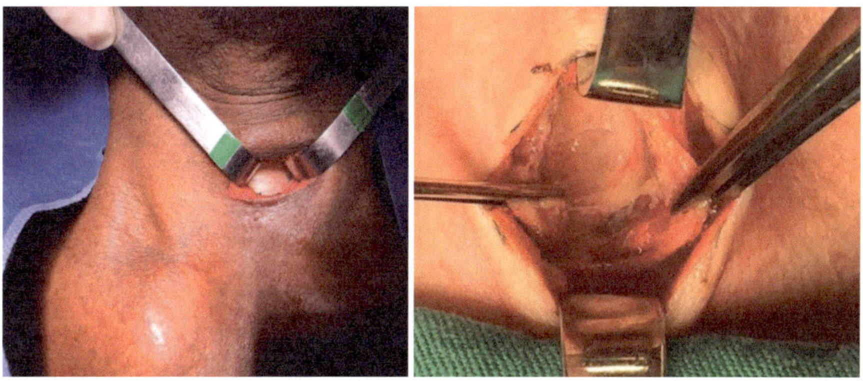

Fig. 24 Exposure of the pretracheal fascia, which provides complete exposure of the trachea

using cauterization for small isthmuses or absorbable thread suturing for larger isthmuses [2, 3, 11, 20, 19, 21, 28].

To expose the trachea, the pretracheal fascia is opened, and the retractors are repositioned if necessary, pulling them cranially (Fig. 24).

At this stage, the patient may complain of worsening respiratory discomfort, which requires rapid and precise action. All instruments, cannulae, aspirators, etc. are needed at this time, along with the collaborative assistance of the ICU team or anesthesiologist. The blunt dissection of the first rings is sufficient to complete the procedure. Lateral dissections will increase the likelihood of vascular or nerve damage. Anesthesia of the tracheal ligament and the trachea follows, using a small amount of local anesthetic without a vasoconstrictor (Fig. 25). In more difficult cases, where the structure to be sectioned is in doubt, the puncture will also serve to identify the trachea [2, 11, 17].

Tracheostomy

The tracheal opening is the critical phase of the procedure. After verifying all of the aforementioned steps, the cannula is chosen according to the previously established purpose, which is discussed in other chapters. Assessments of the integrity of the cannula and the testing of the cuffs, subcannulae, guides, etc. are crucial activities.

The cannula to be used depends on the size of the observed trachea, the indicated purpose, and the characteristics of the cannula itself. Because the cannula or cannulae to be used may have been considered prior to the procedure, a range of differently sized cannulae should be available. Generally, once the trachea is opened, the tracheostomy size should equal two thirds to three fourths of the tracheal diameter [12].

Many tracheal opening methods have been described, which may explain the low morbidity demonstrated between them [2, 3, 11, 12]. They may be grouped as follows: (1) vertical incisions; (2) horizontal incisions; (3) combined incisions; (4) incisions with resection rings; and (5) incisions with a tracheal flap [17, 19, 20, 21, 26] (Figs. 26, 27, 28, and 29).

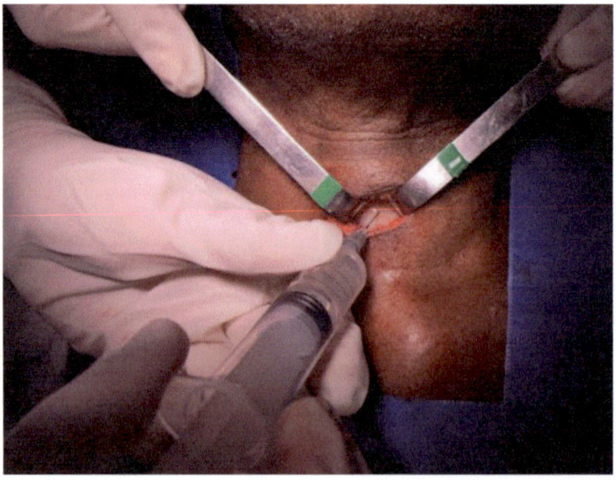

Fig. 25 Infiltration of the intertracheal ligament with lidocaine

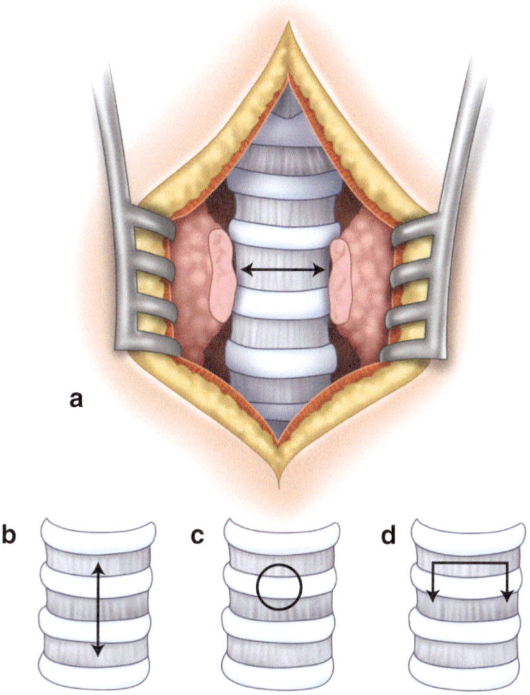

Fig. 26 Possible tracheal openings

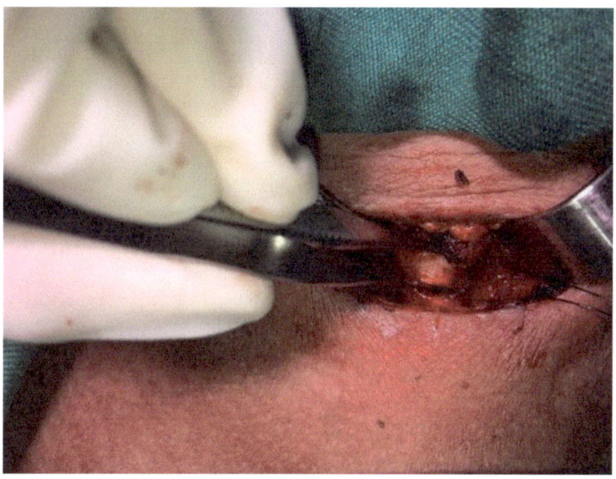

Fig. 27 Tracheal flap preparation: a cold scalpel incision is made in the intercartilaginous ligament and lateral opening

In general, the simplest incisions that allow passage of the cannula and cause the least anatomical and physiological changes are the most recommended. Thus, vertical and horizontal incisions should be the initial choice because they distort these precepts to a lesser extent [13, 14]. No difference in the degree of stenosis as a function of these incisions has been shown [15, 16]. Another important factor to be considered in initially defining the incision is the probable time the patient will

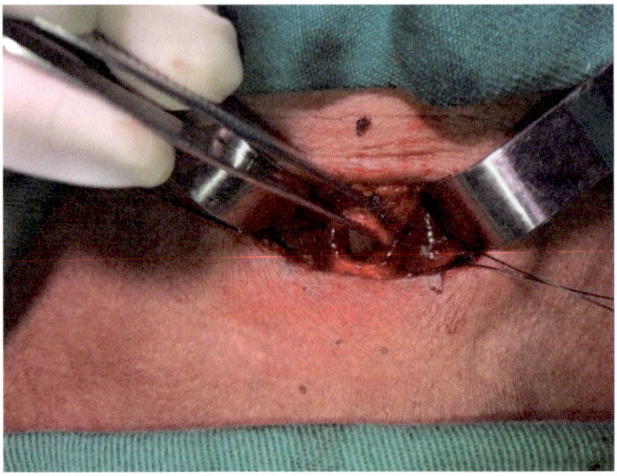

Fig. 28 Tracheal flap preparation: wide exposure facilitates illumination for cannula passage

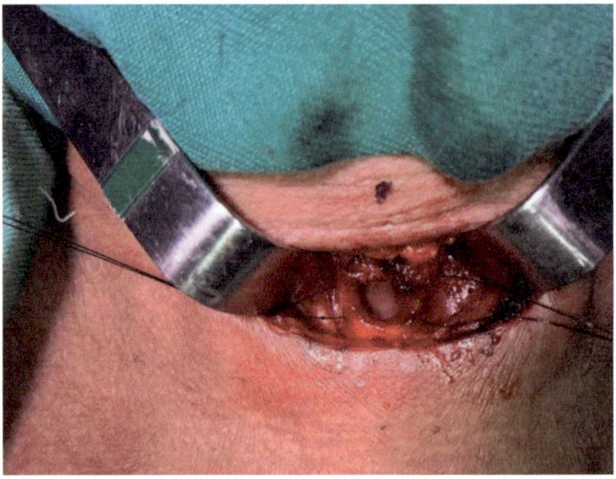

Fig. 29 Bilateral tracheal stay sutures, which aid in fixing the trachea and increase the safety of the procedure

remain with the device. For pathologies that require the tracheostomy long term, combined incisions with or without flaps attached to the skin are appropriate [17].

In our surgical practice, we perform the horizontal tracheal incisions at the height of the third/fourth tracheal ring, directly through the tracheal ligament, sparing any damage to the cartilage. We thereby create the opening necessary for passage of the tracheostomy; however, we may encounter slight vertical resistance when opening the rings because we do not open them completely.

The tracheal incision should be made carefully, at the height of the third to fourth ring [2, 3, 11]. In exclusively horizontal incisions, the ligament is opened, which facilitates postdecannulation healing [11]. The cold scalpel is used to make the first punctiform opening, followed by expansion, preferably using Metzenbaum scissors (Figs. 30 and 31).

The opening should be sufficient for passage of the cannula and must occupy two thirds to three quarters of the diameter of the trachea [12] (Fig. 32).

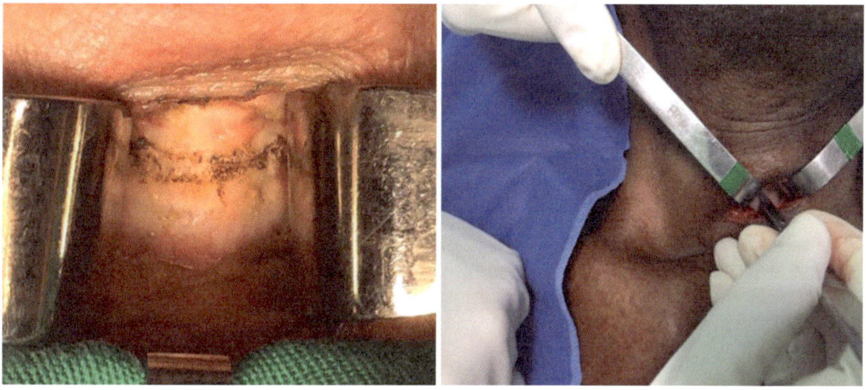

Fig. 30 Marking of the tracheal opening at the ligament level, followed by punctiform opening using a cold scalpel in the preanesthetized ligament

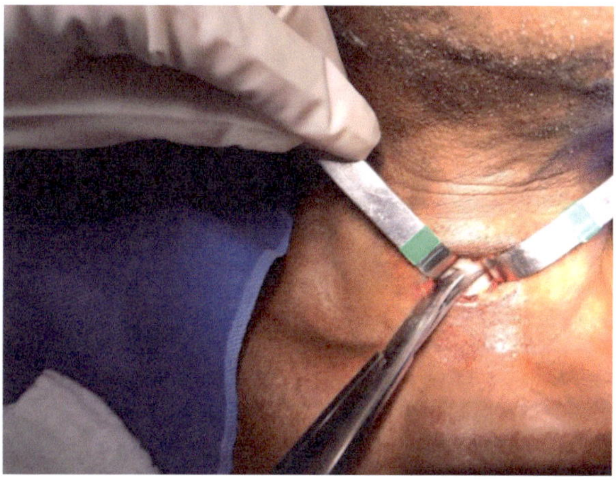

Fig. 31 Tracheal opening expansion using Metzenbaum scissors along the preanesthetized ligament

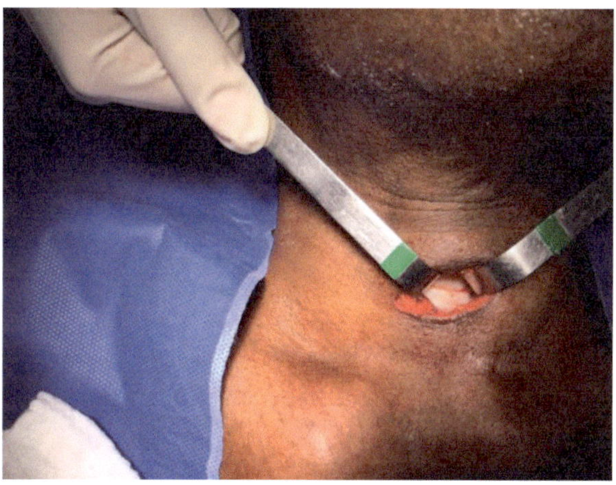

Fig. 32 Tracheostomy performed via the intertracheal ligament. Note the precise coaptation of the edges and minimal tracheal injury

At this stage, a tracheal aspirator must be available for the removal of tracheal secretions and blood from the tracheal wall. The electrosurgical knife may also be useful to cauterize any larger peritracheal vessels. If an electrosurgical knife is used at this stage with the patient under mechanical ventilation, the anesthetist or intensivist should be requested to turn off the oxygen flow to prevent combustion in the airway due to the flammable characteristics of oxygen [2, 3]. Surgical repair may then proceed using nonabsorbable sutures in both the upper and lower rings, which facilitate greater firmness for the passage of the cannula and thereafter in cases of inadvertent cannula loss or when exchange is required [2, 11]. In all cases, the handling of the trachea should be minimal and as delicate as possible because of potential consequent and critical early and late complications. A maneuver that allows false paths to be avoided is to follow the passage of the previously chosen cannula, entering perpendicular to the trachea and followed by counterclockwise rotational movement toward the mediastinum [3, 11] (Figs. 33, 34, and 35).

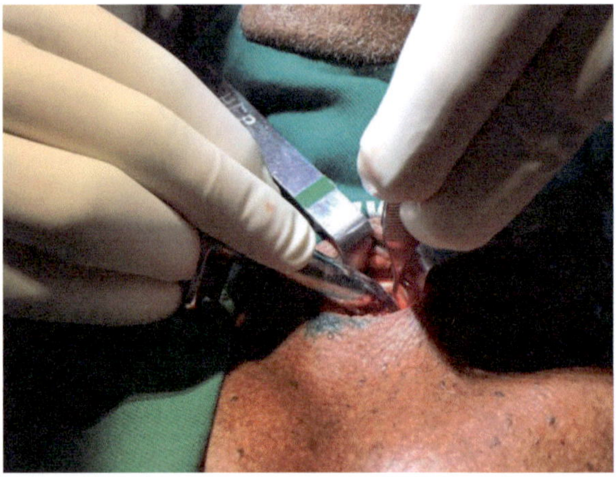

Fig. 33 Passage of the tracheal cannula. Note the stay suture in the tracheal ring and the positioning of the cannula to begin the maneuver

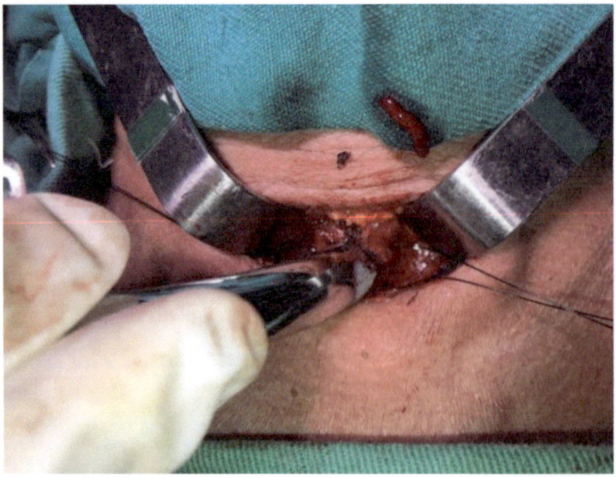

Fig. 34 The cannula is moved counterclockwise in a cautious and continuous introductory maneuver

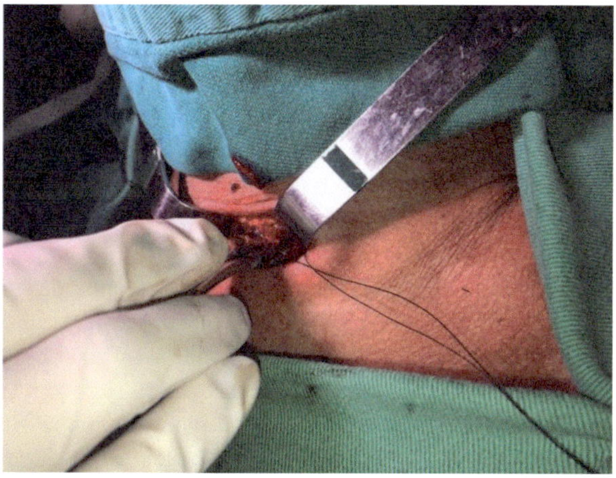

Fig. 35 Final stage of the maneuver, with the cannula tip aimed anteriorly to the trachea

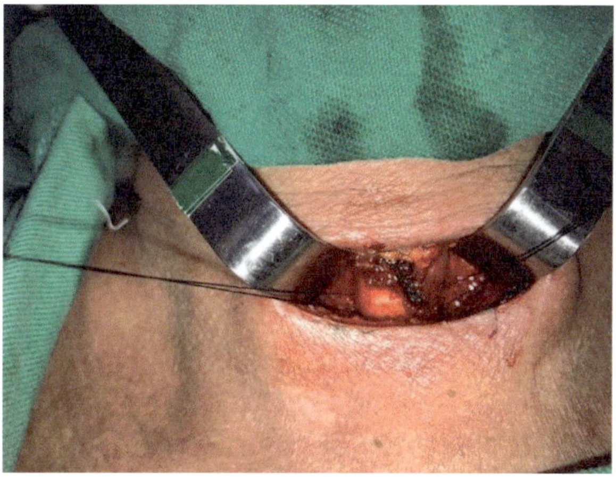

Fig. 36 Lateral tracheal stay sutures ensure greater safety during passage of the cannula

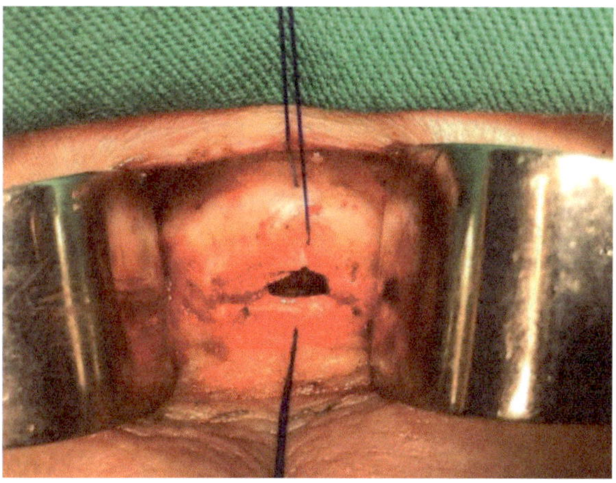

Fig. 37 Stay sutures on the upper and lower edges ensure better countertraction

In cases such as the aforementioned, the creation of the tracheal opening may require removal of the anterior wall of the second and third tracheal rings, which creates a portal for positioning of the cannula. In this scenario, stay sutures lateral to or higher and lower than the portal are used as countertraction points, increasing the safety of the procedure [26] (Figs. 36 and 37).

A tracheal incision with the creation of a tracheal flap is the last technique to be described. Although this is similar to the previous method, here a flap of the superior or inferior trachea is retained, to which the skin is fixed [26, 27]. The tracheocutaneous fistula formed by these last two techniques appears more stable when the flap is directly sutured to the skin, which permits cannula removal or replacement with greater safety [26]. This technique was first described in the 1960s by Bjorg, by whose name the tracheal flap used today is known [29].

In elective tracheostomy of intubated patients, attention must be directed to certain concerns before opening the trachea. First, depending on the mechanical ventilation used, the patient should be sedated as previously described and preoxygenated, which will ensure an apnea period without major complications; second, when incising the trachea, caution must be exercised to not puncture the endotracheal tube balloon; third, the patient may be maintained in apnea and disconnected from mechanical ventilation due to proper patient preoxygenation that will permit sufficient time for passage of the cannula; fourth, careful retraction of the endotracheal tube should proceed until the tube has passed completely through the tracheostomy; and, finally, the cannula is passed through with the endotracheal tube maintained in place, which will be removed after ensuring satisfactory ventilation.

In emergency tracheostomies, because a secured airway is the main objective, part of this stage (or some of these stages) may be disregarded or streamlined; in certain cases, they might be performed only at the next stage. An article published by Chevalier Jackson in 1909 explains the difficulties in performing emergency tracheostomy. According to this author, the trachea should be opened using more of a direct puncture than an incision maneuver with no time for disinfection or hemostasis [18].

Review of the Procedure/Fixing of the Cannula

After passage of the cannula, adequate ventilatory flow must be assessed, which may be determined by simple observation, capnography, or oximetry. The airway is then carefully aspirated to remove secretions and blood [17, 20, 22]. Finally, diligent hemostatic review and suturing of the skin incision should ensue. The suturing must not be made airtight and cause the appearance of subcutaneous emphysema [2, 3, 19].

Fixation of a metal cannula may be achieved using laces tied around the neck; they should always be tied with the head flexed to avoid loosening, using caution when handling the cannula to ensure its position [2, 3, 11, 20] (Fig. 38). Plastic cannulae may be fixed similarly to laces or fixed by direct anchoring to the skin; however, the latter method may restrict vertical movement of the laryngotracheal

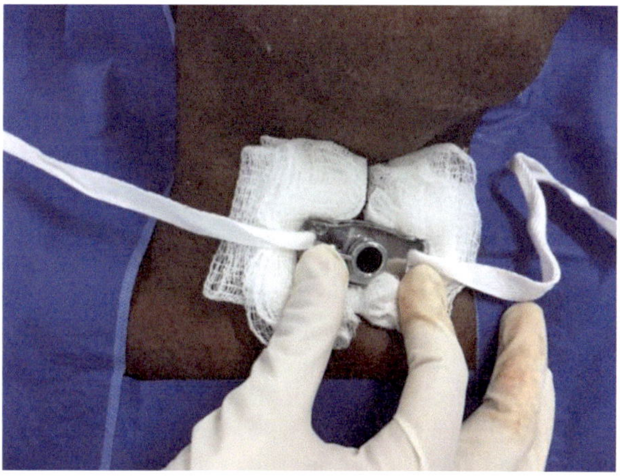

Fig. 38 Cannula fixation by laces tied around the neck. The skin is protected by interposing gauze

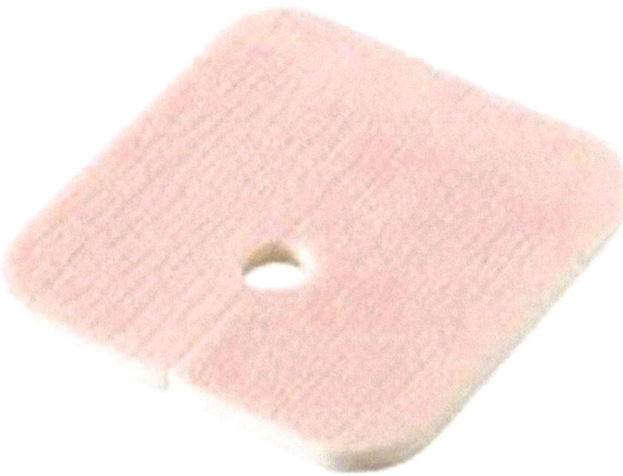

Fig. 39 Polyamide plate to enhance adaptation and contact protection between the skin and cannula

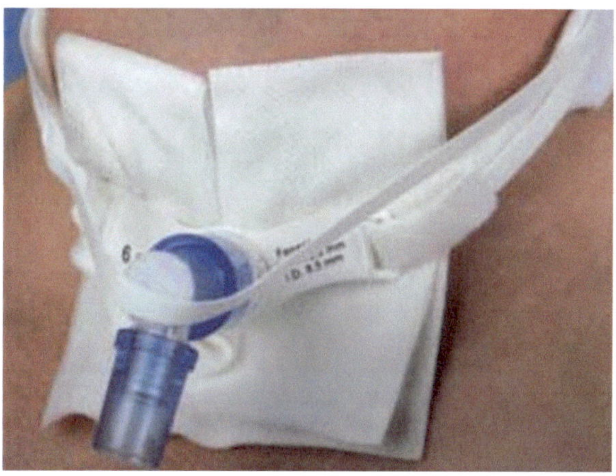

Fig. 40 Final view of fixation and contact protection between the skin and cannula with polypropylene cannulae use. Note the accessory used to prevent aspiration of water when the patient showers

complex, which increases the risk of complications. However, this method is useful in transtumoral tracheostomy, in hostile necks, and in children [20]. Gauzes are interposed between the cannula and the incision to help absorb secretions and reduce friction of the device against the skin, which may cause ulceration [2, 3, 20, 22] (Figs. 39 and 40).

Conclusions

As described, conventional tracheostomy is an age-old surgical procedure. Although the technique has remained virtually unchanged over time, the introduction of new instruments, monitoring, and perioperative multidisciplinary care have made the surgery safe and routine.

A detailed technical description is undoubtedly crucial to standardization. Whether tracheostomy is performed by inexperienced professionals or the most qualified, this chapter prioritizes the anticipation of possible complications and demystifies the technique, making it accessible to all. Consent was obtained from any indivdual participant for whom identifying information is included in this article.

References

1. Frost E. Tracing the tracheostomy. Ann Otolaryngol. 1976;85:618–24.
2. Meirelles RC. Traqueostomia técnica cirúrgica [Tracheostomy surgical technique]. Int Arch Otorhinolaryngol. 1998;2(1):9–15.
3. Ricz HMA, Filho FVM, et al. Traqueostomia [Tracheostomy]. Fundamentos clínica cirúrgica. 2011;44(1):63–9.
4. Gurunluoglu R, Gurunluoglu A. Paul of Aegina: landmark in surgical progress. World J Surg. 2003;27(1):18–25.
5. Portal Educação [Education Portal], Google Analytics. http:www.portalmedico.org.br/pareceres/2009/15_2009.htm.
6. Portal Educação [Education Portal], Google Analytics. http:www.portalmedico.org.br/pareceres/crmam/2011/9_2011.pdf.
7. Portal Educação [Education Portal], Google Analytics. http:www.portalmedico.org.br/pareceres/crmsc/1999/644_2002.htm.
8. Portal Educação [Education Portal], Google Analytics. http:www.portalmedico.org.br/pareceres/CFM/2002/47_2002.htm.
9. Portal Educação [Education Portal], Google Analytics. http:www.portalmedico.org.br/pareceres/CRMDF/2015/12_2015.pdf.
10. Portal Educação [Education Portal], Google Analytics. http:www.portalmedico.org.br/pareceres/crmmg/2015/5563_2015.pdf.
11. Dias F L, Noronha M J R. Traqueostomias—indicações e técnicas [Tracheostomy—indications and techniques]. 1993;9:63–74.
12. Heffner JE, Miller S, Sahn SA. Tracheostomy in the intensive care unit. Chest. 1986;90(2):269–74.
13. Smith MM, Sauders GK, Leib MS, Simmons EJ. Evaluation of horizontal and vertical tracheotomy healing after short-duration tracheostomy in dogs. J Oral Maxilofac. 1995;53(3):289–94.
14. Lulenski GC, Batsakis JG. Tracheal incision as a contributing factor to tracheal stenosis. Ann Oto Rhinol Laringol. 1975;84:781783.

15. Bryant LR, Juyia D, Greenberg S, Huye JM, Schecter FG, Albert HM. Evaluation of tracheal incisions of tracheostomy. Am J Surg. 1978;135:675–9.
16. Tommerup B, Borgeskov S. Endoscopic evaluation at follow-up after Bjork tracheostoma. Scand J Thorac Cardiovasc Surg. 1983;17:181–4.
17. Engels PT, Bagshan SM, Meier M, Brindley PG. Tracheostomy: from insertion to decannulation. Can J Surg. 2009;52:421–33.
18. Jackson C. Tracheotomy. Laryngoscope. 1909;19:285–90.
19. Hardy KL. Tracheostomy: indications, techniques and tubes. Am J Surg. 1973;126:300–10.
20. Futran ND, Dutcher PO, Roberts JK. The safety and efficacy of bedside tracheostomy. Otolaryngol Head Neck Surg. 1993;109(4):707–11.
21. Durbin CG Jr. Techniques for performing tracheostomy. Respir Care. 2005;59:488–96.
22. Mitchell RB, Hussey HM, et al. Clinical consensus statement: tracheostomy care. Otolaryngol Head Neck Surg. 2013;148(1):6–20.
23. De Leyn P, Bedert L, Delcroix M, et al. Tracheostomy: clinical review and guidelines. Eur J Cardiothorac Surg. 2007;32:412–21.
24. Albertin PW. Tracheotomy versus intubation. A 19th century controversy. Ann Otol Rhinol Laryngol. 1984;93:333–7.
25. Cheung NH, Napolitano LM. Tracheostomy: epidemiology, indications, timing, technique, and outcomes. Respir Care. 2014;59(6):895–919.
26. Durbin CG. Tracheostomy: why, when and how? Respir Care. 2010;55(8):1056–68.
27. Heffner JE. Tracheotomy application and timing. Clin Chest Med. 2003;24:389–98.
28. Calhoun KH, Weiss RL, Scott B, et al. Management of the thyroid isthmus in tracheostomy: a prospective and retrospective study. Otolaryngol Head Neck Surg. 1994;111:450–2.
29. Bjorg VO. Partial resection of the only remaining lung with the aid of respirator treatment. J Thorac Cardiovasc Surg. 1960;39:179–88.

Percutaneous Tracheostomy Indications and Surgical Technique

Lucio Pereira and Catherine Lumley

Introduction

Tracheostomy is a procedure used to obtain a surgical airway. It has been performed for over 3000 years. This operative technique was standardized by Chevalier Jackson, but the modern era only started in the 1960s, when the surgical technique, indications, and complications were better described.

The surgical airway can be temporary (in cases where the upper airway obstruction or respiratory abnormality can be reversed) or permanent. The procedure is indicated for an upper airway obstruction caused by tumors, infection, obstructive sleep apnea, or trauma; and in cases of prolonged intubation, as an aid in handling secretions and to facilitate ventilator support. A summary of the indications for tracheostomy can be seen in Table 1.

Even though airway obstruction is the most dramatic indication for a surgical airway, most procedures are performed for prolonged intubation in patients admitted to an intensive care unit (ICU). It is estimated that 20–38% of ICU beds are filled with mechanically ventilated patients [1]. An average of 100,000 tracheostomies for this reason are performed each year in the USA [2].

Airway access for mechanical ventilation is initially provided by endotracheal intubation. The perfect timing for tracheostomy in patients requiring mechanical ventilation is still controversial. Some of the advantages of tracheostomy over endotracheal intubation include less trauma to the larynx, vocal cords, and arytenoids; decreased airway resistance; and improvements in airway hygiene and patient comfort. Patients expected to require ventilation for less than 10 days are usually

L. Pereira, M.D. (✉)
Department of Otolaryngology, Hofstra Northwell School of Medicine, Long Island Jewish Medical Center, New Hyde Park, NY, USA
e-mail: pereiralucio@hotmail.com

C. Lumley, M.D.
Department of Otolaryngology–Head and Neck Surgery, Georgetown University, Washington, DC, USA

T.P. de Farias (ed.), *Tracheostomy*, https://doi.org/10.1007/978-3-319-67867-2_5

Table 1 Indications for tracheostomy

Upper airway obstruction with any of the following:
Stridor
Air hunger
Retractions
Obstructive sleep apnea with documented arterial desaturations
Bilateral vocal cord paralysis
Previous neck surgery or throat trauma
Previous neck irradiation
Prolonged or expected prolonged intubation
Inability of patient to manage secretions, including the following:
Aspiration
Excessive bronchopulmonary secretions
Facilitation of ventilation support
Inability to intubate
Adjunct to manage head and neck surgery
Adjunct to manage significant head and neck trauma

managed by endotracheal intubation alone. Tracheostomy is considered if the patient will require intubation for more than 14–21 days. The reported rate of stenosis following intubation ranges from 0.9% to 8.3% [3]. This is a result of injury due to pressure at the level of the glottis and arytenoid cartilages by the endotracheal tube. Despite the recognition of this problem and improvements in endotracheal tube design and maintenance, prolonged intubation should still be avoided, and tracheostomy should be a solution in most cases.

Open tracheostomy is the gold-standard technique and can be done in a wide variety of patient conditions and clinical scenarios. The surgical procedure is safe and has stood the test of time. Although it can be done at the bedside, the vast majority of such procedures are done in the operating room (OR) and require a specialized surgical team, OR time, and coordination between the ICU and surgical teams. Transportation of a critical patient from the ICU to the OR needs to be taken into account as well, as it demands coordination, and patients can become unstable on their way to the OR.

Percutaneous tracheostomy can be performed at the bedside, obviating the need to transfer the patient to the OR, which can release OR resources. It also allows physicians without surgical training to perform the procedure, making it easier to schedule the procedure and allowing it to be performed in a more timely fashion.

Percutaneous Tracheostomy

In an attempt to find an easier tracheostomy method that could be done at the bedside and avoid transporting critically ill patients to the OR, several authors have described alternative surgical techniques using a percutaneous method. A percutaneous technique for tracheostomy was first described in 1955 by Shelden et al. [4]. This was a blind technique using a cutting trocar guided by a slotted needle to gain access to the trachea (Fig. 1). This method was abandoned because it resulted in several complications,

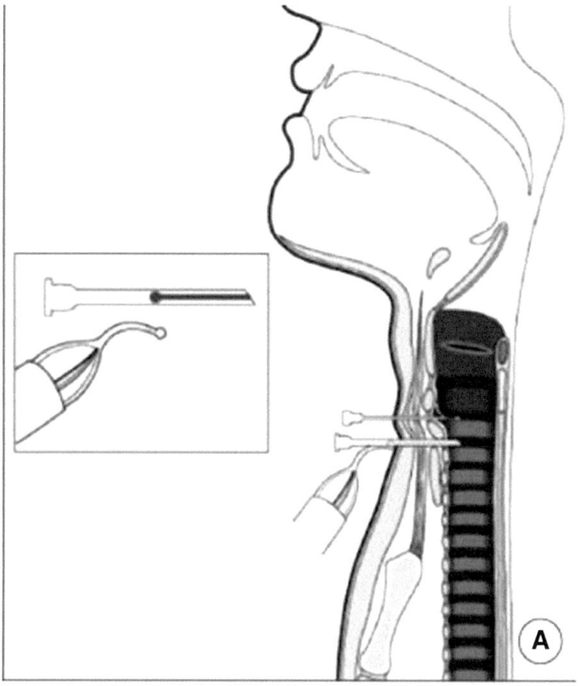

Fig. 1 Shelden technique. The ball-tipped cutting blade is passed through the lateral opening and advanced along the slot

including injury to the carotid and esophagus. Three decades later, Ciaglia et al. published their series using the Seldinger technique [5]. This method introduced the use of fiberoptic bronchoscopy to visualize the tracheal puncture, making the procedure safer. Other authors—such as Schachner (Rapitrach, 1989), Griggs et al. (1990), Fantoni and Ripamonti (1997), and Frova and Quintel (2002)—developed their own techniques for percutaneous tracheostomy. These techniques have been described using a variation of the Seldinger technique [6]. In 1990, Griggs et al. dilated the trachea using curved forceps, which were passed over the guide wire in the trachea. The forceps were then opened and provided force to dilate the trachea and anterior soft tissue. The tracheostomy tube was then passed over the guide wire [7] (Fig. 2). Fantoni and Ripamonti reported a translaryngeal tracheostomy set in 1997 involving a unique cannula to pass into and dilate the trachea retrograde from the lumen out to the skin. This required a guide wire to be passed through a needle in the trachea out through the mouth in order to load the specially designed cannula, which was then pulled back through the oral cavity, larynx, and trachea to pierce through the skin of the neck [8] (Fig. 3). In 2002, Frova and Quintel described a new technique using a screw-like dilator in order to decrease the need for increased pressure applied when introducing the first dilator and therefore decrease the risk of posterior tracheal wall lesion. This was done under fiberoptic guidance and using transillumination. After successful puncture of the trachea, the guide wire was inserted into the trachea. They then placed a hydrophilically coated dilation screw with threads (PercuTwist, Rusch, Kernen, Germany) into the incision, which was turned clockwise and advanced by rotation to

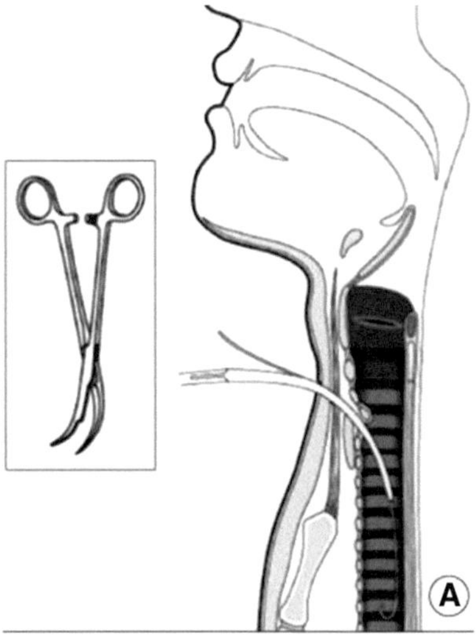

Fig. 2 (**a**) Griggs technique. The trachea is located by aspirating air, using a 14-gauge cannula. The guide wire is then introduced into the trachea, followed by a 14-French dilator. Fully closed metal tracheal dilating forceps are passed over the guide wire and opened just enough to accept the tracheostomy tube

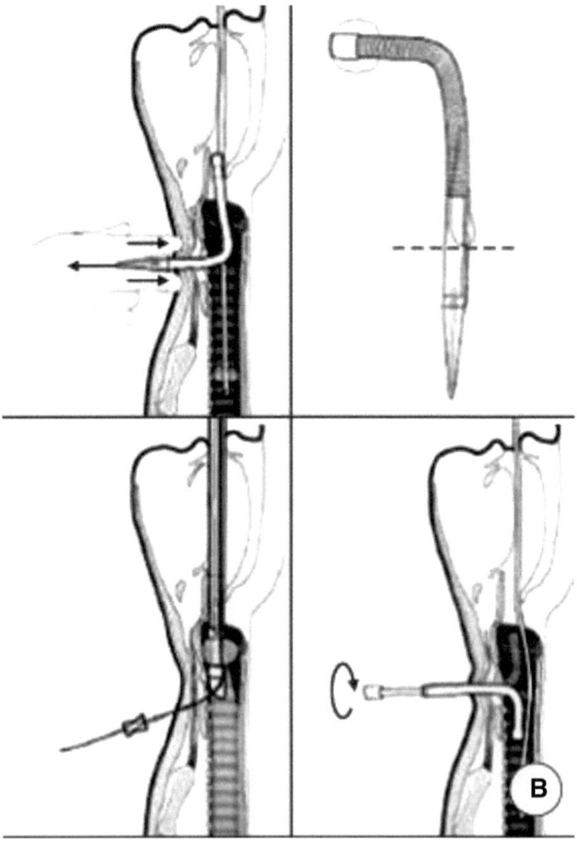

Fig. 3 Fantoni's technique, with retrograde dilation of the trachea from the lumen to the skin

dilate the trachea [9] (Fig. 4). With all of these percutaneous tracheostomy methods, there has been no evidence showing superiority of any one method.

Alvaro Sanabria [6] did a systematic review comparing different percutaneous tracheostomy techniques. He reviewed studies comparing the Ciaglia Blue Rhino, Ciaglia multiple dilator, Blue Dolphin, Griggs dilating forceps, and PercuTwist, but could not find statistically significant differences in outcomes.

Percutaneous tracheostomy was initially viewed with skepticism by surgeons, who were under the impression that it was associated with a higher rate of complications. Several hundred articles have been published on this subject, and many of them have tried to compare open tracheostomy and the percutaneous technique. Three meta-analyses have been performed and concluded that there is no clear difference in terms of complications [10–12]. Dulguerov et al., in their meta-analysis from 1999, showed a higher incidence of perioperative complications associated with percutaneous tracheostomy and a higher rate of postoperative complications with open surgical tracheostomy [11]. Freeman et al. found that the percutaneous technique is easier to perform and has low incidence rates of peristomal bleeding and postoperative infection [12]. Higgins and Punthakee showed that percutaneous tracheostomy is more cost effective and provides greater feasibility in terms of bedside capability and nonsurgical operation [10].

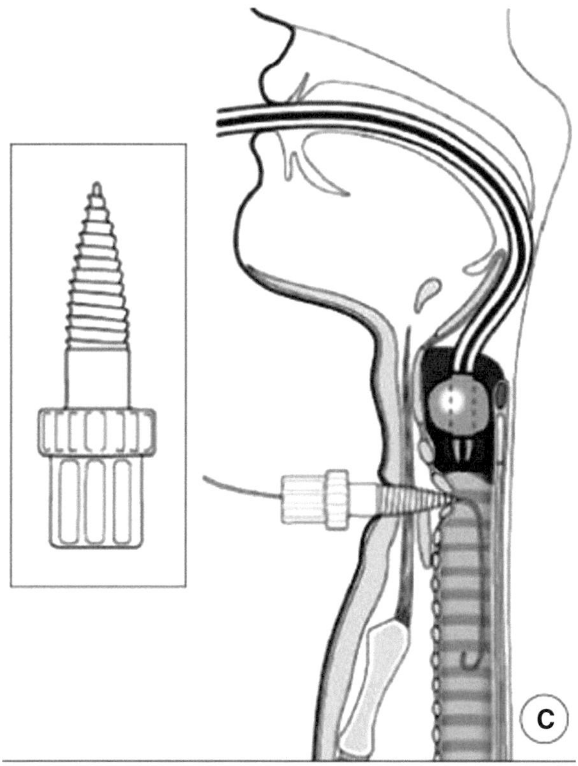

Fig. 4 PercuTwist technique. Note the presence of the dilation screw with threads

The indications for percutaneous tracheostomy are the same as those for standard open tracheostomy (Table 1).

Absolute contraindications to percutaneous tracheostomy include emergent tracheostomy and tracheostomy in infants and children. Relative contraindications include local conditions that can distort the anatomy and the pathway from the skin to the airway. Examples include patients with poor neck landmarks, a large neck mass, a high innominate artery, previous neck surgery, limited neck extension, an active infection over the tracheostomy site, a history of difficult intubation, uncorrectable coagulopathy, and a positive end-expiratory pressure (PEEP) >15 cm H_2O.

Procedure

Several percutaneous techniques are available in the market, such as Ciaglia, Griggs, PercuTwist, Rapitrach, and others. The single-dilator technique is faster with no significant difference in the complication rate [13].

The Ciaglia technique is usually performed using the Cook Blue Rhino single-dilator kit (Cook Medical, Bloomington, IN, USA). A flexible bronchoscope should be available to visualize the introduction and the dilation of the anterior tracheal wall. An open tracheostomy set should also be in the room for use in the rare event that this procedure needs to be converted into an open procedure. A second physician trained in flexible bronchoscopy should be present in order to perform the bronchoscopy.

The patient is sedated, and the neck is extended over a shoulder roll. Use of muscle relaxants prevents the patient from moving and biting the bronchoscope. A bite block can be used to facilitate introduction of the scope.

The patient is then prepped and draped in the standard fashion for a tracheostomy. The landmarks should be palpated, including the thyroid notch, cricothyroid membrane, cricoid cartilage, trachea, and sternal notch. The skin is then injected with 1% lidocaine with a 1:100,000 epinephrine solution.

A direct laryngoscopy is performed to ensure that there is no airway distortion and that the cuff of the endotracheal tube is at the vocal cord level.

A horizontal 2 cm incision is made immediately below the inferior border of the cricoid cartilage, or between the cricoid and the sternal notch (Fig. 5). Tonsil clamps can be used to perform blunt dissection down to the level of the pretracheal fascia. When present, the thyroid isthmus should be pushed down (inferiorly) during this part of the procedure. Transillumination can be done using the bronchoscope to indicate the best site to place the introducer needle.

The flexible bronchoscope is withdrawn and protected by the endotracheal tube prior to needle insertion. The needle is inserted at the inferior edge of the light reflex, which should correspond to the space between the first and second or second and third tracheal rings (Fig. 6). The insertion is visualized through the scope and directed inferiorly to avoid damage to the posterior tracheal wall. Insertion into the

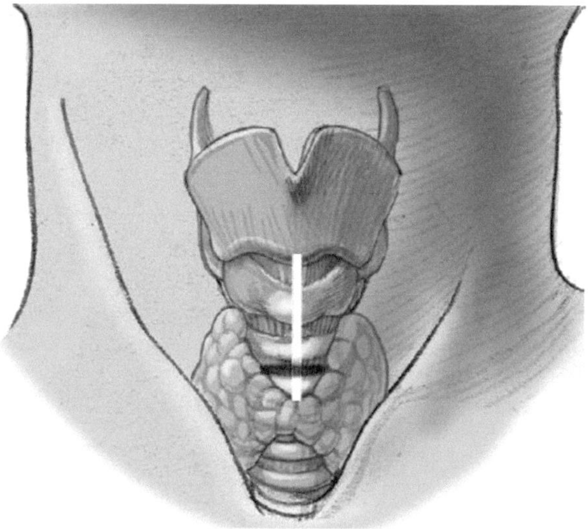

Fig. 5 Transverse incision below the level of the cricoid cartilage

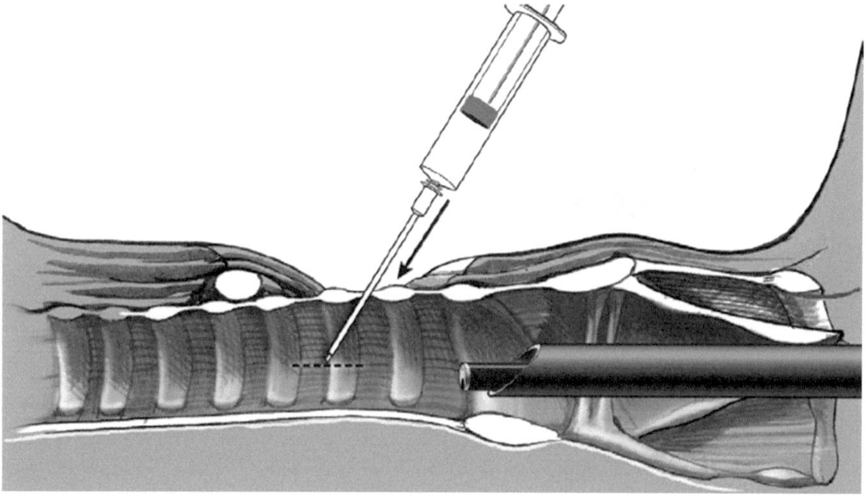

Fig. 6 Placement of the introducer needle

trachea can also be verified by aspiration on the syringe, resulting in air bubble return. The needle is withdrawn, and the cannula is kept in the tracheal lumen.

A J-tipped guide wire is passed through the cannula under direct visualization. After confirmation of proper placement of the guide wire (Fig. 7), the cannula can be removed, leaving the wire in place. At this point, using the bronchoscope, one should confirm that the wire is in the correct position, entering the anterior wall between the 11 and 1 o'clock positions, and goes all the way to the carina without passing through the endotracheal tube opening.

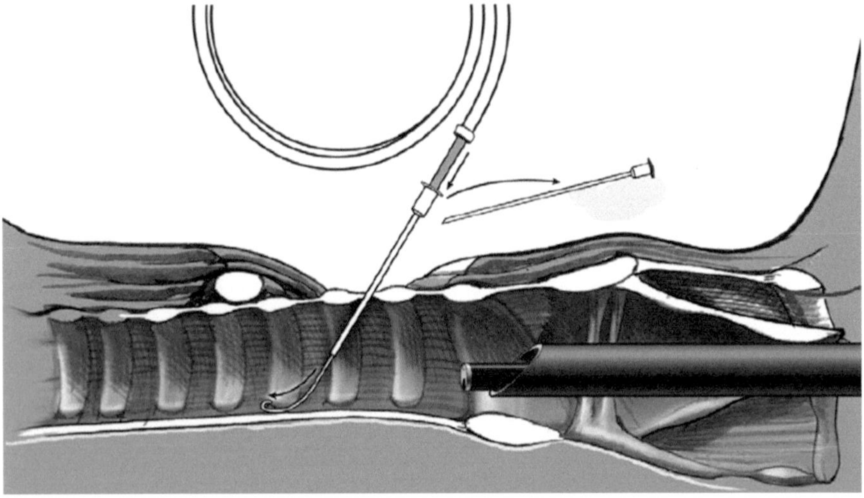

Fig. 7 The guidewire is placed into the trachea through the introducer

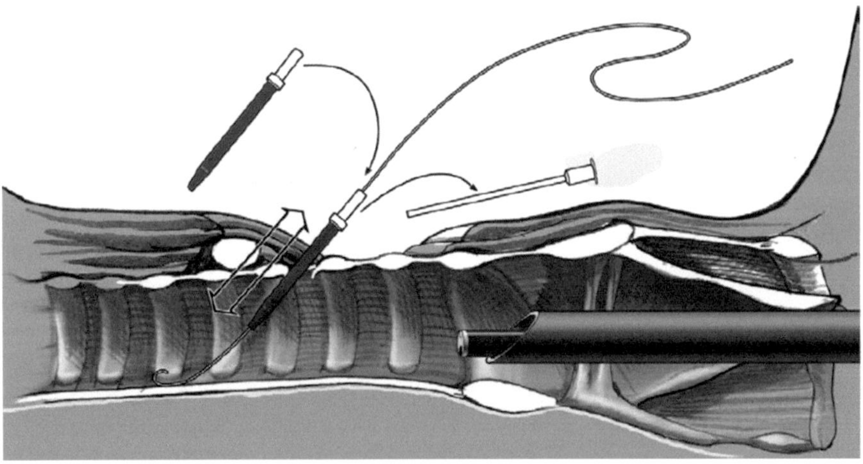

Fig. 8 Introduction of the 8-French dilator

After confirmation of proper placement of the guide wire, the tract is initially dilated with a short 8-French or 11-French catheter (Fig. 8). An 8-French guiding catheter with a safety ridge, to avoid damage to the posterior tracheal wall, is introduced over the guide wire (Fig. 9).

The dilator is used to further dilate the tract to the point where it will accommodate the tracheostomy cannula. The dilator is loaded onto the guide wire/guiding catheter complex. The tip of the dilator should be at the level of the safety ridge. It should be carefully advanced, taking care not to pass the 40-French mark below the level of the skin. While introducing the dilator, moving the complex in and out will help to accomplish good dilation of the soft tissues and anterior tracheal wall (Fig. 10).

Once the tract is dilated, the next step is the placement of the tracheostomy tube. The size of the tracheostomy tube will dictate which dilator will be used for this step. A number 6 cuffed Shiley tube will be used with a 26-French dilator, while a Number 8 Shiley will require a 28-French dilator. The tracheostomy tube is mounted on the appropriate dilator and loaded onto the guide catheter. Now it can be

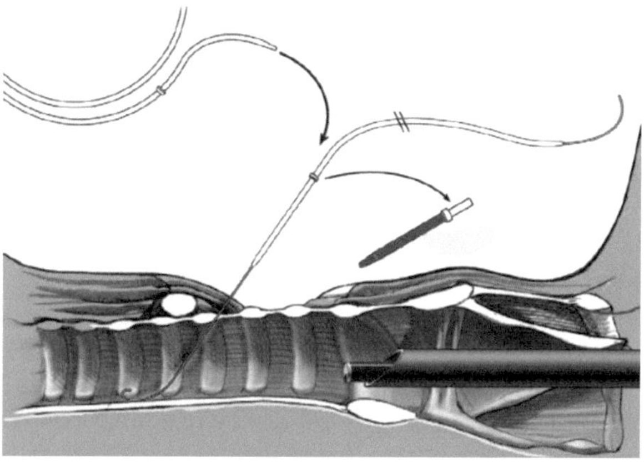

Fig. 9 After removal of the 8-French dilator, the 8-French guiding catheter is placed into the trachea

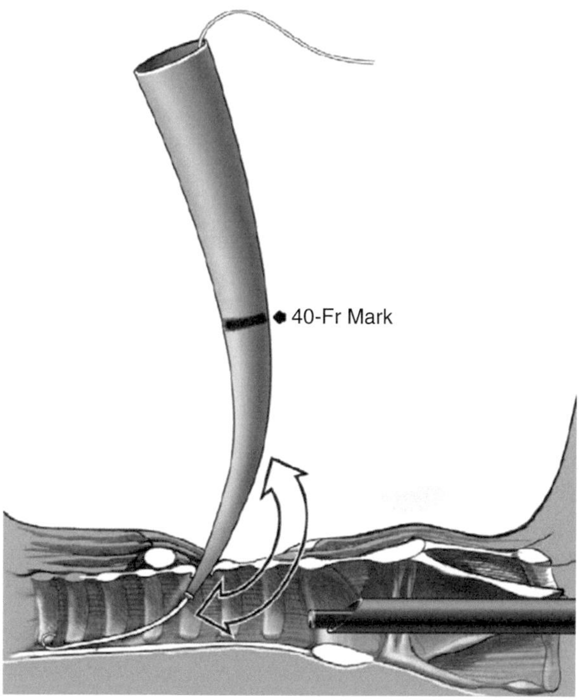

Fig. 10 The dilator is introduced. Note that the 40-French (40-Fr) mark is not supposed to get below the skin level

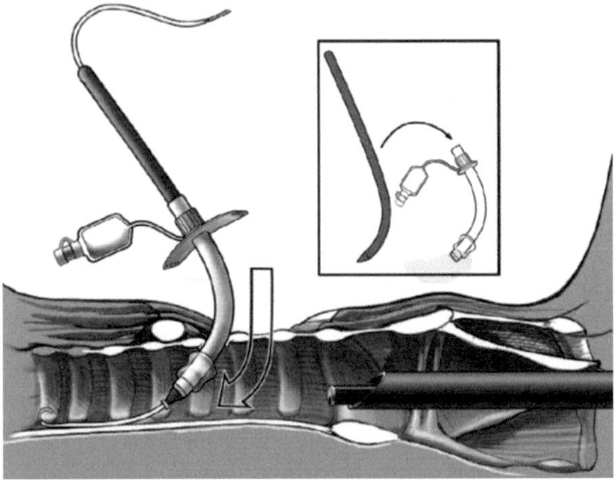

Fig. 11 The tracheostomy cannula/guiding catheter complex is introduced into the trachea

introduced into the trachea under direct visualization (Fig. 11). The dilator, guide wire, and guide catheter are removed, and the proper placement of the cannula is confirmed by the presence of end-tidal CO_2. The bronchoscope is removed from the endotracheal tube and passed through the tracheostomy tube to make sure the tube is in a good position. The tube is then secured in a standard fashion. This can be done by using 2–0 silk stitches on each side of the flange.

Another adjuvant that can be used to improve the safety of the procedure is ultrasound (US). By using US, the physician can visualize the path of the needle and the insertion into the trachea, as well as the placement of the dilator and cannula in real time. Vascular structures and the thyroid isthmus can also be visualized and avoided using this technique, which can be particularly useful in obese patients. Identification of landmarks can be difficult in these patients, and obesity is a relative contraindication to the procedure. US can guide the needle into the trachea; at the same time it helps to avoid injury to vessels and the thyroid, making it safe to perform percutaneous tracheostomy in this population [14]. In a recent article, Gobatto et al. [15] reviewed 60 percutaneous tracheostomies performed at their institution. Eleven procedures were done under bronchoscopy guidance and 49 were done using US guidance. The US-guided procedure was found to be quicker (12 versus 15 min, $p = 0.028$), and the complication rate was not significantly different.

Postoperative Care

Care for a patient with a fresh percutaneous tracheostomy is similar to standard open tracheostomy postoperative care. The tube needs to be secured to the skin to avoid dislodgement, which can cause immediate respiratory distress and airway obstruction. The obturator used to introduce the tracheostomy cannula should be at the bedside in case of tube dislodgement and need for reinsertion. A postoperative chest X-ray is still recommended, even though some studies show that the incidence of positive findings requiring intervention is low [16]. Yeo at al. [17] reviewed the literature from 1960 to 2012 and found that only 0.7% and 1.8% of the chest X-rays performed in surgical and percutaneous tracheostomy cases, respectively, necessitated intervention. Aggressive tracheostomy care is indicated to avoid obstruction of the cannula with mucus plugs or blood clots. If the patient had the tracheostomy for an upper airway obstruction and is off the ventilator after the procedure, the cuff can be deflated the day after the surgery. A tracheal suction catheter is inserted below the distal opening of the cannula, and the cuff can be safely deflated. This will avoid all of the secretions accumulated above the cuff entering the distal tracheobronchial tree. If the patient is still on the ventilator, the cuff should stay inflated. The tracheostomy tract takes longer to mature in comparison with standard open tracheostomy. This may be related not to granulation tissue formation or epithelialization of the tract, but to the time during which the anterior wall needs to be stented in order to remain patent for the tube exchange. Standard tracheostomy tubes are usually changed by postoperative day 5, but percutaneous tracheostomy tubes should not be changed until 10 days after the procedure.

Complications

As with any other new surgical procedure, new and unpredictable complications can arise. With experience, the complications are identified and techniques are modified to avoid specific complications.

The original technique described by Shelden et al. [4] was associated with severe complications such as carotid artery and esophageal lesions. With the introduction of the Seldinger technique, the complication rate declined [18, 19], but some published series still showed a high rate of complications [20]. With the evolution of the technique and better understanding of the potential complications, the method has been shown to be reliable and safe in the hands of experienced surgeons and when used in selected cases. Massick et al. [21] prospectively analyzed the first 100 cases done in a community hospital and observed a reduction in the overall complication rate after the first 20 procedures. The learning curve was also studied by Petiot et al. [22]. They studied 85 consecutive patients who underwent US-guided percutaneous tracheostomy from 2010 to 2014 and found that 50 US-guided percutaneous tracheostomies are needed to achieve an acceptable complication rate.

The rate of complication depends on the type of percutaneous tracheostomy technique, its indications, and whether it is done with bronchoscopy guidance or not, although there are studies showing equivalent results without the use of a bronchoscope [23]. The Rapitrach technique is associated with a higher incidence of complications than the Seldinger technique [24]. It was originally described as a technique for emergency cases and uses a guide wire followed by the introduction of a tracheotome. The jaws of the tracheotome are opened in the trachea, and the tube is inserted between the jaws. This technique is associated with tracheostomy tube cuff perforation and tracheal wall damage.

In a meta-analysis comparing percutaneous and standard open tracheostomy, Higgins and Punthakee [10] showed that the complication rates are similar, with a trend favoring the percutaneous technique. In a retrospective study, Bhatti et al. [25] divided their group of 318 percutaneous tracheostomies, using the Ciaglia Cook Blue Rhino kit, into two groups. In the first 159 cases, the complication rate was 7.5%, while in the second group, comprising the most recent 159 patients, the complication rate was 4.4%. Diaz-Reganon et al. performed a prospective study on 800 consecutive percutaneous tracheostomies [26]. Their complication rate was 4%, and the most common complication was bleeding.

Other possible intraoperative complications include paratracheal insertion, injury of the anterior jugular vein, displacement of the tracheal tube, pneumothorax, desaturation, posterior tracheal wall perforation, thyroid injury, and subcutaneous emphysema. Postoperative complications include bleeding, infection, pneumothorax, tracheostomy tube displacement and, rarely, trachea–innominate fistula. This latter serious complication was found in 0.35% of cases from a total of 572 patients undergoing the procedure [27]. While the incidence rates of intraoperative and early surgical complications have been extensively described in the literature, late complications can be more difficult to identify and evaluate. Since most patients are critically ill, there is a high mortality rate and many patients are lost to follow-up. In their paper comparing rates of tracheal stenosis between percutaneous and standard tracheostomy, Koitschev et al. [28] found suprastomal stenosis greater than or equal to 50% in 23% of patients submitted to percutaneous tracheostomy and 7.3% of patients submitted to standard tracheostomy. There are a few mechanisms associated with the development of tracheal stenosis. Fracture and displacement of tracheal rings during the dilation of the anterior tracheal wall, dynamic collapse of the lateral tracheal wall [29], and bacterial infection leading to local inflammation can contribute to the development of this complication. There is also evidence that the tracheal stenosis caused by percutaneous tracheostomy occurs earlier and is significantly closer to the vocal cords (subglottic) than stenosis caused by standard open tracheostomy [30].

Cost

Percutaneous tracheostomy is associated with a US$456 reduction in cost, a 4.6 min reduction in procedure time, and use of fewer assistants in comparison with standard open tracheostomy, according to the meta-analysis done by Higgins and Punthakee [10]. On average, there is one less person present for the percutaneous procedure, as typically the open procedures involve trainees, which may account for the increased operative time and increased staff numbers [10]. Freeman et al. [31] performed a prospective randomized controlled trial to evaluate the cost effectiveness of percutaneous versus open tracheostomy. Patient groups were well matched based on the severity of illness and primary diagnosis. This study found that costs were statistically significantly lower for a percutaneous tracheostomy procedure than for an open tracheostomy in terms of both equipment/supply and professional charges. The total hospital charge the patients incurred for percutaneous tracheostomy on average was US$1569, compared with an open procedure mean cost of US$3172. This cost difference leads to a savings of roughly US$1600 health care dollars, according to this study. In addition to the decrease in charges, Freeman et al. noted that the average time for their bedside percutaneous procedure was 20.1 min versus 41.7 min in the open procedure group, leading to a decrease in over 20 min of procedure time. Therefore, percutaneous tracheostomy, when indicated, may be more cost effective than open surgical tracheostomy by obviating the need for OR facilities and personnel.

Conclusion

Tracheostomy is one of the most common procedures performed in the intensive care unit. Open tracheostomy can be used in most cases requiring a surgical airway but is associated with a higher cost, delay in performing the procedure after the recommendation for tracheostomy is established, and possible problems associated with transportation of a critically ill patient to the OR. Percutaneous tracheostomy is a good alternative with similar complication rates in experienced hands. Complications are comparable to those of the open technique, and it can be performed by the ICU team shortly after the decision for placement of a surgical airway is made. Late complications are difficult to identify and study, since the patient population is critically ill and follow-up can be a problem. Some of the late complications could also be due to the primary disease, traumatic and prolonged intubation, or lack of proper care after the procedure. Proper set-up (including having a tracheostomy set available) and patient selection are vital for the success of the procedure. Bronchoscope and US guidance should be considered in most cases, especially until the team is more experienced with the procedure, as a learning curve is prominent in the first 20–50 cases. During this period, selection of the right patient is extremely important, and clinicians should err on the side of being more conservative with the indications. Performing a percutaneous tracheostomy in patients who can be easily intubated, in case of losing the airway during the procedure, is good practice and should be considered until the team is more experienced with this procedure.

References

1. Wunsch H, Wagner J, Herlim M, Chong DH, Kramer AA, Halpern SD. ICU occupancy and mechanical ventilator use in the United States. Crit Care Med. 2013;41:2712–9.
2. Yu M. Tracheostomy patients on the ward: multiple benefits from a multidisciplinary team? Crit Care. 2010;14:109.
3. Andrews MJ, Pearson FG. Incidence and pathogenesis of tracheal injury following cuffed tube tracheostomy with assisted ventilation: analysis of a two-year prospective study. Ann Surg. 1971;173:249–63.
4. Shelden CH, Pudenz RH, Freshwater DB, Crue BL. A new method for tracheotomy. J Neurosurg. 1955;12:428–31.
5. Ciaglia P, Firsching R, Syniec C. Elective percutaneous dilatational tracheostomy. A new simple bedside procedure; preliminary report. Chest. 1985;87:715–9.

6. Sanabria A. Which percutaneous tracheostomy method is better? A systematic review. Respir Care. 2014;59:1660–70.
7. Kost KM. Percutaneous tracheostomy: comparison of Ciaglia and Griggs techniques. Crit Care. 2000;4:143–6.
8. Fantoni A, Ripamonti D. A non-derivative, non-surgical tracheostomy: the translaryngeal method. Intensive Care Med. 1997;23:386–92.
9. Frova G, Quintel M. A new simple method for percutaneous tracheostomy: controlled rotating dilation. A preliminary report. Intensive Care Med. 2002;28:299–303.
10. Higgins KM, Punthakee X. Meta-analysis comparison of open versus percutaneous tracheostomy. Laryngoscope. 2007;117:447–54.
11. Dulguerov P, Gysin C, Perneger TV, Chevrolet JC. Percutaneous or surgical tracheostomy: a meta-analysis. Crit Care Med. 1999;27:1617–25.
12. Freeman BD, Isabella K, Lin N, Buchman TG. A meta-analysis of prospective trials comparing percutaneous and surgical tracheostomy in critically ill patients. Chest. 2000;118:1412–8.
13. Johnson JL, Cheatham ML, Sagraves SG, Block EF, Nelson LD. Percutaneous dilational tracheostomy: a comparison of single- versus multiple-dilator techniques. Crit Care Med. 2001;29:1251–4.
14. Guinot PG, Zogheib E, Petiot S, Marienne JP, Guerin AM, Monet P, et al. Ultrasound-guided percutaneous tracheostomy in critically ill obese patients. Crit Care. 2012;16:R40.
15. Gobatto AL, Besen BA, Tierno PF, Mendes PV, Cadamuro F, Joelsons D, et al. Comparison between ultrasound- and bronchoscopy-guided percutaneous dilational tracheostomy in critically ill patients: a retrospective cohort study. J Crit Care. 2015;30:220 e213–27.
16. Hoehne F, Ozaeta M, Chung R. Routine chest X-ray after percutaneous tracheostomy is unnecessary. Am Surg. 2005;71:51–3.
17. Yeo WX, Phua CQ, Lo S. Is routine chest X-ray after surgical and percutaneous tracheostomy necessary in adults: a systemic review of the current literature. Clin Otolaryngol. 2014;39:79–88.
18. Friedman Y, Fildes J, Mizock B, Samuel J, Patel S, Appavu S, et al. Comparison of percutaneous and surgical tracheostomies. Chest. 1996;110:480–5.
19. McHenry CR, Raeburn CD, Lange RL, Priebe PP. Percutaneous tracheostomy: a cost-effective alternative to standard open tracheostomy. Am Surg. 1997;63:646–51. discussion 651-642
20. Wang MB, Berke GS, Ward PH, Calcaterra TC, Watts D. Early experience with percutaneous tracheotomy. Laryngoscope. 1992;102:157–62.
21. Massick DD, Powell DM, Price PD, Chang SL, Squires G, Forrest LA, et al. Quantification of the learning curve for percutaneous dilatational tracheotomy. Laryngoscope. 2000;110:222–8.
22. Petiot S, Guinot PG, Diouf M, Zogheib E, Dupont H. Learning curve for real-time ultrasound-guided percutaneous tracheostomy. Anaesth Crit Care Pain Med. 2016.
23. Jackson LS, Davis JW, Kaups KL, Sue LP, Wolfe MM, Bilello JF, et al. Percutaneous tracheostomy: to bronch or not to bronch—that is the question. J Trauma. 2011;71:1553–6.
24. Leinhardt DJ, Mughal M, Bowles B, Glew R, Kishen R, MacBeath J, et al. Appraisal of percutaneous tracheostomy. Br J Surg. 1992;79:255–8.
25. Bhatti N, Mirski M, Tatlipinar A, Koch WM, Goldenberg D. Reduction of complication rate in percutaneous dilation tracheostomies. Laryngoscope. 2007;117:172–5.
26. Diaz-Reganon G, Minambres E, Ruiz A, Gonzalez-Herrera S, Holanda-Pena M, Lopez-Espadas F. Safety and complications of percutaneous tracheostomy in a cohort of 800 mixed ICU patients. Anaesthesia. 2008;63:1198–203.
27. Dempsey GA, Grant CA, Jones TM. Percutaneous tracheostomy: a 6 yr prospective evaluation of the single tapered dilator technique. Br J Anaesth. 2010;105:782–8.
28. Koitschev A, Simon C, Blumenstock G, Mach H, Graumuller S. Suprastomal tracheal stenosis after dilational and surgical tracheostomy in critically ill patients. Anaesthesia. 2006;61:832–7.

29. Christenson TE, Artz GJ, Goldhammer JE, Spiegel JR, Boon MS. Tracheal stenosis after placement of percutaneous dilational tracheotomy. Laryngoscope. 2008;118:222–7.
30. Raghuraman G, Rajan S, Marzouk JK, Mullhi D, Smith FG. Is tracheal stenosis caused by percutaneous tracheostomy different from that by surgical tracheostomy? Chest. 2005;127:879–85.
31. Freeman BD, Isabella K, Cobb JP, Boyle WA 3rd, Schmieg RE Jr, Kolleff MH, et al. A prospective, randomized study comparing percutaneous with surgical tracheostomy in critically ill patients. Crit Care Med. 2001;29:926–30.

Percutaneous Tracheostomy: Pearls and Pitfalls, and How to Create a "Hand-On" Training Program Course

Marianne Yumi Nakai, Marcelo Benedito Menezes, Norberto Kodi Kavabata, Alexandre Baba Suehara, Antonio Augusto T. Bertelli, William Kikuchi, and Antonio José Gonçalves

Introduction

Tracheostomy is one of the oldest surgical procedures known to mankind. Egyptian tablets dating back to 3600 BC illustrate what could be the origin of this procedure. Tracheostomy was originally an emergency procedure for clearing the upper airways. However, in the 1940s, during the poliomyelitis epidemic, it gained great importance and began to be used in the maintenance of airways. Chevalier Jackson (1865–1958) was responsible for improving and standardizing the surgical technique of tracheostomy that is still used today.

In 1955, Shelden et al. described the first percutaneous tracheostomy technique. Nevertheless, this procedure became popular only after 1985 when Ciaglia et al. described percutaneous tracheostomy using the Seldinger method, using a guide wire and multiple dilators.

Currently, tracheostomy is one of the most common procedures in intensive care units (ICUs), widely recommended for patients with prolonged orotracheal intubation. Its use improves pulmonary hygiene, reduces the use of sedatives, enables oral feeding, and prevents glottic lesions and subglottic stenosis. Nonetheless, defining the timing of tracheostomy still remains controversial. Meta-analyses indicate that early tracheostomy (up to 2 weeks) significantly reduces the use of sedatives, the time of mechanical ventilation, pneumonias associated with mechanical ventilation, and the length of stay in the ICU. Although it does not affect mortality, early tracheostomy is being increasingly indicated, especially for patients with prolonged intubation [1, 2].

The transport of critical patients represents a great risk and is responsible for most complications in the ICU. In one third of the cases, equipment failure during transport (ventilator, infusion pump, monitor, etc.) occurs and up to 70% of the

M.Y. Nakai, M.D. • M.B. Menezes, M.D. • N.K. Kavabata, M.D. • A.B. Suehara, M.D.
A.A.T. Bertelli, M.D. • W. Kikuchi, M.D. • A.J. Gonçalves, M.D. (✉)
Departamento de Cirurgia da Irmandade da Santa Casa de Misericórdia de São Paulo,
Faculdade de Ciências Médicas da Santa Casa de São Paulo, São Paulo, SP, Brazil
e-mail: dr.goncalves@uol.com.br

T.P. de Farias (ed.), *Tracheostomy*, https://doi.org/10.1007/978-3-319-67867-2_6

patients exhibit adverse effects, such as changes in heart rate, hypotension, hypertension, increased intracranial pressure, arrhythmias, and alterations in the respiratory rate [3].

Percutaneous tracheostomy is a safe and effective technique to perform bedside in the ICU [4, 5].

Percutaneous Dilatational Versus Conventional Tracheostomy: Scientific Evidence for Use

Tracheostomy is a safe, low-risk procedure, associated with low surgical morbidity when it is performed using the traditional technique in the operating room (OR). The bedside procedure appears to be safe too, when it is conducted by an expert team, and it presents the lowest costs among all alternative techniques for tracheostomy [6]. In the OR, costs are higher because they include OR time, anesthesiologist time, drug costs, and the need for a team to transport the patient from the ICU to the OR. The advantage of this option is the totally controlled environment in case of an emergency. Those who defend the bedside procedure consider the transportation of a critical patient an unnecessary risk in addition to rising costs [7]. Percutaneous dilatational tracheostomy (PDT) appears to be an alternative, allowing the procedure to be performed at the bedside easily and more quickly, with low risks and results similar to those obtained by open tracheostomy (OT) [8].

Authors have compared OT—in general, performed in an OR—with PDT, using different dilatational kits [5, 8, 9]. Despite this, there are still doubts about the better procedure. It is correct that any technique is less expensive when it is performed at the bedside. The complication rates are low and, regardless of which method is used, they depend mostly on the experience and preference of the surgical team. The differences relate to major and minor bleeding, timing of surgery, presence of intraoperative technical difficulties, postoperative inflammation, infection of the stoma, decannulation and cannula obstruction, late consequences, scar quality, tracheal stenosis, and death [5, 7, 9].

Differences between the different dilatational kits should be considered too. Each instrument for dilatation has its own difficulties and they can present inherent complications [9]. The majority of published papers refer to progressive dilatation with sequential dilators or with an unique conical dilator. The use of dilator forceps, hydrostatic balloons, and a rotative "PercuTwist®" have been referred to only in isolated papers, not in systematic reviews. With regard to OT, data on transportation problems are sparse and fewer papers including the bedside procedure appear in systematic reviews.

Unfavorable anatomy can be a contraindication for PDT. If it is not possible to palpate the median-line structures of the neck (thyroid and cricoid cartilages, tracheal rings, sternal notch), an OT should be preferred, avoiding "blind surgery" with the risk of vascular or pleural lesions [5, 10]. In our opinion, bedside OT can be indicated in most patients, as long all necessary equipment and good lighting are available. Reviewing our recent statistics, from 2013 to 2015, we performed 534 bedside OTs, with six minor bleeding events, one decannulation, one posterior tracheal wall lesion, and one death. ICUs have restriction protocols for open surgical procedures performed under their jurisdiction, but we found no literature supporting this restriction concerning tracheostomy. There are major risks of stomal inflammation and infection with OT compared with PDT, but these risks are not dependent on the location where the surgery is performed [5].

Coagulopathy is another reason for OT to be preferred. Obviously, this situation is not ideal for any surgery, but in OT the conditions for bleeding control are better than in PDT, especially with the possibility of clamping and tying small vessels and other maneuvers and materials to avoid or stop bleeding.

All of the studies we have consulted agreed that PDT is faster than OT, independently of whether it is performed at the bedside or in an OR. The presence of technical difficulties (problems with the point of puncture of the trachea, failure in progression of a guide wire, or decannulation during bronchoscopy) were considered exclusive to PDT [5, 9–11]. Major or minor bleeding events did not differ between techniques, although this evaluation was very subjective. Major bleeding was rare with both techniques. Minor bleeding events was evaluated based on the use of knots or electrocautery, which are not used in PDT.

One meta-analysis [9] showed that stomal infection and inflammation were more frequent in patients undergoing OT, but this did not impact on the survival of patients or compromise their general condition. PDT (performed at the bedside) appeared to involve lower costs than OT performed in the OR. This did not seem to be the case when OT was performed in the ICU. The scar was smaller in patients undergoing PDT, probably related to a smaller skin incision and the fact that retractors were not used [5, 9].

Cannula obstruction and decannulation in the first 48 h after surgery are more frequent with PDT. Some authors have related this to better nursing care in patients undergoing OT, with a larger incision and consequent greater ease for repositioning the cannula. In our experience, this problem relates more to ICU expertise with tracheostomized patients than to the method. The patient should not be moved in the first 24 h and, if it is necessary, extreme care with the cannula is needed.

In a recent meta-analysis [11], mortality was analyzed as the final outcome. No difference was found. That suggests no impact of technical difficulties, the timing of the procedure, or cannula problems on survival.

The PDT learning curve appears to require around 20 procedures. When this point is reached, the number of technical difficulties and complications decreases significantly [12]. With regard to OT, we found no recent studies about the learning curve, but probably this is true for OT too. The presence of a senior surgeon should contribute to reducing problems, whichever technique is used.

When OT performed at the bedside or in the OR are compared, bedside OT presents advantages for all parameters. This result generally is affected by bias, because patients treated in the OR can present more clinical problems before the procedure or more technical difficulties have been foreseen.

The mortality in patients undergoing PDT is 1 in 600. To minimize it, is important that bronchoscopy is used to guide the procedure, and special care is required in cannula fixation, besides adequate nursing training [11].

Thus, we can keep in mind that percutaneous tracheostomy is a safe, faster procedure with lower rates of stoma-related complications, but may be associated with more frequent technical difficulties when compared with the traditional open procedure. The learning curve must be respected and selection of candidates for the percutaneous technique must be judicious in order to avoid technical problems in its accomplishment. By any technique, tracheostomy presents risks, and the person who performs it must be able to resolve its potential trans- and postoperative complications.

Basic Surgical Technique

The percutaneous tracheostomy technique involves puncture of the airway with passage of a guide wire (using the Seldinger technique), dilatation of the trachea, and introduction of the tracheostomy cannula. Unlike the conventional technique, there is no dissection of structures in the percutaneous technique, so it is considered a "blind" technique.

To reduce the risk of complications, it is recommended to use bronchoscopy or ultrasound to guide the puncture.

Bronchoscopy allows internal visualization (via the airway) of the entire procedure and diagnosis of pretracheostomy lesions (tracheoesophageal fistula, glottic lesions, tracheal stenosis, etc.); assists in the correct positioning of the puncture (between the third and fourth tracheal rings and on the midline); prevents an accidental rise of the guide wire; prevents injury to the posterior wall during dilatation; allows checking of the final placement of the tracheostomy cannula; and allows postprocedural airway hygiene.

Ultrasound in turn does not allow visualization of the internal part of the procedure, but allows observation of all of the external structures, which is not possible with bronchoscopy. The main advantage of ultrasound guidance is the prevention of inadvertent puncture of important vessels. However, this technique also allows guidance for correct placement of the puncture and visualization of the descent of the guide wire. The other advantages of bronchoscopy do not apply to ultrasound.

It should be emphasized that anatomical knowledge of the cervical region is essential for performing the technique safely, whether guided by ultrasound or bronchoscopy. The ability to identify the anatomical parameters of the neck allows prediction of the degree of difficulty of the tracheostomy and aids in choosing the method to guide the procedure.

Puncture of the trachea should preferably be performed between the third and fourth tracheal rings, although it can also be performed between the second and third rings. It is absolutely contraindicated to puncture the first tracheal ring due to the risk of cricoid injury during dilation and subsequent subglottic stenosis. The greater the distance between the lower edge of the cricoid and the external furcula, the greater the space for its puncture and, therefore, the simpler the procedure.

Palpation of the cricoid and trachea without difficulty indicates that no important structure is probably in the path of the puncture. In these cases, the use of bronchoscopy is the best choice. When palpation is not possible, ultrasound is more appropriate because it precisely locates the puncture site and prevents vascular lesions.

Currently, the only absolute contraindication for performing percutaneous tracheostomy is emergency tracheostomy. The other contraindications are essentially the same as those of the conventional procedure, i.e., obesity, thyroid goiter, blood dyscrasia, hemodynamic instability, etc.

Percutaneous tracheostomy can be performed by any qualified physician, bearing in mind the limitations of each professional. The physician should feel comfortable with palpation of the structures of the neck and be able to identify difficulties and potential risks of complications. Professionals who do not have the training to perform surgical tracheostomy should avoid performing the percutaneous technique in cases with higher risk of technical difficulties or complications: unfavorable anatomy, history of neck surgery, thyroid goiter, limited cervical extension, etc.

Description of the Technique Guided by Bronchoscopy, Using the Ciaglia Blue Rhino® Kit

The stages of the technique are detailed in Figs. 1, 2, 3, 4, 5, 6, 7, 8, 9, 10, 11, 12, 13, and 14.

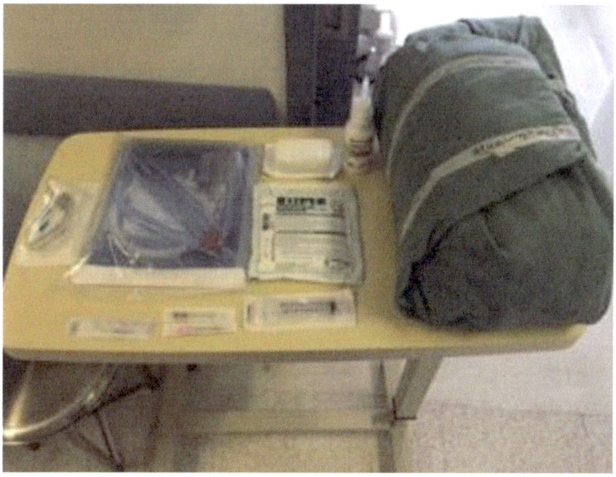

Fig. 1 Stage 1—material preparation: Ciaglia Blue Rhino® kit, apron and sterile fields, tracheostomy cannula, small surgical box

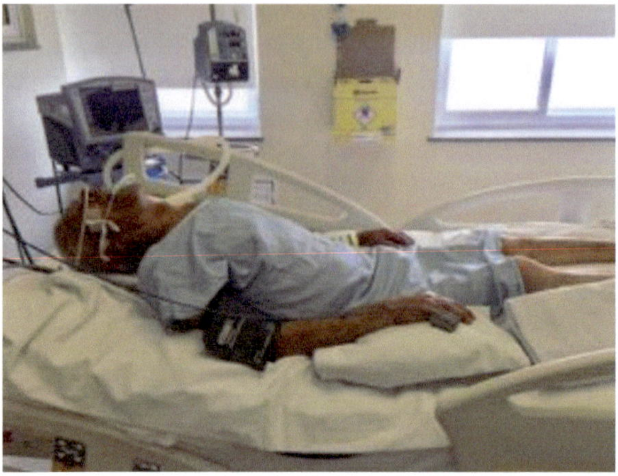

Fig. 2 Stage 2—patient preparation: patient sedation, semi-Fowler's positioning (semi-seated with cervical extension)

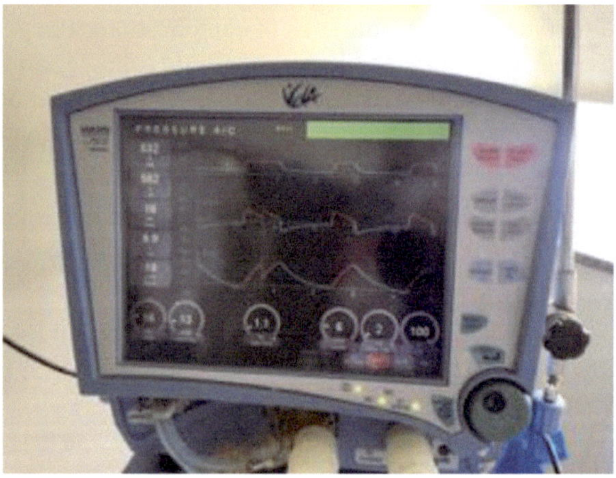

Fig. 3 Stage 3—ventilator adjustment: fraction of inspired oxygen (FiO_2) 100%, controlled assisted mode

Percutaneous Dilatational Tracheostomy Kits

There are several different kits on the market for performing percutaneous tracheostomy. All of them involve an initial tracheal puncture, using the Seldinger technique, with guide wire placement and initial dilatation, followed by the main dilatation and passage of the tracheostomy cannula.

The main kits available are described below.

Single Progressive Plastic Dilator (Ciaglia Blue Rhino®, Cook®)

This kit (see Fig. 15) represents an evolution of the kit initially developed by Ciaglia when the percutaneous tracheostomy technique was described [13]. The previous kit had multiple progressive plastic dilators and required multiple steps in the dilation process until the orifice in the trachea reached the same size as the chosen

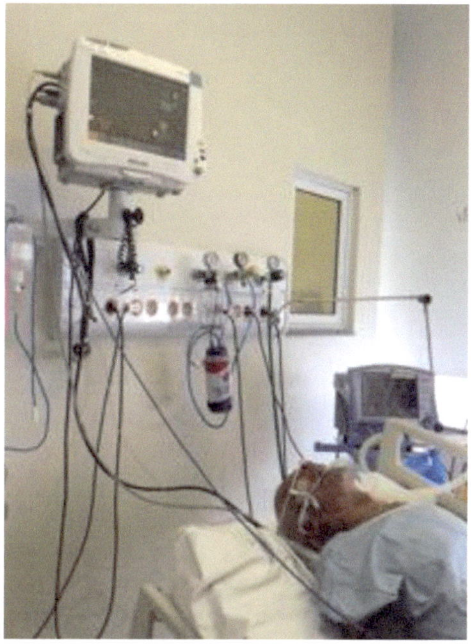

Fig. 4 Stage 4—monitoring: checking that the patient is properly monitored (oximeter, cardioscope, Arterial Blood Pressure)

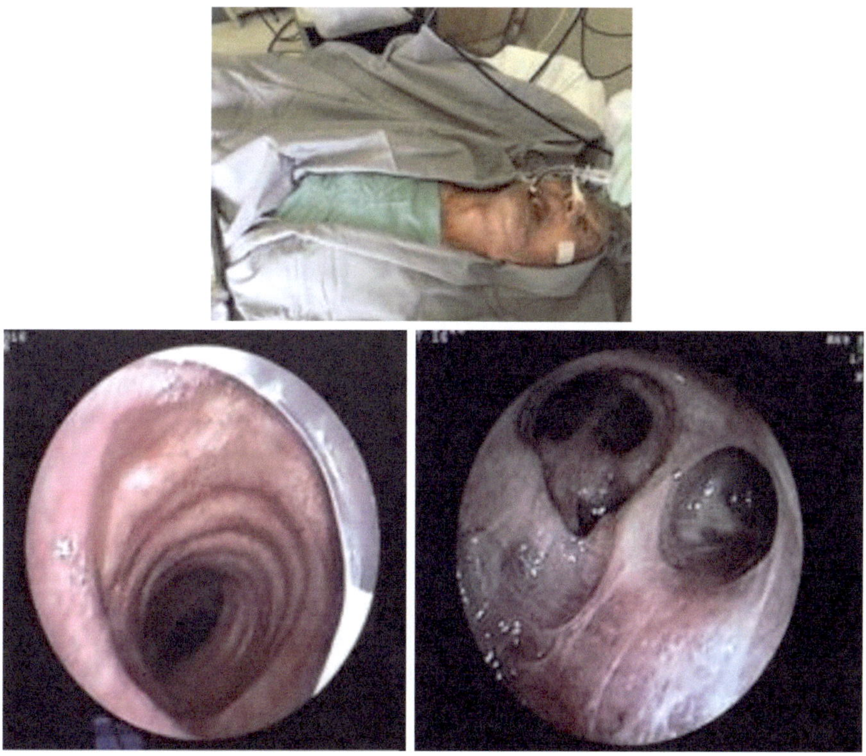

Fig. 5 Stage 5—bronchoscopy: entry of the bronchoscope through the orotracheal tube and positioning of the cannula in the subglottic region

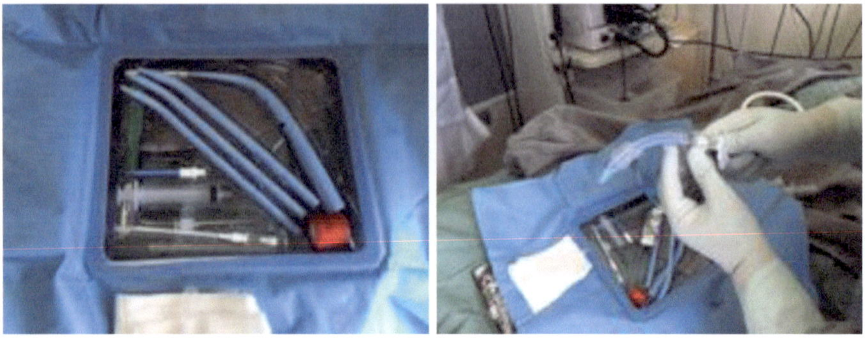

Fig. 6 Stage 6—kit preparation: kit opening, cannula choice (preferably no. 08), mounting of the cannula on the guide rail

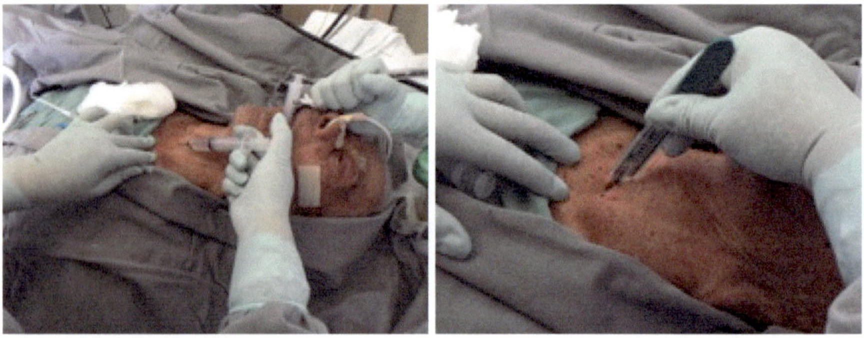

Fig. 7 Stage 7: palpation of anatomical parameters (cricoid and furcula), local anesthesia with xylocaine 2%, vertical incision 2 cm between the cricoid and furcula

cannula. Through use of a unique blue plastic dilator with the shape of a rhinoceros horn—hence the name given to the kit—the process became simpler, since after the initial dilation, this dilator is introduced through the guide wire with another plastic guide for reinforcement. As this dilator has a thin tip and a progressively larger caliber toward its base, the tracheal orifice increases in size as the dilator is introduced. It has black reference marks so the doctor knows how far to insert it (depending on the chosen cannula), as well as a safety mark that represents the maximum safe dilation. After this step, three different cannula introducers (which engage the plastic guide wire assembly) are available, depending on the size of the cannula chosen by the surgeon. This kit is perhaps the most widely used nowadays due to its versatility, since it allows the use of cannulae of different calibers and models. When compared with the Portex® kit, it has the peculiarity of requiring a tracheal puncture on the midline, since this type of dilator does not allow side compensation of the dilation. Studies that have shown that up to 30% of tracheostomies done with this kit are accompanied by tracheal ring fractures, but there seems to be no relation between this fact and other complications such as tracheal stenosis [14].

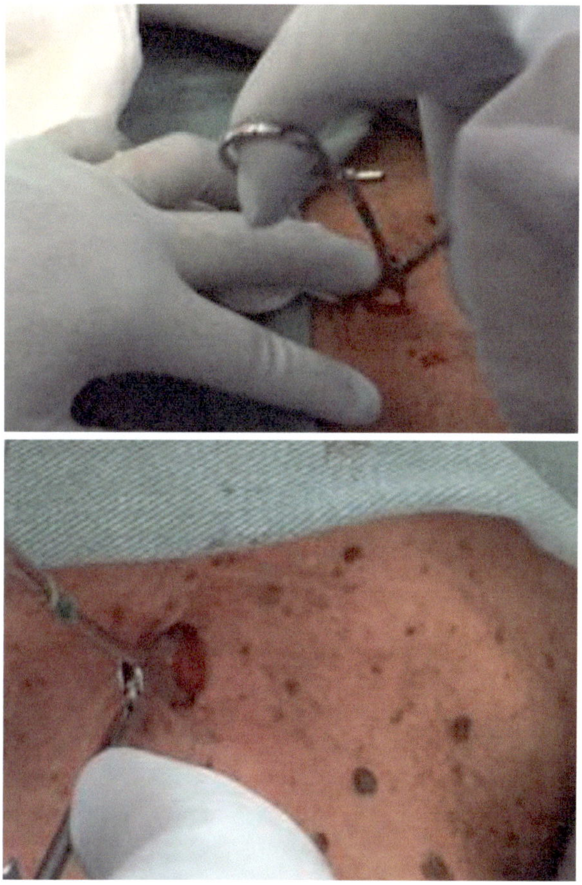

Fig. 8 Stage 8: Divulsion of the subcutaneous tissue immediately under the skin in the midline of the neck, visualization of the bronchoscope light between the second and third tracheal rings

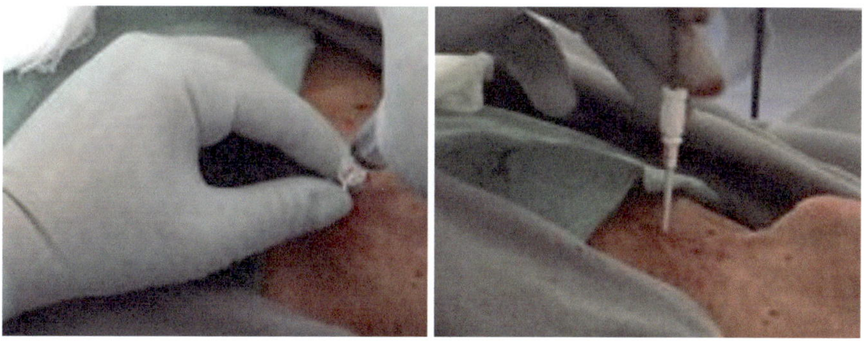

Fig. 9 Stage 9: puncture between the second and third rings on the midline

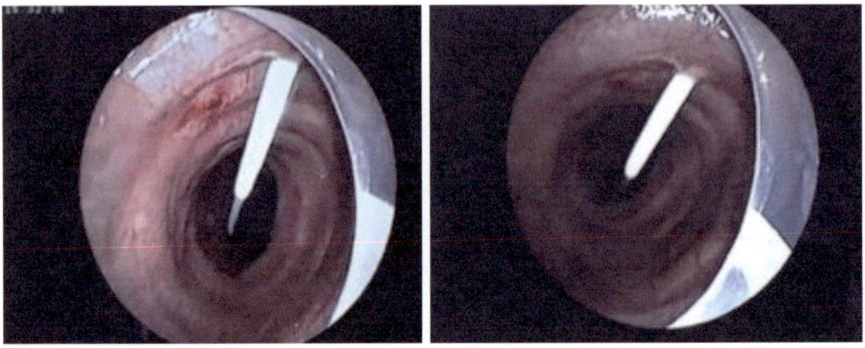

Fig. 10 Stage 10: guide wire path

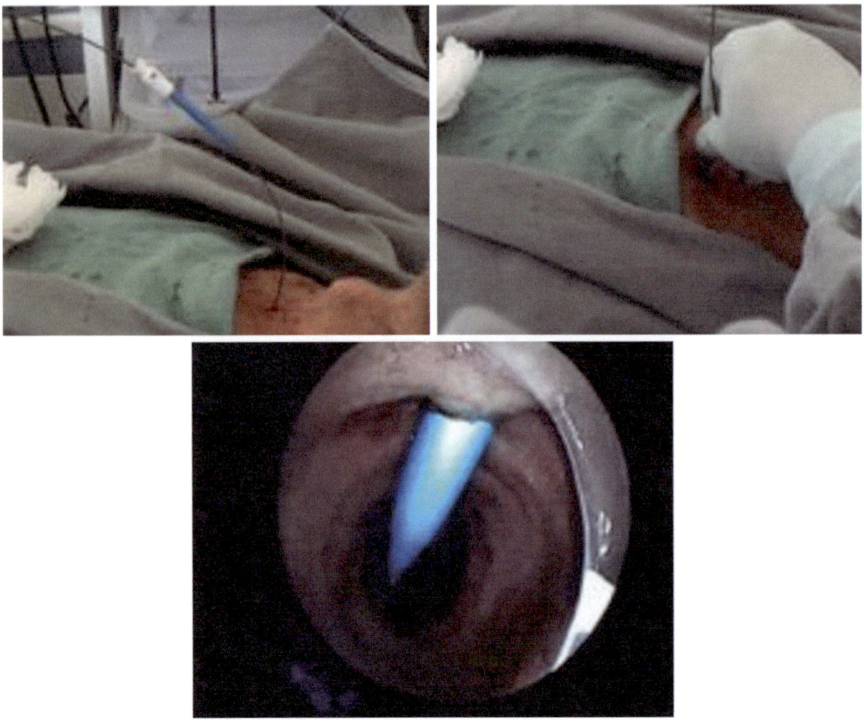

Fig. 11 Stage 11: dilatation with a 14-French dilatator

Dilation by Metallic Forceps (Griggs® Forceps, Portex®)

This kit (see Fig. 16) has metal dilator forceps with a hole in the tip. After puncture, guide wire passage, and initial dilation, the forceps are connected to the guide wire through the orifice and can be led to the tracheal lumen. After the dilation performed with clamp opening to the size of the chosen cannula, the cannula (which has its own introducer and is included in the kit) is placed [15]. The introducer of the cannula is

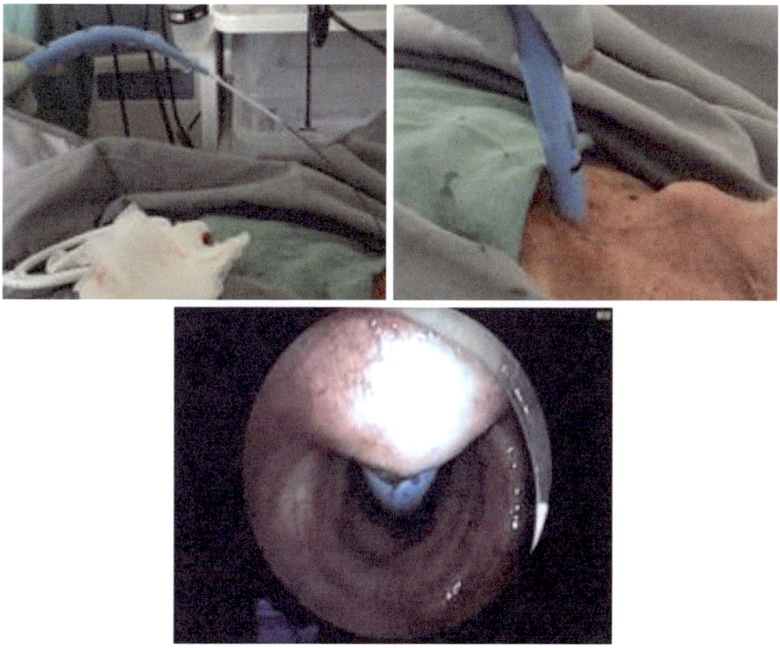

Fig. 12 Stage 12: dilatation with a progressive dilatator

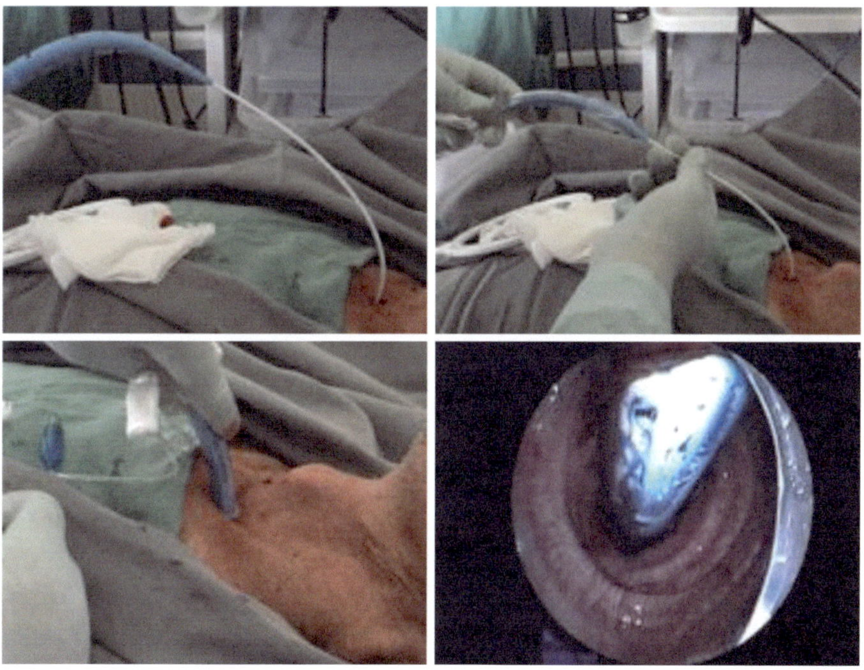

Fig. 13 Stage 13: removal of the progressive dilatator (keeping the guide wire), insertion of the tracheostomy tube mounted in the guide rail

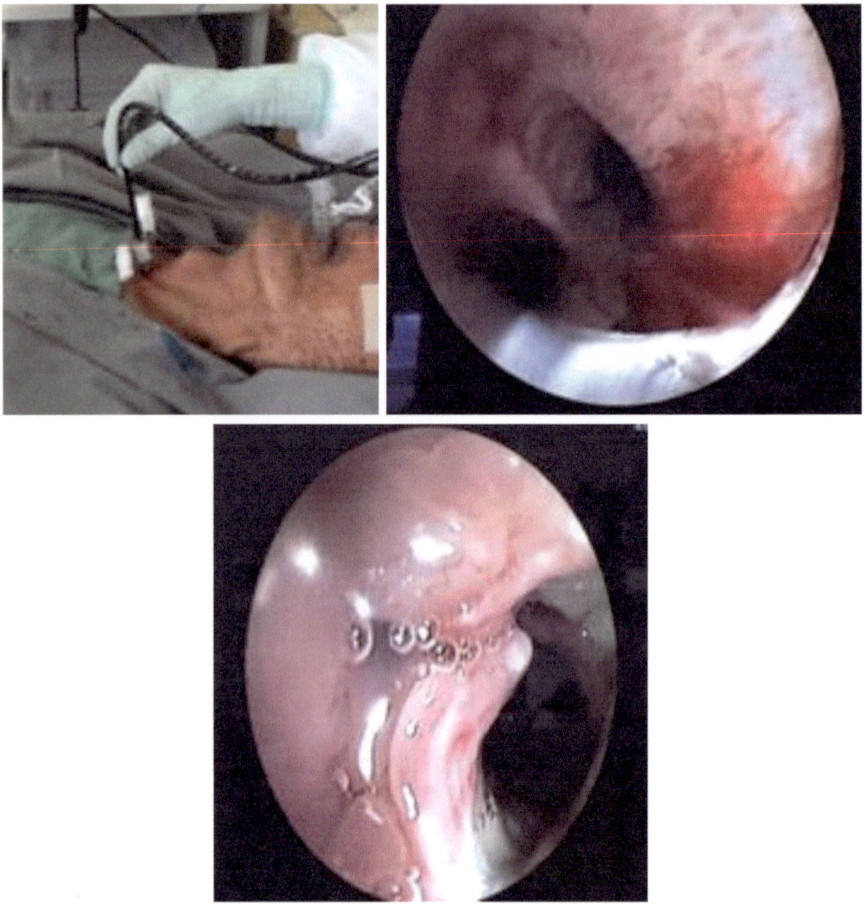

Fig. 14 Stage 14: checking of the tracheostomy tube position, airway aspiration, glottic lesion diagnosis caused by the orotracheal tube

unique because it has one orifice and does not attach to other cannulae models, so the doctor must use the cannula included in the kit or another one of the same brand that also has this kind of introducer. It has the advantage of compensating the dilation to one side, through the unequal opening of the clamp, allowing correction of a paramedian puncture. In addition, the metal clamp can be reused after sterilization, and the kit can be purchased without the tweezers, which may reduce costs.

Balloon Dilator Through Water Pressure (Dolphin BT®, Cook®)

More recently the percutaneous tracheostomy balloon kit (see Fig. 17) was introduced, based on other types of dilatation systems used in other specialties. Unlike other dilatation systems, it has controlled dilatation through pressure measurement inside the balloon, which is inflated with saline during the procedure. Just behind the balloon is the introducer attached to the cannula,

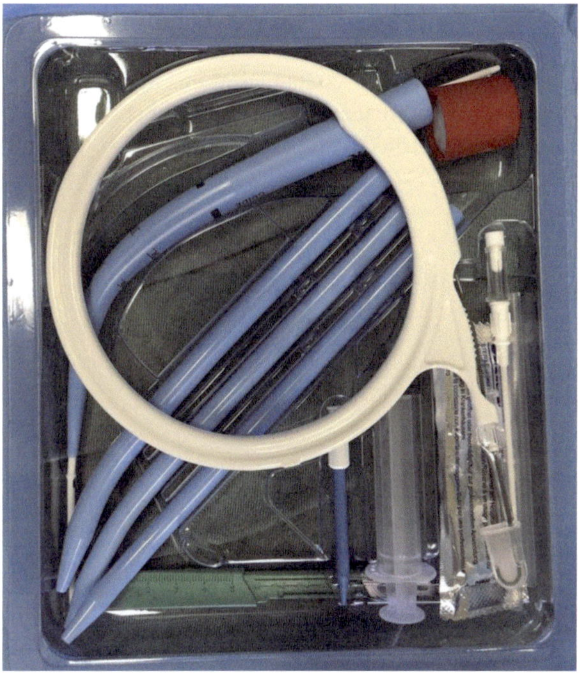

Fig. 15 Ciaglia Blue Rhino® (Cook®) tracheostomy kit with a single progressive dilator in rhino horn format; note the three introducers of differently-sized cannulae in the middle

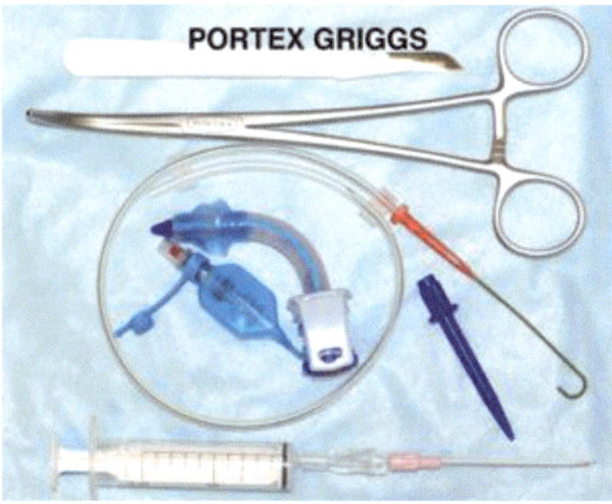

Fig. 16 Percutaneous tracheostomy kit with Griggs® forceps; note the hole in the tip of the forceps for guide wire attachment

which eliminates the step of removing the dilator and introducing the cannula, making the process easier.

Exactly as in the other kits, the procedure starts with a tracheal puncture (using the Seldinger technique) followed by guide wire placement; initial dilatation; positioning of the system with the balloon, introducer, and cannula; dilatation; and introduction of the cannula. The procedure has been shown to be safe and has the advantages of a more controlled dilation (although it is mechanical) independent of the surgeon strength, and tamponade power of the compression made by the balloon [16].

Screw Rotating Plastic Dilator (PercuTwist®, Rush®)

The rotational dilator contained in this kit (see Fig. 18) is introduced into the trachea after puncture using the Seldinger technique, as with other kits. Tracheal dilation is accomplished by progressively rotating the dilator until the tracheal aperture

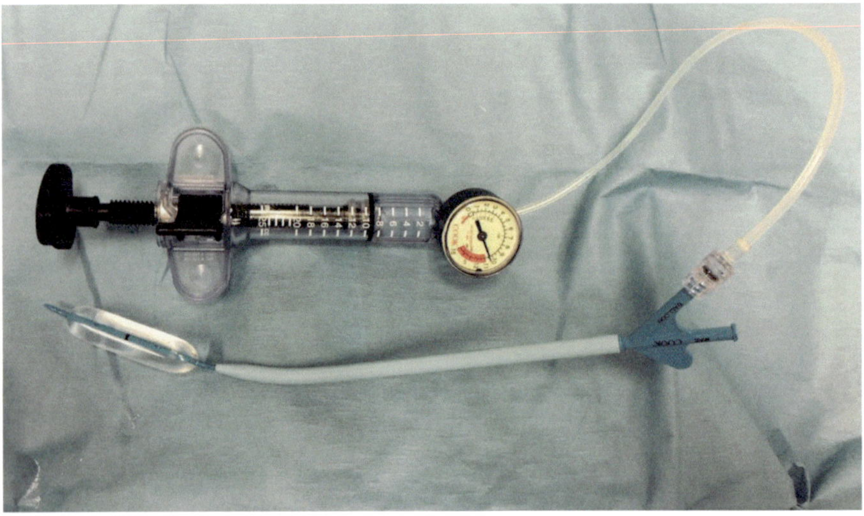

Fig. 17 Dilator balloon kit connected to a manometer; the tracheostomy cannula is located just behind the balloon

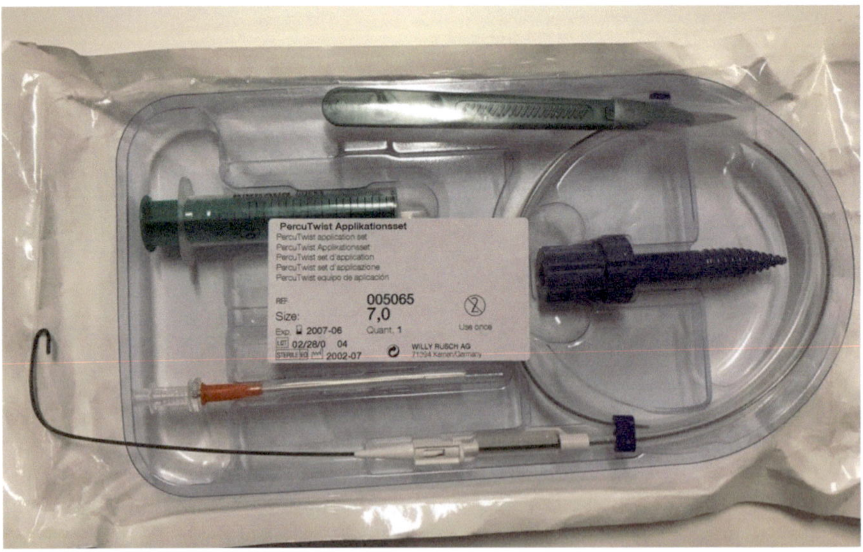

Fig. 18 PercuTwist® kit with a rotational screw dilator

reaches the size of the chosen cannula. Some studies have shown that this kit may cause more trauma than others and can lead more frequently to posterior tracheal wall injuries [17].

Role of Ultrasound in Percutaneous Dilatational Tracheostomy

One of the challenges of performing PDT is to define the right place to make the puncture, in order to make the tracheostomy between the second and the fourth tracheal rings. Due to edema and/or subcutaneous emphysema in ICU patients, palpation of landmarks for the puncture can be difficult. An abnormal physical examination such as the presence of a goiter, a short neck, tracheal deviation, or obesity can also make palpation of the anatomical features difficult or even impossible.

To perform PDT, therefore, it is necessary to use ultrasound equipment with a high-frequency linear transducer (10–14 MHz), which allows an evaluation from the superficial structures to 5 cm deeper [18].

Cartilage appears hypoechoic (dark) on ultrasound. The anterior border of the airway creates a hyperechoic (white) line, due to the acoustic impedance difference between the soft tissue and the air, which produces an intense wave reflection (Figs. 19 and 20). The posterior tracheal wall cannot be evaluated because the air inside the tracheal lumen does not allow the return of the ultrasound wave. The use of the Doppler function can also determine if there is any vessel in the path.

The transducer is initially applied in the transversal orientation to locate the airway and to identify possible risks and difficulties (Figs. 21 and 22). Then, over the midline of the trachea, the transducer is turned to the longitudinal position, with the directional indicator oriented toward the patient's head. The thyroid isthmus is identified to avoid puncturing it, and the tracheal rings from the cricoid are counted (Fig. 19). At that moment, the endotracheal tube is searched for, which is shown as a parallel hyperechoic line (Fig. 20), and it is pulled so that the tube stays cephalad to the puncture site.

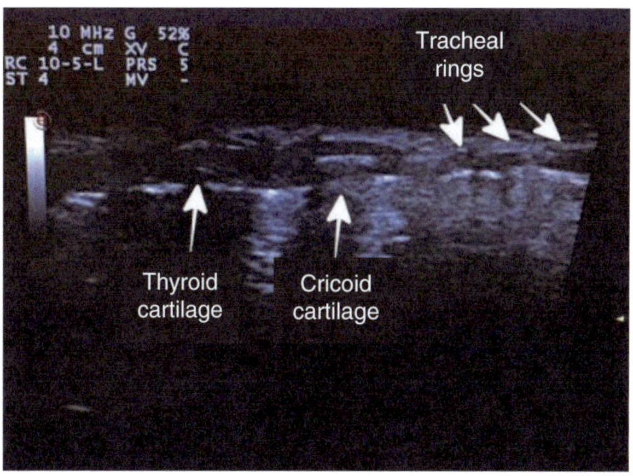

Fig. 19 Longitudinal ultrasound image. The thyroid [*Tireoide*], cricoid [*Cricoide*] and tracheal rings [*Anéis traqueais*] are shown as hypoechoic (*dark*) structures. The air–mucosal interface produces the hyperechoic (*white*) line

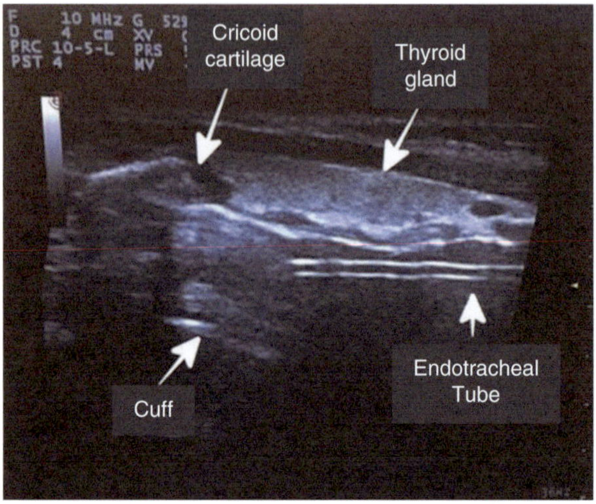

Fig. 20 Longitudinal view. The double parallel hyperechoic line corresponds to the anterior wall of the endotracheal tube (*Tubo*). In this case, for better visualization of the tube, the cuff was inflated with distilled water. *Cricoide* cricoid, *Glandula Tireoide* thyroid

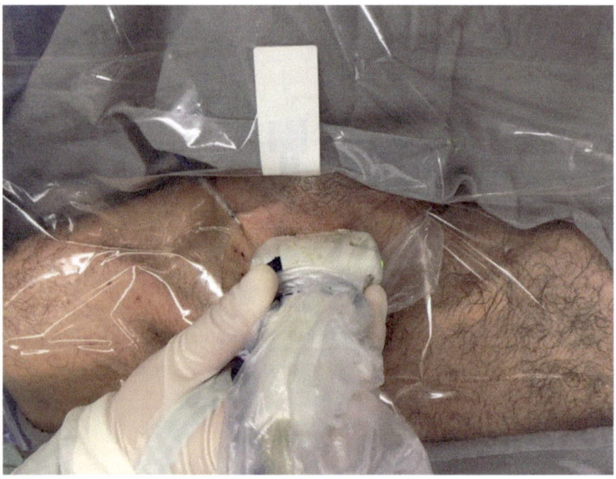

Fig. 21 Use of ultrasound to identify cervical structures

The transducer is turned back to the transversal position, just next to the needle, to guide the puncture on the midline of the trachea, which is shown by an acoustic shadow. The needle must be inserted perpendicularly to the skin and, after that, slightly turned caudally so that the guide wire can be introduced correctly (Fig. 23).

After introduction of the guide wire, the technique specified for the available PDT kit is followed.

Ultrasound evaluation for performing PDT allows:

- Identification of the thyroid isthmus, avoiding its puncture and consequent bleeding [19]
- Identification of vascular structures, anatomical alteration, tracheal deviation

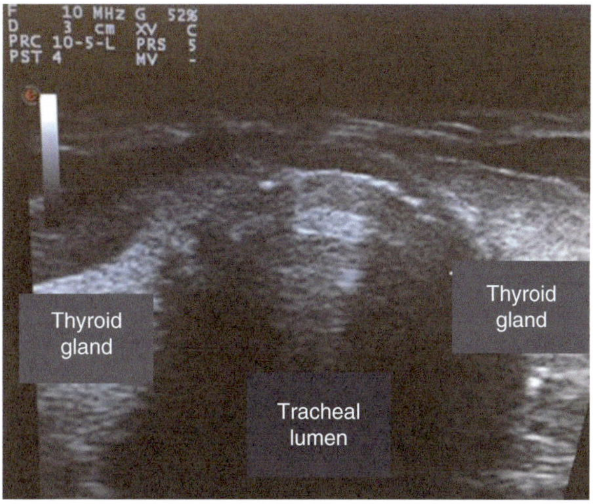

Fig. 22 Ultrasound transverse view to identify cervical structures and the depth of the tracheal lumen (*Luz Traqueal*) from the skin, and to measure the tracheal diameter for the tube selection. *Tireoide* thyroid

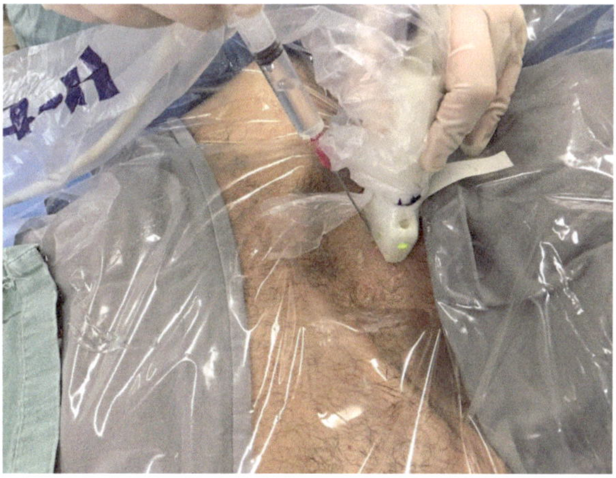

Fig. 23 Tracheal puncture on the midline

- Tracheal lumen measurement for better tube selection
- Positioning of the puncture on the midline between the tracheal rings

This way, the site of the puncture previously determined by the physical examination using palpation landmarks has changed 20–24% after the use of ultrasound, according to some reports [20–22].

Studies comparing bronchoscopy-guided and ultrasound-guided PDT have not shown statistically significant differences between these techniques in terms of mortality, number of punctures, bleeding, hypoxemia, and technical difficulty [23]. However, the learning curve for the ultrasound-guided technique is steeper than that for the bronchoscopy-guided technique. It is estimated that performance of 50 ultrasound-guided PDTs are required to achieve expertise in the procedure, versus only 20 for bronchoscopy-guided PDT [24].

Tracheostomy Complications and Their Care

Conventional surgical tracheostomy and PDT are considered to be low-complexity and easy procedures, frequently performed in mechanically ventilated patients admitted to ICUs. However, complication rates between 5% and 40% are reported in the literature, and when these procedures are performed in emergency situations, critically ill patients, or small children, the complication rates are 2–5 times higher. Although tracheostomy is considered easy and safe to perform, fatal events can occur, with a mortality rate of almost 2% [25, 26].

In emergency situations when cricothyroidotomy or oral intubation are not possible (Goldenberg et al. [26] retrospectively analyzed 1130 patients, where this occurred in 0.26%), performance of a tracheostomy can be challenging, with immediate and early complication rates of 12.2%, as reported by Costa et al. [27].

In our practice, in addition to emergency situations, cases such as low tracheal stenosis are generally associated with major technical difficulties in accessing the trachea—also requiring consideration of the conditions of tension and stress to which the surgical team is submitted. Carrying out the procedure under local anesthesia—sometimes in a situation where it is impossible for the patient to lie in a supine position with neck extension, along with acute respiratory failure and hypoxia—makes the procedure more difficult. Therefore, in this situation, a well-trained and experienced team may be important to reduce the risk of complications, especially fatal ones.

Tracheostomy complications can be classified according to the severity. "Minor" complications include bleeding with no hemodynamic instability; smaller cartilage lesions; mucosal, skin, and soft tissue damage; pneumothorax or small pneumomediastinum without the need for treatment; intraoperative cardiac rhythm disorders; postoperative hemorrhage arrestable by tamponade or fast surgical revision; subcutaneous emphysema; obstruction/failure or dislocation of the cannula without hypoxia; local wound infection requiring systemic antibiotics and/or diagnosed as an infected stoma; tracheitis; extended granulations; small atelectasis; and other non-life-threatening complications.

"Major" complications include bleeding with hemodynamic instability treated only with surgical site exploration and/or causing a significant fall in hemoglobin; cartilage damage discovered postoperatively; perforation or fissure of the posterior tracheal wall; bilateral recurrent laryngeal nerve injury; pneumothorax or pneumomediastinum requiring surgical drainage; aspiration of blood with extensive atelectasis or decreased oxygen saturation levels; tracheoaortal fissure; respiratory and/or cardiac arrest; and mediastinitis. In the immediate postoperative period, obstruction/failure and/or dislocation of the cannula with loss of airway control are serious problems and relatively common. In the late postoperative period, laryngeal and/or tracheal stenosis are severe complications to be resolved.

In recent years, routine use of low-pressure tracheostomy tubes has minimized this adverse effect.

Another classification is related to the timing of occurrence: "immediate complications" occurring during the surgical procedure until its end (intraoperative); "intermediate complications" (early postoperative) occurring until the first postoperative week; and "late complications." "Immediate complications" such as significant bleeding during tracheostomy are unusual, being more frequent when the procedure is performed in an emergency situation, with an incidence of up to 4%; the vascular structures most commonly involved are the anterior jugular veins, the vessels to the thyroid isthmus, and vascular variants such as the thyroid ima artery. Incorrect positioning of the tracheostomy tube or electrocautery-induced intraoperative burns to tracheal and adjacent structures are other possible complications; the latter is usually related to an incorrect surgical technique. For instance, esophageal lesions may occur during careless opening of the trachea, just as a dissection that deviates from the midline can lead to lesions of the recurrent laryngeal nerve and the cupola of the lung, especially in children. Moreover, fracture of the cricoid cartilage may occur when the tracheostomy is performed in a very high position [26] between the cricoid and the first tracheal ring.

In early complications a hemorrhage may also occur later after the intraoperative time, specially if the tracheostomy has been performed in patients with low blood pressure or increase of venous pressure (coughing or vomiting) may cause subsequent bleeding. Nevertheless, most cases can be treated with a compressive dressing, with a small percentage of patients (0.61% in the series reported by Goldenberg et al. [26]) requiring surgical exploration for hemostasis. Severe infections associated with tracheostomy—such as necrotizing fasciitis, mediastinitis, and clavicular osteomyelitis—are rare but require immediate and aggressive treatment. Transient peristomal tracheitis and cellulitis may also occur and cause mucosal damage, which would increase the likelihood of subglottic stenosis, thus reinforcing the need for adequate local wound care. However, Goldenberg et al. [26] suggest that this occurrence is more related to tracheal damage previously caused by prolonged intubation than damage caused by the tracheostomy itself. Pneumonia and pulmonary abscess after tracheostomy are related to aspiration of infected secretions.

Additionally, among early complications, pneumomediastinum, pneumothorax, and subcutaneous emphysema may occur due to excessive dissection during the surgical procedure with tracheal or pleural lesion, or to blockage of the tracheostomy tube by a blood clot, displacement of the tube, the cannula tip touching the posterior wall of the trachea, or a mucus plug or granulation tissue in a later period. Elevated endotracheal pressure in assisted ventilation is another cause of air dissection along the pretracheal fascia. In adults the incidence of pneumothorax is 0–4% and the incidence of subcutaneous emphysema is 0–9%, but in children the incidence of pneumothorax associated with tracheostomy is higher (10–17%) and it is an important cause of death. In these conditions, tight closure of the surgical wound around the tracheostomy tube should be avoided.

Displacement of the tracheostomy tube out of the airway site has an incidence of 0–7% and can be a fatal event, and factors such as short length of the tube, neck thickness (obesity), tracheostomy position (the level at which it was performed), technique (attachment of the tracheostomy edges to the skin or not), and the tracheostomy tube fixation method may contribute to its occurrence [26].

In "late complications" bleeding may occur; however, this may be due to excessive tracheostomy tube traction on granulation tissue or injury of important blood vessels such as the brachiocephalic artery or, more rarely, an anomalous carotid artery. The incidence of tracheobrachiocephalic artery fistula is 0.4–0.6%, and sudden massive bleeding can occur 3 days to 3 weeks after the occurrence of "sentinel bleeding," with a high mortality rate (80–90%). The main cause of this complication is excessive inflation of the tube cuff for a prolonged period of time and consequent necrosis and erosion of the tracheal cartilage and vessel wall, or compression and necrosis of the tracheal wall induced by the tip of the tracheostomy tube at the level of the brachiocephalic artery, which may occur due to the tracheostomy being performed too low (below the third tracheal ring) or by a high position of the artery, which is commonly observed in elderly patients.

Another late complication is tracheoesophageal fistula, which is rare and occurs due to injury to the posterior wall of the trachea during the tracheostomy procedure, or as a consequence of an overinflated and malpositioned tracheostomy tube cuff, promoting excessive pressure on the posterior wall of the trachea; this, associated with the nasogastric tube in the esophagus, may cause tissue ischemia and necrosis and consequent tracheal and esophagus wall erosion. The incidence of tracheoesophageal fistula is 0.01–1%; however, significant related mortality rate of 70–80% [26] is reported.

Subglottic and tracheal stenosis are severe complications associated with previous endotracheal intubation, high tracheostomy or cricothyroidotomy, and trauma to the airway. Children and head trauma patients are at increased risk for stenosis. The mechanism for this damage is excessive insufflation of the tube cuff associated with long-term tracheal intubation, which promotes ischemia and ulceration of the mucosa, exposing the tracheal cartilage. Stenosis at the level of the stoma may be caused by excessive tube traction or a large stoma, and occurred in 1.86% in the study by Goldenberg et al. [26]; however, these instances were correlated with prolonged tracheal intubation (all patients with stenosis were intubated more than 12 days before the procedure).

Tracheocutaneous fistula is another late complication, caused by epithelialization of the stomal tract in patient with long-term use of a tracheostomy tube, and occurs in 0.53% of patients [26]. It may lead to persistent tracheal secretion with consequent irritation of adjacent skin, disturbances in phonation, and frequent infections.

With regard to improvement and wide performance of the PDT technique, the systematic review and risk factor analysis published by Simon et al. [11] selected 45 publications that described 65 events related to the procedure (including cases from their own institution), analyzing a total of 71 cases, with an incidence of lethal complications of 0.17%. Among the main complications related to death, bleeding and airway complications were the most important, accounting for 38% and 29.6%, respectively. Most bleeding (75%) occurred 1–30 days after tracheostomy (at a mean of 5 days); 59.3% of cases were related to arterial bleeding and, of these, almost 70% originated from a tracheobrachiocephalic artery fistula (tracheoinnominate artery fistula). The potential risk factors for bleeding and subsequent death were nonuse of bronchoscopic guidance during the procedure, a low tracheostomy site, coagulopathy, previous surgery on the neck, previous radiotherapy, obesity, anatomical abnormality, paratracheal misplacement of the tracheostomy tube, a malpositioned tube tip, high cuff pressure, and excessive movement of the neck associated with prolonged intubation.

As for airway complications related to fatal events, tracheal tube displacement (52.4%), airway loss during the procedure (19%), and paratracheal misplacement of the tube (14.3%) were the most common, and the risk factors associated with them were nonuse of bronchoscopy, inexperience of the surgical team in the percutaneous technique, patient obesity, patients with a difficult airway, not stitching the tracheal tube, tracheostomy tube replacement in the early postoperative period, and postoperative care by an inexperienced team.

Other fatal complications were described in the study as tracheal perforation (15.5%), pneumothorax (5.6%), severe bronchospasm (4.4%), cardiac arrest and arrhythmia during the procedure related to clinical cardiac comorbidities (4.4%), and sepsis secondary to mediastinitis (1.5%).

Thus, based on their study, Simon et al. [11] suggested measures to improve the safety of PDT, always considering contraindications for the procedure (anatomic distortion of the neck, the presence of a difficult airway, severe acute respiratory distress syndrome, nontreated coagulopathy, and the presence of an unstable cervical spine), depending on the skill and experience of the surgical team in the percutaneous technique; use of bronchoscopy to guide the entire procedure; avoidance of performing low tracheostomy (below the third tracheal ring); not allowing guide wire folds (thereby avoiding the possibility of perforation of the tracheal wall and adjacent structures, especially the esophagus); and routine use of outer flange tracheal tube sutures to the skin.

In conclusion, tracheostomy is a procedure with a low incidence of complications, especially when performed electively; however, fatal events can occur, above all related to lesions of large vessels and obstructions of the airway.

Therefore, measures that may reduce the occurrence of severe and fatal complications [23, 26] are institution of a surgical training program for improvement of the technique to ensure careful dissection on the midline and performance of the tracheostomy or puncture at the appropriate level (ideally between the first and second or second and third tracheal rings), routine use of bronchoscopy or ultrasound in percutaneous tracheostomy, fixation of the tracheostomy tube outer flange with sutures, and adequate postoperative tracheostomy care by nursing staff who are well trained in manipulation of the tracheostomy tube.

Hands-On Percutaneous Dilatational Tracheostomy Training Program Course

Based on technical and practical experience in teaching residents in head and neck and general surgery, the Head and Neck Service of Santa Casa de São Paulo has developed a percutaneous tracheostomy training program.

This program has been transformed into a training course, with emphasis on hands-on management of bronchoscopy-guided and ultrasound-guided percutaneous tracheostomy. The course started in 2015 and is given in our Experimental Surgery Laboratory Center, with approval from the Ethics Committee on Experimental Animals.

This 9-hour course basically consists of expositive and participatory classes, in which the theoretical content represents 40%, with emphasis on practice in percutaneous tracheostomy in experimental and animal training (porcine) models.

The theoretical part of the course presents the historical evolution of the tracheostomy technique, from its creation as the conventional procedure to the development of the percutaneous puncture and dilation system by Ciaglia, with all variants of percutaneous kits available, and also the indications, contraindications, and complications. Also, there is a video session for step-by-step operation of percutaneous tracheostomy in an intensive care unit environment, performed in the surgeon's day practice.

In the hands-on scenario, there are six simulated workstations available: four with full endoscopic facilities, one with an experimental model device, and one with an ultrasound guidance facility. A maximum of two participants and a devoted tutor are allocated to each workstation. Twelve participants can attend the course.

In the 4-hour training workstation sessions, the student performs the PDT technique, divided into the sequence shown in Figs. 24, 25, 26, and 27:

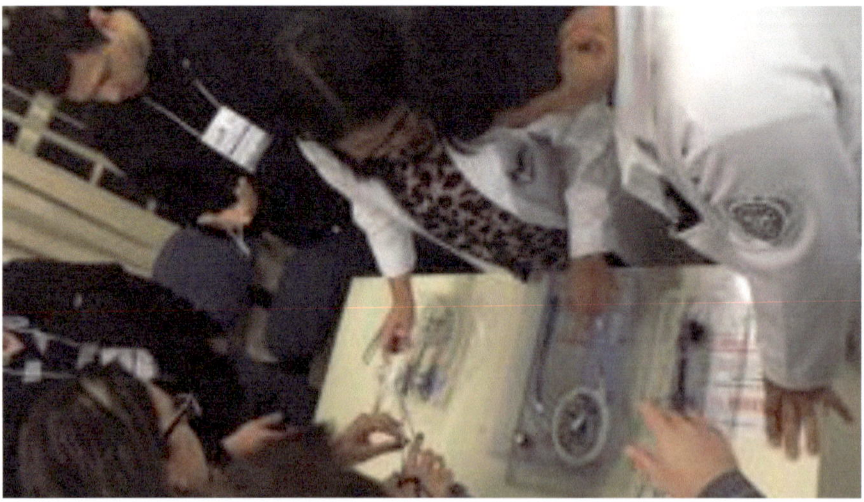

Fig. 24 Presentation of available percutaneous tracheostomy kits

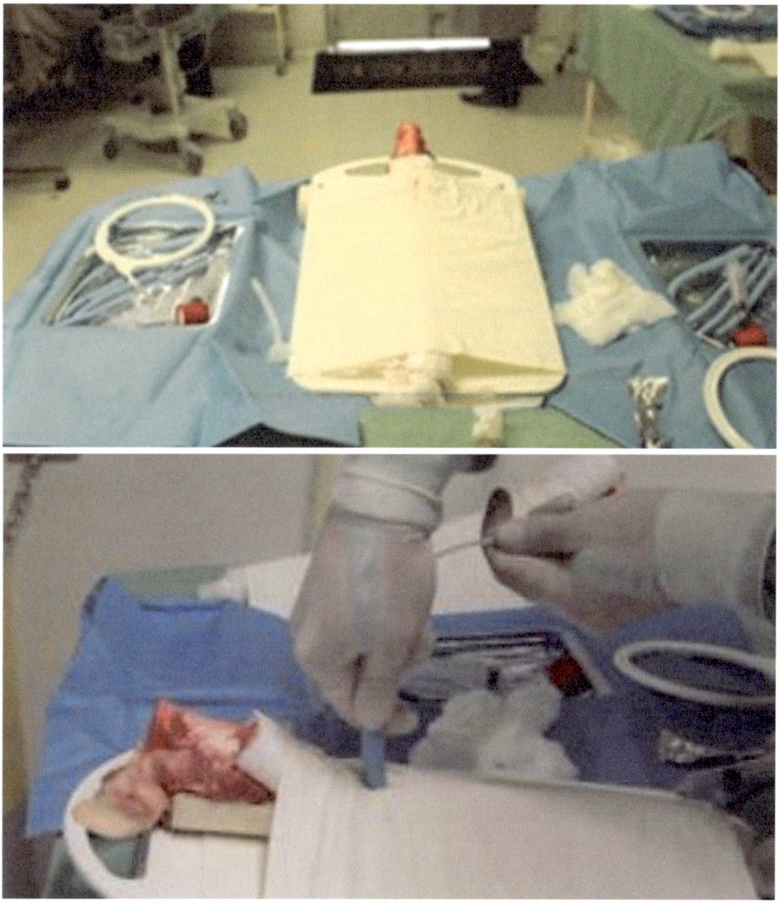

Fig. 25 Operation on the experimental model

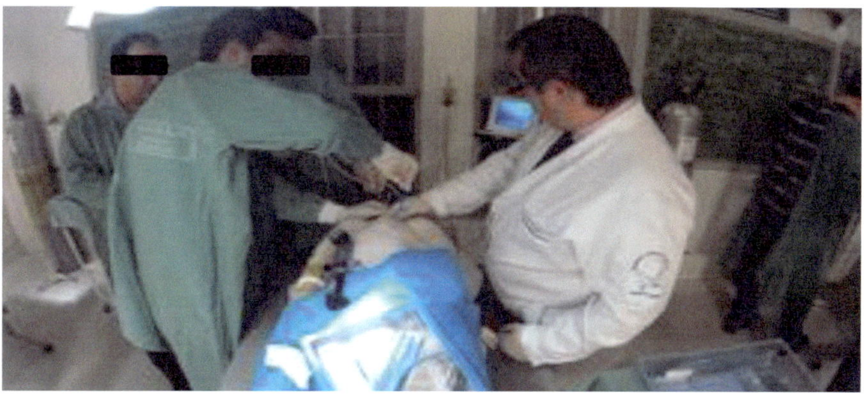

Fig. 26 Workstation training on the animal model (porcine) with endoscopy guidance

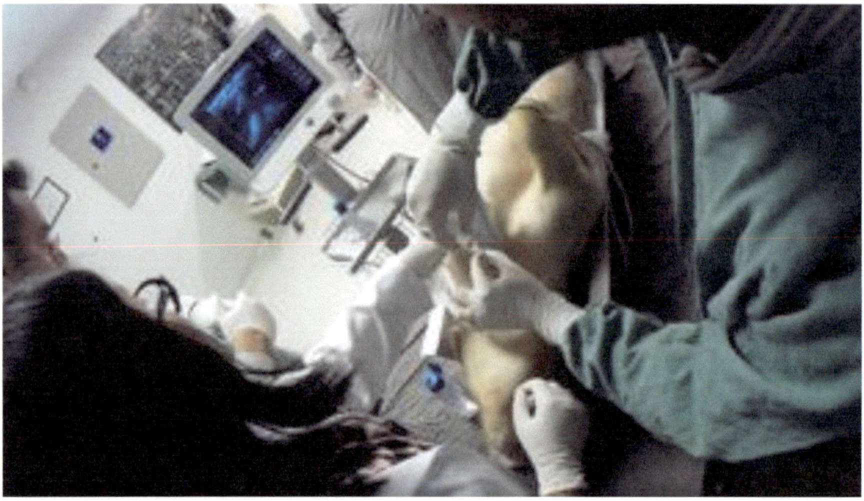

Fig. 27 Ultrasound-guided operation performed on the porcine model

This course has already qualified several surgeons in the practice of the PDT technique.

References

1. Griffiths J, Barber VS, Morgan L, Young JD. Systematic review and meta-analysis of studies of the timing of tracheostomy in adult patients undergoing artificial ventilation. BMJ. 2005;330:1243.
2. Szakmany T, Russell P, Wilkes AR, Hall JE. Effect of early tracheostomy on resource utilization and clinical outcomes in critically ill patients: meta-analysis of randomized controlled trials. Br J Anaesth. 2015;114:396–405.
3. Waydhas C. Intrahospital transport of critically ill patients. Crit Care. 1999;3:R83–9.
4. Dennis BM, Eckert MJ, Gunter OL, Morris JA, May AK. Safety of bedside percutaneous tracheostomy in the critically ill: evaluation of more than 3,000 procedures. J Am Coll Surg. 2013;216:858–65. discussion 865
5. Higgins KM, Punthakee X. Meta-analysis comparison of open versus percutaneous tracheostomy. Laryngoscope. 2007;117:447–54.
6. Durbin CG. Tracheostomy: why, when, and how. Respir Care. 2010;55:1056–68.
7. Perfeito JA, Mata CA, Forte V, Carnaghi M, Tamura N, Leão LE. Tracheostomy in the ICU: is it worthwhile? J Bras Pneumol. 2007;33:687–90.
8. Al-Ansari MA, Hijazi MH. Clinical review: percutaneous dilatational tracheostomy. Crit Care. 2006;10:202.
9. Putensen C, Theuerkauf N, Guenther U, Vargas M, Pelosi P. Percutaneous and surgical tracheostomy in critically ill adult patients: a meta-analysis. Crit Care. 2014;18:544.
10. McCague A, Aljanabi H, Wong DT. Safety analysis of percutaneous dilational tracheostomies with bronchoscopy in the obese patient. Laryngoscope. 2012;122:1031–4.
11. Simon M, Metschke M, Braune SA, Püschel K, Kluge S. Death after percutaneous dilatational tracheostomy: a systematic review and analysis of risk factors. Crit Care. 2013;17:R258.
12. Massick DD, Yao S, Powell DM, et al. Bedside tracheostomy in the intensive care unit: a prospective randomized trial comparing open surgical tracheostomy with endoscopically guided percutaneous dilational tracheotomy. Laryngoscope. 2001;111:494–500.

13. Ciaglia P, Firsching R, Syniec C. Elective percutaneous dilatational tracheostomy. A new simple bedside procedure; preliminary report. Chest. 1985;87:715–9.
14. Ambesh SP, Pandey CK, Srivastava S, Agarwal A, Singh DK. Percutaneous tracheostomy with single dilatation technique: a prospective, randomized comparison of Ciaglia blue rhino versus Griggs' guidewire dilating forceps. Anesth Analg. 2002;95:1739–45, table of contents
15. Griggs WM, Worthley LI, Gilligan JE, Thomas PD, Myburg JA. A simple percutaneous tracheostomy technique. Surg Gynecol Obstet. 1990;170:543–5.
16. Zgoda MA, Berger R. Balloon-facilitated percutaneous dilational tracheostomy tube placement: preliminary report of a novel technique. Chest. 2005;128:3688–90.
17. Byhahn C, Westphal K, Meininger D, Gürke B, Kessler P, Lischke V. Single-dilator percutaneous tracheostomy: a comparison of PercuTwist and Ciaglia Blue Rhino techniques. Intensive Care Med. 2002;28:1262–6.
18. Kristensen MS, Teoh WH, Graumann O, Laursen CB. Ultrasonography for clinical decision-making and intervention in airway management: from the mouth to the lungs and pleurae. Insights Imaging. 2014;5:253–79.
19. Bonde J, Nørgaard N, Antonsen K, Faber T. Implementation of percutaneous dilation tracheotomy—value of preincisional ultrasonic examination. Acta Anaesthesiol Scand. 1999;43:163–6.
20. Kollig E, Heydenreich U, Roetman B, Hopf F, Muhr G. Ultrasound and bronchoscopic controlled percutaneous tracheostomy on trauma ICU. Injury. 2000;31:663–8.
21. Rajajee V, Fletcher JJ, Rochlen LR, Jacobs TL. Real-time ultrasound-guided percutaneous dilatational tracheostomy: a feasibility study. Crit Care. 2011;15:R67.
22. Yavuz A, Yılmaz M, Göya C, Alimoglu E, Kabaalioglu A. Advantages of US in percutaneous dilatational tracheostomy: randomized controlled trial and review of the literature. Radiology. 2014;273:927–36.
23. Gobatto AL, Besen BA, Tierno PF, et al. Ultrasound-guided percutaneous dilational tracheostomy versus bronchoscopy-guided percutaneous dilational tracheostomy in critically ill patients (TRACHUS): a randomized noninferiority controlled trial. Intensive Care Med. 2016;42:342–51.
24. Petiot S, Guinot PG, Diouf M, Zogheib E, Dupont H. Learning curve for real-time ultrasound-guided percutaneous tracheostomy. Anaesth Crit Care Pain Med. 2016.
25. Gillespie MB, Eisele DW. Outcomes of emergency surgical airway procedures in a hospital-wide setting. Laryngoscope. 1999;109:1766–9.
26. Goldenberg D, Ari EG, Golz A, Danino J, Netzer A, Joachims HZ. Tracheotomy complications: a retrospective study of 1130 cases. Otolaryngol Head Neck Surg. 2000;123:495–500.
27. Costa L, Matos R, Júlio S, Vales F, Santos M. Urgent tracheostomy: four-year experience in a tertiary hospital. World J Emerg Med. 2016;7:227–30.

Conventional or Percutaneous Tracheostomy?

Lúcio Noleto, Thiago Pereira Diniz,
and Terence Pires de Farias

Introduction

The term *tracheostomy*, of Greek origin, defines an opening in the trachea that maintains communication with the exterior, usually by means of a cannula. It is one of the most performed procedures in critically ill patients, especially in intensive care units (ICUs). This procedure is one of the oldest in medicine, and is even described in medical books of antiquity [1].

Galen, a renowned Greek physician at the time, performed a tracheostomy for treatment of upper airway obstruction in the second century BC. The first successful tracheostomy, however, is credited to Antonio Brasalova in 1546, an Italian physician, in a patient with a laryngeal abscess [1].

A new technique, similar to percutaneous tracheostomy through blind tracheal cannulation, was started in 1955 by Shelden et al. but, due to some accidents—including fatal ones—this technique did not obtain good acceptance [2]. In 1969, Toye and Weinstein developed a guide and dilator in order to facilitate the passage

L. Noleto, M.D., Ph.D. (✉)
Department of Head and Neck Surgery, University of the State of Piaui, Piaui, Brazil
e-mail: lanoleto@yahoo.com.br

T.P. Diniz, M.D.
Department of General Surgery, University of the State of Piauí, Piauí, Brazil

T.P. de Farias, M.D., Ph.D., M.Sc., Researcher.
Department of Head and Neck Surgery, Brazilian National Cancer Institute—INCA,
Rio de Janeiro, RJ, Brazil

Department of Head and Neck Surgery, Pontifical Catholic University,
Rio de Janeiro, RJ, Brazil

T.P. de Farias (ed.), *Tracheostomy*, https://doi.org/10.1007/978-3-319-67867-2_7

of the cannula [2]. In 1985, Ciaglia et al. described a modification of the open tracheostomy and introduced the Seldinger principle for the percutaneous approach [3]. The first percutaneous tracheostomy system utilized multiple, sequentially larger dilators (Fig. 1). However, in 1999, Ciaglia modified the original procedure for the single progressive dilator method, known today as Blue Rhino (Cook Co., Bloomington, IN, USA) [3, 4]. Other methods of anterograde percutaneous tracheostomy were reported by Griggs (Figs. 2 and 3) in 1990 using rounded-tip forceps dilatation, by Frova and Quintel in 2002 using stomal dilatation with a single screw dilation device (PercuTwist), and by Zgoda and Berger in 2005 and Cianchi et al. in 2010 using a modification of the Blue Rhino device, which employed balloon dilatation [5–7].

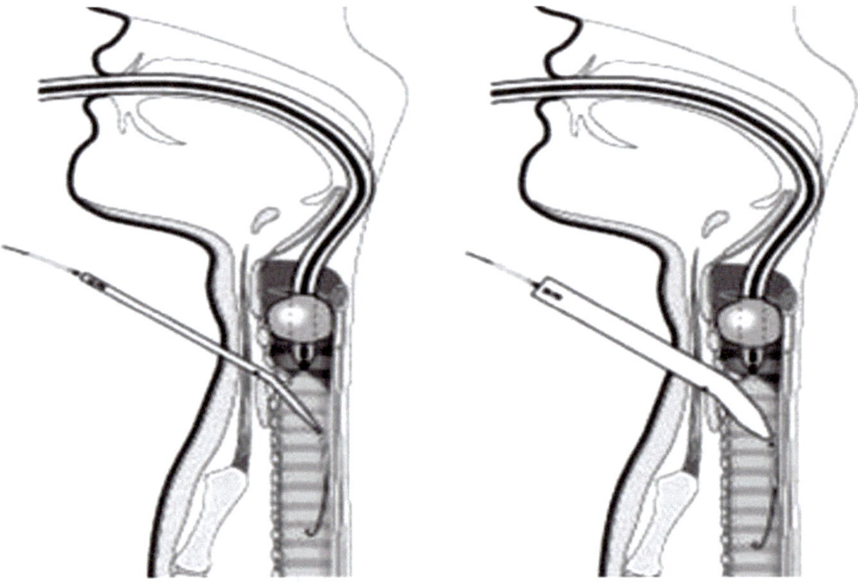

Fig. 1 Passage of progressive dilators through the guide wire

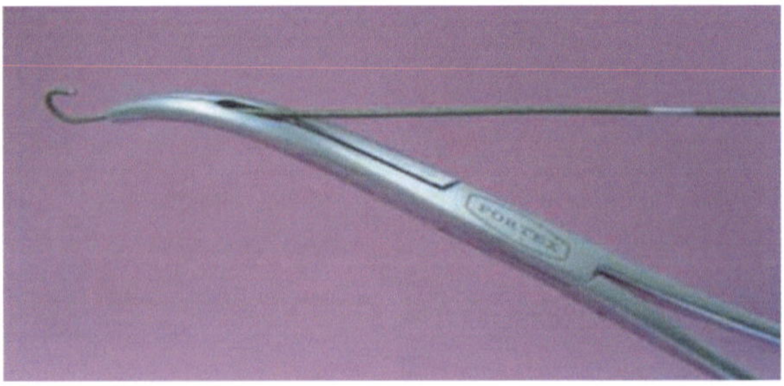

Fig. 2 Griggs forceps. At the end of the clamp there is a hole through which the thread will be inserted

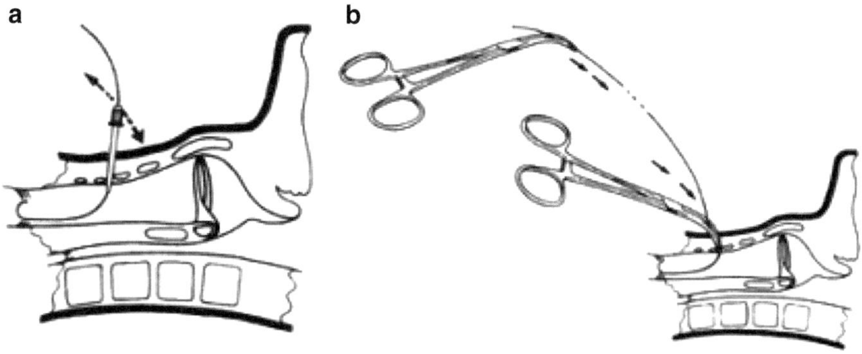

Fig. 3 Demonstration of guide wire passing through the Griggs clamp

Several trials have compared conventional (i.e., surgical) tracheostomy (CT) and percutaneous tracheostomy (PT), and which is the best method is discussed in the literature [8–10]. This chapter discusses general aspects of tracheostomies, such as indications, complications, descriptions of techniques, paralleling the conventional and percutaneous techniques.

Percutaneous Versus Conventional Tracheostomy: Indications and Contraindications

Tracheostomy is considered the airway of choice in patients requiring prolonged ventilatory support or airway protection, as well as facilitating respiratory dynamics and the weaning process of ventilatory support, when indicated [11]. There are basically two scenarios that culminate in the indication for a tracheostomy: elective tracheostomy and emergency tracheostomy. The first, in general, is a patient admitted to an ICU with a prolonged tracheal intubation time, while the second is indicated when there is a need to guarantee the airway in cases of acute respiratory failure due to tracheal obstruction.

Tracheostomy has several advantages over translaryngeal intubation, including better tolerability by the patient, less laryngeal irritation, facilitation of nursing care, increased communication capacity, better breathing, and reduction of dead space. Approximately 5–13% of patients using an orotracheal tube in ICUs will need to spend more than 21 days on mechanical ventilation (MV), i.e., prolonged MV. In these patients, the intensive care team has to make a decision about when to perform a tracheostomy. Currently, most intensivists agree that if a patient needs MV for more than 10–14 days, a tracheostomy is indicated and should be performed under optimal conditions, either in the ICU, in a hospital room, or in a surgical center [12–14]. What the advantages are of performing the procedure at the bedside or in a surgical environment has been a divergent theme and the object of discussion in several trials. Variables such as cost, complications, and other issues will be described next.

Nowadays, tracheostomy is a standard and elective procedure in critically ill patients, and its indications include relief of upper airway obstruction, prevention of upper and laryngeal airway injuries due to prolonged tracheal intubation, the need for easy and frequent access to the lower airway for aspiration and removal of secretions, a decreased level of patient consciousness as well as protective airway reflexes, and severe changes in respiratory physiology. However, prolonged respiratory failure requiring long-term MV is probably the most common indication. In emergency situations, the main indications are tracheal obstructions due to trauma in the postoperative period of cervical surgery where there is inadvertent bilateral recurrent laryngeal nerve damage by benign or malignant tumors, such as tumors that cause extrinsic obstruction of the upper airways and endoluminal tumors—for example, a laryngeal tumor. However, the indications, risks, benefits, timing, and technique of the conventional and percutaneous procedures remain controversial and depend on the clinical condition of the patient—in particular, the respiratory performance status [14].

Tracheostomy contraindications have changed over time. Some causes that were absolute contraindications to the percutaneous method—such as distortion of the anatomical references of the neck by a hematoma, tumor, or previous surgical scar; infection of soft parts of the neck; an obese or short neck making it difficult to identify anatomical repairs; and inability to extend the neck—have been increasingly considered only relative contraindications due to the increased experience of teams with the method [15]. Also, according to De Leyn et al. [15], the only absolute contraindications to PT are the presence of a skin infection at the puncture site and a large prior cervical surgery that completely obscures the cervical anatomy.

Percutaneous Versus Conventional Tracheostomy: Surgical Approach

The anatomical and technical concepts that guide the performance of CT must be respected in PT [16]. The sequence to be followed is practically the same in both techniques, with some differences in the materials and kits used.

(a) *Sedation, analgesia, and muscle blockade:* Tracheostomy is performed under general anesthesia or sedation, although it may be practiced under local anesthesia. If necessary, a muscle blocker may be used. It is important to be assisted by a physician in the ICU or an anesthesiologist in the operating room. In patients with high airway obstruction, for which endotracheal intubation is not feasible, the tracheostomy is performed with local anesthesia and minimal sedation.

(b) *Positioning of the patient:* There are similarities regarding the positioning of the patient. In both techniques, the patient should be positioned in the dorsal position with a cushion under the shoulders to extend the neck. This maneuver provides greater exposure of the trachea. It is worth noting that extension is not possible in cases of cervical spine fracture, cervical arthrosis, recent neck surgery, a short neck, kyphosis, sequelae of radiotherapy, or other alterations.

(c) *Incision and dissection by planes until the trachea is identified:* The incision in the skin can be transverse or longitudinal. The transverse incision is made about 2 cm (one to two fingers) above the sternal furcula, with extension between 2 and 3 cm; the aesthetic result is better. The vertical incision corresponds to the tracheal plane, initiated just below the cricoid cartilage extending approximately 2 cm in the caudal direction. In the conventional technique, in elective situations, transverse incisions are preferred, while percutaneous transection is generally performed longitudinally, with a smaller extension, as described below. In PT, a longitudinal incision of 1.5 cm in length and 1.5 cm below the cricoid cartilage is performed. The subcutaneous tissue and the superficial fascia are opened on the midline by divulsion with Kelly tweezers. The trachea is palpated and the area to be punctured is released by digital blunt dissection to avoid puncturing the isthmus of the thyroid. With the bronchoscope inserted through the orotracheal intubation cannula, it is retracted into the subglottic space. The trachea should be punctured on the midline between the second and third tracheal rings.

(d) *Guide wire passage, dilatation, and passage of the tracheal cannula:* The guide wire is then passed through the needle and directed distally. With the thread in position, the dilation of the path with the dilator begins. From this point, the PT technique will differ depending on the materials or set of dilators used. There are basically two techniques, using either the Blue Rhino set or the Portex set. In the Blue Rhino technique, the guide catheter should be placed on the guide wire to increase its gauge and improve the conduction of the dilator to the tracheal lumen. Thereafter, the trachea is dilated with a single dilator. As soon as the dilation is completed, a tracheostomy cannula placed over a dilator is introduced by the path into the trachea. When the bronchoscopist confirms that the cannula is well positioned, the dilator with the guide catheter and guide wire are withdrawn, the cannula cuff is inflated, and the extension of the respirator is connected to the tracheostomy cannula to ventilate the patient. The incision can be closed with a surgical stitch and the cannula is attached to the neck. In the Portex technique (also called the Griggs technique), the dilatation of the trachea is performed with a metal clamp that has a groove between its rods, such that the clamp slides around the guide wire. Once in the tracheal lumen, the surgeon opens the forceps by dilating the bronchial-guided path. Thereafter, a tracheostomy cannula, which forms part of the kit—the obturator of which is pierced, allowing passage of the guide wire—is introduced into the tracheal lumen. The bronchoscopist performs aspiration of secretions through the tracheostomy cannula and checks for proximal hemostasis through laryngoscopy using the orotracheal intubation cannula as a guide for the fiberoptic bronchoscope, as shown in Figs. 5 and 6.

Percutaneous Versus Conventional Tracheostomy: Complications and Other Issues

As early as 1992, a prospective study on PT concluded that it was a risky procedure with potential for potentially serious complications—namely, severe hemorrhage, a false tracheostomy tube pathway, and death [17]. Since then, the number of studies published in this area has been increasing every year.

Massick et al. [18] demonstrated the existence of an important learning curve in the development of PT, especially in the first 20 patients, with the majority of complications occurring during initial contact with the technique. The complications of PT are classically divided into early and late complications, and some result from the injury of anatomical structures that are in the vicinity of the tracheostomy site. Early complications include hemorrhage, infection, pneumothorax, pneumomediastinum, subcutaneous emphysema, paratracheal insertion of the tracheostomy tube, laceration of the posterolateral wall of the trachea, technical failures, and perioperative hypoxia due to tube obstruction or accidental decannulation [19].

Late complications include development of granulation tissue with consequent tracheal stenosis, difficulty in decannulation, obstruction of the upper airway with respiratory insufficiency after decannulation, tracheoesophageal fistula, tracheomalacia, tracheal–innominate artery fistula, pneumonia, and aspiration [20, 21]. Bleeding is probably the most common perioperative complication, most of which is insignificant due to minimal tissue disruption, the tamponade effect of the tracheostomy tube, and the vasoconstrictive effect of adrenaline when used as a local anesthetic [22, 23].

Among late complications, tracheal stenosis is the most feared and, at the same time, the most difficult to quantify because many patients undergoing PT are severely ill and may die or be discharged before being decannulated. Although there is no ideal method of postoperative evaluation to determine the incidence of late complications after PT, recent studies have used a number of methods, including questionnaires, radiography and tracheal tomography, magnetic resonance imaging, laryngotracheoscopy, and pulmonary function tests [24].

A trial using laryngotracheoscopy and high-resolution computed tomography to assess the incidence of tracheal stenosis in 48 patients undergoing PT revealed a global incidence of tracheal stenosis of 31%, with only 20% of these patients being symptomatic, with a symptomatic tracheal stenosis index of 6%. For comparison with the conventional technique, Anthony Delaney et al. performed a meta-analysis in 2006, surveying 17 studies comparing PT and CT in critically ill patients in the ICU, and concluded that there was in fact a greater tendency, although not significant, toward tracheal stenosis in patients undergoing CT [25].

There are some parameters on which there is agreement in the literature, favoring the percutaneous or surgical technique, as well as indifferent results. It is also worth noting that the indication for the best method should take into account the expertise and experience of the team and the availability of appropriate materials for the procedure.

Time Required to Perform the Procedure

Regarding the procedure time, most trials show a shorter percutaneous execution time, although in some cases there may be technical difficulties, such as difficulty in performing the tracheal puncture, failure of the thread progression guide, and difficulty in introducing the cannula and positioning the puncture centrally and in an adequate tracheal space. In these cases, it seems obvious that there is an increase in the procedure time, thus indicating an advantage of conventional surgery [26].

In a large, prospective, randomized trial, Siamak Yaghoobi and colleagues compared the results of PT and CT in ICU patients. After 4 years of data collection and application of exclusion criteria, 40 patients were allocated to each group. The procedure times—defined by the time interval from the first puncture of the trachea to the end of successful insertion of the tracheostomy tube and connection to the ventilator—were 10.01 ± 2.42 min in the PT group and 15.08 ± 3.16 min in the CT group.

Coagulation Pitfalls

The first measure to be taken before the tracheostomy, as in any other surgical procedure, is to correct coagulopathies. Usually these patients undergo tracheostomy in the operating room. Auzinger et al. published an important prospective study in 60 patients with severe coagulopathy and liver disease, who underwent the percutaneous technique in the ICU, and only one patient experienced significant bleeding, which ceased after the insertion of the cannula. The experience of the team and the correction of blood dyscrasias are determinants of success. It must be emphasized that all of the materials available in the surgical center should be available in the ICU to perform the procedure—for example, electrocautery and surgical wires, which are essential for regular hemostasis [23].

McCormick and Manara [27], in their case report article, showed that although massive hemorrhage during PT occurs only rarely, it can be fatal. One patient died during the procedure due to uncontrollable hemorrhage of the innominate vein. This patient had a prior history of right breast carcinoma treated with mastectomy and radiotherapy, which resulted in extensive fibrosis of the tissues adjacent to the left innominate vein, distorting the normal anatomy. Two other patients did not survive late hemorrhagic complications, which were caused by erosion of the aorta through the tracheostomy tube in one case and were caused by erosion of the innominate vein in the other case. In the postmortem evaluation of both patients, it was pointed out that the unexpectedly low location of the tracheal stoma may have contributed to the event. So, what is the lower limit for performing the puncture or incision? Ideally, it should never be performed below the fourth tracheal ring [28].

Urgent Tracheostomy

Initially considered an absolute contraindication to the percutaneous method, urgent tracheostomy is currently advocated for its safety in obtaining an emergency airway. According to Klein et al., this procedure can be performed in emergency situations, provided it is done by an experienced team. Still speaking of critical patients, individuals with severe respiratory insufficiency and a very unfavorable ventilatory status (positive end-expiratory pressure (PEEP) >10 mmHg and fraction of inspired oxygen (FiO_2) <70%) traditionally undergo the conventional technique. This fact is explained by the possible hypoxemia that may occur during manipulation with the bronchoscope, in which the orotracheal tube is drawn. There has been a report of PT without major problems under these conditions [29].

Morbid Obesity

Patients with morbid obesity undergoing PT present a 2.7-fold higher risk of perioperative complications and a 4.9-fold risk of severe morbidities. For these patients, blunt dissection of the pretracheal tissues is recommended, allowing tracheal palpation. Once PT is chosen, it is important that the neck is extended so that there is palpation of a repair point [30].

Bulky Thyroid Goiter

The presence of a thyroid goiter may make it difficult to palpate and identify cervical structures, but it is not a contraindication to the procedure, especially via the percutaneous method, where there is a greater controversy. Proper cervical extension, puncture at the level of the first tracheal ring, or cervical ultrasonography (USG) aid make PT possible. Even when a transthyroid procedure is performed, dissection is minimal and bleeding is usually self-limited [31].

Cervical Immobility

As a rule, inability to perform cervical hyperextension is considered a contraindication to performance of PT. In the postoperative period of arthrodesis of the cervical spine, it is considered safe to perform the procedure from the seventh postoperative day [10, 11]. In a clinical review, Al-Ansari MA and Hijazi MH [9] reported a 96% success rate and a 7.1% complication rate in patients who did not have the possibility of adequate cervical extension.

Previous Tracheostomy or Cervical Scar

Historically, the presence of a previous tracheostomy has been a relative contraindication to performance of PT. On the other hand, the presence of a previous scar, in a certain way, directs the puncture and possibly there are fewer pretracheal tissues, which would facilitate the procedure. Meyer et al. [32] reported a case series of 14 patients with previous tracheostomy, where the method was successfully performed. Using either technique, one can always find local fibrosis and difficulty opening the tracheal rings, which makes the technique difficult [32].

Costs and Environment for the Procedure

When performed in a hospital room, as long as there is all of the necessary equipment, PT a viable procedure when carried out by a trained surgical team, besides presenting the lowest cost among the alternatives for performing this surgery [14]. When tracheostomy is performed in the operating room, the costs increase significantly due to the time of occupation of the room and the need for a team of professionals to transport the patient, in addition to the presence of the anesthesiologist and any drugs used. Those who defend it cite the advantage of having everything available for cases in which there are operative complications. Those that oppose it, in addition to citing the cost, draw attention to the risk of transporting a critical patient from one sector to another within the hospital [33]. PT appears to be an alternative, facilitating a low-risk bedside procedure with results similar to those obtained with the traditional technique. A trial conducted by Cantais, Kaiser, Le-Goff, and Palmier [41] also demonstrated that PT is a safe procedure to perform at the bedside. In general it seems to be a less traumatic procedure and the cutaneous incision required is less than in the surgical procedure. In addition, the former requires tracheal opening by dilation of the soft tissue space between the tracheal rings rather than a direct cut of a cartilaginous ring. Therefore, a lower incidence of tracheal stenosis at the stoma site would be expected. Several studies have shown significant cost savings in Western countries; however, usually the main limitation is still the high cost of the commercial set, especially in developing countries.

Bacchetta et al. studied 86 patients undergoing tracheostomy after cardiac surgery. The authors concluded that there was no difference in clinical outcomes or complications, but there was a significant reduction in the costs for patients undergoing PT. Although this was a remarkable trial, with socioeconomic reality diverging among different nations, these data should be considered until individualized studies are performed. The percutaneous technique requires the availability of a greater quantity of materials and kits suitable for such a procedure—a fact not observed with the conventional technique, which depends basically on availability of the cannula. Regarding the costs of the procedure, the average cost of the procedure when performed in the ICU is US$1569, compared with US$3172 when performed in the operating room.

Cervical Bronchoscopy and Ultrasonography

Another divergent point in the literature is performance of tracheostomy with bronchoscopy and cervical USG. In an attempt to reduce the incidence of complications, it is possible to use bronchoscopy and cervical USG as ancillary methods in PT. While bronchoscopy (Figs. 4 and 5) may, for example, ensure that the tracheal puncture is made on the midline and at the desired level to help control all steps of the procedure [2], USG allows optimal selection of the intercartilaginous space for insertion of the tracheostomy tube and may also help to define the pre and paratracheal anatomy in order to avoid lesion of pretracheal vascular structures [34]. These

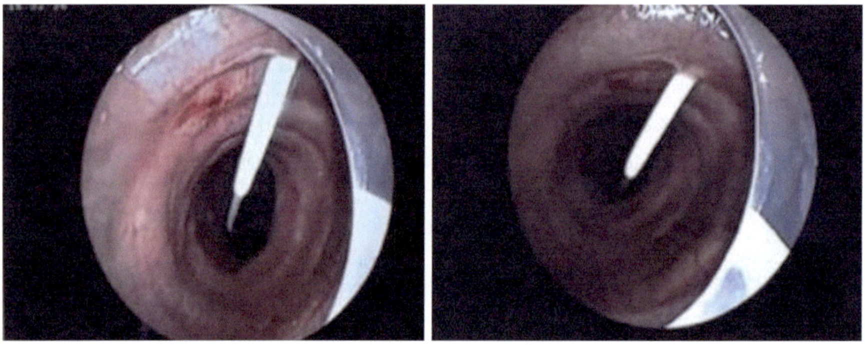

Fig. 4 Bronchoscopic image of guide wire passing during percutaneous tracheostomy

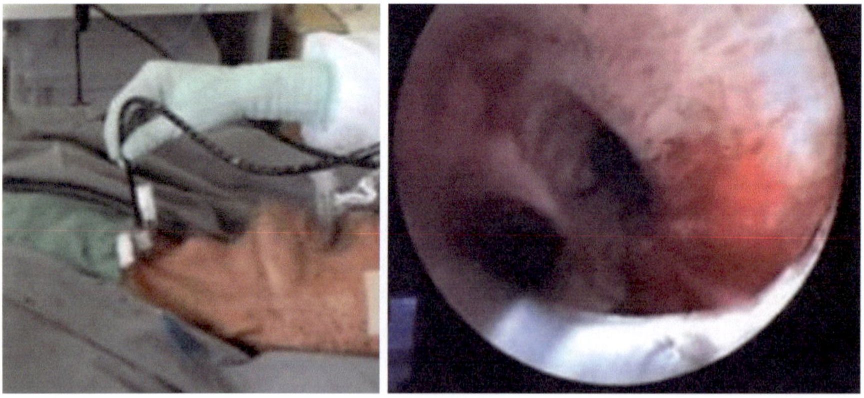

Fig. 5 Introduction of videobronchoscopy through the tracheostomy cannula and verification of the positioning of the cannula. The positioning of the cannula is observed just above the carina

benefits may be especially important when factors that increase the technical difficulty of the procedure—such as obesity, difficult anatomy, and cervical spine–related precautions—are present [28]. Despite the potential benefits, PT techniques do not always include control with bronchoscopy, and its advantages and disadvantages have been widely discussed. While some authors suggest that PT without bronchoscopic guidance is a safe procedure, others argue that bronchoscopy is essential to achieve a low rate of complications, allowing confirmation of the puncture, dilation, introduction, and adjustment of the cannula, as well as aspiration of secretions or clots; others have described the occurrence of complications despite bronchoscopic orientation.

Kost [2] analyzed 500 patients undergoing bronchoscopic PT, who had a complication rate of 9.2%. The rates of complications of PT with and without the assistance of bronchoscopy were compared in a meta-analysis of 23 studies with a total of 2237 patients. In the control group, without bronchoscopy, the incidence of complications was 16.8% (occurring in 233 of 1385 patients), whereas in the bronchoscopy group, the incidence was 8.3% (occurring in 71 of 851 patients) ($p < 0.0001$), representing a significant reduction in complications.

Berrouschot et al. [35] also compared PT with and without bronchoscopic control. The rates of perioperative complications were equivalent (7% versus 6%), but in the group without bronchoscopic control there were more severe complications (two cases of posterior tracheal wall perforation and one death due to tension pneumothorax). The authors concluded that bronchoscopic control not only minimizes the severity of complications but can also prevent major complications, or at least allow them to be immediately discovered and treated. More recently, Jackson et al. [36] also set out to compare the incidence of complications of PT with and without the support of bronchoscopy in a group of 243 patients with traumatic lesions; however, they did not find significant differences and concluded that bronchoscopic orientation is not consistently required but can be used as an adjunct in selected high-risk patients, such as those with cervical spine immobilization, obesity, or difficult cervical anatomy. Although no study has shown that bronchoscopy is indispensable, there are no concerns about undesirable effects when it is used.

Over the past 15–20 years, several studies have advocated the use of USG as an alternative to bronchoscopy to guide PT in real time, or as a complementary tool to evaluate the cervical anatomy prior to puncture (Figs. 6, 7, and 8). Ultrasound delimitation of the cervical anatomy before tracheal puncture can help prevent and/or minimize hemorrhagic complications from lesions of pretracheal vascular structures [28]. It may also help to confirm the correct position of the endotracheal tube when it is withdrawn during PT to the level immediately below the vocal cords, because when the tip of the tube reaches the second tracheal ring, the intensity of the Doppler signal increases greatly due to the presence of turbulent open air [37]. The possibility of ultrasonically measuring pretracheal soft tissue thickness, both in obese patients and in patients with palpable regular cervical anatomy, may aid in selection of the most appropriate tracheostomy tube size and prevent posterior misplacement with possible lesion of the posterior tracheal wall [19].

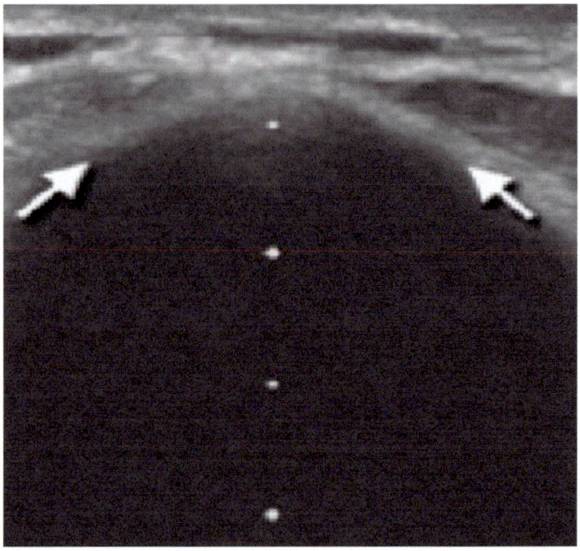

Fig. 6 Typical appearance of the trachea and pretracheal soft tissues. The anterior wall of the trachea contributes to the arch-shaped ultrasound contour (*arrows*) that establishes the border between the more superficial dense soft tissues (hyperechogenic sign) and the air inside the trachea (hypoechogenic sign)

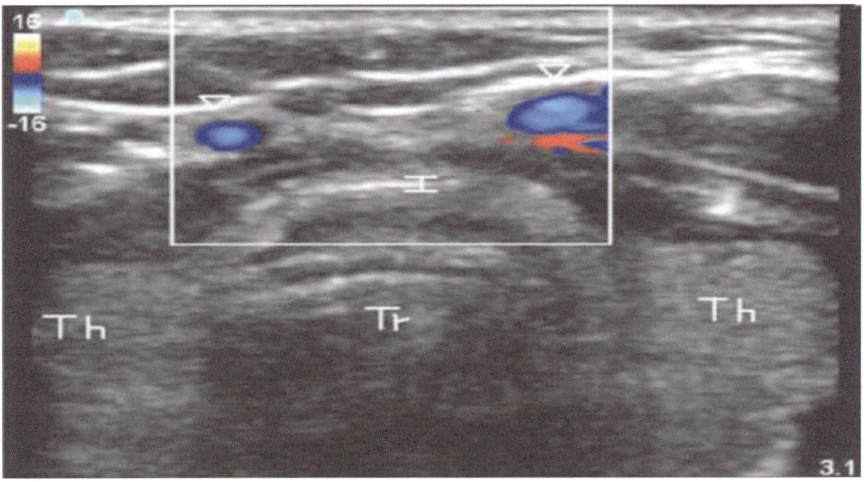

Fig. 7 Axial image of the trachea, showing the tracheal lumen and adjacent structures with pretracheal vein representation (shown by *arrowheads*) [38]. *I* isthmus, *Th* thyroid lobes

More recently, Guinot et al. [38] evaluated the feasibility and complication rate of USG-guided PT in a prospective study of 26 obese patients compared with 24 nonobese patients. The procedure was possible in all patients and there were no surgical conversions or deaths. The overall complication rates were similar in both groups and most complications were minor (hypotension, saturation drop, tracheal cuff puncture, and hemorrhage), with no differences between them.

A trial conducted by Kolling et al., which included 72 patients undergoing bronchoscopy and cervical USG, showed that preoperative USG altered the location of

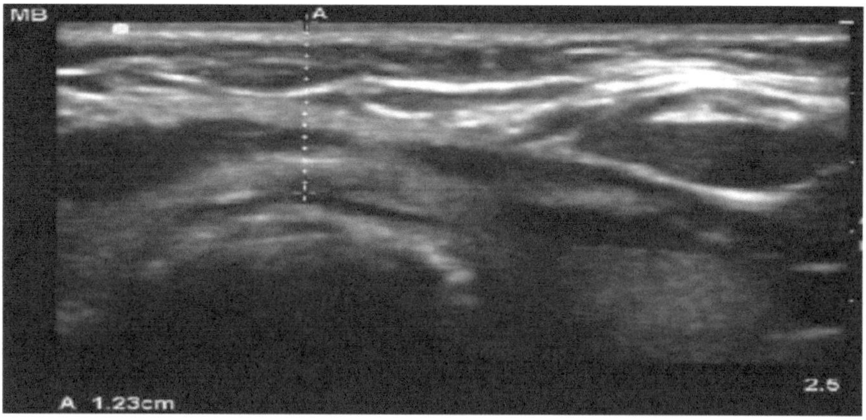

Fig. 8 Cervical ultrasound showing the distance (1.2 cm) between the skin and the second tracheal ring

the previously planned tracheal puncture in 23.6% of the patients to avoid lesion of subcutaneous vessels, as well as leading to conversion to CT due to detection of a goiter with extensive subcutaneous vascularization, although we have already seen in this chapter that a bulky goiter does not contraindicate PT.

In the face of a controversial theme and divergent opinions (about using auxiliary methods or not), it is noted that most of the studies advocate the use of these methods when performing tracheostomies. Therefore, it is believed that if there is availability of bronchoscopy and/or cervical USG, they should be used routinely, as they have a tendency to reduce fatal complications and allow better identification of anatomical structures. It should be recalled that the learning curves for performing the procedure with the aid of such instruments must also be taken into account: around 20 procedures using the bronchoscope and 50 procedures using cervical USG. Unfortunately, it is known that such an arsenal for tracheostomies is not available in most developing countries and is not part of the routine of some services.

Stoma Infection and Scarring

In 2014, Putensen et al. published a meta-analysis in *Critical Care*, evaluating several parameters, among them being infection or inflammation of the stoma. A lower incidence of these events was observed in patients undergoing the percutaneous technique, although none of them resulted in greater impairment of the general state of the patients. It is believed that the size of the incision, as well as the shorter time taken to perform the procedure, are determinants of such an outcome. The scar usually has a better aesthetic result with the percutaneous procedure, probably related to the smaller extension of the skin incision [39].

Cannula Obstruction and Morbidity and Mortality

The occurrence of cannula obstruction and decannulation up to 48 h postoperatively was more frequent in groups undergoing PT. This was due to greater ease in managing the cannula on the part of the multidisciplinary team (especially nurses and physiotherapists) in patients undergoing CT. It is believed, therefore, that it is easier to manipulate a surgical tracheostomy, since it has traditionally been performed for longer, whereas obstruction seems to occur more in patients treated percutaneously, because of the fear that the teams have in manipulating something in which they have less experience, especially with regard to routine aspiration of the cannula. In the most recent meta-analysis, the outcome of mortality in the two groups was evaluated, and there was no difference between them, suggesting that any complications or technical difficulties observed in the studies and related to the procedures have no impact on patient survival. The mean mortality with the percutaneous technique is about one in six hundred procedures performed, which is similar to the mortality observed with the conventional technique [40].

Thus, we observe that both percutaneous and conventional surgical tracheostomy are relatively low-risk approaches, which can be performed in a hospital room, reducing costs and time, and that in trained hands with adequate availability of materials, they are procedures with acceptable morbidity and fewer contraindications over time. Regarding the choice of technique, if there is a possibility and availability of sets for PT, this should be the technique of choice, since it is a less morbid procedure, aesthetically more favorable, and has few contraindications. Even though more trials are necessary to confirm this, it is believed that there will be greater diffusion of the percutaneous approach worldwide, thereby resulting in more teams being trained to perform it. Consequently, more scientific publications will appear on the subject, answering questions that have not yet been convincingly resolved.

References

1. Shelden CH, Pudenz RH, Tichy FY. Percutaneous tracheotomy. J Am Med Assoc. 1957;165(16):2068–70.
2. Kost KM. Endoscopic percutaneous dilatational tracheotomy: a prospective evaluation of 500 consecutive cases. Laryngoscope. 2005;115(10 Pt 2):1–30.
3. Ciaglia P, Firsching R, Syniec C. Elective percutaneous dilatational tracheostomy: a new simple bedside procedure; preliminary report. Chest. 1985;87:715–9.
4. Byhahn C, Lischke V, Halbig S, et al. Ciaglia Blue Rhino: a modified technique of percutaneous dilatational tracheostomy—technique and early results. Anaesthesist. 2000;49:202–6.
5. Griggs WM, Worthley LIG, Gilligan JE, et al. A simple percutaneous tracheostomy technique. Surg Gynecol Obstet. 1990;170:543–5.
6. Fikkers BG, Verwiel JMM, Tillmans RJGH. Percutaneous tracheostomy with the PercuTwist technique not so easy [letter]. Anaesthesia. 2002;57(9):935–6.
7. Zgoda MA, Berger R. Balloon-facilitated percutaneous dilatational tracheostomy tube placement: preliminary report of a novel technique. Chest. 2005;128(5):3688–90.
8. Higgins KM, Punthakee X. Meta-analysis comparison of open versus percutaneous tracheostomy. Laryngoscope. 2007;117:447–54.

9. Al-Ansari MA, Hijazi MH. Clinical review: percutaneous dilatational tracheostomy. Crit Care. 2006;202(9):10.
10. Putensen C, Theuerkauf N, Guenther U, Vargas M, Pelosi P. Percutaneous and surgical tracheostomy in critically ill adult patients: a metaanalysis. Crit Care. 2014;18:544.
11. MacIntyre NR, Cook DJ, Ely EW, Epstein SK, Fink JB, Heffner JE, American College of Chest Physicians; American Association for Respiratory Care; American College of Critical Care Medicine, et al. Evidence-based guidelines for weaning and discontinuing ventilatory support: a collective task force facilitated by the American College of Chest Physicians; the American Association for Respiratory Care; and the American College of Critical Care Medicine. Chest. 2001;120(6 Suppl):375S–95S.
12. Griffiths J, Barber VS, Morgan L, Young JD. Systematic review and meta-analysis of studies of the timing of tracheostomy in adult patients undergoing artificial ventilation. BMJ. 2005;330:1243.
13. Szakmany T, Russell P, Wilkes AR, Hall JE. Effect of early tracheostomy on resource utilization and clinical outcomes in critically ill patients: metaanalysis of randomized controlled trials. Br J Anaesth. 2015;114:396–405.
14. Durbin CG. Tracheostomy: why, when, and how? Respir Care. 2010;55(8):1056–68.
15. Boles J-M, Bion J, Connors A, Herridge M, Marsh B, Melot C, et al. Weaning from mechanical ventilation. Eur Respir J. 2007;29(5):1033–56.
16. De Leyn P, Bedert L, Delcroix M, Depuydt P, Lauwers G, Sokolov Y, et al. Tracheotomy: clinical review and guidelines. Eur J Cardiothorac Surg. 2007;32(3):412–21.
17. Wang MB, Berke GS, Ward PH, Calcaterra TC, Watts D. Early experience with percutaneous tracheostomy [abstract]. Laryngoscope. 1992;102(2):157–62.
18. Massick DD, Powell DM, Price PD, Chang SL, Squires G, Forrest LA, et al. Quantification of the learning curve for percutaneous dilational tracheotomy. Laryngoscope. 2000;110(2 Pt 1):222–8.
19. Feller-Kopman D. Acute complications of artificial airways. Clin Chest Med. 2003;24(3):445–55.
20. Epstein SK. Late complications of tracheostomy. Respir Care. 2005;50(4):542–9.
21. Norwood S, Vallina VL, Short K, Saigusa M, Fernandez LG, McLarty JW. Incidence of tracheal stenosis and other late complications after percutaneous tracheostomy. Ann Surg. 2000;232(2):233–41.
22. Petros S. Percutaneous tracheostomy. Crit Care. 1999;3(2):R5–R10.
23. Díaz-Reganón G, Minambres E, Ruiz A, González-Herrera S, HolandaPena M, López-Espadas F. Safety and complications of percutaneous tracheostomy in a cohort of 800 mixed ICU patients. Anaesthesia. 2008;63(11):1198–203.
24. Goldenberg D, Ari EG, Golz A, Danino J, Netzer A, Joachims HZ. Tracheotomy complications: a retrospective study of 1130 cases. Otolaryngol Head Neck Surg. 2000;123:495–500.
25. Delaney A, Bagshaw SM, Nalos M. Percutaneous dilatational tracheostomy versus surgical tracheostomy in critically ill patients: a systematic review and meta-analysis. Crit Care. 2006;10(2):R55.
26. McCague A, Aljanabi H, Wong DT. Safety analysis of percutaneous dilational tracheostomies with bronchoscopy in the obese patient. Laryngoscope. 2012;122:1031–4.
27. McCormick B, Manara AR. Mortality from percutaneous dilatational tracheostomy. A report of three cases. Anaesthesia. 2005;60(5):490–5.
28. Muhammad JK, Major E, Wood A, Patton DW. Percutaneous dilatational tracheostomy: haemorrhagic complications and the vascular anatomy of the anterior neck. A review based on 497 cases. Int J Oral Maxillofac Sur. 2000;29(3):217–22.
29. Mallick A, Quinn AC, Bodenham AR, Vucevic M. Use of the Combitube for airway maintenance during percutaneous dilatational tracheostomy. Anaesthesia. 1998;53(3):249–55.
30. Byhahn C, Wilke HJ, Halbig S, Lischke V, Westphal K. Percutaneous tracheostomy: Ciaglia Blue Rhino versus the basic Ciaglia technique of percutaneous dilatational tracheostomy. Anesth Analg. 2000;91(4):882–6.

31. Paran H, Butnaru G, Hass I, Afanasyv A, Gutman M. Evaluation of a modified percutaneous tracheostomy technique without bronchoscopic guidance. Chest. 2004;126(3):868–71.
32. Meyer M, Critchlow J, Mansharamani N, Angel LF, Garland R, Ernest A. Repeat bedside percutaneous dilational tracheostomy is a safe procedure. Crit Care Med. 2002;30(5):986–8.
33. Perfeito JA, Mata CA, Forte V, Carnaghi M, Tamura N, Leão LE. Tracheostomy in the ICU: is it worthwhile? J Bras Pneumol. 2007;33:687–90.
34. Sustić A, Kovac D, Zgaljardić Z, Zupan Z, Krstulović B. Ultrasound-guided percutaneous dilatational tracheostomy: a safe method to avoid cranial misplacement of the tracheostomy tube. Intensive Care Med. 2000;26(9):1379–81.
35. Berrouschot J, Oeken J, Steiniger L, Schneider D. Perioperative complications of percutaneous dilational tracheostomy. Laryngoscope. 1997;107(11 Pt 1):1538–44.
36. Jackson LS, Davis JW, Kaups KL, Sue LP, Wolfe MM, Bilello JF, et al. Percutaneous tracheostomy: to bronch or not to bronch: that is the question. J Trauma. 2011;71(6):1553–6.
37. Reilly P, Sing R, Gibson F, Anderson H, Rotondo M, Tinkoff G, et al. Hypercarbia during tracheostomy: a comparison of percutaneous endoscopic, percutaneous Doppler, and standard surgical tracheostomy. Intensive Care Med. 1997;23(8):859–64.
38. Guinot PG, Zogheib E, Petiot S, Marienne JP, Guerin AM, Monet P, et al. Ultrasound-guided percutaneous tracheostomy in critically ill obese patients. Crit Care. 2012;16(2):R40.
39. Putensen C, Theuerkauf N, Guenther U, Vargas M, Pelosi P. Percutaneous and surgical tracheostomy in critically ill adult patients: a meta-analysis. Crit Care. 2014; 18: 544.
40. Simon M, Metschke M, Braune SA, Püschel K, Kluge S. Death after percutaneous dilatational tracheostomy: a systematic review and analysis of risk factors. Crit Care. 2013;17:R258.
41. Cantais E, Kaiser E, Le-Goff Y, Palmier B. Percutaneous tracheostomy: prospective comparison of the translaryngeal technique versus the forceps-dilational technique in 100 critically ill adults. Crit Care Med. 2002;30(4):815–9.

Pediatric Tracheostomy

Pedro Collares Maia Filho, Marcelle Morgana Vieira de Assis and Terence Pires de Farias

Introduction

The upper age limit used to define the pediatric population varies among experts, with some including adolescents up to the age of 21 years [1, 2] and others only up to the age of 18 years [3]. Furthermore, defining pediatric subpopulations and related terms (newborn, infant, toddler, child) can be confusing [1–3]. To avoid misunderstandings on this subject, this chapter adopts the age classification and definitions detailed in Table 1.

Table 1 Adopted nomenclature for pediatric subpopulations defined by age

Pediatric subpopulation	Approximate age range
Newborn or neonate	Birth to 1 month of age
Premature	<38 weeks' gestational age
Term	>38 weeks' gestational age
Infant	1 month to 2 years
Child	2–12 years
Adolescent or teen	12–18 years
Children	Birth to 18 years
Baby	Birth to 1 year
Toddler	1–3 years

P.C.M. Filho, M.D. (✉)
Head and Neck Surgeon, Department of Home Care, Waldemar de Alcantara General State Hospital, Fortaleza, Brazil
e-mail: pedro_collares@hotmail.com

M.M.V. de Assis, P.T.
Physiotherapist, Department of Home Care, Waldemar de Alcantara General State Hospital, Fortaleza, Brazil

T.P. de Farias, M.D., Ph.D., M.Sc., Researcher.
Department of Head and Neck Surgery, Brazilian National Cancer Institute—INCA, Rio de Janeiro, RJ, Brazil

Department of Head and Neck Surgery, Pontifical Catholic University, Rio de Janeiro, RJ, Brazil

T.P. de Farias (ed.), *Tracheostomy*, https://doi.org/10.1007/978-3-319-67867-2_8

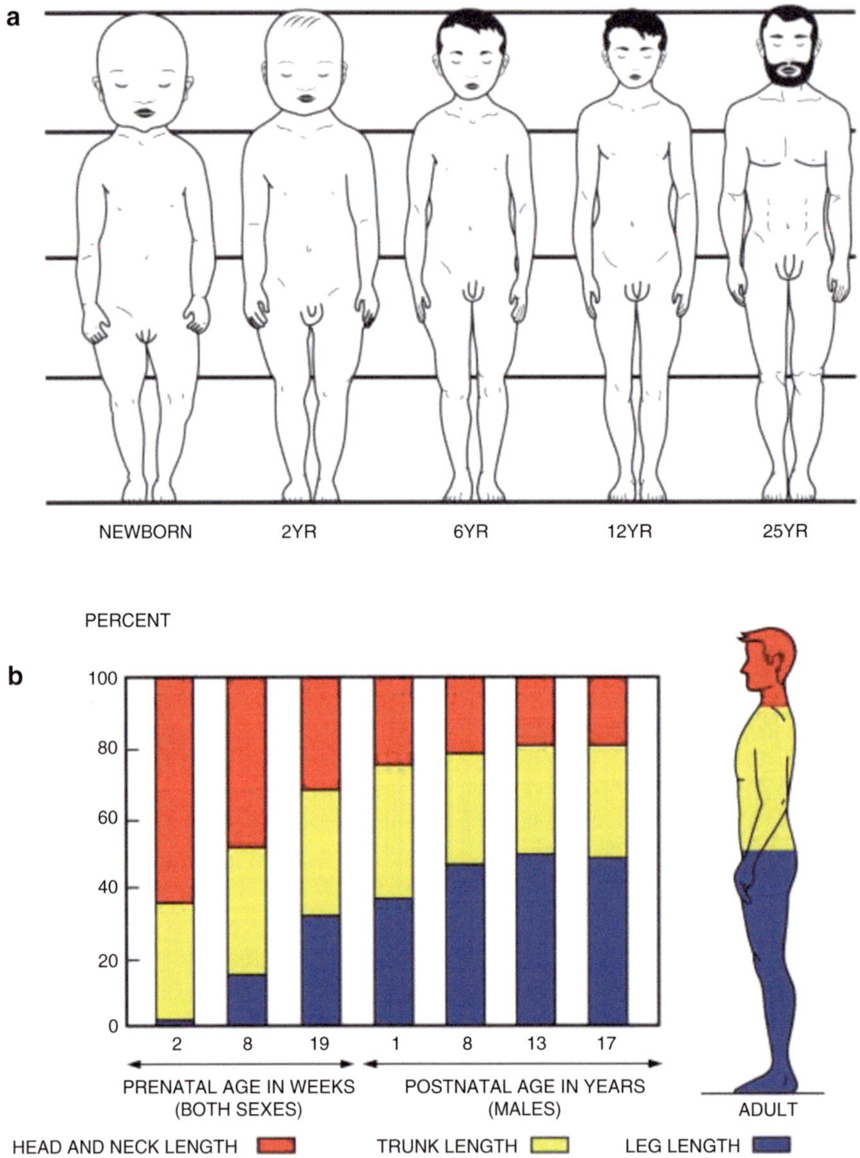

Fig. 1 (**a**) Proportional changes in body segments with age (*top*). (**b**) Percentage distribution of body segments as related to pre- and postnatal development (*bottom*). (Adapted from Huelke [4], with permission)

Children are not small adults. Significant changes from birth to adulthood are developed not only in body size and weight, but also in anatomical proportions (see Fig. 1) and physiological aspects [4, 5].

Regarding the pediatric airway, some anatomical differences need to be highlighted:

- A smaller diameter of airway lumen and a looser mucosal layer make it highly susceptible to trauma and obstruction by edema or secretion [5].
- Children's necks are shorter than adults' necks (see Fig. 1) [5, 6].
- The proportionally larger head predisposes children to upper airway obstruction by natural neck flexion and soft tissue compression, especially in the supine position [5, 7].
- The neonatal tongue has a flat dorsal surface and minimal lateral mobility, and appears large in the small oral cavity [7].
- The larynx is approximately cylindrical in an older child (>8 years old) and in an adult, while the neonate's and infant's larynx is conically shaped (see Fig. 2), widest at the supraglottic level and narrowest at the subglottic level (although some magnetic resonance imaging studies suggest that the narrowest part may be at the glottis, as in adults) [7–10].
- The cricoid ring is functionally the narrowest part of the neonatal airway [5, 7, 10].
- The tracheal length is related to the child's age and height, not to body weight [7, 10].
- The trachea is soft and flexible; furthermore, the airway is small and often very precarious [11].

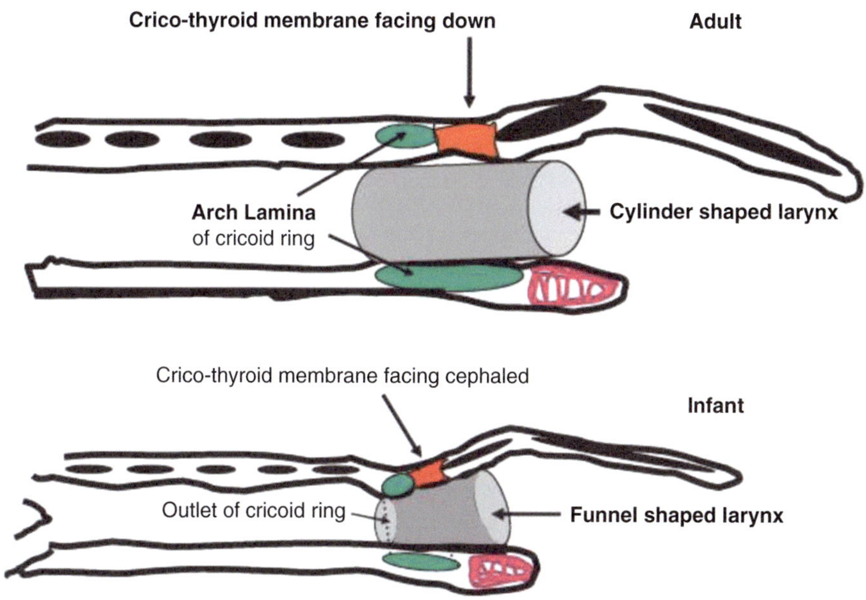

Fig. 2 Differences in the shape of the larynx with age. The outlet of the cricoid ring is the narrowest part of the infant's airway, circularly shaped, permitting an adequate seal with an adequately sized, uncuffed orotracheal tube for ventilation and against aspiration of gastric contents. The cricothyroid membrane is forced into a cephalad-facing position and is particularly exposed to injury—even perforation by intubation. (Reprinted from Holzki et al. [10], with permission)

Over the last 50 years, the indications for pediatric tracheostomy have markedly changed while its frequency has increased, reaching about 5000 procedures per year in the USA [12]. In the past, most children used to need urgent tracheostomy for treating acute airway infections (epiglottitis, diphtheria, croup), usually with subsequent decannulation if the patient survived the disease. Nowadays, chronic conditions (such as neuromuscular illnesses or subglottic stenosis) are the main surgical indications, and most children will be tracheostomized permanently [12–17].

Such a shifted pattern can be explained by medical advances in several fields. Immunization against *Corynebacterium diphtheria* and *Haemophilus influenza* has significantly reduced the incidence of infectious diseases requiring urgent tracheostomy. Furthermore, perinatal care development has increased the chances of surviving previously deadly conditions, such as extremely premature birth or severe congenital diseases. Newborns in this situation usually require prolonged ventilator support [12–18]. Therefore, contemporarily tracheostomized pediatric patients tend to be younger and have chronic conditions.

Considering the distinct anatomical and physiological aspects explained above, it is understandable why pediatric tracheostomy is assumed to be technically more difficult than tracheostomy in adults [17, 18]. It is also important to feature the higher morbidity and mortality rates in children compared with adults [17–19]. Later in this chapter, pediatric tracheostomy complications will be more fully discussed.

Indications

In a recent paper, Campisi et al. summarized general conditions as indications for tracheostomy (both adult and pediatric) [20]:

- Bypass of an acute or chronic upper airway obstruction
- Facilitation of the care of patients requiring long-term ventilatory support
- Protection from aspiration by providing access for tracheobronchial toilet
- Prevention of laryngotracheal stenosis in patients requiring long-term intubation
- Facilitation of weaning from a ventilator by eliminating ventilatory dead space

The study also outlined that common indications for tracheostomy in children include congenital and acquired airway stenosis, neurological conditions requiring long-term ventilation or pulmonary toilet, bilateral vocal fold insufficiency, and infectious compromise of the upper airway [20]. It is also important to note that multifactorial indications (more than one reason for tracheostomy in the same patient) may occur in many cases [21].

Nevertheless, variations based on the pediatric population served by each institution may occur. At the Brazilian National Cancer Institute (INCA), for example, most indications for pediatric tracheostomies are due to tumoral obstruction of the airway (see Fig. 3). Likewise, a large number of oncological tracheostomies would not be expected in a neonatology-specialized hospital.

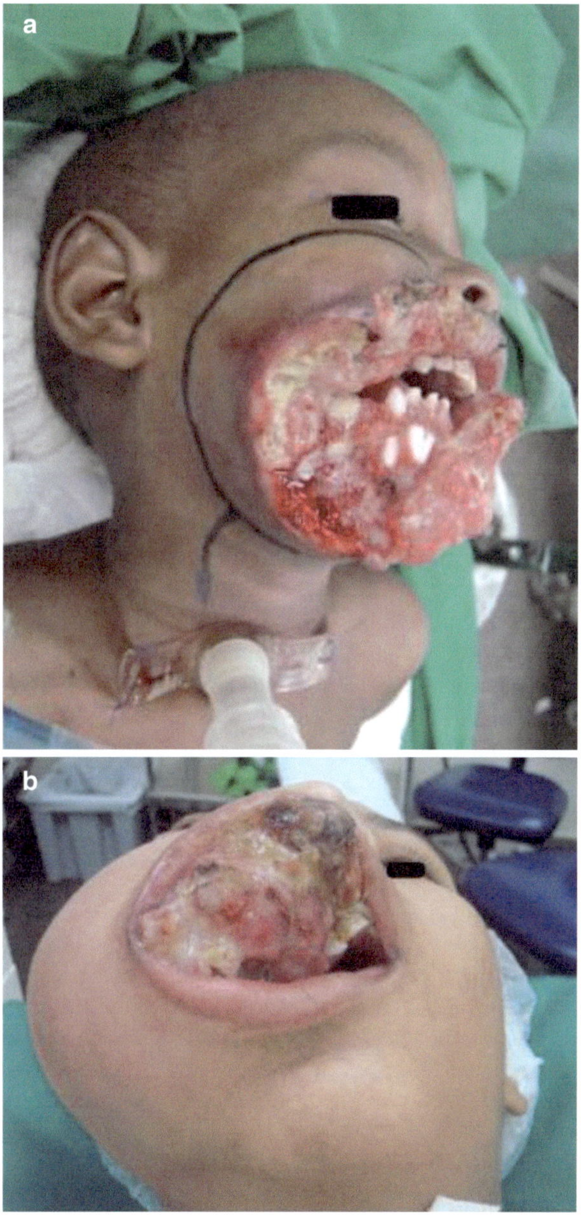

Fig. 3 (**a**) Child and (**b**) adolescent undergoing tracheostomy for tumoral airway obstruction at the Brazilian National Cancer Institute (INCA) in 2016

Injuries related to tracheal tubes (mostly subglottic stenosis) in all age groups have been reported in the literature for decades. In adolescents and adults, these have been mainly associated with overinflated cuffs, while in children they have been linked with oversized tubes [10].

Adults receiving invasive ventilatory support by orotracheal intubation usually have an early indication for a surgical airway (at 2–10 days), especially when

Table 2 Trachsel and Hammer criteria favoring tracheostomy indication in children

Children requiring long-term ventilation/ pulmonary toilet	Children with upper airway obstruction
Young age with a high risk of midfacial deformation from mask pressure	Low chance of definitive, spontaneous resolution within a reasonable time (weeks)
Ventilator dependency for most of the day (more than 12 hours per day)	Low probability that surgery can definitely correct the cause
Inability to cope with a mask (full face or nasal mask)	High risk of critical upper airway obstruction with simple respiratory tract infections or minor bleeding (epistaxis)
Recurrent aspirations (gastroesophageal reflux, laryngeal incompetence) with significant benefit from pulmonary toilet	High risk of or previous history of difficulties in airway management in the event of an emergency
Safety measures and local experience highly in favor of invasive ventilation	Difficult-to-control gastroesophageal reflux

Adapted from Trachsel and Hammer [22], with permission

prolonged intubation is anticipated, with an intention to avoid laryngeal damage [9]. Some studies have also related it to lower mortality in comparison with a delayed procedure [6].

However, the timing of tracheostomy in intubated children is controversial (from >14 days to >90 days) [6]. Some infants may tolerate orotracheal tubing for weeks to months without adverse laryngeal effects [6, 9, 22]. Additionally, the higher complication rates, especially in younger pediatric patients, may overcome the benefits of a surgical airway in some pediatric intensivists' judgment. Some have reported that they would consider tracheostomy only after a number of failed extubations [6]. Nevertheless, long intubation periods interfere with children's normal development and may cause laryngotracheal damage [6, 9]. Besides, a surgical airway may allow home care assistance (dehospitalization) for severely impaired children and prevent midfacial hypoplasia [22].

The lack of guidelines makes the indication for intubated pediatric patients still mostly empirical. Trachsel and Hammer have suggested some criteria that might help (see Table 2), but maybe a specialized multidisciplinary team approach (pediatrician, surgeon, nurse, physiotherapist, speech therapist) would be a reasonable way to manage such complex decisions [21, 22].

Preoperative Evaluation

As discussed previously, the current conventional pediatric patient with an indication for tracheostomy can be defined as young (newborn or infant), suffering from a chronic condition usually associated with multiple comorbidities, intubated, and ventilator dependent. Therefore, most cases nowadays should be classified as elective procedures, and careful preoperative evaluation must be done.

The International Pediatric Otolaryngology Group (IPOG) consensus [23] recommends the following:

- The medical history should be taken and a physical examination should be performed, including assessment of anatomical landmarks and neck mobility for intraoperative extension.
- Laboratory investigations, including a complete blood cell count and coagulation studies (international normalized ratio (INR) and prothrombin time (PTT)) should be performed; further investigations may depend on the patient's underlying medical comorbidities.
- Patients and their caregivers should be provided with adequate information and education regarding the nature of the procedure and its benefits, risks, and expected postoperative course.
- Emotional support should be provided to patients and their families as appropriate.
- When appropriate, a preoperative evaluation by a communication and/or feeding specialist in speech and/or feeding rehabilitation should be performed.

It is also advisable to check if a range of tracheostomy tube sizes and models are available before starting the procedure. Later in this chapter, the options of pediatric tubes will be discussed.

Surgical Procedure and Techniques

Although adult tracheostomy has routinely been done at the bedside in an intensive care unit (ICU), pediatric tracheostomy is usually performed in an operating room (OR), with general anesthesia and anesthesiologist support [6, 11]. We do agree with this, considering that it is a technically difficult procedure that carries high complication rates. Adolescents and older children may be an exception to this recommendation, and bedside tracheostomies have been performed in this age group, including by a percutaneous technique [6, 24].

Steps in the Conventional Technique

1. *Positioning* (see Fig. 4): Supine position with the neck in extension, using a cylindrical pillow or a rolled sheet under the shoulders. That may be the key to a successful tracheostomy in general and may be the most important step in pediatrics. As already explained, young children have a short neck with a tendency to keep it flexed, naturally obstructing and "hiding" the airway. The right positioning increases neck and trachea exposure, bringing the trachea closer to the surface. Head support must be provided to avoid cervical spine injury.
2. *Neck examination*: Once the patient is positioned, cervical surface landmarks must be identified (palpation of the thyroid cartilage, cricoid cartilage, and suprasternal notch). These landmarks are often difficult to palpate in children, though [11]. At this moment, care must be taken to identify prominent vascular pulsations suggestive of a high-riding innominate artery [20]. The surgical site can then be prepared and draped in sterile fashion.

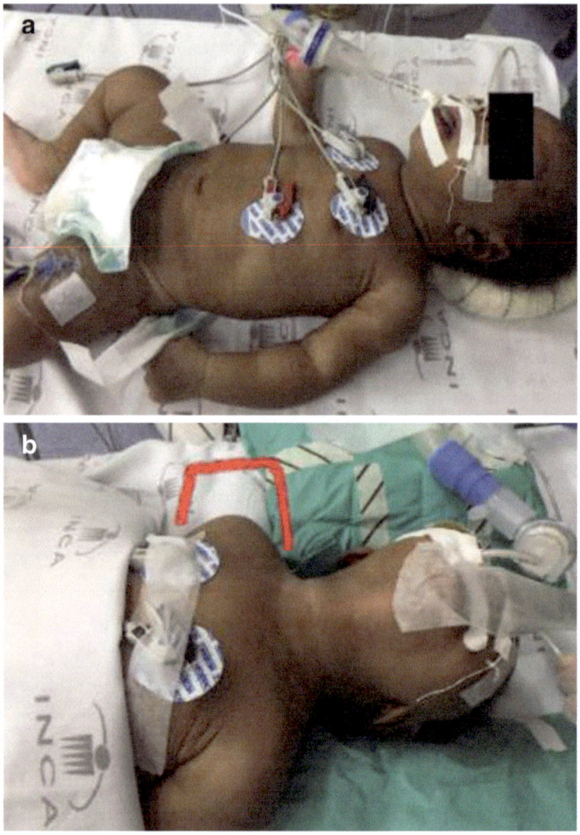

Fig. 4 Positioning an infant for tracheostomy. (**a**) *Top:* patient in a supine position without neck extension. (**b**) *Bottom:* patient correctly positioned, with neck extension. Part of the rolled sheet can be seen under the right shoulder (*outlined in red*). Observe the marked improvement of neck exposure and notice that the back of the head is fully supported

3. *Skin incision* (see Fig. 5a): In our routine practice, we prefer a 3 cm horizontal skin incision, halfway between the cricoid cartilage and the sternal notch (at the second and third tracheal ring level). For us, vertical incisions go against cervical skin tension lines and do not provide much better exposure than horizontal incisions. In our opinion and of other authors, there is no reason for using vertical skin incisions in an elective procedure [20]. Surveys among surgeons report an approximate 60% preference for horizontal skin incisions [25]. On the other hand, some authors recommend vertical skin incisions for emergency procedures, providing fast access to the trachea and minimizing the risk of vascular injury and excessive bleeding [15, 20]. Others claim that vertical incisions may offer an improved anatomical orientation—especially in infants, whose important anatomical landmarks, such as the cricoid and thyroid cartilages, may not be easily palpable—and may reduce the risk of pneumothorax by minimizing the need for dissection lateral to the trachea [25].
4. *Dissection until the thyroid gland space* (see Fig. 5b): Two skin flaps (one superior and other inferior) are made through horizontal dissection of the subcutaneous fat and platysma, reaching the strap muscles. At this point, the dissection turns in a vertical direction, separating the strap muscles along the midline raphe, with the auxiliary surgeon providing lateral retraction until the thyroid gland space is entered.

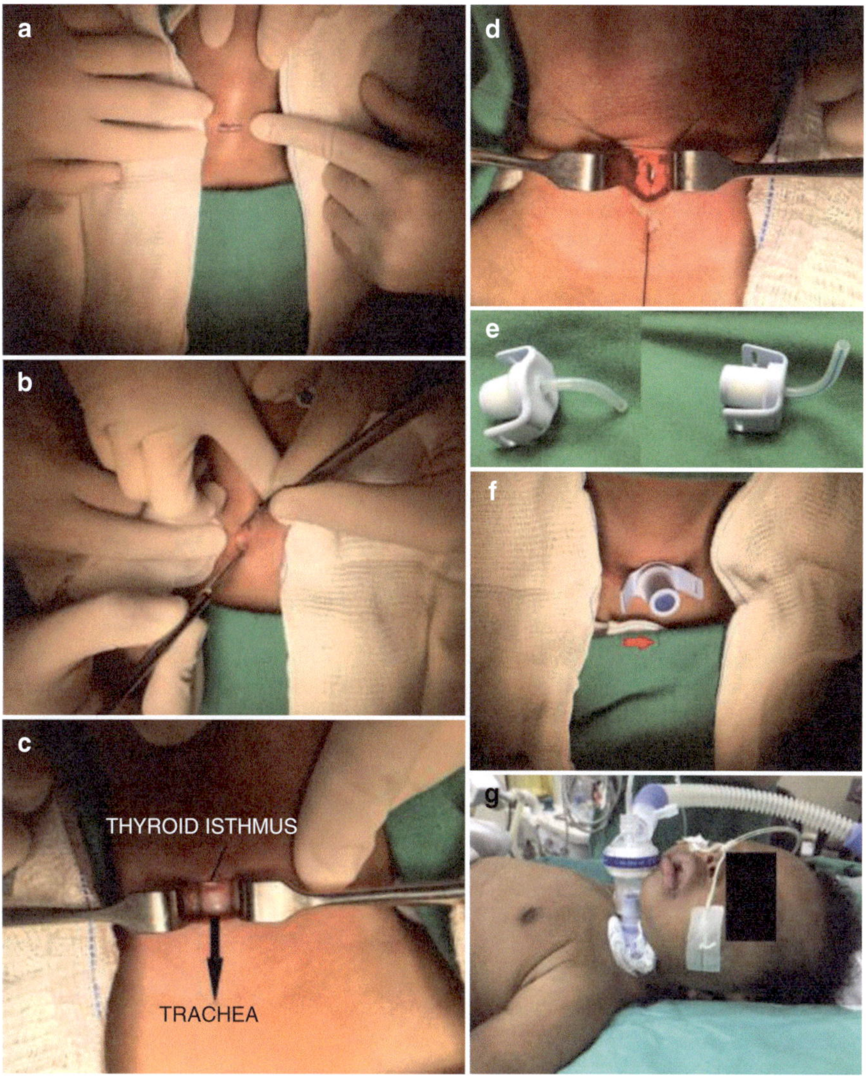

Fig. 5 Infant undergoing conventional tracheostomy for prolonged ventilatory support. (**a**) Horizontal skin incision. (**b**) Horizontal subplatysmal dissection. (**c**) Vertical dissection with lateral retractors. (**d**) Vertical tracheostomy with three absorbable suture fixation points. (**e**) Uncuffed tracheal tube. (**f**) Tube positioned; note the stay suture below the tube (*red arrow*) used for traction of the inferior tracheostomy border during the first tube change. (**g**) Tube fixated with ties around the neck

5. *Trachea exposure and hemostasis* (see Fig. 5c): Pretracheal fat tissue is dissected laterally and superiorly, while blood vessels below the isthmus are controlled and the thyroid gland is pushed up with retractors, exposing the anterior tracheal wall. Eventually, the isthmus needs to be divided vertically (and sutured hemostatically) for better exposure of the tracheal rings. Some authors advocate rou-

tine isthmus division, despite greater operative tissue traumatization and the resulting risks [15]. Kremer et al. maintain that there is a risk of chondritis on the first or second tracheal cartilage ring, which is caused by the upward pull on the cannula, if the isthmus has not been cut. In addition, they consider it a definite advantage to bisect the isthmus, for this enables installation of the cannula without force and helps avoid not only damage to the front and rear walls of the trachea, but also faulty installation of the cannula in the mediastinum and uncontrolled tissue damage [15]. Bleeding control must be reviewed before opening the trachea, and a Valsalva maneuver should be performed by the anesthesiologist to help evidence occult lower pressure bleeding. It is worth remembering that normal blood volume in pediatrics is only about 85 mL/kg [5] and that multiple combined diseases are the rule in those patients. Therefore, little blood waste may be "a lot" in such conditions, and minimum losses must be achieved.

6. *Tracheostomy* (see Fig. 5d and Fig. 6): Once the trachea is fully exposed, a cricoid hook is used to pull the cricoid superiorly. This stabilizes the laryngotracheal complex—an essential step prior to making an incision in the trachea [20]. Many types of incision are used for opening the anterior wall of the trachea: vertical; horizontal (between two cartilaginous rings); with part of a ring resection (oval window); Björk flap (inferior stalked to a skin cartilage flap—developed in 1960); and H-shaped incisions (horizontal incision associated with both superior and inferior flaps). *None of these types has achieved a consensus (most authors report no differences in the frequency or severity of complications among types of tracheal fenestration performed), although specific complications and advantages have been more frequently related to specific types of tracheostomy* (see Table 3). *The tracheal incision can be made vertically or* horizontally according to the surgeon's preference, since it is between the second and fourth tracheal ring-because placement of the incision and insertion superior to the second ring may predispose the patient to developing subglottic stenosis [20]. Regardless of the type of incision, *in children it is advisable to use fixation sutures at the borders of the tracheostomy, reducing the chance of tube false passage*. Some prefer maturation of the tracheal borders to the skin

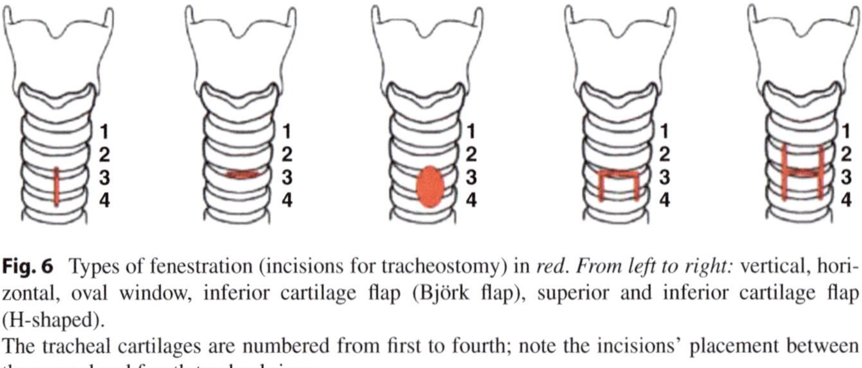

Fig. 6 Types of fenestration (incisions for tracheostomy) in *red*. *From left to right:* vertical, horizontal, oval window, inferior cartilage flap (Björk flap), superior and inferior cartilage flap (H-shaped).
The tracheal cartilages are numbered from first to fourth; note the incisions' placement between the second and fourth tracheal rings

Table 3 Advantages and complications specifically related to each type of tracheostomy (tracheal incision)

Type of tracheostomy	Reported advantages	Reported complications
Vertical	–	Deformation of the anterior tracheal wall and pressure lesions on the cartilage [15]
Horizontal	Less suprastomal granulation formation [25]	–
Oval window	–	Tracheomalacia (a large window might destabilize the tracheal wall) [15]
Björk flap	Facilitates placement of a cannula and decreases the risk of pneumomediastinum [15] Reduces the danger of tracheostomal collapse during cannula exchange or during accidental decannulation [15]	Higher incidence of granuloma in the stoma [15] Higher risk of tracheal stenosis [15]

and remove subcutaneous fat from the skin incision for a better fit of the suture. Surveys performed at three time points showed that *most surgeons used stay sutures (85–94%), routine removal of subcutaneous fat (62%), and a vertical tracheal incision (75–87%),* while only 5–10% of responding surgeons made a horizontal tracheal incision [25].

7. *Tracheostomy tube passage* (see Fig. 5e–g): There should not be any resistance while inserting the tube, and correct ventilation must be confirmed by the anesthesiologist. Campisi et al. recommend that the position of the tip of the tracheostomy tube should be verified by flexible bronchoscopy to ensure that the tip is above the carina and that there is no blood or mucus blocking the lower airways [20]. Although bronchoscopy is not our routine practice, we do recommend postoperative chest radiography (see Fig. 7), also for excluding other complications (pneumothorax).

Pearls and Pitfalls

Campisi et al. [20] propose certain considerations and modifications for the standard tracheostomy procedure in pediatric patients to minimize the risk of complications:

- If possible, maintain spontaneous respiratory effort. This is particularly beneficial in the setting of acute airway compromise and after the tracheostomy (step 4) due to the resultant airway leak and difficulty of effective ventilation.
- Preselect—and have available in the surgical set—an appropriately sized tracheostomy tube and a second tube that is one size smaller in case of inability to insert the tube.

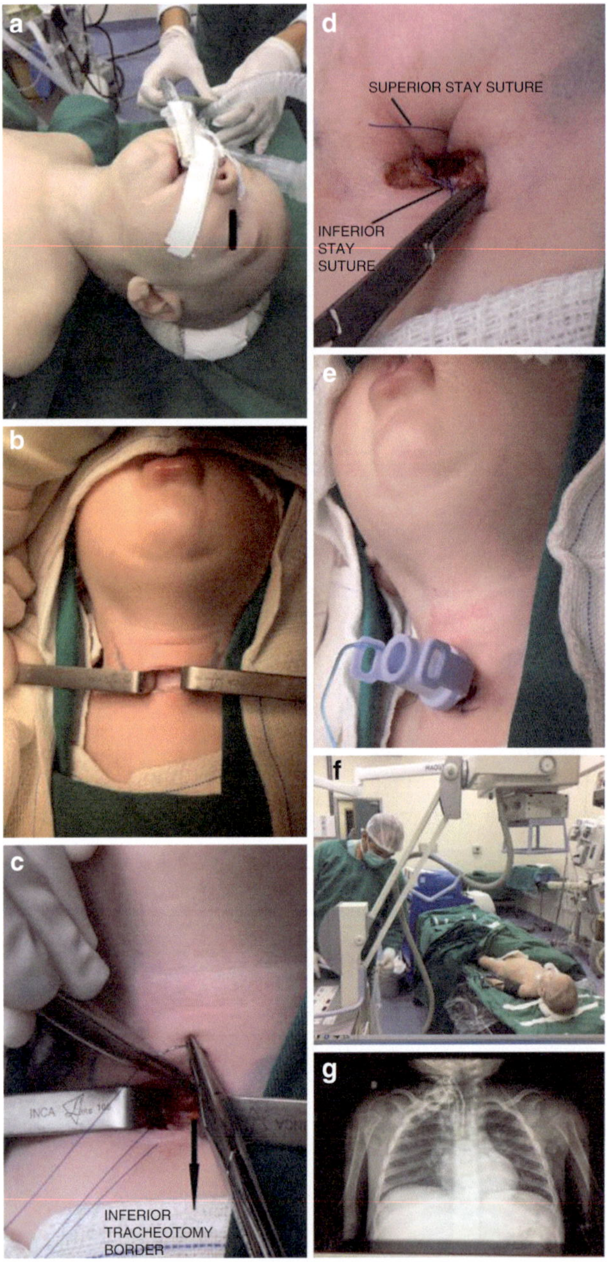

Fig. 7 Child undergoing conventional horizontal tracheostomy. (**a**) Patient positioned with neck extension. (**b**) Horizontal skin incision and dissection. (**c**) Horizontal fenestration and positioning of stay sutures on the inferior and superior borders of the trachea. (**d**) Stay sutures matured in the skin. (**e**) Cuffed tracheal tube, size 4.5 mm, inside the maturated tracheostomy. (**f**) Tracheostomy concluded and postoperative chest radiography in the operation room. (**g**) Chest radiography showing the position of the tube and no signs of pneumothorax

- Excise peristomal subcutaneous adipose tissue and suture the edges of the tracheostomy to the skin to mature the tracheostoma (maturation sutures).
- Place vertically oriented stay sutures on either side of the vertical tracheostomy around a tracheal ring. When pulled, stay sutures approximate the tracheostomy edges to the skin surface. This will facilitate the insertion of the tracheostomy tube and the reinsertion of a tube if it is accidentally decannulated. The stay sutures should be taped to the chest wall and labeled as "left" and "right."
- *Do not remove any tracheal cartilage to create the tracheostomy. Cartilage sparing is the key to the prevention of suprastomal collapse and tracheomalacia.*
- Meticulous hemostasis is important to prevent hemorrhage and the need to return to the OR.

Recently, the IPOG published a consensus document [23] recommending the following intraoperative considerations:

- Use of stay sutures is important in case of accidental decannulation. Consider 4-0 Prolene, nylon, or Vicryl. Consider color coding (to distinguish left from right) or labeling of "left" and "right."
- You may consider maturing the stoma (see Fig. 7) in case of accidental decannulation in the small infant or neonate.
- Suggestions for fixation of the tracheostomy tube in place include Velcro ties without skin suturing; Velcro ties without skin suturing but with consideration of suturing the Velcro to itself so it cannot be opened; cotton ties; skin suturing; trach gauze, Exu-Dry, or Mepilex dressing under the flanges ± under the neck ties.
- Consider flexible tracheoscopy at the end of the case in order to assess the distance from the tip of the tracheostomy tube to the carina, as well as the presence of distal compression/obstruction. Consider a complete airway examination during the same anesthetic either prior to the tracheostomy or after the tracheostomy tube is in place.
- Consider antibiotic prophylaxis until the first tracheostomy tube change in all patients.
- The timing of the first tracheostomy tube change should be at the discretion of the surgeon. Among IPOG members, this varies between 3 and 7 days, with the majority performing the change between 5 and 7 days.

Oncological Tracheostomy: Technical Peculiarities

Skin Incision: Adjustments must be made in cases of large cervical tumors with airway displacement, so the skin incision will be properly positioned. Diagnostic imaging examinations may help in planning the incision (see Fig. 8). Besides, larger incisions should be considered (see Fig. 9).

Trachea Exposure and Hemostasis: When indicated for treatment of oncological obstructive conditions, especially in transtumoral tracheostomies, anomalous large blood vessels (collateral circulation) and friable tumoral masses are potentially causes of severe bleeding (see Figs. 8 and 9). Achieving bleeding control may be a challenge. Besides anesthesiologist support (blood transfusion reservation, invasive

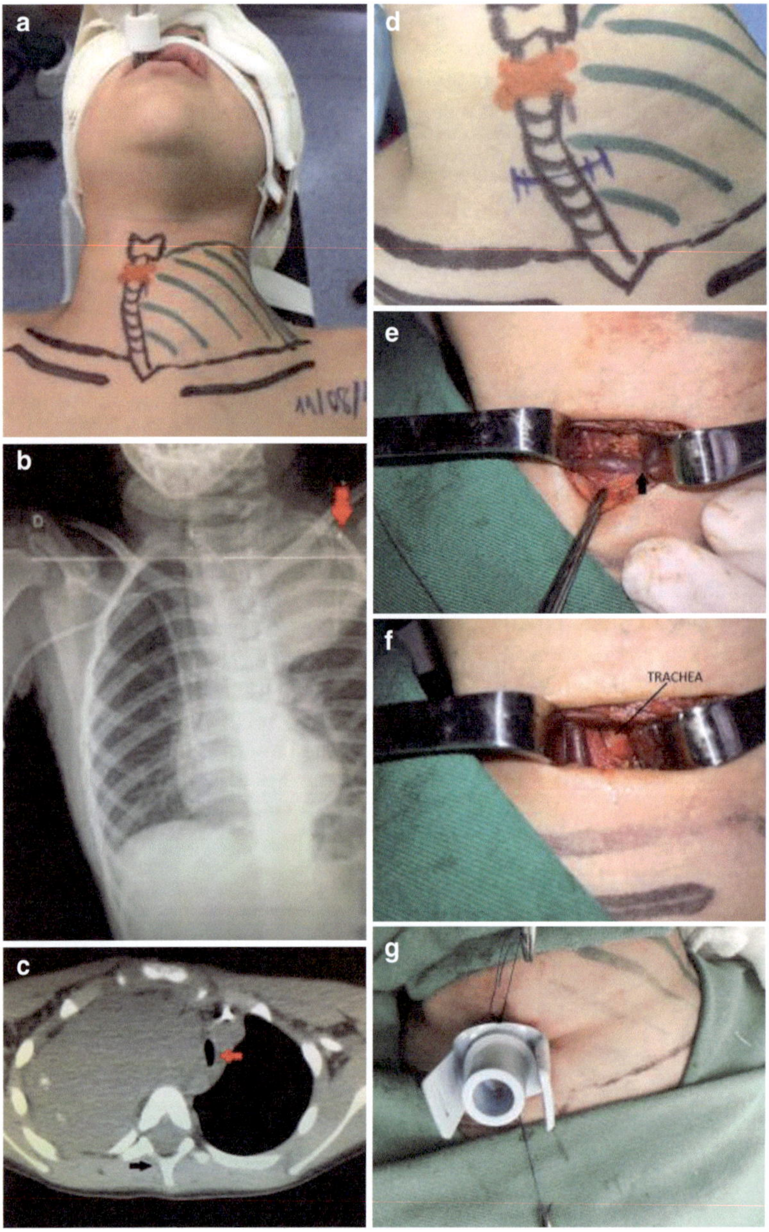

Fig. 8 Child undergoing oncological tracheostomy. (**a**) Patient with left cervical mass, airway deviated to the right. (**b**) Chest radiography showing a large left cervicothoracic mass (*red arrow*). (**c**) Tomography showing a large tumor pushing the trachea (*red arrow*) toward the right; note the position of the spinal vertebra (*black arrow*) as a reference for the central position. (**d**) Planed incision (*blue line*). (**e**) Note the large venous blood vessel (*black arrow*) crossing in front of the trachea. (**f**) Trachea more visible after blood vessel removal. (**g**) Tracheal tube positioned; note the two stay sutures for traction of the superior and inferior tracheostomy borders

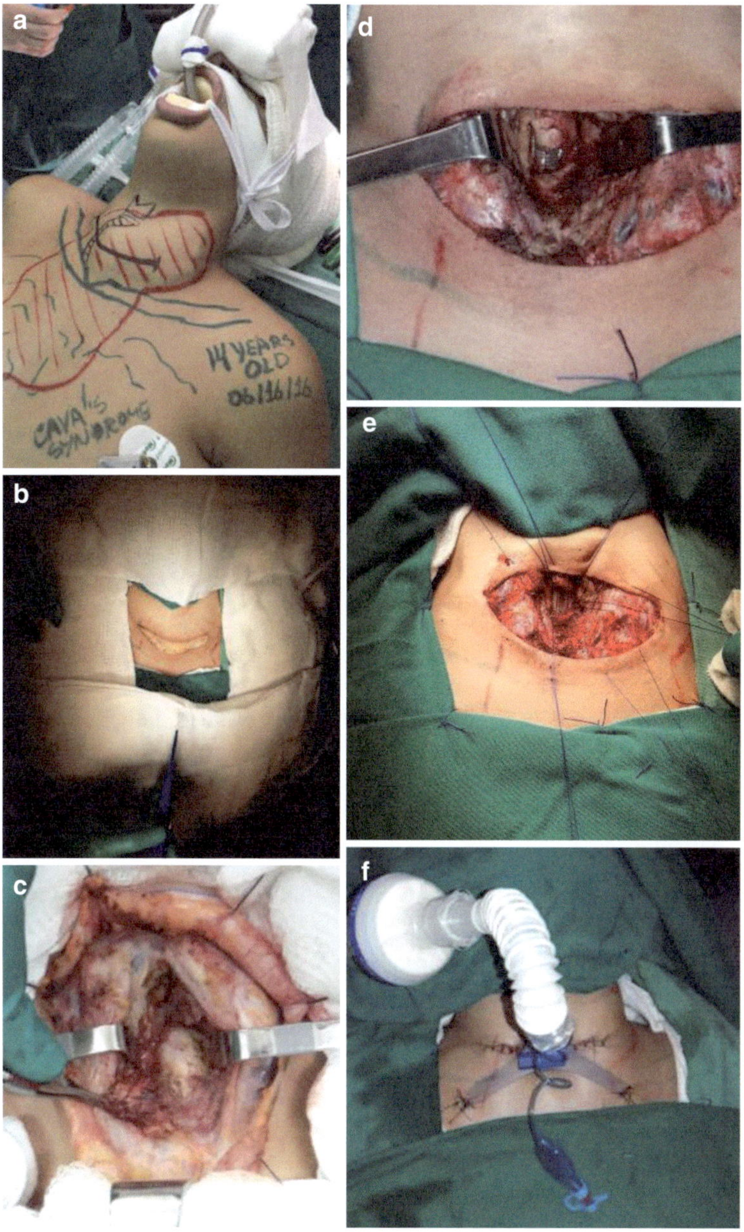

Fig. 9 Adolescent undergoing transtumoral tracheostomy. (**a**) Left cervical mass with extension to the mediastinum, presenting with signs of superior vena cava syndrome. Note the airway deviated to the right and the planed incision (*black line*). (**b**) Large horizontal incision. (**c**) Trachea exposed after tumor parts covering the trachea were removed (transtumoral approach). (**d**) Note the H-shaped tracheostomy incision with the wire-reinforced orotracheal tube still inside the tracheal lumen. (**e**) Suture points prepared for skin maturation of the H-shaped tracheal incision. (**f**) Tracheostomy concluded; a cuffed tracheal tube was used, fixated with suture points in the skin. The large skin incision around the tracheostomy was sutured

cardiovascular monitoring), use of hemostatic substances and special devices (harmonic scalpel) is welcomed, if they are available.

Tracheostomy and Stay Sutures: For such dramatic situations, it is advisable to perform tracheal incisions that can be submitted to maturation sutures on the skin. The purposes are to isolate the airway from bleeding and to try to avoid tumor growth inside the tracheostomy lumen (see Figs. 8 and 9). *In older children, we prefer horizontal incisions, just as in adults.*

Percutaneous Tracheostomy

Percutaneous tracheostomy is seldom used in children, especially younger ones. Nevertheless, some authors are starting to try some percutaneous techniques even in young pediatric patients, and are reporting successful experiences, but done in an OR setting [24]. The procedure still has not been safely recommended for bedside practice, though.

Another chapter in this book specifically addresses the subject of percutaneous tracheostomy.

Pediatric Tracheostomy Tube Choices

Choosing the right tracheostomy tube for children demands a thoughtful evaluation, considering:

- The purpose of the tracheostomy
- The patient's anatomy
- Associated diseases
- Conditions for tracheostomy care

The decision must embrace:

- The material (metal or plastic—polyvinyl chloride (PVC), silicone, polyurethane)
- The size/diameter
- The type (cuffed/uncuffed, with/without inner cannula, with/without speech devices or fenestra, Montgomery T-tube)

As metallic tubes are not designed to connect to ventilator devices, children who need invasive ventilatory support should not use this kind of tube. The metal interferes with tomography imaging quality and cannot be used during magnetic resonance examinations. Patients receiving neck radiation therapy also are not supposed to use this this kind of tube, to prevent skin injury. On the other hand, metallic tubes are a good choice for domiciliary use because they deteriorate slowly (allowing long-term use without changes needed) and have an inner cannula (with a lower risk of obstruction and an easier cleaning process).

Plastic devices are perfect for connecting invasive ventilatory support. They are softer—especially the silicone ones—which is ideal for the fragile anatomy of younger children's airway. They can be used during neck radiation therapy and radiological examinations with minimum interference. The cuffed ones provide better tracheal sealing, avoiding air leakage from a high-pressure invasive ventilator and providing better protection against bronchoaspiration, although that is hardly necessary and should be avoided because of increased risk of tracheal injury [20]. Newborns do not use a cuff because their narrow trachea cannot fit it. The uncuffed cannulae for such patients already have a minimum diameter for reasonable ventilation flow, almost sealing the tracheal lumen. [9] A cuffed option in this situation either would markedly reduce the diameter of the tube and ventilatory flow or would injure such a delicate airway. The disadvantages of plastic tubes are that usually they do not have an inner cannula, they are more easily obstructed by mucus plugs, and they need to be changed within shorter periods of time.

Deciding on the size/diameter of pediatric tracheal tubes can be confusing. Table 4 gives a valuable guide to the types and sizes recommended for different patient ages.

Unfortunately the chart in Table 4 provides too much information to memorize, particularly if it is not part of routine use. A more simple alternative is to memorize the formulas described below: [27]

- The Cole formula for uncuffed tubes is:
  Internal diameter (in mm) = 4 + (age in years/4)
- The Motoyama formula for cuffed tubes in children aged 2 years or older is:
  Internal diameter (in mm) = 3.5 + (age in years/4)
- The Khine formula for cuffed tubes in children younger than 2 years is:
  Internal diameter (in mm) = 3 + (age in years/4)

However, the size of the patient may be inconsistent with the chronological age, and hence the parameters mentioned above will not apply [20]. Various studies have reported failure with age-based formulas (up to 60%), but they are still more precise than weight-based ones [27–29]. Use of the width of the fifth fingernail, although less often accurate than the age-based formula, may be an option when age information is not available [28].

In addition to the diameter, the length and curvature of the tube change according to the tracheostomy tube size. As such, the length and curvature must also be considered when selecting a tracheostomy tube [20]. Ideally, the length of the tube should extend at least 2 cm beyond the stoma with the tip no closer than 1–2 cm to the carina [30]. The tube should fit perfectly inside the trachea, without pressure points, which can evolve into granulomas, stenosis, or perforation fistulas. Silicone tubes are the best option for avoiding these complications.

Table 4 Sizing chart for the pediatric airway
Reprinted from Tweedie et al. [26], with permission

			Preterm-1 month		1-6 months	6-15 months	18months -3yrs	3-6 years	6-9 years	9-12 years	12-14 years
	Trachea (Transverse Diameter mm)		5		5-6	6-7	7-8	8-9	9-10	10-13	13
PLASTIC	Great Ormond Street	ID (mm)		3.0	3.5	4.0	4.5	5.0	5.5	6.0	7.0
		OD (mm)		4.5	5.0	6.0	6.7	7.5	8.0	8.7	10.7
	Shiley	Size		3.0	3.5	4.0	4.5	5.0	6.5	6.0	6.5
		ID (mm)		3.0	3.5	4.0	4.5	5.0	6.5	6.0	6.5
		OD (mm)		4.5	5.2	5.9	6.5	7.1	7.7	8.3	9.0
		Length (mm) Neonatal		30	32	34	36				
	*Cufted Tube Available	Paediatric		39	40	41*	42*	44*	45*		
		Long Paediatric						50*	52*	54*	56*
	Portex (Blue Line)	ID (mm)		3.0	3.5	4.0	4.5	5.0	6.0	6.0	7.0
		OD (mm)		4.2	4.9	5.5	6.2	6.9	6.9	8.3	9.7
	Portex (555)	Size		2.5	3.0	3.5	4.0	4.5	6.0	5.5	
		ID (mm)		2.5	3.0	3.5	4.0	4.5	6.0	5.5	
		OD (mm)			5.2	5.9	6.5	7.1	7.7	8.3	
		Length Neonatal		30	32	34	38				
		Paediatric		30	36	40	44	48	50	52	
	Bivona	Size	2.5	3.0	3.5	4.0	4.5	5.0	5.5		
		ID (mm)	2.5	3.0	3.5	4.0	4.5	5.0	5.5		
		OD (mm)	4.0	4.7	5.3	6.0	6.7	7.3	8.0		
	All sizes available with Fome Cuff, Aine Cuff & TTS Cuff	Length Neonatal	30	32	34	36					
		Paediatric	38	39	40	41	42	44	46		
	Bivona Hyperflex	ID (mm)	2.5	3.0	3.5	4.0	4.5	5.0	6.5		
		Usable Length (mm)	55	60	65	70	75	80	85		
	Bivona Fiextend	ID (mm)	2.5	3.0	3.5	4.0	4.5	5.0	6.5		
		Shaft Length (mm)	38	39	40	41	42	44	46		
		Flextend Lenght (mm)	10	10	16	15	17.5	20	20		
	TracoeMini	ID (mm)	2.5	3.0	3.5	4.0	4.5	5.0	5.5	6.0	
		OD (mm)	3.6	4.3	5.0	5.6	6.3	7.0	7.6	8.4	
		Length (mm) Neonatal (360)	30	32	34	36					
		Paediatric (355)	32	36	40	44	48	50	55	62	
SILVER	Alder Hey	FG		12-14	16	18	20	22	24		
	Negus	FG			16	18	20	22	24	26	28
	Chevater Jackson	FG		14	16	18	20	22	24	26	28
	Shafteld	FG		12-14	16	18	20	22	24	26	
		ID (mm)		2.9-3.6	4.2	4.9	6.0	6.3	7.0	7.6	
	Cricoid (AP Diameter)	ID (mm)		3.6-4.8	4.8-5.8	5.8-6.5	6.5-7.4	7.4-8.2	8.2-9.0	9.0-10.7	10.7
	Branchoscope (Statrz)	Size		2.5	3.0	3.5	4.0	4.5	5.0	5.0	6.0
		ID (mm)		3.5	4.3	5.0	6.0	6.6	7.1	7.5	7.5
		OD (mm)		4.2	5.0	5.7	6.7	7.3	7.8	8.2	8.2
	Endotracheal Tube (Portex)	ID (mm)	2.5	3.0	3.5	4.0	4.5	5.0	6.0	7.0	8.0
		OD (mm)	3.4	4.2	4.8	5.4	6.2	6.8	8.2	9.6	10.8

Postoperative Care

Since tracheostomies in children are mostly used as a long-term artificial airway, long-term caregiving concepts have had to be developed. Children with chronic tracheostomies face the potential hazards of airway compromise, and optimal care is aimed at reducing this risk [31–33].

Postoperative care of patients undergoing tracheostomy is often underemphasized. Perhaps the most critical event after tracheostomy is the tube change, although many other aspects of tube care are critical (e.g., suctioning, hygiene, humidity, emergency protocol training).

Tracheostomy Tube Changes

For optimal management of patients with tracheostomy tubes, it is imperative to know when to change the tube. There are several indications for tube changing, such as those listed by White et al. [34]:

- First change: 7–14 days after placement
- To reduce the size of the tube (as part of weaning from mechanical ventilation and to facilitate vocalization and swallowing)
- Routine change as part of ongoing airway management (every 60–90 days)
- Malpositioned tube due to incorrect length or size
- Patient–ventilator asynchrony with a tracheostomy tube problem suspected
- Cuff leak
- Tube or flange fracture
- To allow passage of a bronchoscope (larger tube)
- To change the type of tube (e.g., need for a tube with an inner cannula)

The frequency of tube changes also depends on the material of the tube and the presence of infection and/or secretions. PVC, which is most widely used for pediatric tracheostomy tubes, can allow tubes to stay in place for several weeks. Additionally, it is important to observe the conditions of the removed tube (tracheobronchial secretions adhered to the walls, for example) and the individual characteristics of the patient (the amount of mucus production and general health factors).

The first tracheostomy tube change is performed once the tracheostomy tract has matured. The indications for the first tracheostomy tube change include downsizing the tube to improve patient comfort, to reduce pressure on the tracheal mucosa by reducing the tube external diameter, and to facilitate speech. Some patients may need adjustment of the original tracheostomy tube size or length [35]. Conventional practice recommends changing the first tube 7–14 days following placement in adults [36]. However, there are no data to support this specific time frame, which is suggested to allow stable endotracheal–cutaneous tract formation. In children, a much shorter changing time might be reasonable [37].

There is little evidence to guide when to change a long-term tracheostomy tube. Some reasons often considered to support routine tracheostomy tube changes include:

- Prevention of granulation tissue formation around the tracheostomy tube [38]
- Prevention of tube blockage from excessive secretions
- Facilitation of weaning or speech by changing the size or type of tracheostomy tube

Based on the American Thoracic Society guideline for long-term tracheostomy child care, flexible PVC tubes may be used for 3–4 months before they stiffen. Alternatively, a metal tracheostomy tube may be used indefinitely, as long as there is no cracking of the soldered joint [30]. There appears to be considerable variability in practice from one institution to another [34].

Both authors of this chapter work in a local reference institution for patients in home care mechanical ventilation program. The program has a current capacity of 30 children and is always full, as there is a perpetual waiting list for dehospitalization in our public health system.

The protocol adopted by our multidisciplinary team program recommends a routine plastic tube change every 2 months. For metal tubes (which are used in only about 25% of our pediatric patients), the recommendation is a routine change every 3 months (the average time for tube material oxidation and "peeling" appearance).

Registering the date of each change, the reason (routine or not), the conditions of the removed tube, the size of the new tube, and the status of the tracheostoma (granulomas, infection, stenosis) is done systematically. It is also imperative to document in the medical records if the change happened without problems or difficulties. Otherwise, the difficulties must be detailed.

For tube changes, precautions must be taken regarding:

- The positioning of the patient (see Fig. 10)
- Availability of spare tubes (different sizes)
- Availability of a surgical tray and intubation material
- Airway aspiration before and after the change, including during cuff deflation (aspiration of secretions accumulated above the cuff)

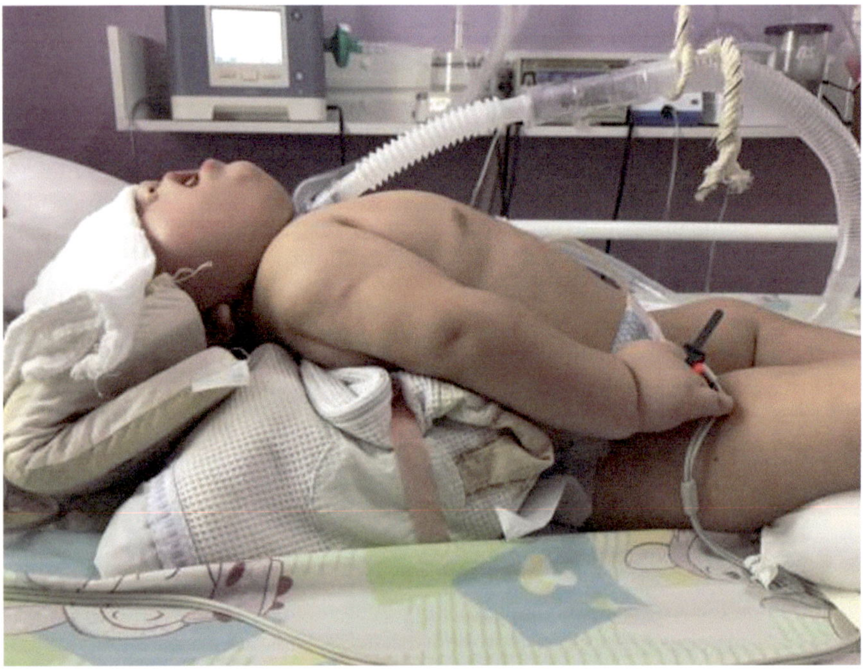

Fig. 10 Child positioned (with neck extension) for tube changing in a home care program

Fixation of the Tube

Various materials such as Velcro ties, twill tapes, silk ribbons, elastic straps with hooks, and stainless steel chains are available to secure the tube in place. How well the tie is secured is the most important aspect of choosing a tracheostomy tie—not the material. In children, especially in those with tracheostomies for bypassing an obstructed upper airway, preventing accidental decannulation is vital [39].

There is a risk of tracheostomy dislodgement during the tie placement, and it is important that one person maintain the airway by securing the tracheostomy tube in place, while the other person secures the tie. There is no consensus on the fit of the tie. The tie must be tight enough to secure the tube and loose enough to avoid skin breakdown and vascular obstruction [30].

Tracheostomy tie changes should be performed as required, if they become wet or soiled (e.g., due to secretions), to maintain skin integrity [34].

Tube Hygiene

An essential component of tracheostomized child management is maintaining and ensuring a patent airway by suctioning [39]. Techniques for suctioning are designed to efficiently clear the airway of mucus while avoiding the potential hazards of suctioning. The techniques described in the nursing and respiratory care literature recommend suctioning the patient if they are critically ill and has an artificial airway [40–45]. Suctioning for a child with a tracheostomy should be done in the most effective and least traumatic way possible [39].

Cuff

The indications for cuffed tracheostomy tubes are rather limited in pediatric patients. However, when they are indicated, modern high-volume/low-pressure cuffs are nowadays usually preferred to the traditional low-volume/high-pressure ones to minimize the risks of airway trauma [46].

However, cuff pressure and volume have to be monitored to remain at "just sealed" or "minimum occlusion" pressures/volumes in order to prevent ischemia of the airway mucosa.

Humidification

The upper airway works as a filter, heater, and humidifier of the inspired air. When the upper airway is bypassed, as in intubated or tracheostomized patients, unheated, nonhumidified air is inhaled [39].

A significant humidity deficit can result in pathological changes in the structure and function of the airways. These changes include loss of ciliary action, damage to mucous glands, disorganization of airway epithelium and basement membranes, cellular desquamation, and thickening of mucous secretions [47]. The ultimate consequences include deterioration of pulmonary function and an increased risk of infection.

Heat and humidity may be added to the inspired gas by different methodologies. Heated humidifiers, usually employed during mechanical ventilation in ICUs or mechanical ventilation in home care, are efficient and safe but are also costly and inconvenient. Nebulizers combine efficacy and safety with low cost in comparison with heated humidifiers. However, the necessary equipment, including a gas flow generator and tubing, makes them inconvenient for active children.

Factors such as efficacy, safety, cost, convenience, and the child's respiratory status should be considered for each individual application. An ideal device for every application is not currently available [30].

Home Care Routines and Emergency Care

Family education and many other factors beyond the purpose of this discussion are the key to successful transition from hospital to home-based care. Parents and/or caregivers who will take a tracheostomized child home should learn how to perform routine tracheostomy care and how to identify and manage tracheostomy complications [9].

The home care teaching should begin even before the actual tracheostomy. It should be individualized to the child and family, taking into account unique ethnic and language needs. A rooming-in period before discharge, affording the family the opportunity to implement the care plan, should be encouraged. In addition, a day pass may be considered.

All home care equipment, including portable equipment, should be used in the hospital before discharge. A child with a tracheostomy, whether in an institutional or home environment, should be cared for only by individuals who have been trained. The physician who was responsible for the decision to place a tracheostomy is also responsible for ensuring that adequate training for the parents and/or other caregivers is available. Before discharge home, two adults who will be consistent caregivers should be trained by the multidisciplinary health care team [9].

In our protocol, when hospital discharge is decided upon, the child is transferred to an intermediate care unit, where the parents, family members, or caregivers stay by the bed, learning all of the care needed by the child, from bathing to handling and tracheostomy care. After checking the clinical conditions for discharge, the patient is referred for evaluation and training by the home care team. The child with clinical stability, suitable social conditions, and suitable and trained caregivers is then scheduled to be discharged from hospital to home-based care.

Decannulation, Complications, and Mortality

Tracheostomized children are complex patients. It has already been pointed out that tracheostomized children present more acute complications related to anatomical surgical difficulties in comparison with adults. Furthermore, most of them will not be able to decannulate, because of multiple associated diseases. Children with neurological impairment have poor prospects for decannulation [19, 48]. Because of that, late complications related to long-term tracheostomy use are also expected. Complication rates as high as 77% and up to 3.6% specific mortality have been reported (the overall mortality, including deaths not related to the procedure, may reach 42%) [19, 49].

Examples of early complications (within 7 days of the procedure) are bleeding, accidental decannulation, mucus plugging, pneumothorax/pneumomediastinum, and subcutaneous emphysema [19, 50]. They are less common than late complications [49].

Examples of late complications (after 7 days) are peristome/suprastomal granulation (see Fig. 11), tracheal stenosis, tracheomalacia, infection, stomal breakdown,

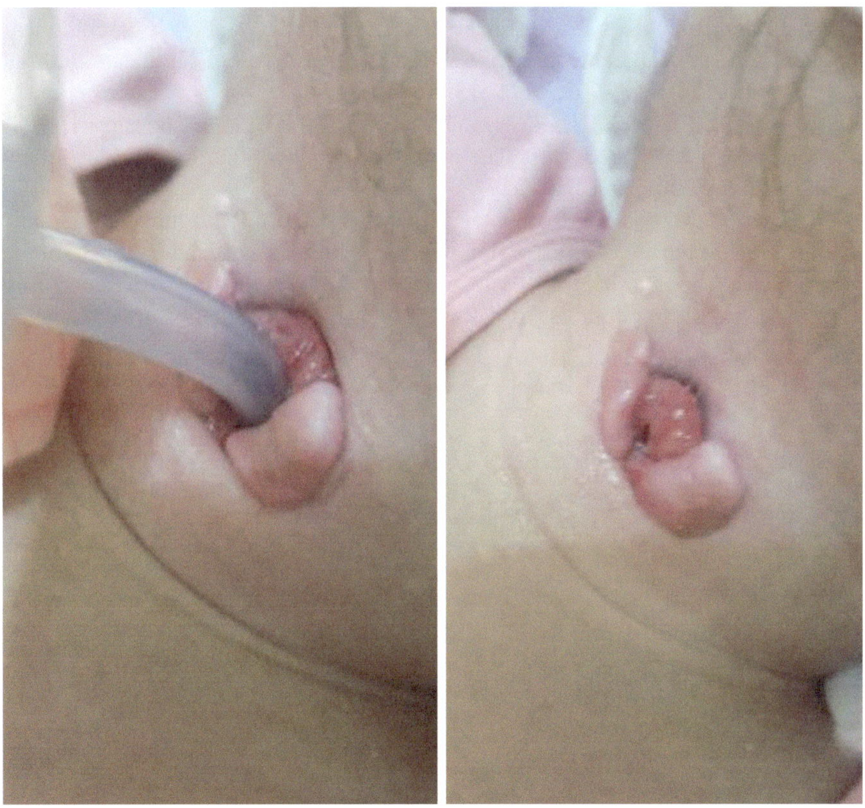

Fig. 11 Child receiving home care ventilator support with a stomal granuloma, better evaluated during a tube change. This is the most common complication in tracheostomized children but is mostly harmless. It may cause stomal stenosis and self-limited bleeding

and tracheoesophageal fistula [19, 50]. That is why the guideline for children requiring chronic tracheostomy care recommends airway evaluation with either a rigid or flexible bronchoscopy every 6–12 months, searching for early detection of airway complications, ensuring appropriate tracheostomy tube size and position, and determining readiness for decannulation [30].

In children, the most common tracheostomy-related cause of death has been reported to be cannula obstruction, followed by cannula misplacement and accidental decannulation [50].

Recommended Reading Campisi P, Forte V. Pediatric tracheostomy. Seminars in Pediatric Surgery 2016;25(3):191–5.

- Deutsch ES. Tracheostomy: pediatric considerations. Respiratory Care 2010;55(8):1082–90.
- Oberwaldner B, Eber E. Tracheostomy care in the home. Paediatric Respiratory Reviews 2006;7(3):185–90.
- Eber E, Oberwaldner B. Tracheostomy care in the hospital. Paediatric Respiratory Reviews 2006;7(3):175–84.
- Kremer B, Botos-Kremer AI, Eckel HE, Schlöndorff G. Indications, complications, and surgical techniques for pediatric tracheostomies—an update. Journal of Pediatric Surgery 2002;37(11):1556–62.
- Tweedie DJ, Skilbeck CJ, Cochrane LA, Cooke J, Wyatt ME. Choosing a paediatric tracheostomy tube: an update on current practice. Journal of Laryngology and Otology 2008;122(2):161–9.
- Sherman JM, Davis S, Albamonte-Petrick S, Chatburn RL, Fitton C, Green C, et al. Care of the child with a chronic tracheostomy. This official statement of the American Thoracic Society was adopted by the ATS Board of Directors, July 1999. American Journal of Respiratory and Critical Care Medicine 2000;161(1):297–308.
- Strychowsky JE, Albert D, Chan K, Cheng A, Daniel SJ, De Alarcon A, et al. International Pediatric Otolaryngology Group (IPOG) consensus recommendations: Routine peri-operative pediatric tracheotomy care. Int J Pediatr Otorhinolaryngol. 2016;86:250-5.

References

1. Age & Stages by American Academy of Pediatrics. 2017. https://www.healthychildren.org/English/ages-stages/Pages/default.aspx?nfstatus=401&nftoken=00000000-0000-0000-0000-000000000000&nfstatusdescription=ERROR%3A+No+local+token.
2. Guidance for Industry and FDA Staff: Pediatric Expertise for Advisory Panels [Internet]. 2003. https://www.fda.gov/downloads/MedicalDevices/DeviceRegulationandGuidance/GuidanceDocuments/ucm082188.pdf.
3. Knoppert D, Reed M, Benavides S, et al. Paediatric Age Categories to be Used in Differentiating Between Listing on a Model Essential Medicines List for Children. 1st ed. [ebook] World Health Organisation (WHO). 2007. p.4. Available at: http://archives.who.int/eml/expcom/children/Items/PositionPaperAgeGroups.pdf [Accessed 29 Oct. 2017]

4. Huelke DF. An overview of anatomical considerations of infants and children in the adult world of automobile safety designs. Annu Proc Assoc Adv Automot Med. 1998;42:92–113.
5. Macfarlane F. Paediatric anatomy and physiology and the basics of paediatric anaesthesia. Association of Anaesthetists of Great Britain and Ireland. 2005. http://wwwaagbiorg/node/914.
6. Mok Q. Tracheostomies in paediatric intensive care: evolving indications and changing expectations. Arch Dis Child. 2012;97(10):858–9.
7. Schmidt AR, Weiss M, Engelhardt T. The paediatric airway: basic principles and current developments. Eur J Anaesthesiol. 2014;31(6):293–9.
8. Litman RS, Weissend EE, Shibata D, Westesson PL. Developmental changes of laryngeal dimensions in unparalyzed, sedated children. Anesthesiology. 2003;98(1):41–5.
9. Deutsch ES. Tracheostomy: pediatric considerations. Respir Care. 2010;55(8):1082–90.
10. Holzki J, Laschat M, Puder C. Iatrogenic damage to the pediatric airway. Mechanisms and scar development. Paediatr Anaesth. 2009;19(Suppl 1):131–46.
11. Cochrane LA, Bailey CM. Surgical aspects of tracheostomy in children. Paediatr Respir Rev. 2006;7(3):169–74.
12. Lewis CW, Carron JD, Perkins JA, Sie KC, Feudtner C. Tracheotomy in pediatric patients: a national perspective. Arch Otolaryngol Head Neck Surg. 2003;129(5):523–9.
13. Schweiger C, Manica D, Becker CF, Abreu LS, Manzini M, Sekine L, et al. Tracheostomy in children: a ten-year experience from a tertiary center in southern Brazil. Braz J Otorhinolaryngol. 2016;
14. Hadfield PJ, Lloyd-Faulconbridge RV, Almeyda J, Albert DM, Bailey CM. The changing indications for paediatric tracheostomy. Int J Pediatr Otorhinolaryngol. 2003;67(1):7–10.
15. Kremer B, Botos-Kremer AI, Eckel HE, Schlöndorff G. Indications, complications, and surgical techniques for pediatric tracheostomies—an update. J Pediatr Surg. 2002;37(11):1556–62.
16. Gergin O, Adil EA, Kawai K, Watters K, Moritz E, Rahbar R. Indications of pediatric tracheostomy over the last 30 years: has anything changed? Int J Pediatr Otorhinolaryngol. 2016;87:144–7.
17. Serra A, Cocuzza S, Longo MR, Grillo C, Bonfiglio M, Pavone P. Tracheostomy in childhood: new causes for an old strategy. Eur Rev Med Pharmacol Sci. 2012;16(12):1719–22.
18. Dal'Astra AP, Quirino AV, Caixeta JA, Avelino MA. Tracheostomy in childhood: review of the literature on complications and mortality over the last three decades. Braz J Otorhinolaryngol. 2017;83(2):207–14.
19. Wilcox LJ, Weber BC, Cunningham TD, Baldassari CM. Tracheostomy complications in institutionalized children with long-term tracheostomy and ventilator dependence. Otolaryngol Head Neck Surg. 2016;154(4):725–30.
20. Campisi P, Forte V. Pediatric tracheostomy. Semin Pediatr Surg. 2016;25(3):191–5.
21. Yaneza MM, James HL, Davies P, Harrison S, McAlorum L, Clement WA, et al. Changing indications for paediatric tracheostomy and the role of a multidisciplinary tracheostomy clinic. J Laryngol Otol. 2015;129(9):882–6.
22. Trachsel D, Hammer J. Indications for tracheostomy in children. Paediatr Respir Rev. 2006;7(3):162–8.
23. Strychowsky JE, Albert D, Chan K, Cheng A, Daniel SJ, De Alarcon A, et al. International Pediatric Otolaryngology Group (IPOG) consensus recommendations: routine peri-operative pediatric tracheotomy care. Int J Pediatr Otorhinolaryngol. 2016;86:250–5.
24. Gollu G, Ates U, Can OS, Kendirli T, Yagmurlu A, Cakmak M, et al. Percutaneous tracheostomy by Griggs technique under rigid bronchoscopic guidance is safe and feasible in children. J Pediatr Surg. 2016;51(10):1635–9.
25. Song JJ, Choi IJ, Chang H, Kim DW, Chang HW, Park GH, et al. Pediatric tracheostomy revisited: a nine-year experience using horizontal intercartilaginous incision. Laryngoscope. 2015;125(2):485–92.
26. Tweedie DJ, Skilbeck CJ, Cochrane LA, Cooke J, Wyatt ME. Choosing a paediatric tracheostomy tube: an update on current practice. J Laryngol Otol. 2008;122(2):161–9.
27. Shibasaki M, Nakajima Y, Ishii S, Shimizu F, Shime N, Sessler DI. Prediction of pediatric endotracheal tube size by ultrasonography. Anesthesiology. 2010;113(4):819–24.

28. King BR, Baker MD, Braitman LE, Seidl-Friedman J, Schreiner MS. Endotracheal tube selection in children: a comparison of four methods. Ann Emerg Med. 1993;22(3):530–4.
29. Eipe N, Barrowman N, Writer H, Doherty D. A weight-based formula for tracheal tube size in children. Paediatr Anaesth. 2009;19(4):343–8.
30. Sherman JM, Davis S, Albamonte-Petrick S, Chatburn RL, Fitton C, Green C, et al. Care of the child with a chronic tracheostomy. This official statement of the American Thoracic Society was adopted by the ATS Board of Directors, July 1999. Am J Respir Crit Care Med. 2000;161(1):297–308.
31. Shinkwin CA, Gibbin KP. Tracheostomy in children. J R Soc Med. 1996;89(4):188–92.
32. Carr MM, Poje CP, Kingston L, Kielma D. Heard C. Complications in pediatric tracheostomies. Laryngoscope. 2001;111(11 Pt 1):1925–8.
33. Alladi A, Rao S, Das K, Charles AR, D'Cruz AJ. Pediatric tracheostomy: a 13-year experience. Pediatr Surg Int. 2004;20(9):695–8.
34. White AC, Kher S, O'Connor HH. When to change a tracheostomy tube. Respir Care. 2010;55(8):1069–75.
35. Schmidt U, Hess D, Kwo J, Lagambina S, Gettings E, Khandwala F, et al. Tracheostomy tube malposition in patients admitted to a respiratory acute care unit following prolonged ventilation. Chest. 2008;134(2):288–94.
36. De Leyn P, Bedert L, Delcroix M, Depuydt P, Lauwers G, Sokolov Y, et al. Tracheotomy: clinical review and guidelines. Eur J Cardiothorac Surg. 2007;32(3):412–21.
37. Deutsch ES. Early tracheostomy tube change in children. Arch Otolaryngol Head Neck Surg. 1998;124(11):1237–8.
38. Yaremchuk K. Regular tracheostomy tube changes to prevent formation of granulation tissue. Laryngoscope. 2003;113(1):1–10.
39. Oberwaldner B, Eber E. Tracheostomy care in the home. Paediatr Respir Rev. 2006;7(3):185–90.
40. Chang V. Protocol for prevention of complications of endotracheal intubation. Crit Care Nurse. 1995;15(5):19–20.
41. Glass CA, Grap MJ. Ten tips for safer suctioning. AJN. 1995;95(5):51–3.
42. Carroll P. Safe suctioning prn. RN. 1994;57(5):32–8.
43. Branson RD, Campbell RS, Chatburn RL, Covington J. Endotracheal suctioning of mechanically ventilated adults and children with artificial airways. Int Anesthesiol Clin. 1996;34(1):73–80.
44. Runton N. Suctioning artificial airways in children: appropriate technique. Pediatr Nurs. 1991;18(2):115–8.
45. Hodge D. Endotracheal suctioning and the infant: a nursing care protocol to decrease complications. Neonatal Netw. 1991;9(5):7–15.
46. Newth CJ, Rachman B, Patel N, Hammer J. The use of cuffed versus uncuffed endotracheal tubes in pediatric intensive care. J Pediatr. 2004;144(3):333–7.
47. Van Oostdam J, Walker D, Knudson K, Dirks P, Dahlby R, Hogg J. Effect of breathing dry air on structure and function of airways. J Appl Physiol. 1986;61(1):312–7.
48. Tsuboi N, Ide K, Nishimura N, Nakagawa S, Morimoto N. Pediatric tracheostomy: survival and long-term outcomes. Int J Pediatr Otorhinolaryngol. 2016;89:81–5.
49. Eber E, Oberwaldner B. Tracheostomy care in the hospital. Paediatr Respir Rev. 2006;7(3):175–84.
50. Das P, Zhu H, Shah RK, Roberson DW, Berry J, Skinner ML. Tracheotomy-related catastrophic events: results of a national survey. Laryngoscope. 2012;122(1):30–7.

Tracheostomy and Obesity

André Leonardo de Castro Costa, Marcus Antônio de Mello Borba, Daniela Silva Santos, and Terence Pires de Farias

Epidemiology

The Obesity Medicine Association defines obesity as "a chronic, relapsing, multifactorial neurobehavioral disease, wherein an increase in body fat promotes adipose tissue dysfunction and abnormal fat mass physical forces, resulting in adverse metabolic, biomechanical, and psychosocial health consequences" [1].

Being overweight or obese—defined as having excess body weight in relation to height according to the World Health Organization (WHO)—is associated with genetic, behavioral, socioeconomic, and environmental factors.

A.L. de Castro Costa, M.D., M.Sc. (✉)
Department of Stomatology, Federal University of Bahia, Salvador, Bahia, Brazil

Department of Head and Neck Surgery, Aristides Maltez Hospital, Salvador, Bahia, Brazil

Department of Head and Neck Surgery, Portuguese Hospital, Salvador, Bahia, Brazil
e-mail: costaalc@gmail.com

M.A. de Mello Borba, Ph.D.
Faculty of Medicine, Department of Experimental Surgery and Surgical Specialties, Federal University of Bahia, Salvador, BA, Brazil

Department of Head and Neck Surgery, Portuguese Hospital, Salvador, BA, Brazil

Department of Head and Neck Surgery, Aristides Maltez Hospital, Salvador, BA, Brazil

D.S. Santos, M.D.
Depattment of Head and Neck Surgery, Portuguese Hospital, Salvador, BA, Brazil

T.P. de Farias, M.D., Ph.D., M.Sc., Researcher.
Department of Head and Neck Surgery, Brazilian National Cancer Institute—INCA, Rio de Janeiro, RJ, Brazil

Department of Head and Neck Surgery, Pontifical Catholic University, Rio de Janeiro, RJ, Brazil

T.P. de Farias (ed.), *Tracheostomy*, https://doi.org/10.1007/978-3-319-67867-2_9

Table 1 Common classifications of body weight in adults and children

	Age	Indicator	Normal weight	Overweight	Obese
Adults[b]	≥20 years	BMI (kg/m^2)	18.50–24.99	≥25.00	≥30.00[a]
				Preobese[c]: 25.00–29.99	Class 1: 30.00–34.99
					Class 2: 35.00–39.99
					Class 3: ≥40.00
Children					
International					
WHO 2006[d]	0–6 months	BMI Z or WH Z	>–2 to ≤2 SDs	>2 to ≤3 SDs	>3 SDs
			At risk of overweight: >1 to ≤2 SDs		
WHO 2007[e]	5–19 years	BMI Z	>–2 to ≤1 SD	>1 to ≤2 SDs	>2 SDs
IOTF[f]	2–18 years	Growth curve for BMI at age 18		BMI = 25	BMI = 30
US[g]	2–19 years	BMI percentile	≥5th to <85th	≥85th to <95th	≥95th

BMI body mass index, *CDC* Centers for Disease Control and Prevention, *IOTF* International Obesity Task Force, *SD* standard deviation, *WH* weight-for-height, *WHO* World Health Organization, *Z* z score

[a]Per WHO 2000 classifications, in BMI as kg/m^2 [139]. These categories, if not the exact terminology, of adult weight status have been adopted by other major health organizations, including the US National Heart, Lung, and Blood Institute and National Institute of Diabetes and Digestive and Kidney Diseases

[b]In the USA, typically "class" is referred to as "grade." Obesity has an unofficial cut point of BMI ≥27 kg/m^2 in Asian populations

[c]Preobesity has an unofficial cut point of 23 to <27 kg/m^2 in Asian populations

[d]Per the WHO 2006 classifications, BMI Z are BMI z scores, and WH Z are WH z scores, based on age- and sex-specific growth standards for children aged 0–60 months. In children aged <2 years, weight-for-length is used

[e]Per the WHO 2007 classifications, BMI Z are BMI z scores based on age- and sex-specific growth standards and references for children aged 5–19 years

[f]Per Cole et al. [140], for the IOTF, based on age- and sex-specific curves defined to pass through BMIs of 25 or 30 kg/m^2 at the age of 18 years, for children aged 2–18 years

[g]Per the CDC 2000 classifications, BMI percentiles are based on age- and sex-specific growth references for children aged 2–19 years

The criteria currently most widely used for classifying weight-to-height is the body mass index (BMI: the body weight in kilograms, divided by squared height in meters) (Table 1) in adults, which ranges from underweight or wasting (<18.5 kg/m^2) to severe or morbid obesity (≥40 kg/m^2). Children have many specific and geographical criteria, which are also detailed in Table 1 [2, 3].

In 2013, an estimated one in three adults worldwide was overweight or obese, and adult obesity exceeded 50% in several countries around the globe.

While the prevalence of adult obesity in the developed world seems to have stabilized, the global prevalence of obesity in children and adolescents, as well as adult obesity in developing countries, is still increasing. In addition, some developed countries continue to observe an increasing prevalence of extreme classes of obesity [2].

More than half of the Brazilian population (56.9%)—about 82 million people—were classified as overweight or obese in 2013 [4]. In this same year, it was reported that obesity affected one in five Brazilians aged 18 years or older, most of whom were women (24.4% versus 16.8% of men). Over a 10-year period, obesity among women aged 20 years or older rose from 14.0% in 2003, according to the Household Budgets Survey, to 25.2% in 2013, according to the National Health Survey. Among men, this rate grew more modestly, from 9.3% to 17.5%. The accumulation of abdominal fat was also more frequently found in the female sex, affecting 52.1% of women and 21.8% of men [5].

Causes of Obesity

Obesity is a multifactorial disease, which includes endocrine, immune, environmental, neurobehavioral, and genetic/epigenetic components, and affects numerous organ systems, increasing the risks of hypertension, thromboembolic events, asthma, obstructive sleep apnea, stroke, nerve entrapment, psychosocial dysfunction, and a host of other cardiometabolic disorders.

Indications for Tracheostomy in Obese Patients

Tracheostomy, a procedure commonly performed in the management of critically ill patients, is increasingly becoming indicated in obese patients.

Recently, a study demonstrated that prolonged ventilation and obstructive sleep apnea are the main indications for tracheostomy in this population [6].

Percutaneous Versus Open Surgical Techniques

Obese critically ill patients are at greater risk for requiring intubation and prolonged mechanical ventilation; in some cases, it is necessary to perform a tracheostomy.

Tracheostomy is one of the most common surgical procedures performed in critically ill patients. The prevalence reported in studies around the world varies between 10% and 20% [7].

The relative contraindications to percutaneous tracheostomy include obesity and a short neck. In an analysis from Oslo of more than 1000 patients undergoing percutaneous tracheostomy, no risk of complications was found in obese patients. BMI was recorded in 311 patients from 2006 to 2009. The rate of complications

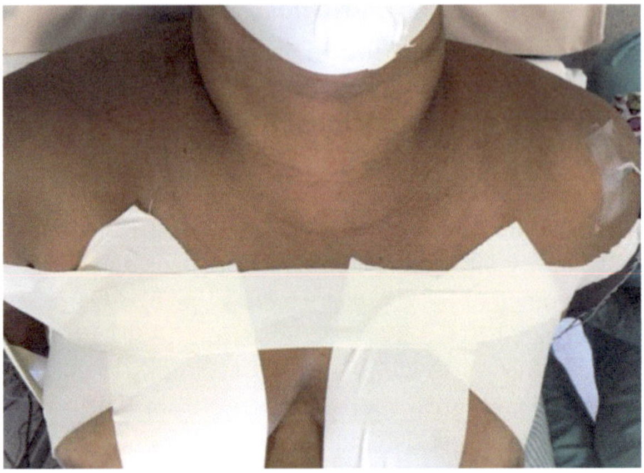

Fig. 1 Exposure of the trachea before performing an open tracheostomy procedure

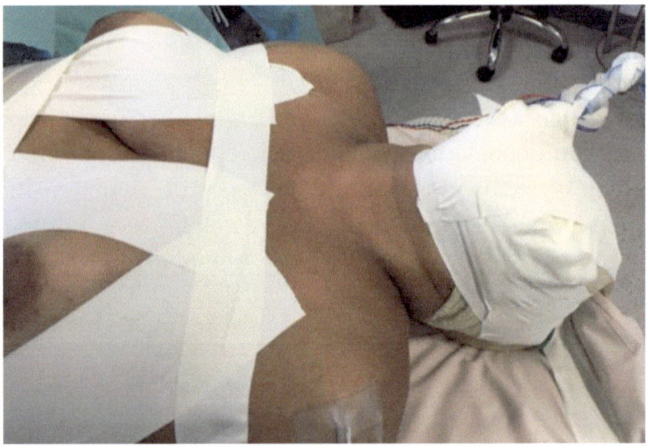

Fig. 2 Exposure of the trachea before performing an open tracheostomy procedure

(of all kinds) in patients with a BMI of 30 or higher (n = 541) was 12.2% compared with 13.0% in nonobese patients (odds ratio [OR] 0.9, 95% confidence interval [CI] 0.3–2.5). The 90-day mortality rates were 30% (95% CI 25–35) and 26% (95% CI 21–31), respectively ($p > 0.05$). The median duration of the percutaneous tracheostomy procedure was 10 min in obese patients and 9 min in nonobese individuals [8].

The decision to perform percutaneous tracheostomy in a patient with obesity should take into account factors such as the individual patient's neck anatomy and the experience of the performing physician. In addition, the practitioner must be prepared to convert to an open surgical technique if complications arise during percutaneous tracheostomy.

Sometimes, unusual positions may be required to adequately expose the trachea, as seen in Figs. 1 and 2, prior to the tracheostomy procedure.

Types of Tubes

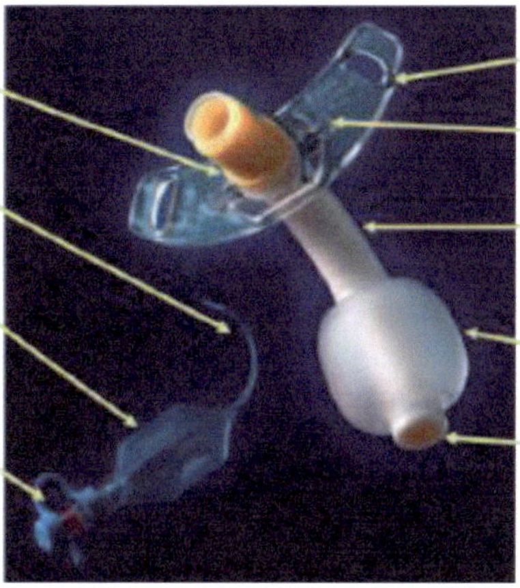

Fig. 3 Components of standard tracheostomy tubes

Tracheostomy tubes are used to facilitate the administration of positive pressure ventilation, to provide a patent airway in patients prone to upper airway obstruction, and to provide access to the lower respiratory tract for airway clearance. They are available in a variety of sizes and styles from several manufacturers. The inner diameter, outer diameter, and any other distinguishing characteristics (percutaneous, extra length, fenestrated) are marked on the flange of the tube as a guide to the clinician. Some features are relatively standard among typical tracheostomy tubes (Fig. 3) [9].

In obese patients, due to the thick layer of fat between the skin and the trachea (Fig. 4), the cannula should have some characteristics to facilitate better adaptation, like an adjustable lenght, for example (Fig. 5) If you don't have this device you can remove the addipose tissue between the trachea and the skin or put a suture to mobilize and closer the trachea to the skin. These maneuvers may facilitate the tracheostomy tube adjustment and are easier to perform during an open procedure.

Complications

Surgery is technically more difficult in obese patients than in nonobese patients, and is associated with higher complication rates arising from difficulties in accessing the airway due to anatomy or other medical and anatomical concerns in obese patients.

In particular, obese patients requiring tracheostomy face an increased risk of complications, primarily related to potentially fatal airway events, such as obstruction, accidental decannulation, and tracheostomy tube displacement. The most likely cause of these events is increased pretracheal soft tissue thickness (PTSTT),

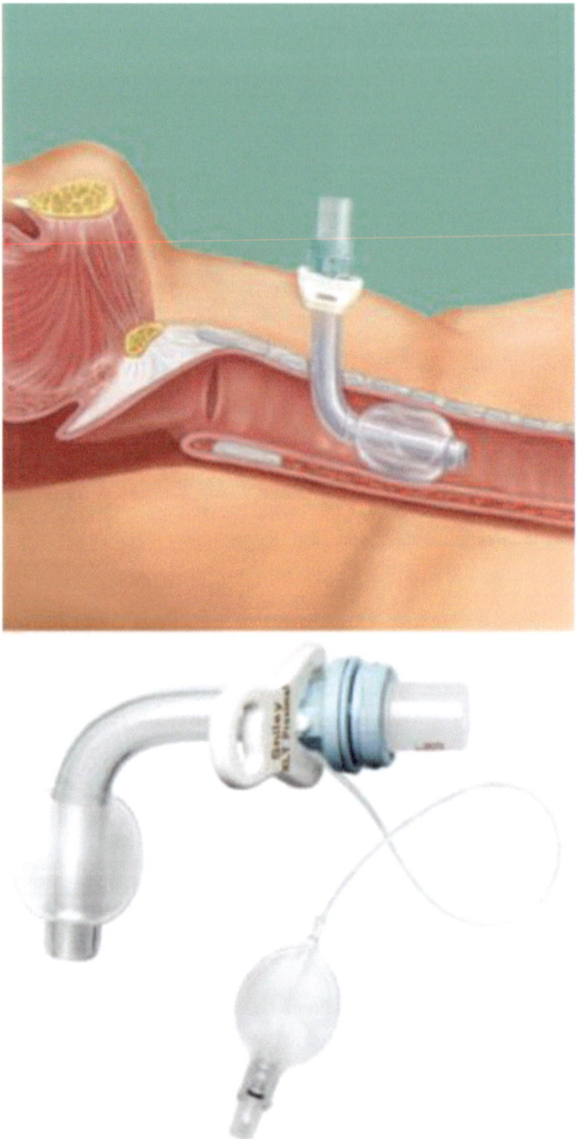

Fig. 4 Thick layer of fat in the neck and an adjustable tracheostomy tube

which effectively reduces the intratracheal length of the tracheostomy tube. Agitation, straining, and coughing may all result in decannulation or displacement of the tube into pretracheal soft tissues. Reinsertion of the tube may prove difficult as a result of thick pretracheal tissue, which can lead to creation of a false passage.

The use of ultrasound and fiberoptic bronchoscopy have decreased the incidence of complications related to percutaneous tracheostomy in obese patients [7], but neither modality is very feasible or cost effective. Both require specific equipment and trained specialists, and must sometimes be performed in a timely manner. Some

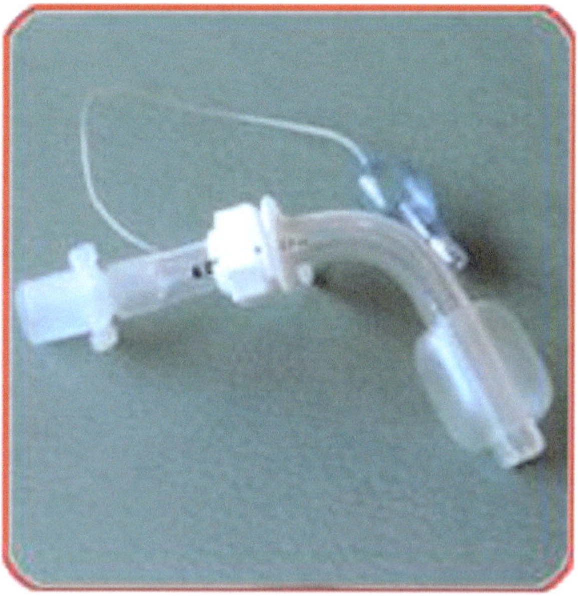

Fig. 5 Thick layer of fat in the neck and an adjustable tracheostomy tube

authors [10] have suggested a practical combination of arm and neck circumference measurements performed in the supine position to provide an equivalent correlation that can be used to select a suitable tracheostomy tube. Neck circumference is an anthropometric measurement that has been significantly correlated with BMI [6].

According to Cordes et al. [6], a relative risk calculation revealed a 2.823 greater risk of tracheostomy complications in obese patients. Analysis of variance (ANOVA) analysis revealed that BMI significantly influenced the procedure duration ($p < 0.0001$), yet multiple regression analysis found no significant association between a greater number of predicted complications and the procedure duration.

References

1. American Society of Bariatric Physicians. Obesity algorithm. 2016. http:// media.clinicaladvisor.com/documents/55/obesityalgorithm_13552.pdf. Accessed 23 Jan 2016.
2. Hruby A, Hu FB. The epidemiology of obesity: a big picture. PharmacoEconomics. 2015;33(7):673–89. https://doi.org/10.1007/s40273-014-0243-x.
3. Wang Y, Lim H. The global childhood obesity epidemic and the association between socio-economic status and childhood obesity. Int Rev Psychiatry. 2012;24(3):176–88. https://doi.org/10.3109/09540261.2012.688195.
4. Brasil. 2015a. http://teen.ibge.gov.br/noticias-teen/8354-como-vai-a-saude-dos-brasileiros.html. Accessed 3 Mar 2017.
5. Brasil. 2015b. http://saladeimprensa.ibge.gov.br/noticias.html?view=noticia&id=1&idnoticia=2965&busca=1&t=pns-2013-dois-anos-mais-metade-nascimentos-ocorreram-cesariana. Accessed 3 Mar 2017.
6. Cordes SR, Best AR, Hiatt KK. The impact of obesity on adult tracheostomy complication rate. Laryngoscope. 2015;125(1):105–10. https://doi.org/10.1002/lary.24793.

7. Romero CM, Cornejo RA, Ruiz MH, Galvez LR, Llanos OP, Tobar EA, et al. Fiberoptic bronchoscopy-assisted percutaneous tracheostomy is safe in obese critically ill patients: a prospective and comparative study. J Crit Care. 2009;24(4):494–500.
8. Rosseland LA, Laake JH, Stubhaug A. Percutaneous dilatational tracheotomy in intensive care unit patients with increased bleeding risk risk or obesity. A prospective analysis of 1000 procedures. Acta Anaesthesiol Scand. 2011;55(7):835–41.
9. Hess DR, Altobelli NP. Tracheostomy tubes. Respir Care. 2014;59(6):956–971.; discussion 971-3. https://doi.org/10.4187/respcare.02920.
10. Szeto C, et al. A simple method to predict pretracheal tissue thickness to prevent accidental decannulation in the obese. Otolaryngol Head Neck Surg. 2010;143(2):223–9. https://doi.org/10.1016/j.otohns.2010.03.007.

Oncological Tracheostomy

Carlos Eduardo Santa Ritta Barreira,
Marina Azzi Quintanilha, Terence Pires de Farias,
Jose Gabriel Miranda da Paixão, Juliana Fernandes
de Oliveira, Fernando Luiz Dias, and Paulo Jose
de Cavalcanti Siebra

Introduction

The prevalent reasons why tracheostomy is performed depends on each institution's policies. In general hospitals, most tracheostomies are performed due to prolonged intubation in intensive care units; in cancer centers they are performed mostly to manage the symptoms of growing head and neck cancers or in preparation for major surgeries to treat these tumors. Patients with tumors of the oral cavity, pharynx, or larynx, or other neck masses, may suffer airway narrowing, swallowing disorders, decreased mouth opening, dysphagia, and aspiration during disease progression. Airway intervention may occur before, during, or after the proposed treatment, and the timing to perform it has a profound impact on the patient's life. Although tracheostomy performance is part of head and neck surgical routine, literature regarding this theme is scarce, especially with regard to the indications and head and neck patient management (Figs. 1 and 2).

C.E.S.R. Barreira, M.D., Ph.D. (✉) • M.A. Quintanilha, M.D.
Department of Head and Neck Surgery, Santa Luzia Hospital, Brasília, DF, Brazil
e-mail: csantaritta@yahoo.com.br

T.P. de Farias, M.D., Ph.D., M.Sc., Researcher.
Department of Head and Neck Surgery, Brazilian National Cancer Institute—INCA,
Rio de Janeiro, RJ, Brazil

Department of Head and Neck Surgery, Pontifical Catholic University of Rio de Janeiro,
Rio de Janeiro, RJ, Brazil

F.L. Dias, M.D., Ph.D., M.Sc., F.A.C.S.
Head and Neck Surgery Department, Brazilian National Cancer Institute—INCA,
Rio de Janeiro, RJ, Brazil

Head and Neck Department, Pontifical Catholic University of Rio de Janeiro, Rio de Janeiro,
RJ, Brazil

J.G.M. da Paixão, M.D. • J.F. de Oliveira, M.D. • P.J. de Cavalcanti Siebra
Department of Head and Neck Surgery, Brazilian National Cancer Institute – INCA,
Rio de Janeiro, RJ, Brazil

T.P. de Farias (ed.), *Tracheostomy*, https://doi.org/10.1007/978-3-319-67867-2_10

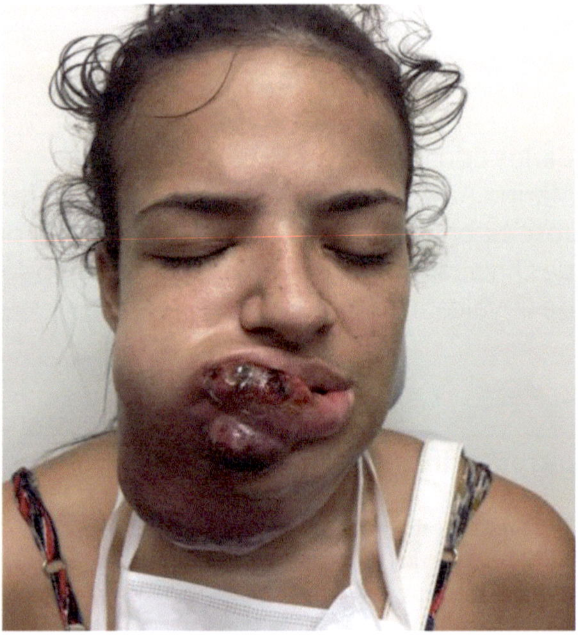

Fig. 1 Patient with decreased mouth opening and swallowing disorder

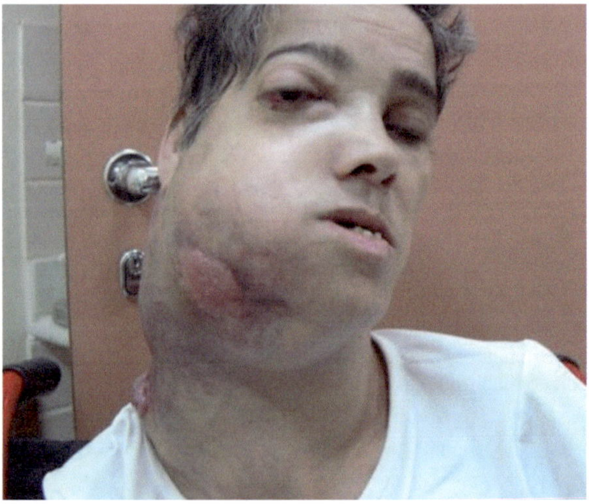

Fig. 2 Growing neck mass and narrowing airways

Indications in Oncological Patients

The management of airways in patients with head and neck tumors needs special attention by medical staff. In those cases, most tracheostomies are indicated to ensure optimal breathing conditions by preventing the growing tumor from

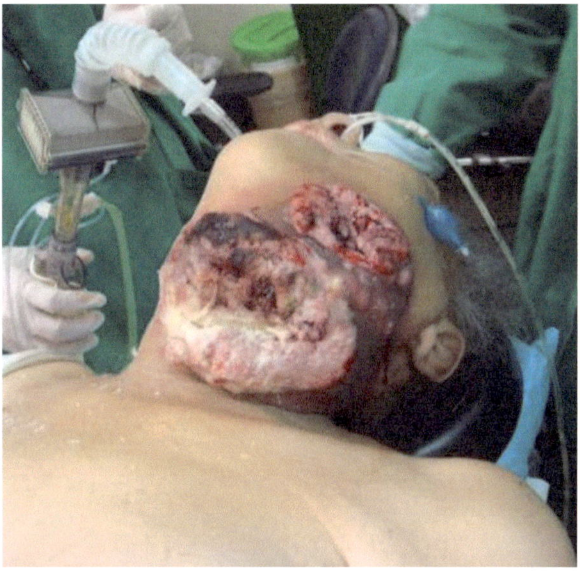

Fig. 3 Tracheostomy indication due to risk of airway blockage

blocking the airway, providing clearance of upper respiratory tract secretions, or protecting against or minimizing the risk of bronchoaspiration. The risk of airway blockage is a life-threatening condition and should be considered the most important indication to perform an elective tracheostomy in patients with head and neck tumors. This risk may be identified by any of the following respiratory signs and symptoms: inadequate ventilation; uncomfortable breathing; dyspnea; or nocturnal dyspnea, orthopnea, or stridor. Stridor [1] and these other signs are not common until an obstruction of greater than 50% occurs. Patients with compromised airways should undergo tracheostomy as soon as possible, in order to prevent the need for an emergency approach (Fig. 3).

During preparation for major surgery, patients may need definitive airway protection until complete recovery. Tracheostomies should be indicated when surgical conditions may lead to severe edema, risk of respiratory tract structure collapse, or bronchoaspiration. The risk of narrowing of the airway by edema should be considered in oral or laryngopharyngeal cancer resections. Although it is not easy to predict or measure the severity of edema and its consequences for respiratory conditions, two factors that play pivotal roles in determining airway protection are tumor localization and stage. Mandibulectomies, partial laryngectomies, and large reconstructions of the aerodigestive tract may lead to abnormal function and airway obstruction postoperatively. Swallowing disorders due to these surgeries may cause bronchoaspiration by secretion or bleeding. If there is a possibility of a postoperatively compromised airway, elective tracheostomy should be considered as a safe course of treatment [2]. In the UK, a national survey showed that 69% of maxillofacial surgical units perform elective tracheostomy routinely in patients with free flap reconstruction following ablative head and neck surgery [3] (Figs. 4 and 5).

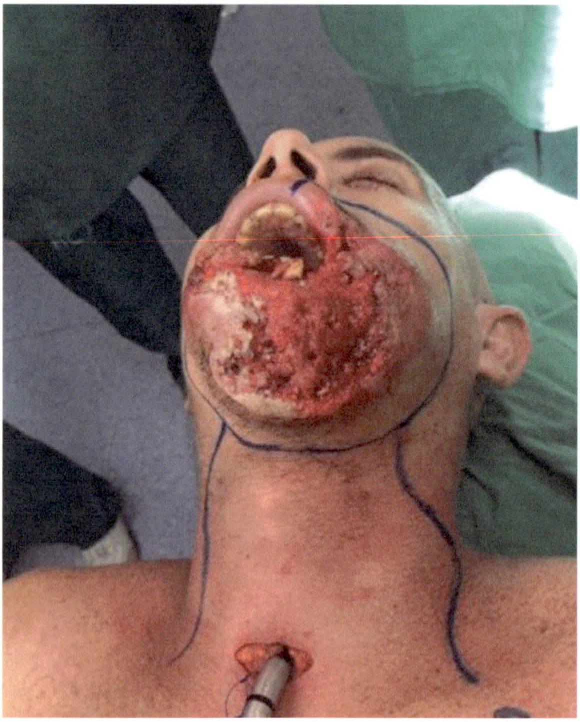

Fig. 4 Preparation for major surgery

Craniofacial surgeries are other major procedures that need respiratory attention in postoperative care. In addition to the aforementioned indications to protect airways and assist patient recovery, tracheostomy is indicated to avoid pneumocephalus [4]. It can occur as a complication due to positive air pressure in upper airways, collecting air or gas in the intracranial cavity. Fliss et al. reported a tension pneumocephalus incidence of 5.6% in skull base reconstructions after anterior subcranial tumor resection [5] (Figs. 6 and 7).

Emergency Tracheostomy in Oncological Patients

Patients with a delayed diagnosis and/or receiving treatment for head and neck tumors can suffer acute obstruction of the upper airways, and urgent tracheostomy can be frequently indicated in these situations [6, 7]. Urgent surgical airway intervention occurs with high stress levels and critical conditions, exposing patients to a higher risk of hypoxia and cardiopulmonary arrest. Research shows that the occurrence of complications is increased 2- to 5-fold in urgent situations [8–10] (Fig. 8).

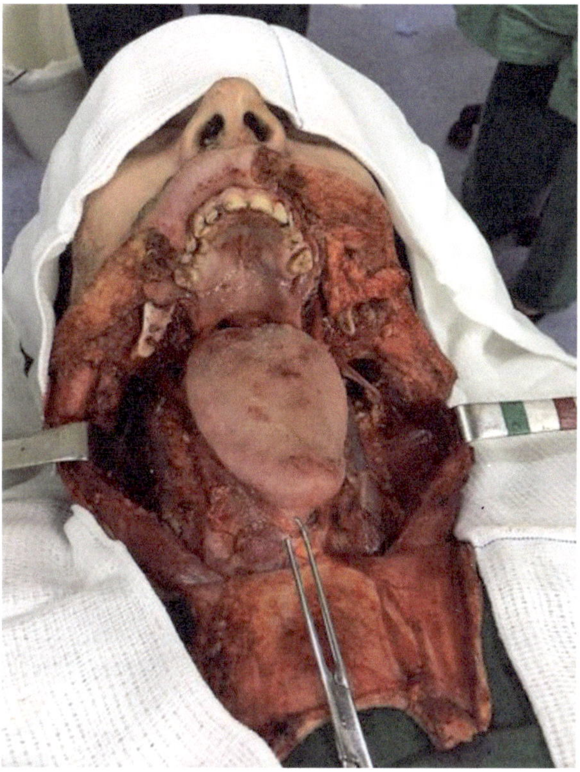

Fig. 5 After mandibulectomy and detachment of tongue muscles, leading to superior airway collapse

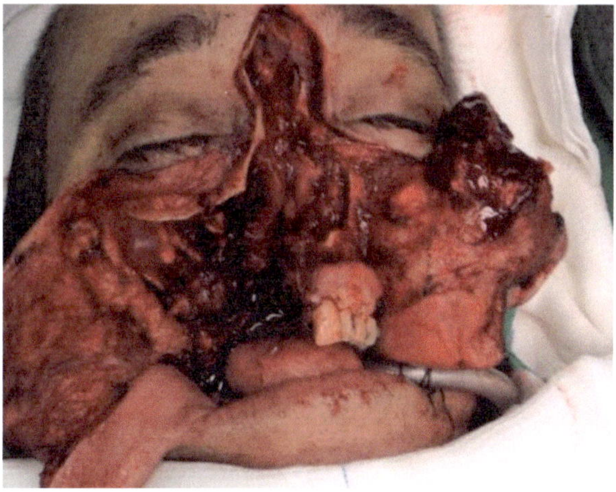

Fig. 6 Craniofacial surgery, showing potential communication between the central nervous system and the upper aerodigestive tract

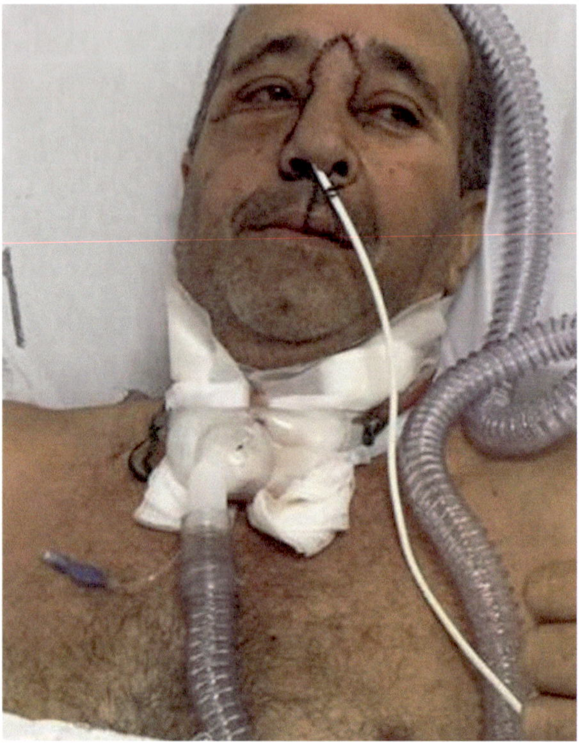

Fig. 7 After craniofacial surgery, with tracheostomy indicated to avoid positive air pressure in upper airways

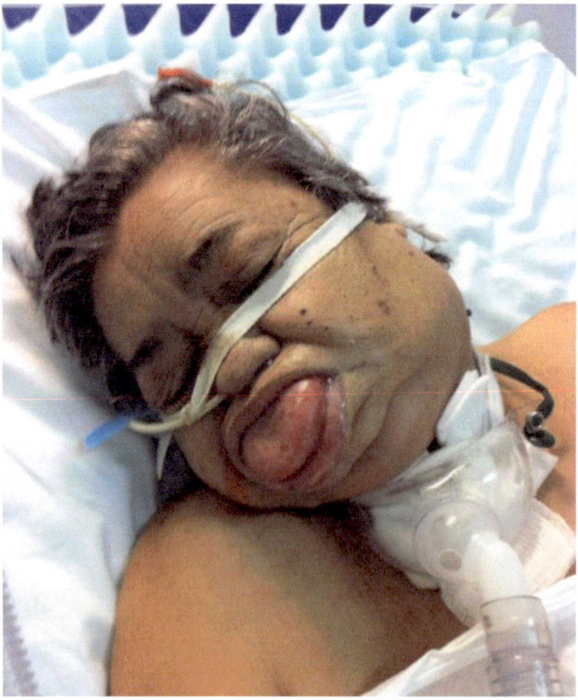

Fig. 8 Severe edema due to oropharyngeal tumor; tracheostomy was performed to secure the airway

Table 1 Tracheostomy indications in patients with head and neck tumors

Context	Signs and symptoms
Elective tracheostomy	Progressive airway narrowing
	Swallowing disorder
	Decreased mouth opening
	Aspiration
	Preparation for major surgery
Emergency tracheostomy	Acute airway obstruction Inadequate ventilation Uncomfortable breathing Dyspnea Nocturnal dyspnea, orthopnea, or stridor

Due to obstruction caused by tumor growth, orotracheal intubation—even for bronchoscopy—can be very difficult to execute, and a cricothyrotomy procedure should be avoided because of the possibility of tumor violation and contamination of surrounding tissues. Due to these peculiarities, emergency tracheostomy in patients with head and neck cancer is frequently performed on awake patients under local anesthesia. This procedure should be considered a safe and effective method to ensure airway patency in these patients [6, 11, 12] (Table 1).

Tracheostomy in Oral and Oropharyngeal Cancer

Patients with oral cancer may be eligible for tracheostomy at any stage of treatment, due to either the risk of airway blockage or a critical emergency of acute obstruction. Whether or not to perform tracheostomy may be a thorny decision for medical staff, as there are many factors influencing the difficulty of predicting airway maintenance, and because it has a profound impact on the patient's life—not only because of psychological aspects or nursing care, but also because it may increase the complication rate. Chest infection rates in patients undergoing major head and neck surgery may increase from 11% to 20% in tracheostomized patients [13].

Surgeons should evaluate surgical defects, resected structures, and functional loss and its consequences. The patient's clinical condition and pathological findings are important in making a decision. As a consensus, elective tracheostomy is considered the most effective and definitive method to ensure airway safety, and it is recommended for patients with a high risk of airway obstruction [2, 14, 15] (Figs. 9, 10, and 11).

In an attempt to clarify and provide criteria for indication for elective tracheostomy in patients with oral and oropharyngeal tumors, some authors have developed scoring systems based on multiple findings. Kruse-Lösler et al. [16] developed a system that predicts the likelihood of postoperative respiratory failure. They identified the following significant parameters for indication for tracheostomy: tumor size, tumor localization, multimorbidity, alcohol consumption, and pathologic chest X-ray findings. Kruse-Lösler considered the size and the localization to be the main significant factors

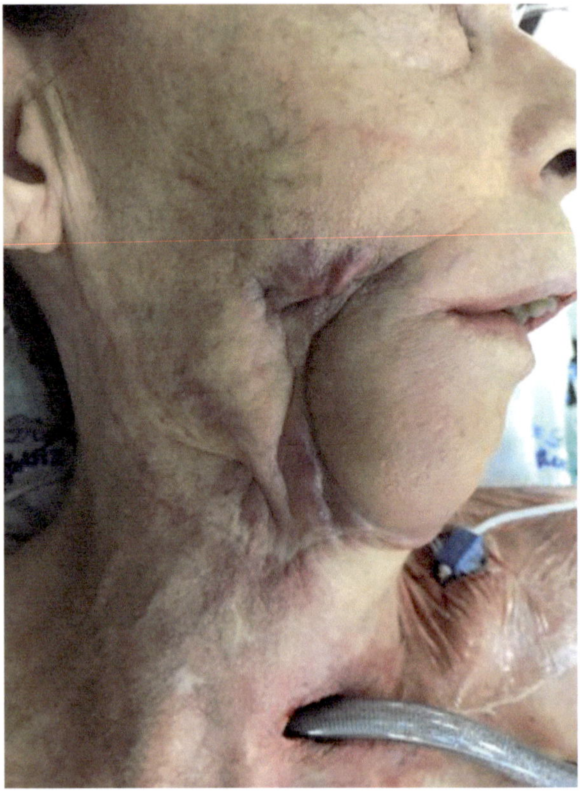

Fig. 9 Recurrent oral cavity tumor; tracheostomy was performed to prepare for the procedure

influencing the indication for tracheostomy. The patient's general medical condition, which includes cardiorespiratory disease and the level of alcohol consumption, were also considered important parameters. Based on different score values (Table 2), Kruse-Lösler recommended elective tracheostomy in patients with seven or more points [16].

However, the scoring system devised by Kruse-Lösler et al. lacked consideration in regard to surgical factors [15]. Indeed, there were no considerations for technical surgical details or the reconstructive methods adopted. Cameron et al. described the development of a surgical scoring system based on tumor localization, mandibulectomy, neck dissection, and reconstruction [14]. Thus, Cameron et al. evaluated important surgical aspects to predict the need for tracheostomy, the decision to perform mandibulectomy and neck dissections, and the use of bulky reconstructive flaps. Cameron describes that a threshold score of 5 gives acceptable sensitivity and specificity, and good positive predictive value (PPV) and negative predictive value (NPV). Cameron's complete scoring system is shown in Table 3. The authors pointed out that this scoring system has the potential to assist clinicians in the decision regarding airway management; it is not intended to replace clinical judgment.

Lee et al. proposed a retrospective study to investigate the usefulness of a tracheostomy scoring system in decision making for postoperative airway management in oral

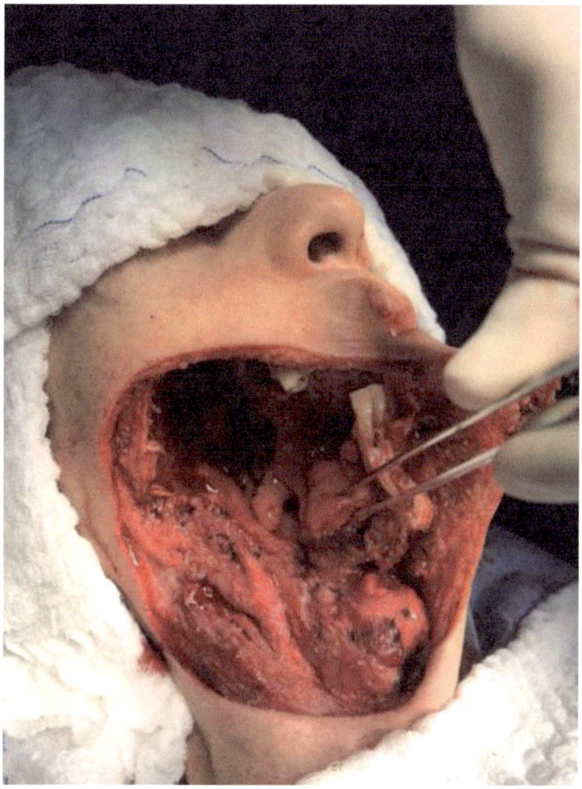

Fig. 10 After resection, showing a major tridimensional defect of the upper aerodigestive tract

cancer patients, and concluded that both Cameron's and Kruse-Lösler's systems cannot be absolute guidelines in all cases. Using these scoring systems was not sufficient to make a decision on whether to perform an elective tracheostomy after oral cancer surgery, but it could be helpful in predicting the severity of the airway obstruction after surgery [2] (Fig. 12).

Kim et al. [15] noted the insufficiency of Cameron's considerations about tumor size and the patient's systemic health condition, and suggested a new scoring system for elective tracheostomy, covering both surgical and systemic factors. This scoring system considers a score of 5 as a relevant cutoff to determine that an elective tracheostomy is indicated [15] (Table 4).

Kruse-Lösler et al. published, for the first time, a scoring system to assist in establishing the indications for elective tracheostomy; they described an easily performed scoring system, enabling comparison of different patients and using well-defined criteria. Since this publication, some authors have tried to develop new scoring systems to solve limitations. These systems are aimed at better prediction of airway safety regarding patients undergoing oral and oropharyngeal resections. At present, there are no scoring systems able to replace clinical experience regarding whether or not to perform a tracheostomy.

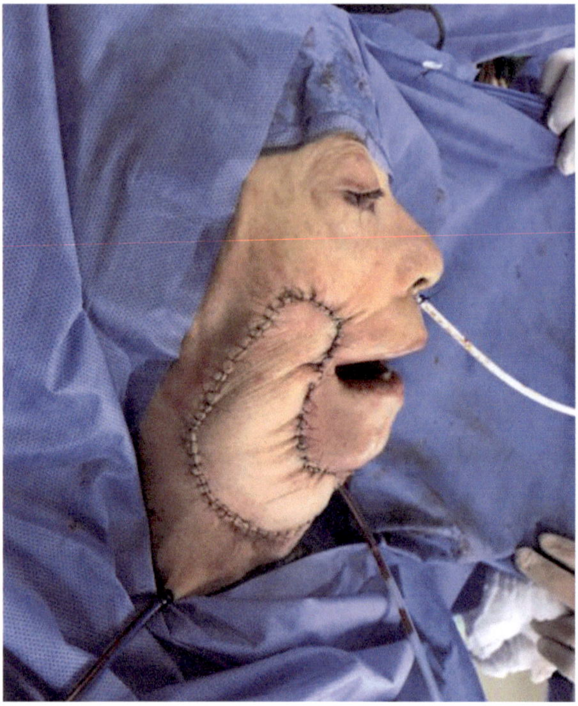

Fig. 11 After free flap reconstruction, requiring tracheostomy due to important functional loss

Table 2 Scoring system devised by Kruse-Lösler et al. for elective tracheostomy in oral cancer

Parameter	0 points	1 point	2 points	3 points	4 points	Points value
Tumor localization	-	Anterior second premolar	Posterior second premolar	-	-	1–2
Tumor size	-	T1	T2	T3	T4	1–4
Chest X-ray findings	Normal	Pathological findings	-	-	-	0–1
Multimorbidity	No	Yes	-	-	-	0–1
Alcohol use	No	<100 g/day	>100 g/day	Hard drinks	-	0-3
Total						2–11

Acta Anaesthesiol Scand [16]

Tracheostomy in Laryngeal and Pharyngeal Cancer

Tracheostomy in Organ Preservation

Transglottic carcinoma—a term designated to clarify tumor growth patterns (involvement of both true and false vocal cords), created by McGavran and associates—can be treated by total laryngectomy. Mittal et al. do not consider

Table 3 Scoring system devised by Cameron et al. to guide airway management after major head and neck surgery

Scoring factor			Score
Tumor site	Cutaneous		0
	Mouth	Buccal mucosa	0
		Maxilla	0
		Mandibular alveolus	1
		Anterior tongue	1
		Floor of mouth	2
	Oropharynx	Soft palate	3
		Anterior pillar	3
		Tonsillar pillar	4
		Posterior tongue	4
		Hypopharynx	4
Mandibulectomy		No	0
		Yes	1
Bilateral neck dissection		No	0
		Yes	3
Reconstruction		None	0
		Radial forearm free flap	2
		Other	3

Int. J. Oral Maxillofac. Surg. 2009

conservative surgery and exclusive radiation an effective course of treatment for transglottic tumors. According to their retrospective study, temporary or permanent tracheostomy stands among the most frequent complications in patients undergoing vocal conservation surgery followed by irradiation or not. The need for permanent tracheostomy is also an important prognostic factor in 5-year survival [17].

Pretreatment tracheostomy has been related to a higher risk of stomal recurrence and a poor prognosis [17]. Nevertheless, Modlin and Ogura found no difference in stomal recurrence between patients who did and those who did not undergo pre-treatment tracheostomy [18].

Organ preservation, an evolution in advanced laryngeal cancer treatment, originated from the Veteran Affairs study in 1991 and the Radiation Therapy Oncology Group 91-11 study in 2003, which determined primary chemoradiation as being standard treatment for advanced tumors. Its use imposed an increase in functional complications and a decrease in overall survival in older patients and those with T4 disease [19]. According to O'Neill et al., 19% of patients who underwent total laryngectomy and 22% of patients who underwent organ preservation had a tracheostomy prior to treatment.

Jefferson et al. demonstrated that persistent tracheostomy was associated with pretreatment tracheostomy, subglottic tumor extension, three-dimensional conformal radiotherapy, and postradiotherapy cervical lymphadenectomy in larynx primaries, and pretreatment tracheostomy and feeding tube dependency in hypopharynx primaries. Tracheostomy was not associated with worse local control. Furthermore, organ preservation may not restore prelaryngeal deficits. Normally these reports assess swallowing—not airway—impairment and factors associated with tracheostomy dependence [20].

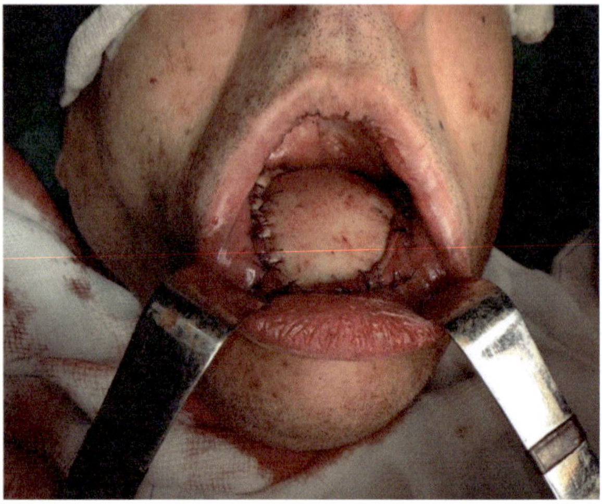

Fig. 12 Total glossectomy followed by bulky flap reconstruction, with expected important swallowing function loss and airway structure collapse

Table 4 Scoring system devised by Kim et al. for elective tracheostomy in oral cancer

Oral cancer	Scoring factor	Subsection	Score
	TNM stage	I	0
		II	1
		III	2
		IV	3
	Reconstruction	No reconstruction	0
		Soft tissue free flap	1
		Soft + hard tissue free flap	2
	Chest PA	No pathological finding	0
		Pathological finding	1
	Number of systemic diseases	None	0
		1–2	1
		≥3	2

Elective tracheostomy scoring system for severe oral disease patients. J Korean Assoc Oral Maxillofac Surg 2014
PA posterior–anterior X-ray, *TNM* Tumor–Node–Metastasis scoring system

Organ preservation is indicated not only for laryngeal cancers but also for laryngopharyngeal and hypopharyngeal cancers.

Tracheostomy in Organ Preservation Laryngeal Surgery

Organ preservation laryngeal surgery is a procedure encompassing partial laryngeal removal and functional preservation (speech, swallowing, and respiration), with local control and cure and without the need for a permanent tracheostomy [21]. The aim is to preserve airflow through the larynx and laryngeal sphincter function, preventing the need for a permanent tracheostomy [22].

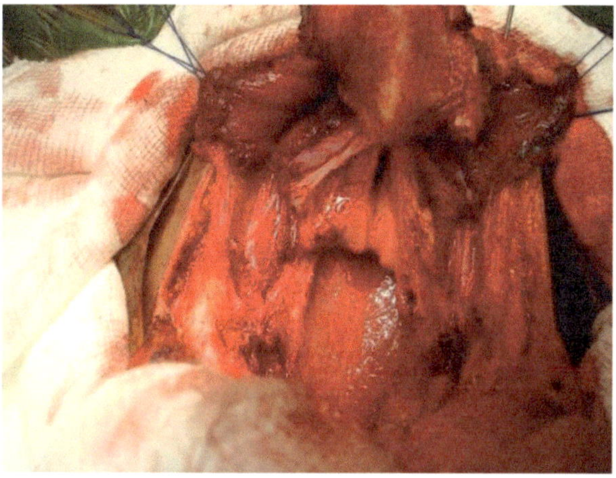

Fig. 13 Supraglottic laryngectomy

Vertical Partial Laryngectomy

Vertical partial laryngectomy stands for a range of procedures, from cordectomy to extended hemilaryngectomy. The extent of surgery determines whether tracheostomy is necessary.

Horizontal Partial Laryngectomy

Supraglottic Laryngectomy

In this technique, described by Alonso in 1939, tracheostomy is part of the surgical procedure and the aim is to perform decannulation as soon as possible, with safety. The technique is executed with the concern being to avoid anastomosis tension, in the same fashion as supracricoid laryngectomy (Fig. 13).

Supracricoid Laryngectomy

Supracricoid laryngectomy was first described as an organ preservation surgery technique aimed at achieving functional and oncological results; therefore, the need for a permanent tracheostomy is avoided. A temporary tracheostomy is mandatory. The trachea must be released inferiorly (cervicomediastinally), avoiding recurrent laryngeal nerve injury. Tracheostomy should be performed as distal from cricoid as possible, since the anastomosis (cricohyoidoepiglottopexy [CHEP] or cricohyoidopexy [CHP]) should bear no tension. Complications such as aspiration and pneumonia are causes of failed decannulation [21].

The cricoarytenoid unit is a functional laryngeal structure after supracricoid laryngectomy. Normally, patients bearing two arytenoids accomplish earlier decannulation than patients undergoing one arytenoid resection and may accomplish better functional results [21–24]. Postoperative radiotherapy normally imposes longer and more arduous rehabilitation regarding functional results [22]. The protocol for decannulation varies according to institutional practice. All patients undergo progressive decannulation with downsizing of the tracheostomy tube, applying a cuffless tracheostomy tube and capping the tracheostomy tube, with laryngoscopy control [22, 23, 25] (Figs. 14 and 15).

Near-Total Laryngectomy

This technique, described by Pearson in 1980, is indicated for patients with advanced laryngeal–hypopharyngeal tumors restricted to one side of the larynx–hypopharynx. A shunt between the trachea and pharynx is created through neopharynx closure, and tracheostomy is paramount. The intrinsic laryngeal musculature with ipsilateral nerve preservation controls the shunt, pumping air from the lung to the pharynx. There is no need to perform tracheostomy as distal from cricoid as possbile. The procedure gives the patient a physiological voice at the expense of requiring a permanent tracheostomy [26, 27] (Figs. 16 and 17).

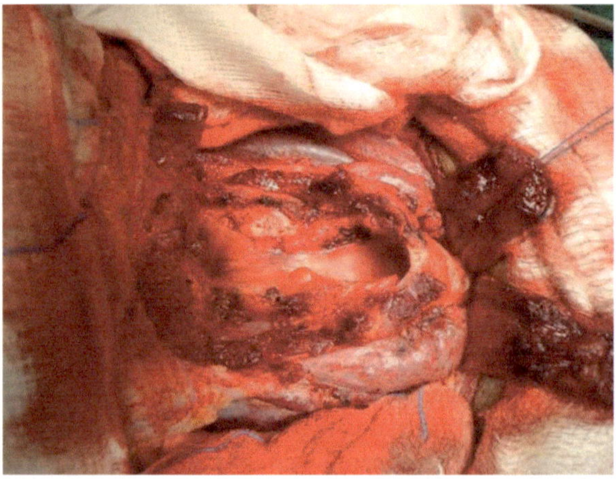

Fig. 14 Supracricoid laryngectomy

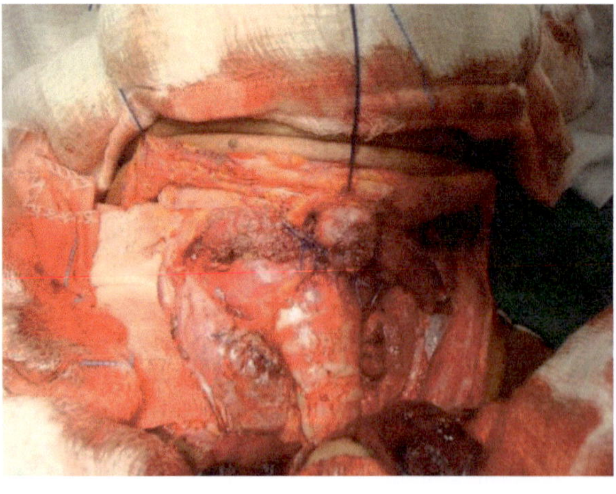

Fig. 15 Cricohyoidoepig lottopexy

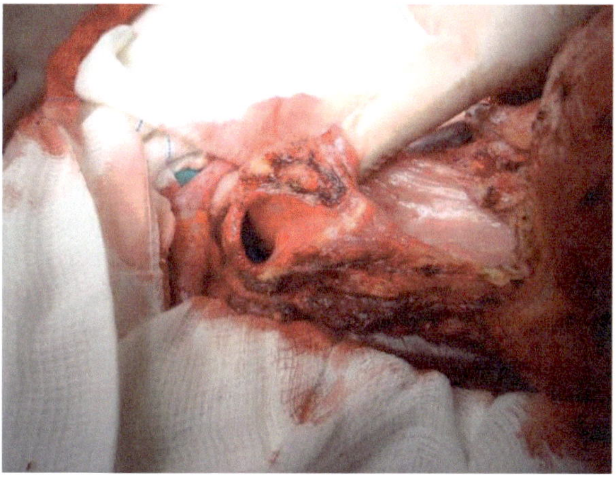

Fig. 16 Near-total laryngectomy

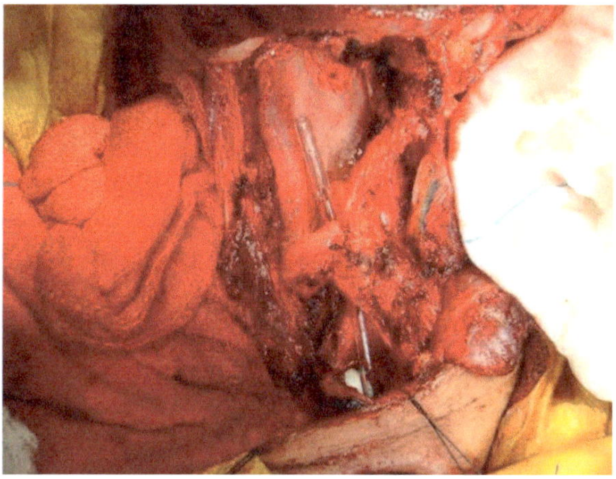

Fig. 17 Shunt in near-total laryngectomy

Endoscopic Technique

Normally, the endoscopic technique obviates the need for a tracheostomy.

Total Laryngectomy

Patients have to live with a permanent tracheostomy when total laryngectomy is performed. The indications for tracheostomy prior to oncological surgical treatment are due to airway blockage by tumor growth and/or laryngeal edema, as clarified before in the indications in oncological patients. Care should be taken to avoid tumor violation and spillage concerning subglottic laryngeal lesions and not to perform tracheostomy so distal from cricoid preventing tensionless stoma maturation to the skin.

Questionnaires (Quality of Life)

Questionnaires are used to assess the patient's quality of life. There are several questionnaires available, and they represent a tool for subjective assessment from the patient's perspective. These questionnaires are not necessarily head and neck cancer specific but may evaluate language, speech, and communication. The World Health Organization's International Classification of Functioning, Disability and Health (ICF), issued in 2001; the Voice Handicap Index; and the North American questionnaires Functional Assessment of Cancer Therapy and University of Washington Quality of Life Questionnaire are some examples. Undoubtedly, patients who bear a tracheostomy have some level of impairment and some loss of quality of life [28]. The pictures presented in this chapter were taken after patient's consent and with purpose to learn and to be used exclusivelly in this context.

References

1. Hollingsworth HM. Wheezing and stridor. Clin Chest Med. 1987;8:231–40.
2. Lee HJ, Kim JK, Choi SY. The evaluation of a scoring system in airway management after oral cancer surgery. Maxillofac Plast Reconstr Surg. 2015;37:19.
3. Marsh M, Elliott S, Anand R, Brennan PA. Early postoperative care for free flap head & neck reconstructive surgery—a national survey of practice. Br J Oral Maxillofac Surg. 2009;47:182–5.
4. Cantù G, Solero CL, Pizzi N, et al. Skull base reconstruction after anterior craniofacial resection. J Craniomaxillofac Surg. 1999;27:228.
5. Fliss DM, Gil Z, Spektor S. Skull base reconstruction after anterior subcranial tumor resection. Neurosurg Focus. 2002;5:1–7.
6. Altman KW, Waltonen JD, Kern RC. Urgent surgical airway intervention: a 3-year county hospital experience. Laryngoscope. 2005;115:2101–4.
7. Yuen HW, Loy AH, Johari S. Urgent awake tracheotomy for impending airway obstruction. Otolaryngol Head Neck Surg. 2007;136:838–42.
8. Gillespie MB, Eisele DW. Outcomes of emergency surgical airway procedures in a hospital-wide setting. Laryngoscope. 1999;109:1766–9.
9. Pracy P, Gleeson M, editors. Tracheostomy. In: Scott-Brown's otorhinolaryngology: head and neck surgery, Holder Arnold. Florida: CRC Press; 2008. p. 2292–303.
10. Goldenberg D, Ari EG, Golz A, Danino J, Netzer A, Joachims HZ. Tracheotomy complications: a retrospective study of 1130 patients. Otolaryngol Head Neck Surg. 2000;123:495–500.
11. Costa L, Matos R, Júlio S, et al. Urgent tracheostomy: four-year experience in a tertiary hospital. World J Emerg Med. 2016;7:227–30.
12. Fang CH, Friedman R, White PE, et al. Emergent awake tracheostomy—the five-year experience at an urban tertiary care center. Laryngoscope. 2015;125(11):2476–9.
13. Castling B, Telfer M, Avery S. Complications of tracheostomy in major head and neck cancer surgery; a retrospective study of 60 consecutive cases. Br J Oral Maxillofac Surg. 1994;32:3–5.
14. Cameron M, Corner A, Diba A, Hankins M. Development of a tracheostomy scoring system to guide airway management after major head and neck surgery. Int J Oral Maxillofac Surg. 2009;38(8):846–9.
15. Kim YH, Kim MY, Kim CH. Elective tracheostomy scoring system for severe oral disease patients. J Korean Assoc Oral Maxillofac Surg. 2014;40:211–9.
16. Kruse-Lösler B, Langer E, Reich A. Score system for elective tracheotomy in major head and neck tumour surgery. Acta Anaesthesiol Scand. 2005;49:654–9.
17. Bharat M, Marks JE, Ogura JH. Transglottic carcinoma. Cancer. 1984;53:151–61.

18. Modlin B, Ogura JH. Post-laryngectomy tracheal stomal recurrences. Laryngoscope. 1969;(2):239–50.
19. O'Neill CB, O'Neill JP, Atoria CL, Baxi SS, Henmann MC, Ganly I, Elkin EB. Treatment complications and survival in advanced laryngeal cancer: a population-based analysis. Laryngocope. 2014;124:2707–13.
20. Jefferson GD, Wenig BL, Spiotto MT. Predictors and outcomes for chronic tracheostomy after chemoradioation for advanced laryngohypopharyngeal cancer. Laryngoscope. 2016;126:385–91.
21. Chawla S, Carney AS. Organ preservation surgery for laryngeal cancer. Head Neck Oncol. 2009;1:12.
22. Farrag TY, Koch WM, Cummings CW, Goldenberg D, Abou-Jaoude PM, Califano JA, Flint PW, Webster K. Supracricoid laryngectomy outcomes: the Johns Hopkins experience. Laryngoscope. 2007;117:129–32.
23. Laccourreye H, Laccourreye O, Weinstein G, Menard M, Brasnu D. Supracricoid laryngectomy with cricohyoidopexy: a partial laryngeal procedure for selected supraglottic and transglottic carcinomas. Laryngoscope. 1990;100:735–41.
24. Leszezynska M, wierzbicka M, Tokarski M, Szyfter W. Attempt to improve functional outcomes in supracricoid laryngectomy in T2b and T3 glottic cancers. Eur Arch Otorhinolaryngol. 2015;272:2925–31.
25. Bron L, Brossard E, Monnier P, Pasche P. Supracricoide partial laryngectomy with cricohyoidoepiglottopexy and cricohyoidopexy for glottic and supraglottic carcinomas. Laryngoscope. 2000;110:627–34.
26. Arain A, Ghaffar S. Preliminary report—near total laryngectomy for SCC larynx. J Pak Med Assoc. 2011;61(6):607–10.
27. Maamoun SI, Amira G, Younis A. Near total laryngectomy: a versatile approach for voice restoration in advanced T3 and T4 laryngeal cancer: functional results and survival. J Egypt Natl Canc Int. 2004;16(1):15–21.
28. Tchiesner U. Preservation of organ function in head and neck cancer. GMS Curr Top Otorhinolaryngol Head Neck Surg. 2012;11:1–18.

Mediastinal Tracheostomy

Paulo José de Cavalcanti Siebra, Ruiter Diego de Moraes Botinelly, Terence Pires de Farias, Alexandre Ferreira Oliveira, and Fernando Luiz Dias

Introduction

Mediastinal tracheostomy (MT) is the construction of a stoma on the anterior chest by using the intrathoracic trachea when there is insufficient length for reanastomosis with the remaining trachea or for a traditional suprasternal tracheostomy. This procedure requires a laryngectomy (if not done previously) associated with removal of the upper sternum, the medial third of the clavicles, and eventually the proximal third of the first and second ribs, to provide access to the intrathoracic trachea [1–3]. Few surgeons or institutions have extensive experience of this procedure, due to its rarity, complexity, and association with high morbidity. In the literature, there are some case series with small sample sizes, but with acceptable results [4].

P.J. de Cavalcanti Siebra, M.D. • R.D. de Moraes Botinelly, M.D. (✉)
Head and Neck Surgeon, Fellow of Head and Neck Surgery at Brazilian National Cancer Institute, Rio de Janeiro, RJ, Brazil
e-mail: pj_siebra@hotmail.com; ruiterdiegob@hotmail.com

T.P. de Farias, M.D., Ph.D., M.Sc., Researcher.
Department of Head and Neck Surgery, Brazilian National Cancer Institute—INCA, Rio de Janeiro, RJ, Brazil

Department of Head and Neck Surgery, Pontifical Catholic University, Rio de Janeiro, RJ, Brazil
e-mail: terencefarias@yahoo.com.br

A.F. Oliveira, M.D., Ph.D.
Department of Surgery, Federal University of Juiz de Fora, Juiz de Fora, MG, Brazil

F.L. Dias, M.D., Ph.D., M.Sc., F.A.C.S.
Head and Neck Surgery Department, Brazilian National Cancer Institute—INCA, Rio de Janeiro, RJ, Brazil

Head and Neck Department, Pontifical Catholic University of Rio de Janeiro, Rio de Janeiro, RJ, Brazil

T.P. de Farias (ed.), *Tracheostomy*, https://doi.org/10.1007/978-3-319-67867-2_11

History

In 1942, Watson planned a procedure for the treatment of a squamous cell carcinoma 4 cm above the carina. The patient had undergone a laryngectomy followed by radiotherapy 15 years previously. A "V" portion of the sternum was resected and skin flaps were mobilized to allow closure of the tracheostomy margins [23].

In 1952, Kleitsch removed a patient's upper sternum and inserted a polyethylene tube for MT [21]. In the same year, Minor, after removal of a recurrent carcinoma in a tracheostoma, fashioned skin flaps into the shape of a tube through a sternal opening to connect with the trachea [22]. In 1959, Waddell and Cannon pulled a tracheal segment on the right of the ascending aorta and anastomosed it with a skin tube created with flaps from the anterior chest region through an opening in the sternum. Of the four patients who underwent this procedure, two died of massive bleeding [17].

In 1962, Sisson et al. resected a large piece of skin along with a tumor and removed the notch and the heads of both clavicles in surgery for recurrence of laryngeal carcinoma in the stoma. Skin flaps were mobilized to the superior closure of the stoma and the lower failure was covered with skin grafts. After undergoing the procedure, two patients died from postoperative bleeding by the innominate artery, and the pectoralis muscle (PM) flap began to be interposed between the trachea and the innominate artery [15].

In 1966, Grillo fashioned a large bipedicled total thickness flap from the skin of the anterior chest region through two main horizontal incisions in an effort to eliminate the tension in the tracheocutaneous anastomosis responsible for poor healing and the threat of bleeding from the innominate artery. This flaps reaches the terminal stump of the trachea in the mediastinum, which was accessed by removing the notch and sternal portions of both clavicles and the first and second costal cartilages. The stoma emerged at the center of the flap, requiring only a simple suture [19].

Indications

The patient must be carefully selected for this procedure due to its complexity, potential for complications, degree of deformity, and postoperative sequelae. The reconstruction of the alimentary tract should be taken into consideration as, according to necessity, there will be a considerable increase in the complexity of the surgery. Thus, a good preoperative evaluation becomes crucial. The patient needs a good performance status with good heart and lung function, and must be well nourished and psychologically prepared for the deformities and sequelae of the resection and reconstruction. A history of abdominal surgery influences the type of reconstruction. A history of cervical radiotherapy compromises the tracheal circulation, which increases the risk of ischemia and makes it more difficult to access the large vessels of the neck for a microsurgical anastomosis [5, 6].

According to Conti et al., the main indications for MT are malignant neoplasms of the subglottic region extending to the proximal trachea, a recurrence in stoma after laryngectomy, and a well-differentiated thyroid carcinoma with tracheal

Table 1 Indications for mediastinal tracheostomy

Indication
Malignant neoplasm of the subglottic region, extending to the proximal trachea
Recurrence of stoma after total laryngectomy
Well-differentiated thyroid carcinoma with tracheal invasion

invasion, after either curative or palliative resection (Table 1). The recommended minimum length of the residual trachea for this procedure is 5.0 cm. The same authors also recommend chemotherapy and radiation associated with tracheal stenting for cases of cervical esophageal cancer with tracheal invasion; the 3-year survival rate is just 11% after a radical procedure.

The presence of metastases is not an absolute contraindication to this procedure. However, in these cases, other methods for palliation with less morbidity should be considered, such as radiotherapy or stent placement [4].

The main contraindications to MT are invasion or involvement of the great vessels, distal trachea invasion of 3.0–4.0 cm above the carina, column or prevertebral fascia invasion, and the presence of disease in the bronchial lumen [7].

Description of the Procedure and Perioperative Care

The most commonly used incisions are the collar incision and the bipedicled/apron incision. In cases of recurrence in a previous tracheostoma, the peritracheostoma skin should be resected (Fig. 1).

In the case of a collar incision, a platysmal subcutaneous flap is made to expose the larynx, trachea, sternocleidomastoid, and carotid sheaths. The lower flap permits better exposure of the anterior thoracic wall. Using a surgical saw, a resection is done of the middle third of the clavicle, sternal notch, and cartilaginous limit of the first two ribs, with preservation of bilateral internal thoracic arteries (Figs. 2 and 3). The need to extend the resection to the second rib depends on the length of the remaining trachea. With this, the surgeon has a good view of the upper mediastinal structures.

Prior to use of the saw, digital dissection of the posterior wall of the sternum is recommended.

The trachea is divided obliquely to facilitate skin suturing (Fig. 4). The inferior portion is reintubated and the superior portion is resected along with the affected structures (Fig. 5). After that, the trachea is released from the esophagus by blunt dissection, with preservation of the vascularization (Fig. 6). When the tracheal stump causes compression of large vessels, it is transposed inferiorly through the innominate artery to decrease the distance from the skin and to prevent anastomosis tension, reducing the risk of peristomal dehiscence, mediastinitis, and rupture of large vessels (Fig. 7).

For closure of the defect and fashioning of the tracheocutaneous anastomosis, use of myocutaneous flaps is recommended to protect the large vessels and avoid tension

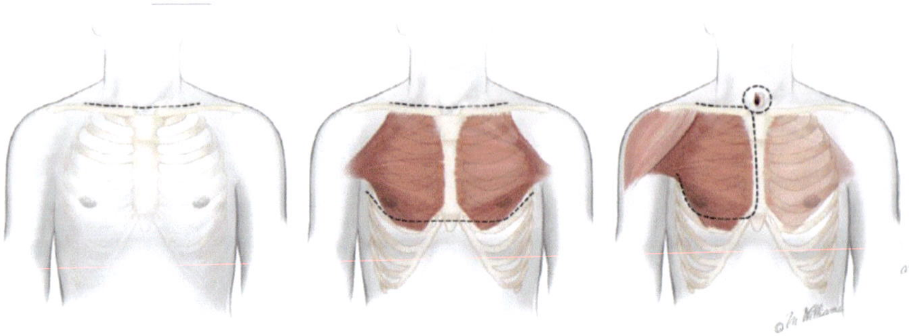

Fig. 1 Most commonly used skin incisions. (Reproduced from Sugarbaker et al. [24], with permission. Copyright Mcgraw-Hill Education. All rights reserved)

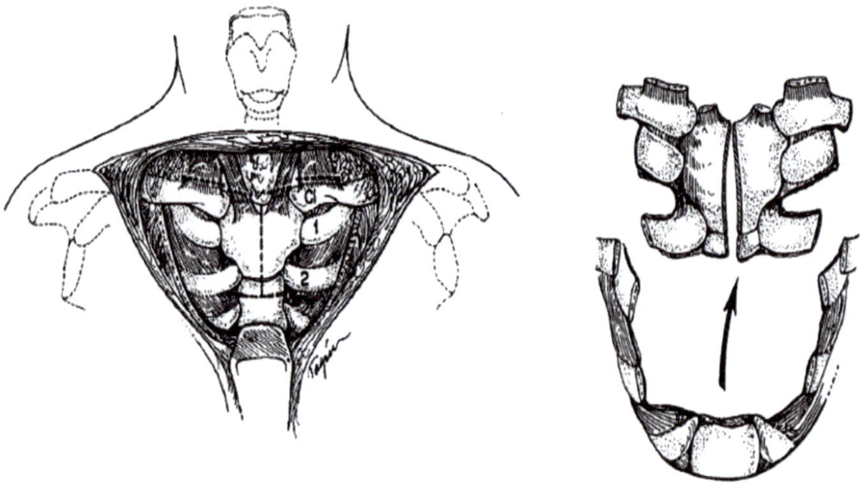

Fig. 2 The inferior skin flap is elevated and the upper sternum is divided to facilitate evaluation for resectability

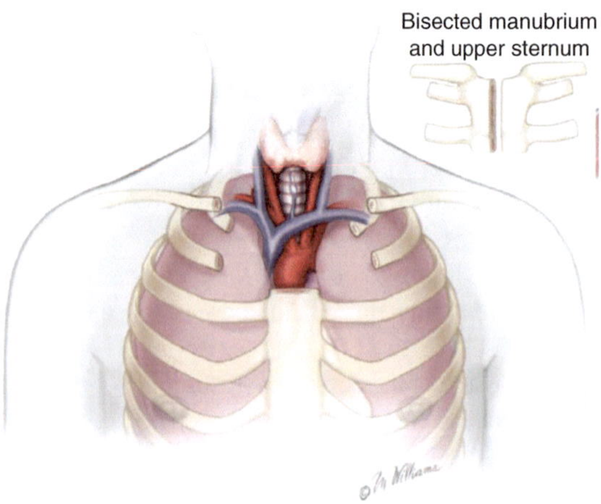

Fig. 3 The Manubrium is bisected and the upper sternum is removed. (Reproduced from Sugarbaker et al. [24], with permission. Copyright Mcgraw-Hill Education. All rights reserved)

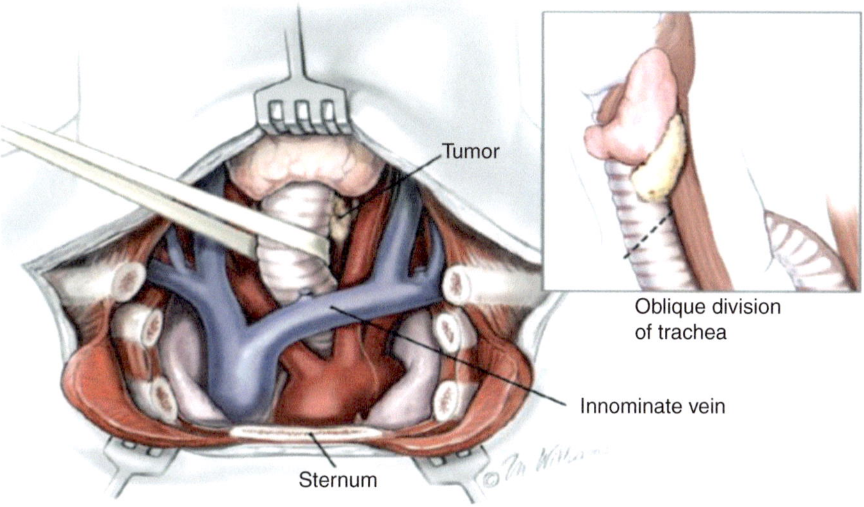

Fig. 4 Tumor site and trachea, divided obliquely. (Reproduced from Sugarbaker et al. [24], with permission. Copyright Mcgraw-Hill Education. All rights reserved)

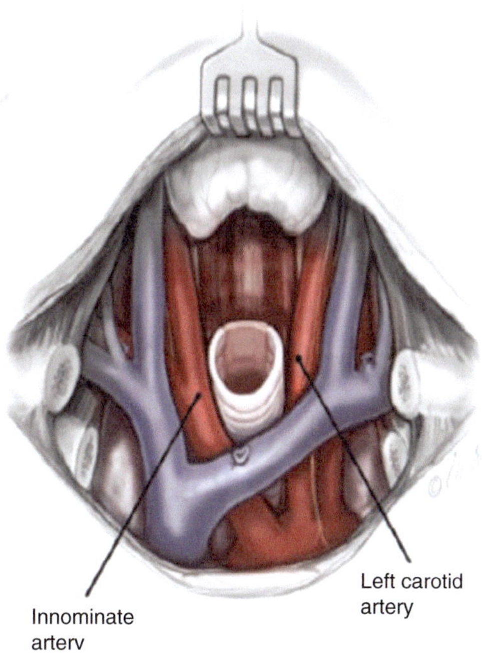

Fig. 5 The inferior portion is reintubated and the superior portion is resected along with the affected structures. Tracheal relocation. (*Left:* reproduced from Sugarbaker et al. [24], with permission. Copyright Mcgraw-Hill Education. All rights reserved)

between the tissues. Sisson et al. described the importance of separating the innominate artery from the trachea by using a PM flap, thereby reducing the occurrence of vessel rupture and fistula. For Orringer, the most important factor to avoid this disastrous

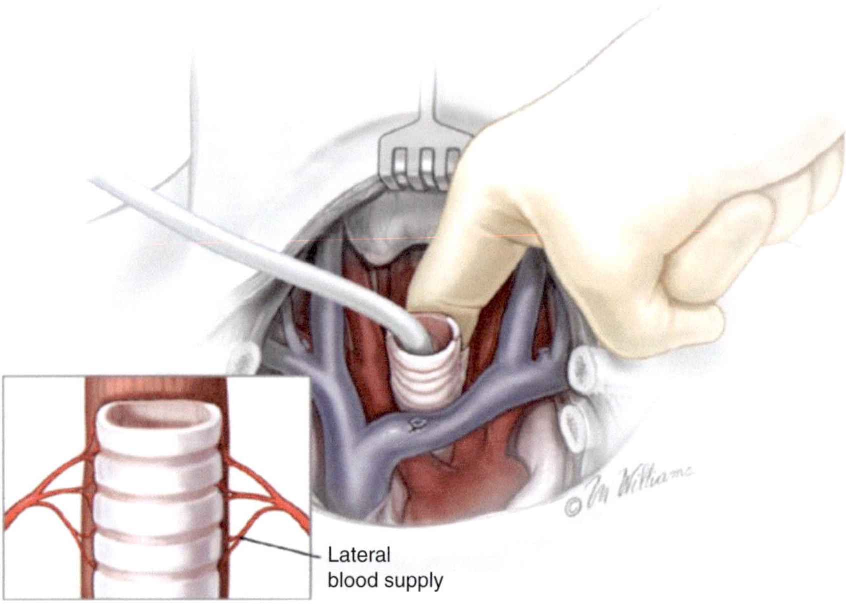

Fig. 6 Releasing the trachea from the esophagus by blunt dissection, with preservation of the vascularization. (Reproduced from Sugarbaker et al. [24], with permission. Copyright Mcgraw-Hill Education. All rights reserved)

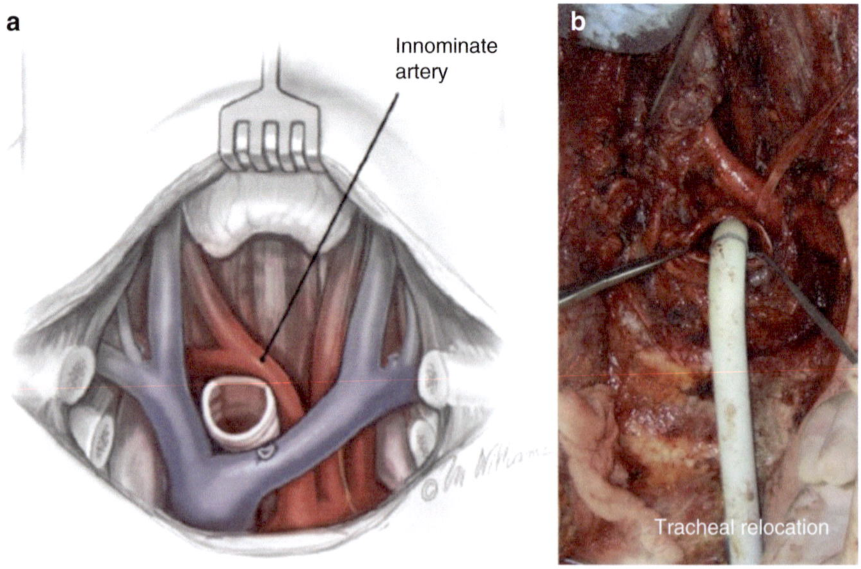

Fig. 7 Prevention of anastomosis tension by transposing the trachea inferiorly. Schematic drawing (**a**). Tracheal relocation-in vivo view [4] (**b**). (Reproduced from Sugarbaker et al. [24], with permission. Copyright Mcgraw-Hill Education. All rights reserved)

complication was considered to be a tension-free reconstruction; thus, a myocutaneous flap can be used, such as the deltopectoral flap and thoracoacromial flap ("nipple flap").

The pectoralis major is the preferable flap because it is able to provide a wide quantity of myocutaneous tissue according to the defect to be reconstructed. Its blood supply originates from the descending branch of the acromioclavicular artery—a branch of the subclavian artery, which usually originates in the middle third of the clavicle and has a flow direction toward the nipple. Other flaps, such as deltopectoral and bipedicled flaps, may also be used (Fig. 8) [8].

For development of the flap, the main reference points are outlined on the skin: the sternal notch, xiphoid process, clavicle, and its middle third (origin of the vascular pedicle). The defect must be measured, and a similar area of skin is drawn between the nipple and sternum (Figs. 9 and 10).

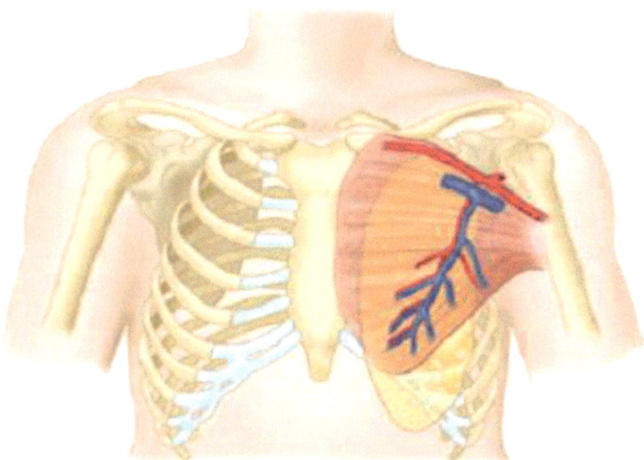

Available skin surface

Pectoralis major muscle and descending branches of acromiothoracic vessels

Fig. 8 Available skin surface and wide myocutaneous tissue

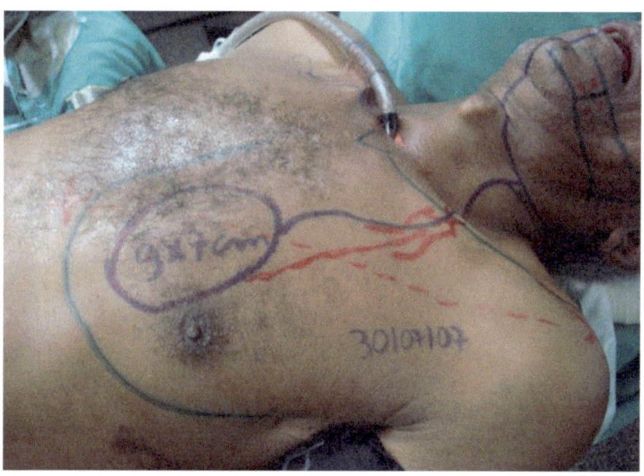

Fig. 9 Main reference points for the major pectoralis flap outlined

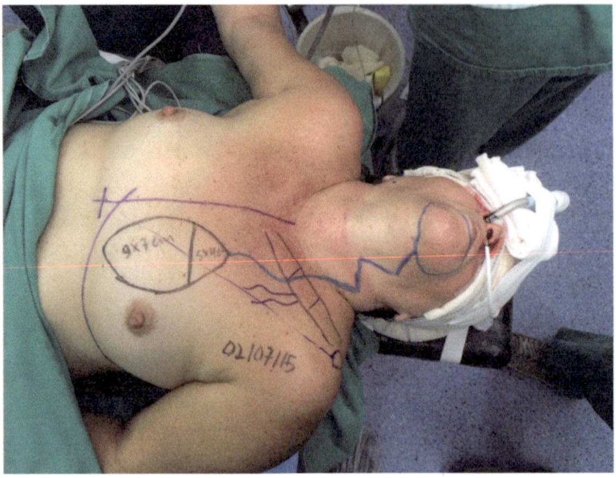

Fig. 10 Another example of the Pectoralis Major Flap reference points

The incision of the donor area is performed, with elevation of the skin flaps medially and laterally to the flap (Fig. 11). The medial insertion of the muscle into the sternum is released, with ligation of perforating branches of the internal thoracic artery, and the lateral edge of the muscle is released from the pectoralis minor muscle. Elevation of the flap is initiated medially with deepening of the incision to the level of the ribs and cranial release from the ribs and intercostal muscles, through blunt dissection and electrocautery use, to the site of origin of the pedicle vessels (middle third of the clavicle). The lateral limit of the muscle is incised, preserving the pedicle (visible below the flap). The flap is mobilized to the defect area and for coverage of the large mediastinal vessels. The tracheostoma is created by transposing the trachea through the interior of the flap (Fig. 12) [8].

Prior to manufacture of the tracheocutaneous anastomosis, sutures may be placed between the trachea and the subcutaneous tissues to ensure better stability. Drains should be positioned below the flap, and a interrupted suture is made between the skin and the tracheal stump.

The donor area is covered with the medial and lateral skin flaps, created during PM dissection. In cases where these remnants do not present sufficient approximation, it is possible to place cutaneous grafts in the uncovered areas (Figs 13 and 14).

For tracheocutaneous anastomosis and closure, the muscles must be reapproximated and the trachea attached to the subcutaneous tissue to ensure better support. As the skin is closed, the tracheocutaneous anastomosis is initiated. Local flaps—such as the deltopectoral flap, PM flap, and bipedicled flap—are used to cover the

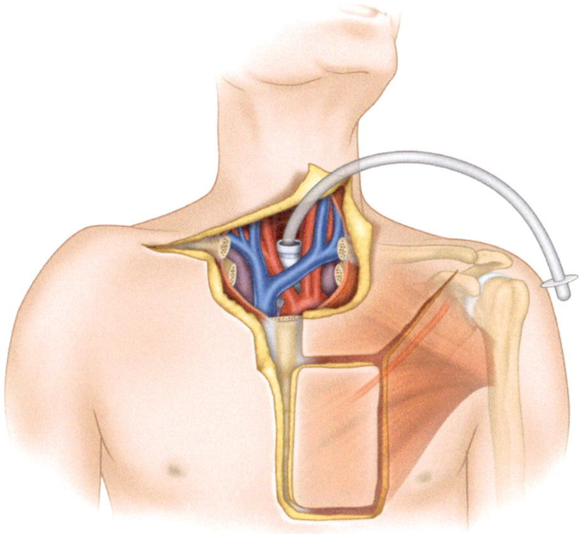

Fig. 11 Incision of the donor area

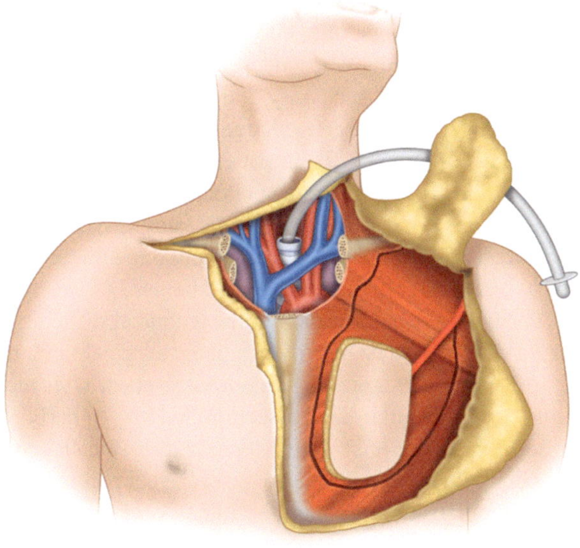

Fig. 12 Pectoralis major flap dissection

defect generated by resection and to avoid stress on the structures. Drains are placed beneath the flap, and an interrupted suture is fashioned (Figs. 12, 13, and 14).

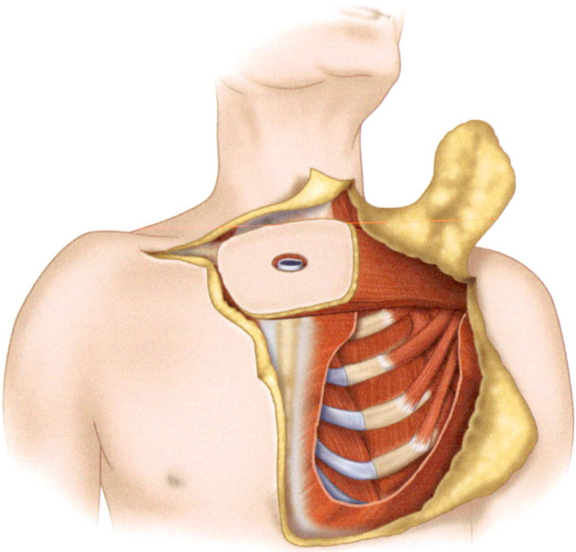

Fig. 13 Transposing the trachea trough the Flap

The main ways to reconstruct the alimentary tract are transposition of intra-abdominal organs (stomach, jejunum, colon) or use of microsurgical flaps (jejunum or myocutaneous flaps) [5].

The decision must take into account several factors—the main one is of reconstruction. In patients who undergo total esophagectomy in addition to laryngotracheal resection, it is necessary to transpose the intra-abdominal organs. Elevation of the stomach is often preferred, due to the reduction in surgical time and the need for fewer anastomoses [5, 9]. In patients who have already undergone gastric surgery, such as a gastrostomy, the next choice may vary between a long colon segment and the jejunum. When only a pharyngectomy is performed, without the need for a full esophagectomy, a microsurgical jejunal flap or a tubed myocutaneous flap (from the radial forearm or anterior thigh) can be used [5, 6, 10, 11].

There are several reasons for the technical difficulties and major morbidity associated with MT: (1) a heavily irradiated surgical field, usually impairing the healing of soft tissue coverage; (2) paradoxical chest wall movements induced by manubrium and clavicular head resection, leading to early respiratory failure and stoma or flap dehiscence [12]; and (3) fistulization, which occurs in 65% of patients requiring complementary pharyngeal–esophageal reconstruction [13, 14].

Postoperative care should be intensive. Immediate postoperative intensive care unit (ICU) placement is recommended in patients undergoing esophagectomy and microsurgical anastomoses. The major cause of mortality after surgery is primary

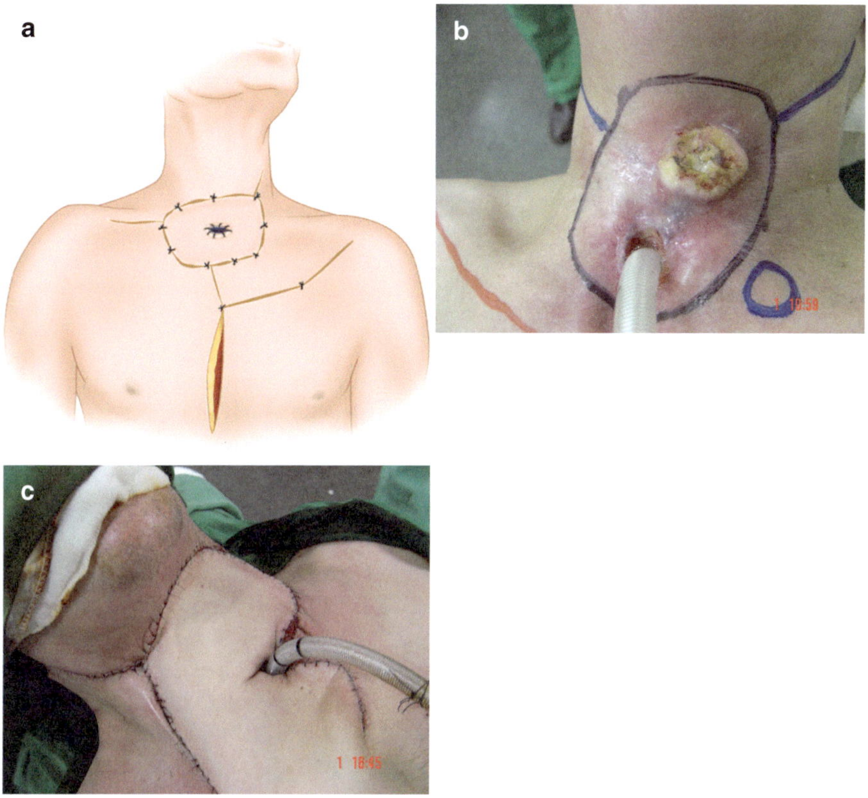

Fig. 14 (**a**) Reconstruction of the donor area with skin flaps and final aspect. (**b**) Example of Extensive Laringeal Recurrence. (**c**) Underwent Mediastinal Tracheostomy

rupture of the innominate artery with fatality rates of 33–55% [15–17]. To prevent these complications, it is crucial to preserve the blood supply to the tracheal stump and to protect the brachiocephalic artery, to fill the dead space, and to create a tracheostomy with tension-free sutures on the skin flap, using, for example, the omentum OR pectoralis major [2]. Other complications are alimentary tract fistula from anastomosis, ischemia of the trachea, skin flap loss, chylothorax, and hypoparathyroidism. Lung incarceration after anterior MT is also a described complication [12].

Nevertheless, MT can offer acceptable terms of palliation and quality of life, similar to those of patients undergoing routine laryngectomy. Bone resection (manubrium, clavicle, sternum, first and second ribs) can generate an area of instability in the anterior chest with pulmonary herniation and increased susceptibility to pneumonia [9] (Table 2).

Table 2 Complications of mediastinal tracheostomy

Complication
Rupture of the innominate artery
Alimentary tract fistula
Ischemia of trachea
Skin flap loss
Chylothorax
Hypoparathyroidism

Case Report

The patient was a 52-year-old male and a smoker who presented in August 2013 with otalgia, odynophagia, dysphagia, and hoarseness, which had started 6 months prior to admission. Laryngoscopy revealed a tumor affecting the arytenoids, interarytenoid space, postcricoid region, aryepiglottic left fold, and left pyriform sinus, with extension to the superior esophageal sphincter and cervical esophagus confirmed by MRI scanning and computed tomography (CT). The left hemilarynx was paralyzed, and there was destruction of the cricoid and thyroid cartilages. The cervical lymph nodes were not clinically affected. Positron emission tomography (PET) CT did not establish disease at other sites. The patient was clinically staged as T4aN0M0. As the patient refused radical surgical treatment, he underwent an induction scheme with three doses of Taxol/platinum/5-fluorouracil (TPF) on days 1, 22, and 43, with an excellent response. As a result, we decided to continue conservative treatment with intense modulated radiation therapy (IMRT) (7000 cGy) associated with cetuximab.

At week 12 after treatment, the laryngoscopy and PET CT scan showed a complete response. The patient remained on monthly control but did not attend regular consultations.

Fourteen months after his initial treatment, the patient presented again with otalgia and noisy breathing, and with associated dysphagia. The laryngoscopy showed ulceration throughout the postcricoid region. Digestive endoscopy showed a 3 cm–long involvement of the cervical esophagus with tracheal invasion.

Endoscopic gastrostomy was performed and rescue surgical treatment was indicated, which was again refused by the patient. Cetuximab was initiated in a maintenance scheme.

After 2 months, the patient returned with hoarseness and dyspnea, and an urgent tracheostomy was required. In August 2015, the patient underwent a total laryngopharyngoesophagectomy, with colonic retrosternal transposition for alimentary tract reconstruction, associated with resection of the affected trachea and fashioning of a tracheostomy (Figs. 1, 2, and 3). A left deltopectoral flap was used to cover the colon and to avoid cutaneous tension (Figs. 15 and 16).

In the postoperative period, the patient presented with a colon–pharyngocutaneous fistula and severe cervical infection, which caused tracheostomy dehiscence and collapse of the tracheal stump to the mediastinum. The fistula was primarily closed, but without success.

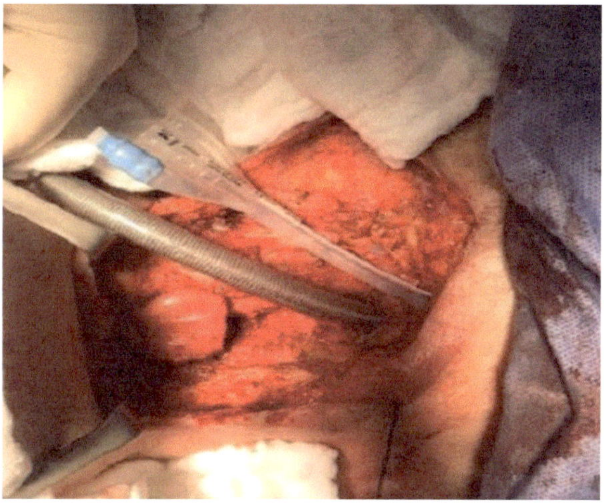

Fig. 15 Distal trachea containing the endotracheal tube after resection of the lesion. The Foley catheter is inserted into the colon

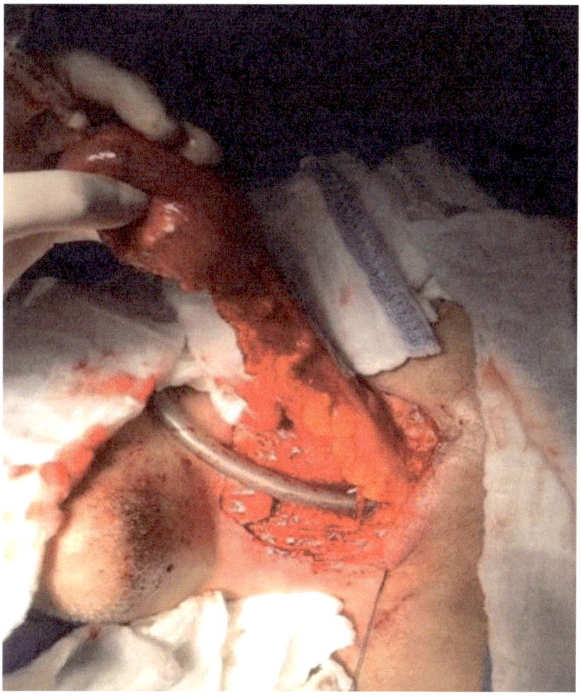

Fig. 16 Retrosternal colon transposition

After extended hospitalization in the ICU, the administration of a large variety of antibiotics and infectious process resolution, great difficulty of cannula exchange and airway patency persisted due to the depth of the tracheal stump position.

In November 2015, MT was indicated. It occurred with resection of 50% of the manubrium, removal of the clavicular heads, and transposal of the tracheal stump inferiorly through the innominate artery. The colon–pharyngocutaneous fistula was again primarily closed. The left PM flap was used for mediastinal vessel coverage and a right deltopectoral flap was used to reinforce the neck coverage (Figs. 17 and 18).

The patient was evaluated with a colon–pharyngocutaneous fistula that needed to be closed twice during hospitalization with resuturing of the edges, but with no complications of MT. The patient was discharged for ambulatory control in the third postoperative month after the first surgery (Fig. 19).

Currently, 10 months after the rescue surgery and 7 months after MT, there is no evident disease and no surgical complications. The patient presented with just a single episode of moderated pneumonia, which needed a short hospitalization for systemic antibiotic therapy.

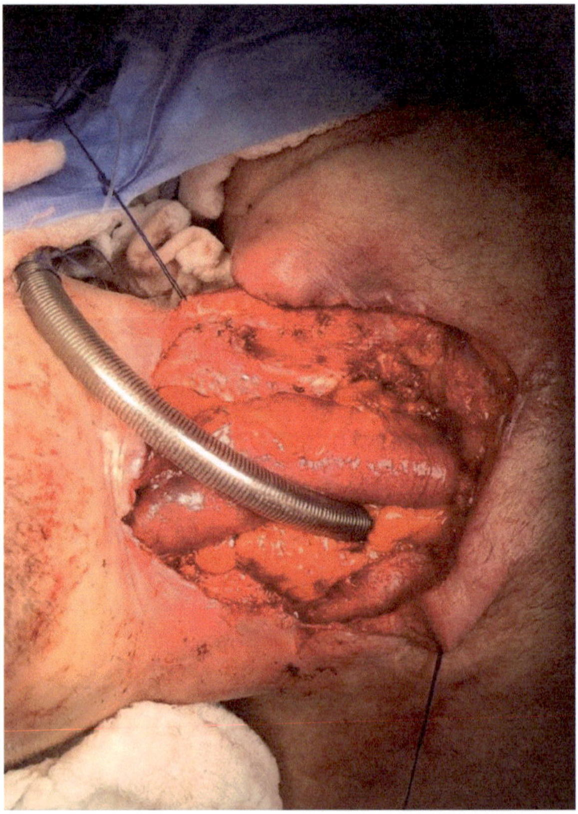

Fig. 17 Colon–pharyngeal anastomosis of the neck with good extension

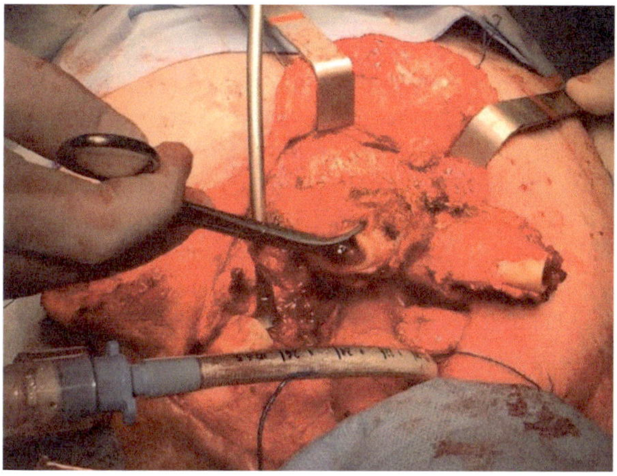

Fig. 18 Resection of the manubrium and clavicular heads

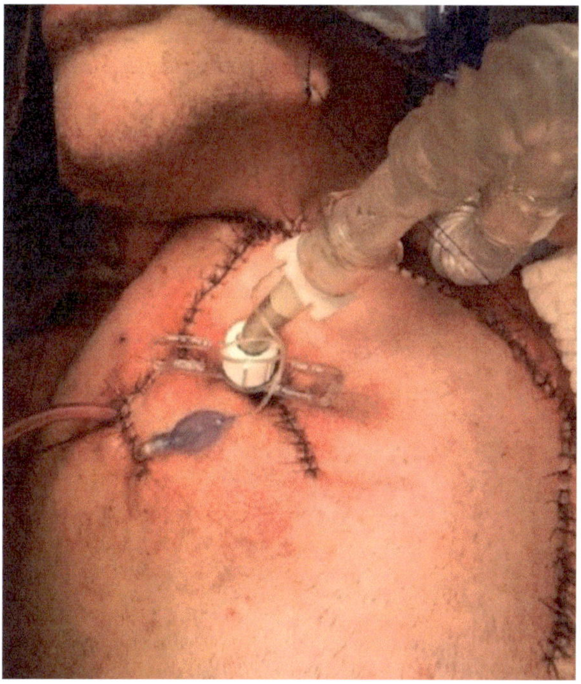

Fig. 19 Deltopectoral flap

Discussion and Outcomes

In our reported case, the first treatment planned was a radical surgical resection because there was locally advanced cancer. However, the patient refused this treatment plan, leading to completion of a chemotherapy regimen of induction (TPF) associated with concurrent radiotherapy with cetuximab. This treatment consisted of three cycles 21 days apart (75 mg/m^2 Taxol on day 1, 35 mg/m^2 platinum on days 1 and 2, and 750 mg/m^2 5-fluorouracil on days 1–5) as an adjunct to radiotherapy with the intention to preserve organs with control comparable to that of surgical treatment. An advantage of this treatment is a better laryngeal preservation rate than that achieved with exclusive use of radiotherapy. In addition, replacement of cisplatin by cetuximab has lower levels of toxicity when performed concurrently with radiation therapy. A laryngopharyngoesophagectomy would be the gold standard treatment in this case, but the patient declined it.

MT consists of a procedure that is usually indicated for re-establishment of an alternative airway after resection of advanced tumors, especially after laryngopharyngectomy associated with esophagectomy, and after resection of recurrence in the tracheostoma [4]. In the presented case, the indication was not because of a tumor, but as a way of solving a surgical complication of the first procedure: anastomotic dehiscence with migration of the remaining trachea into the mediastinum.

The current literature shows small series of cases, often obtained over decades. However, these studies show the degrees of morbidity and mortality associated with this procedure as well as the techniques used to protect the artery and innominate vein.

Orringer studied 44 patients who underwent MT, ten as a palliative procedure and another 34 (72%) for airway reconstruction after cervical exenteration (pharyngolaryngectomy with esophagectomy). Of the latter, 31 had alimentary tract reconstruction by gastric transposition and three by transposition of the colon. A perioperative mortality rate of 14% (six deaths) was observed, all in patients who underwent cervical exenteration. Only nine patients (32%) had a postoperative course without complications. The length of stay ranged from 10 to 51 days (median 26.2 days). Only one patient had a rupture of the innominate artery, in which the trachea was not transposed down the artery. Orringer reported that the critical factor to avoid fatal complications was elimination of tension between the structures, which could be achieved with implementation of the trachea below the innominate artery.

In the work of Kamiyama et al. [20], 40 patients undergoing pharyngolaryngectomy with total esophagectomy were studied. MT was performed in nine cases (22.5%), and of these, four (44%) had complications related to the tracheostomy. Of the 31 patients who underwent traditional tracheostomy, only four (12.5%) had complications related to ostomy. Survival at 5 years was 48.6% and perioperative mortality was 5% (two deaths: one by bleeding due to brachiocephalic vein injury and the other due to injury of the innominate artery).

Berthet [9] evaluated 12 patients undergoing MT, all for recurrence in stoma after laryngectomy. In all 12 surgeries, relocation of tracheal segments remaining below the innominate artery and a myocutaneous flap to cover the tracheostomy were necessary. Reconstruction of the alimentary tract was required in four patients (three with gastric transposition and one with primary closure). There was one death in the postoperative period (8.3%), due to a vascular fistula. The length of hospital stay varied between 13 and 86 days. Survival at 5 years was 53%. The author concluded that despite the surgical risks, long-term survival after total resection of the lesion is acceptable.

Grillo [19] and Mathisen described modifications in the MT and cervical exenteration techniques. They performed a prophylactic ligation of the innominate artery in all patients with some degree of tension between the tracheal stump and the mediastinal vessels under electroencephalographic monitoring. Prior to surgery, all patients underwent arteriography to assess the cerebral vasculature and the patency of the Willis polygon. The authors also used the omentum to cover the artery stumps and to separate them from the trachea, and gave preference to a bipedicled flap for cutaneous coverage of the tracheostoma. They performed MT in 14 cases in a series of 18 patients who underwent cervical exenteration. The innominate artery had to be divided in seven of these patients. Of these seven, only one had hemiplegia, which was treated through a bypass to the left subclavian artery. Alimentary tract reconstruction was performed, preferably by choice of the colon, transposing it through a substernal tunnel. In this study, the colon was used for reconstruction in ten patients, while the stomach was used only in three. There was one death in the study due to anastomotic leakage in a reconstruction with a gastric tube, which resulted in mediastinal sepsis. The median survival was 10 months, and six patients survived for more than 4 years. The authors describe functional results equivalent to laryngectomy and recommend this procedure for palliation only in cases with a survival prediction longer than 6 months.

Chan et al. [18] studied 38 patients with cervical–mediastinal tumors who underwent MT. There was no artery ligation in any case. Of these 38, 31 (81.6%) required repositioning of the trachea below the innominate artery to prevent tension and 14 patients required a PM flap for tracheostoma closure. Digestive tract reconstruction was necessary in 34 cases, of which eight had a primary closing of the neopharynx. A jejunum free flap was used in eight cases, the gastric tube was transposed in 12, and a tubed PM flap was made in six patients. The authors described in-hospital mortality of 5.3% (two deaths) due to bleeding of the great vessels. There was a leakage from the gastrointestinal anastomosis in six patients (three who underwent gastric transposition and three who had reconstruction with a tube-shaped PM). Eleven patients (28.9%) had ischemia or partial necrosis of the terminal portion of the trachea. During follow-up, 18 patients (47.4%) had stenosis of the tracheostoma. In these cases, a history of leakage from the anastomosis or tracheal ischemia was statistically significant as a risk factor for tracheostoma stenosis ($p = 0.34$ and $p = 0.26$, respectively). The PM flap was considered a protective factor, inasmuch as tracheostoma stenosis occurred in just one patient (7.1% of those who underwent it). The survival rates were 80.6% at 1 year and 55.6% at 5 years. The authors recommended not skeletonizing the terminal stump of the trachea to prevent its ischemia.

In a study involving 13 patients undergoing MT, Conti et al. described two in-hospital deaths (one for bleeding of the innominate artery) and only five cases with no complications. The average hospital stay was 29 days, ranging from 12 to 101 days. The survival rates at 3 and 5 years were 57% and 43%, respectively. Worse outcomes were observed in patients operated on for esophageal carcinoma or for laryngeal carcinoma recurrence.

In the existing literature, when a complete resection of the esophagus occurs, the main options are the gastric pull-up, colonic transposition, and transposition of the jejunum, with the choice depending on the service experience and the specific conditions of the patient (previous gastrostomy, prior laparotomy, and previous colonic or jejunal surgery). When the gastric pull-up is chosen, there is the possibility of distal ischemia or gastric stump ischemia, which rarely happens with the colon. Furthermore, the colon can provide a large segment for reconstruction, but at the expense of increased intra-abdominal anastomoses. In cases where only the cervical esophagus is resected, the microsurgical jejunal flap is a good option, as are tubed myocutaneous flaps (e.g., the anterolateral thigh flap and forearm flap) [5, 6, 11].

MT is an important option for airway reconstruction where there is an insufficient length of trachea to perform the traditional procedure in the cervical region. There was a decrease in the incidence of innominate artery rupture after the use of flaps for coverage and fashioning of a tension-free trachea–skin anastomosis [4]. Although it has a high rate of complications, MT continues to be viable in well-selected patients, as observed in our case report.

To conclude, MT is an exceptional procedure due to the morbidity and risks it presents and should be performed only in patients with an excellent general condition. It may also be indicated as a palliative treatment in selected cases. This report shows the feasibility of its use associated with laryngopharyngoesophagectomy for a locally advanced tumor. The surgeon should be aware of the possibility of esophagectomy, with several options for gastrointestinal transit reconstruction.

References

1. Gomez-Caro A, Gimferrer JM, Macchiarini P. Technique to avoid innominate artery ligation and perform an anterior mediastinal tracheostomy for residual trachea of less than 5 cm. Ann Thorac Surg. 2007;84:1777–9.
2. Grillo HC, Mathisen DJ. Cervical exenteration. Ann Thorac Surg. 1990;49:401–9.
3. Orringer MB. Anterior mediastinal tracheostomy with and without cervical exenteration. Ann Thorac Surg. 1992;54:628–37.
4. Conti M, Benhamed L, Mortuaire G, Chevalier D, Pinçon C, Wurtz A. Indications and results of anterior mediastinal tracheostomy for malignancies. Ann Thorac Surg. 2010;89(5):1588–95.
5. Carlson GW, Schusterman MA, Guillamondegui OM. Total reconstruction of the hypopharynx and cervical esophagus: a 20 year experience. Ann Plast Surg. 1992;29:408–12.
6. de Vries EJ, Stein DW, Johnson JT, et al. Hypopharyngeal reconstruction: a comparison of two alternatives. Laryngoscope. 1989;99:614–7.
7. Maipang T, Singha S, Panjapiyakul C, Totemchokchyakarn P. Mediastinal tracheostomy. Am J Surg. 1996;171:581–6.
8. Jatin Shah 2012 Head and Neck Surgery and Oncology, 4th Edition. ISBN978–0–323-05589-5.
9. Berthet JP, Garrel R, Gimferrer JM, Paradela M, Marty-Ané CH, Molins L, Gómez-Caro A. Anterior mediastinal tracheostomy as salvage operation. Ann Thorac Surg. 2014;98(3):1026–33.
10. Goldberg M, Freeman J, Gullane PJ, et al. Transhiatal esophagectomy with gastric transposition for pharyngolaryngeal malignant disease. J Thorac Cardiovasc Surg. 1989;97:327–33.
11. Goligher JC, Robin IG. Colon in reconstruction after pharyngectomy: use of left colon for reconstruction of pharynx and esophagus after pharyngectomy. Br J Surg. 1954;42:283–90.
12. Gomez-Caro A, Gimferrer JM, Molins L. Lung Incarceration after anterior mediastinal tracheostomy. Ann Thorac Surg. 2013;95:1795–7.

13. Patel UA, Moore BA, Wax M, et al. Impact of pharyngeal closure techniqueon fistula after salvage laryngectomy. JAMA Otolaryngol Head Neck Surg. 2013;139:1–6.
14. Paydarfar JÁ, Birkmeyer NJ. Complications in head and neck surgery: a meta-analysis of postlaryngectomy pharyngocutaneous fistula. Arch Otolaryngol Head and Neck Surg. 2003;132:67–72.
15. Sisson GA, Strachley CJ Jr, Johnson NE. Mediastinal dissection for recurrent cancer after laryngectomy. Laryngoscope. 1962;72:1064–77.
16. Terz JJ, Wagman LD, King RE, et al. Results of extended resection of tumours involving the cervical part of the trachea. Surg Gynecol Obstet. 1980;151:491–6.
17. Waddell WR, Cannon B. A technic for subtotal excision of the trachea and establishment of a sternal tracheostomy. Ann Surg. 1959;149:1–8.
18. Chan YW, Yu Chow VL, Lun Liu LH, Ignace Wei W. Manubrial resection and anterior mediastinal tracheostomy: friend or foe? Laryngoscope. 2011;121:1441–5. https://doi.org/10.1002/lary.21.
19. Grillo HC. Terminal or mural tracheostomy in the anterior mediastinum. J Thorac Cardiovasc Surg. 1966;51:422–7.
20. Kamiyama R, Mitani H, Yonekawa H, Fukushima H, Sasaki T, Shimbashi W, Seto A, Koizumi Y, Ebina A, Kawabata K. A clinical study of pharyngolaryngectomy with total esophagectomy: postoperative complications, countermeasures, and prognoses. Otolaryngology Head and Neck Surgery. 2015;153:392–9. first published on June 26, 2015.
21. Kleitsch WP. Anterior mediastinal tracheostomy. J Thorac Surg. 1952;24:38–42.
22. Minor GR. Trans-sternal tracheal excision for carcinoma. J Thorac Surg. 1952;24:88–92.
23. Watson WL. Cancer of the trachea fourteen years after treatment for cancer of larynx. J Thorac Surg. 1942;12:142–50.
24. Sugarbaker DJ, Bueno R, Colson YL, Jaklitch MT, Krasna MJ, Mentzer SJ, Williams M, Adams A. Adult chest surgery. 2nd ed. New York: McGraw-Hill Education; 2015. https://accesssurgery.mhmedical.com/book.aspx?bookID=1317.

Check for updates

Transtumoral Tracheostomy

Dorio Jose Coelho Silva, Ricardo Mai Rocha, Terence Pires de Farias, and Rafael Vianna Locio

Introduction

Tracheostomy is a surgical procedure indicated for maintenance of the airway in patients with severe respiratory insufficiency due either to mechanical obstruction of the upper airways or obstruction resulting from retention of secretions, insufficient ventilation, or both [1]. In this chapter we will mainly pay attention to mechanical obstructions, which are usually due to changes in the anatomy of the larynx, trachea, oropharynx, and hypopharynx, and, in specific cases (and more usually in the specialty of head and neck surgery), are caused by advanced malignant neoplasia. There are several tumors of the upper digestive tract or cervical masses that can compress and deflect the airway (Fig. 1); among these, we highlight those most frequent in our practice: malignant neoplasms of the larynx, anaplastic carcinoma, thyroid lymphoma, and bulky submarining goiters with airway compression [1, 2].

D.J.C. Silva, M.D.
Department of Head and Neck Surgery, Evangelic Hospital of Vila Velha, Vila Velha, Brazil

R.M. Rocha, M.D. (✉)
Assistant Professor of Head and Neck Surgery, Universidade Federal do Espirito Santo, Vitoria, Brazil

Assistant Professor of Head and Neck Surgery, Faculdade Brasileira Multivix, Vitoria, Brazil
e-mail: ricardomai@gmail.com

T.P. de Farias, M.D., Ph.D., M.Sc., Researcher.
Department of Head and Neck Surgery, Brazilian National Cancer Institute—INCA, Rio de Janeiro, RJ, Brazil

Department of Head and Neck Surgery, Pontifical Catholic University, Rio de Janeiro, RJ, Brazil

R. Vianna Locio, M.S., (Medical Student).
Faculdade Pernambucana de Saúde/IMIP — Maternity Childhood Institute of Pernambuco, Recife, PE, Brazil

T.P. de Farias (ed.), *Tracheostomy*, https://doi.org/10.1007/978-3-319-67867-2_12

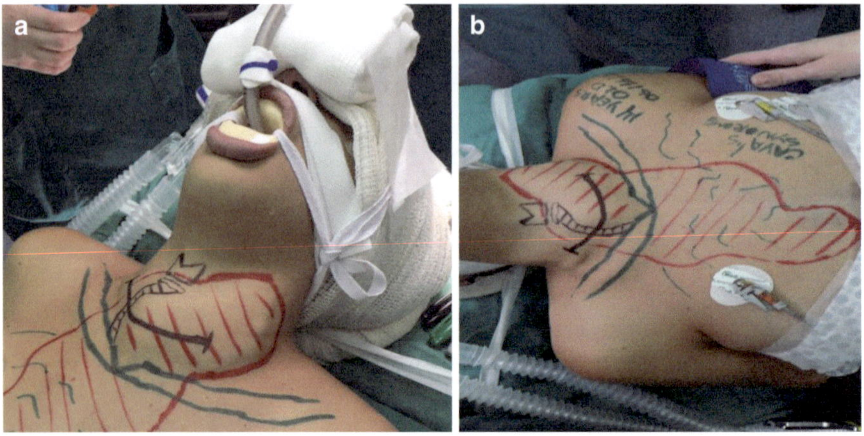

Fig. 1 Large lesion affecting the cervical topography with important tracheal deviation to the right

Anaplastic thyroid carcinoma is a rare neoplasm and highly aggressive, with survival often measured in months. It may be associated with a well-differentiated thyroid neoplasm and long-term goiter. The finding of an association between anaplastic carcinoma and a well-differentiated thyroid tumor is usually made during investigation of the anaplastic carcinoma within a piece of a well-differentiated carcinoma on histological analysis [3, 4].

It is believed that the incidence of anaplastic carcinoma has decreased due to the appearance and improvement of immunohistochemical studies facilitating more accurate diagnosis, iodine supplementation in the diet, and more aggressive treatment of well-differentiated thyroid carcinomas [3, 4].

It is estimated that anaplastic thyroid carcinoma is associated with 1–3% of benign and malignant tumors of the thyroid, although some studies have observed an increase in this ratio primarily related to geographic factors (iodine intake deficiency and endemic goiter) [4].

The age of greatest incidence varies from 50 to 90 years, and it is very rare in patients below 50 years of age (<10%). There is a predominance of females, in a proportion of 3:1 [4].

Many studies have suggested an origin of undifferentiated thyroid carcinoma in thyroid with some diseases such as goiter (80%), adenoma, or even a well-differentiated carcinoma. A strong association between prior history and the histology of this tumor has led many researchers to suspect a malignant transformation from a benign condition or a well-differentiated carcinoma into a highly malignant neoplasm. Approximately 20% of patients with anaplastic thyroid carcinoma presented with a previous history of a well-differentiated thyroid carcinoma, and 20–30% had a coexisting differentiated carcinoma. The commonly associated differentiated carcinoma is papillary, but a follicular tumor may also have this association. Approximately 10% of patients with Hürthle cell carcinoma have foci of anaplastic carcinoma in surgical specimens [5].

As we have seen, anaplastic carcinoma arises from one or another point of dedifferentiation, particularly mutation of the p53 tumor suppressor protein. No precipitating effect has been identified, and the mechanisms that lead to emergence of an undifferentiated tumor from a well-differentiated carcinoma remain uncertain [5].

Almost all patients present with an often palpable and voluminous thyroid mass. However, regional or remote dissemination may be present in up to 90% of cases. The most frequent sites of regional involvement are the perithyroid tissues (fat and muscles), lymph nodes, larynx, trachea, esophagus, pharynx, and large cervical and mediastinal vessels. The lungs are the main sites of distant metastasis (up to 90%), followed by the bones and brain, at a much lower frequency [4, 6].

Usually the first symptom is rapid growth of a cervical mass, occurring in up to 85% of patients. This growth can cause cervical pain and compression (or invasion) of the upper aerodigestive tract, resulting in dyspnea, dysphagia, dysphonia, cough, and sometimes hemoptysis. Up to 50% of patients may have enlarged cervical lymph nodes, and other findings include laryngeal stridor, tracheal deviation, or even signs of compression of the superior vena cava [6].

Imaging diagnosis is important in assessing the extent of disease, in therapeutic planning, and in monitoring of the response to treatment. Thoracic radiography is important in evaluating the presence of pulmonary metastases, as well as evaluation of bone metastases in ribs or spine. Ultrasonography of the neck is important in determining local involvement and regional lymph nodes, as well as suggesting, if there is extrathyroidal extension, that the thyroid tumor is a malignant neoplasm. Computed tomography (CT) of the neck and mediastinum should delineate the extent of the thyroid tumor and identify invasion of large vessels and the upper aerodigestive tract [4].

Several characteristics are important in the prognosis of patients. Patients who have disease confined to the thyroid, or who have disease with local or regional extension, have longer survival than those with distant metastases. Tumor size also seems to be important [7].

Other characteristics that present an adverse prognosis are advanced age at diagnosis, male gender, and presence of dyspnea as the initial symptom [8].

Many patients with anaplastic carcinoma die within a few months, primarily due to local extension and airway obstruction, with a median survival of only 3–4 months [7, 8].

Surgery is rarely indicated in these patients, certainly given the advanced-stage diagnosis in the vast majority of cases; however, if the tumor appears to be confined to the thyroid, surgery should be attempted not only to improve the prognosis but also to facilitate adjuvant treatment [9].

In the most severe cases where neoplastic involvement of the cervical area is already present, we perform a transtumoral tracheostomy. A neoplastic lesion involving a course of surgery can completely distort the anatomy, compromising important structures, and necessitating a more accurate surgical technique requiring care beyond the tracheal site itself [9, 10].

When tracheal deviation is suspected, it is prudent to carry out a follow-up examination to identify where the new airway is located, which is normally unnecessary

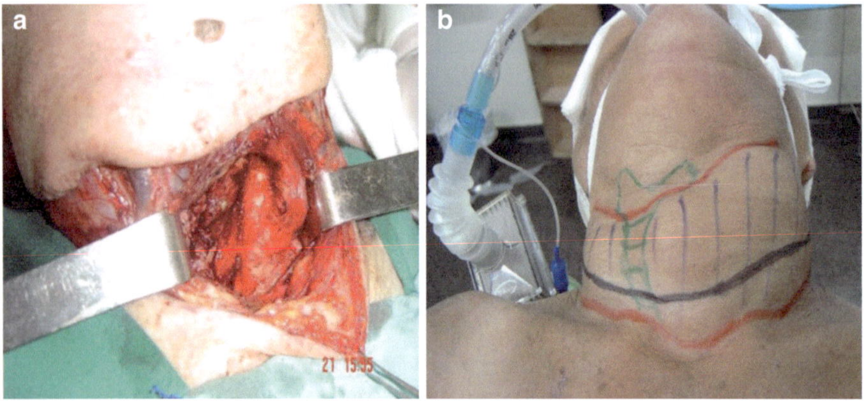

Fig. 2 (**a**) Tracheal deviation visible during surgery. (**b**) Drawing of the tracheal deviation prior to surgery

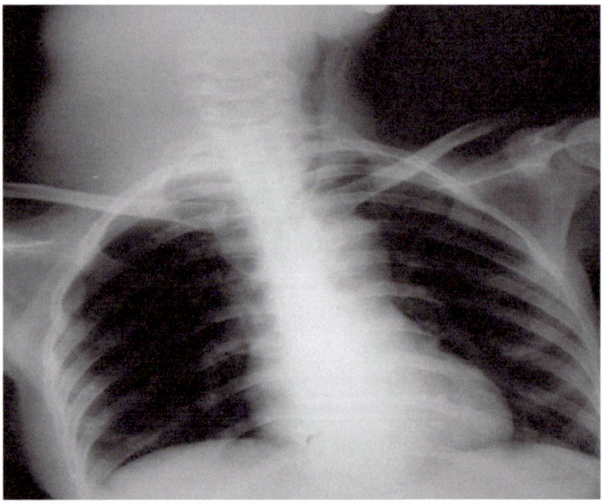

Fig. 3 An X-ray may be useful in identifying the new site of the trachea after deviation by the neoplastic process

during standard tracheostomy (Fig. 2). Depending on the time and the setting for performing the tracheostomy, even a cervical X-ray (Fig. 3) helps in defining the most appropriate access site to avoid wasting surgical time. More accurate examinations such as CT or magnetic resonance imaging (MRI) are obviously more informative, and their indication depends basically on the availability and speed with which they can be performed [11].

At times, there is no way to avoid access via the cricoid or even higher (Fig. 4), via the thyroid cartilage, which, depending on the neoplastic situation, is already literally destroyed by the lesion [1, 2, 12].

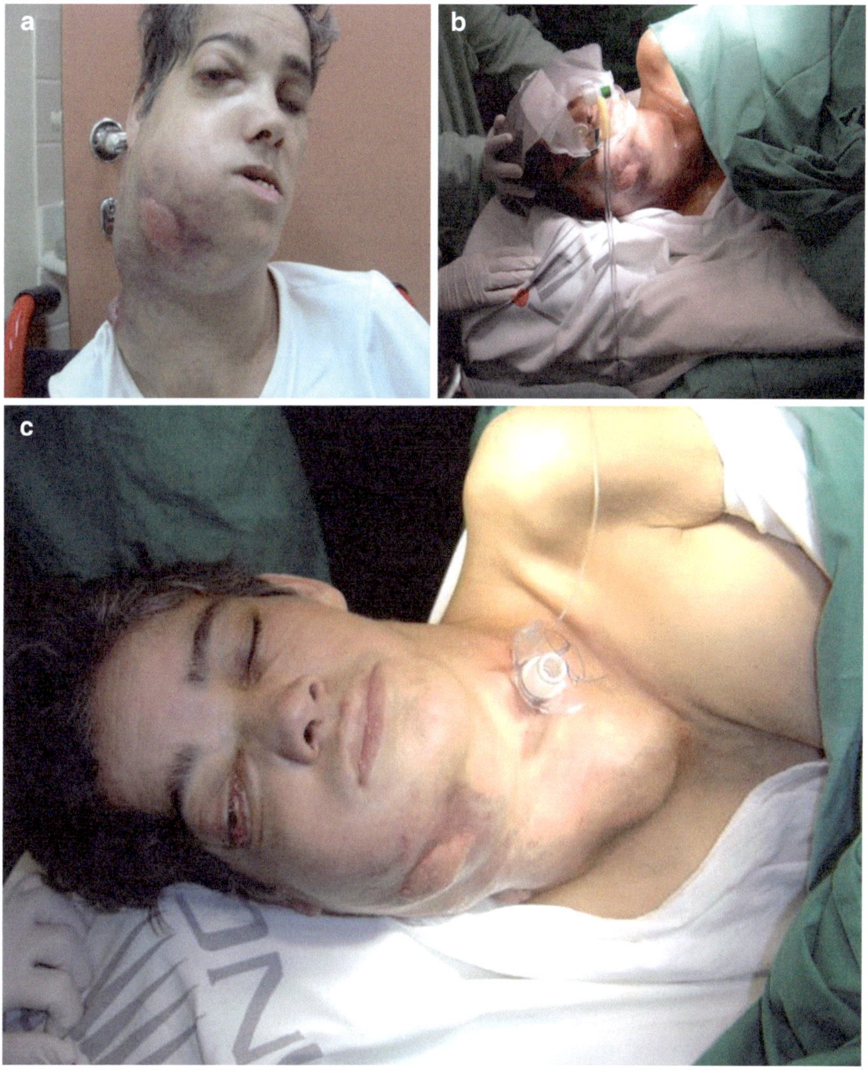

Fig. 4 Significant airway deviation in a patient with a massive cervical desmoid tumor

Because the airway is compromised, the anesthesiologist must have instruments available to facilitate orotracheal intubation and may sometimes use bronchofibroscopy (Fig. 5) for adequate visualization of the airway and to minimize local trauma with a risk of bleeding, which will make it even more difficult to access [1, 5].

The well-known palliative procedure for anaplastic thyroid carcinoma is no longer a rarity in certain oncology centers where the patients are of low socioeconomic status [2, 12, 13].

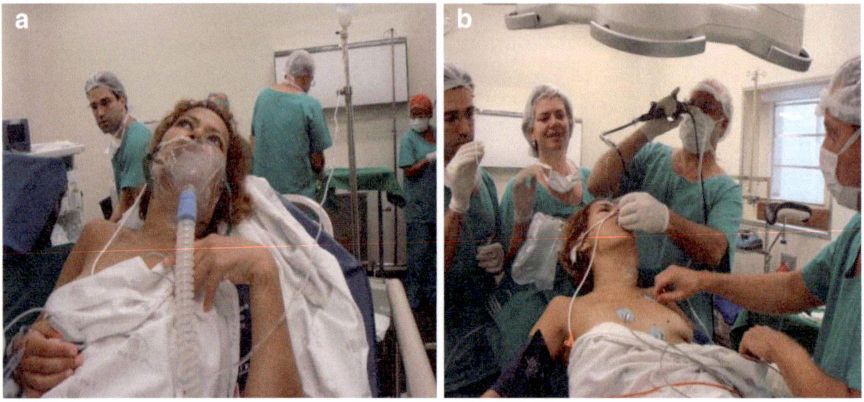

Fig. 5 General anesthesia prior to tracheostomy, via intubation assisted by nasofibroscopy

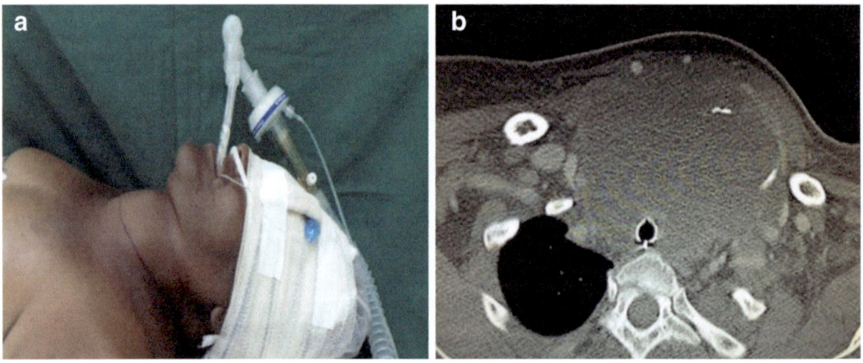

Fig. 6 Lesions of cervical origin with tracheal compression

Transtumoral tracheostomy may be necessary in lesions originating from the upper digestive tract and cervical lesions. The former are lesions of the larynx, hypopharynx, and even the oropharynx. The latter are thyroid lesions (Fig. 6), cervical metastasis of unknown primary tumor [1, 2]. Another significant point, which increases the difficulty of the procedure, is radiation therapy, especially if only recently completed [14].

Patient Approach

The patient being electively treated with a present neoplastic lesion and in whom there is a risk of progression to transtumoral tracheostomy needs to be approached in a precautionary way in order to convince them that performing the procedure before obstructive symptoms occur (Fig. 7) is the best option. The rationale for the procedure and its potentially life-saving justification must be made explicit by the

Fig. 7 Older patients with large cervical masses with an indication for tracheostomy; older age may be a factor in resistance to acceptance of a tracheostomy

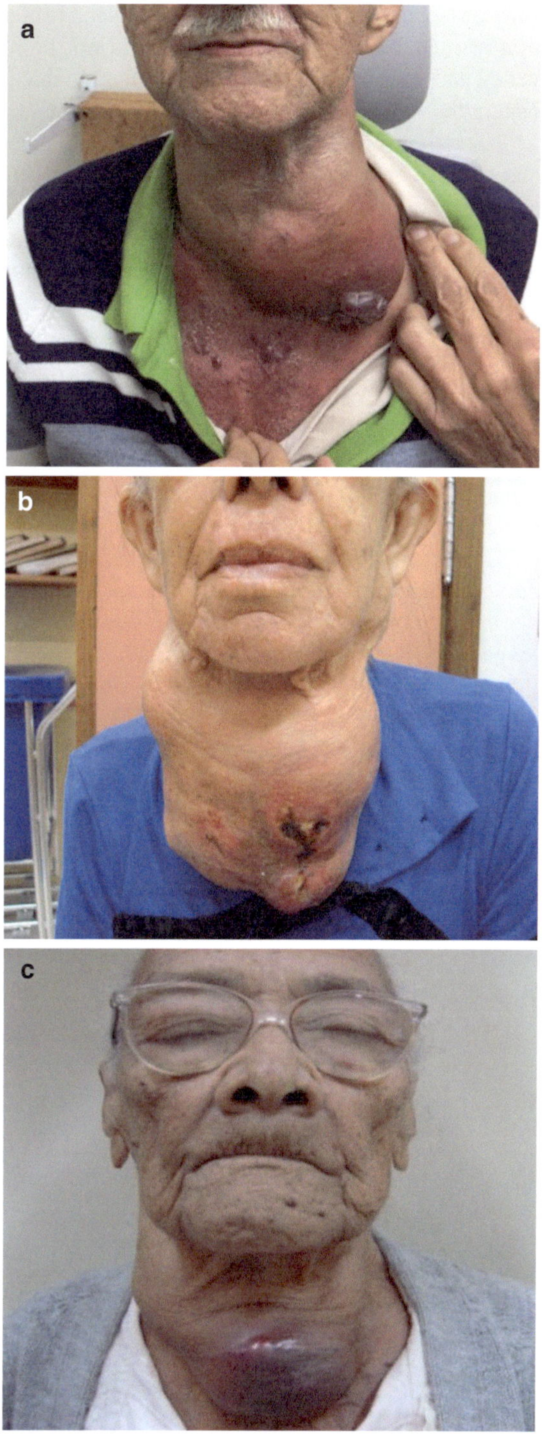

surgeon. Certainly the ethical conduct of the professional, and formal documentation of it in the medical records, should not be neglected. Such time devoted to verbal and documented clarification will undoubtedly be advantageous for the clinician in the future, both in relation to the patient's family and in legal terms.

When there is still no cancer diagnosis, and depending on the family culture and clarification, the justification for the procedure is more difficult. In these cases, it is advisable to follow up with more regular consultations so that even without results of an oncological diagnosis, knowledge of the evolution of the lesion itself provides a sufficient and convincing argument for performing the tracheostomy before any obstructive symptoms occur.

Surgical Technique

General anesthesia is performed by orotracheal intubation, and bronchofibroscopy often facilitates the procedure by reducing the risk of bleeding from airway trauma and allowing better visualization of the lumen.

The patient is placed in dorsal decubitus with the use of a cushion under the shoulders and support under the head, allowing hyperextension of the neck. This maneuver exposes the trachea better, bringing it more anteriorly and showing more of its length (Fig. 8). The support helps to stabilize the head. The surgeon should position the patient while the anesthetist raises his or her chin. The area to be demarcated will have a upper limit of the mandible and a lower limit of the pectoral region [15].

A large horizontal incision (Fig. 9) is performed, and then detachment of myocutaneous flaps is performed in the upper and lower subplots (Fig. 10).

The median raphe formed by the cervical fascia is incised vertically, and the prethyroid muscles (hyoid sternum and thyroid sternum) are folded laterally

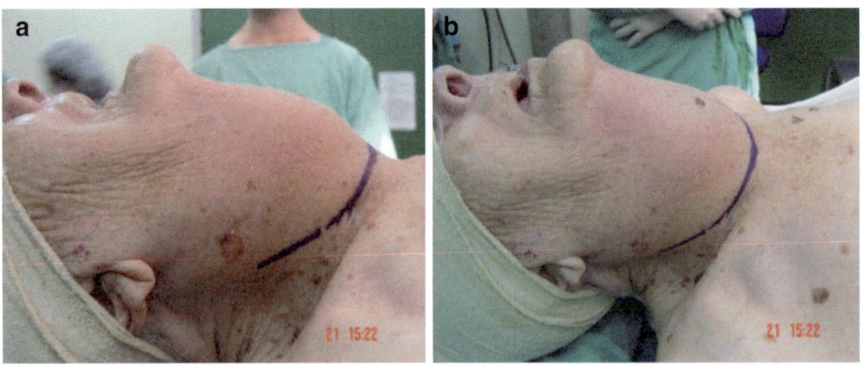

Fig. 8 Positioning of the patient on the surgical table in hyperextension and cranial fixation, when possible, are essential for the procedure

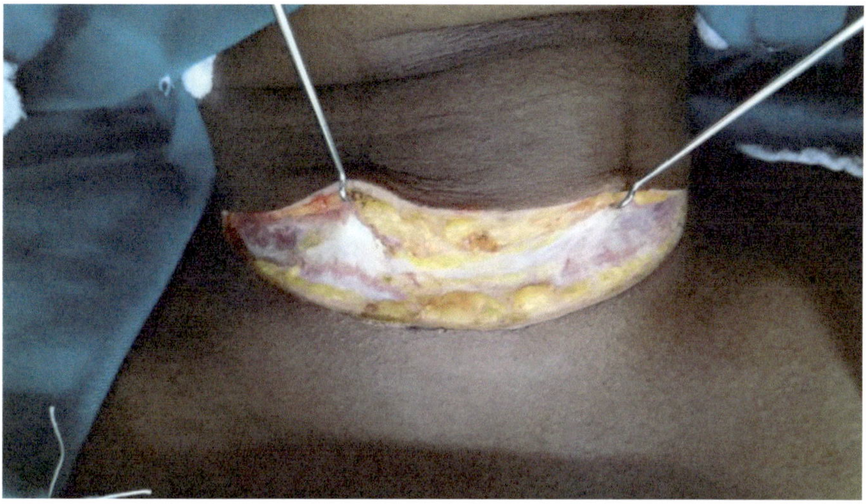

Fig. 9 A large cervical incision is important in transtumoral tracheostomy, even when there is already an understanding of the tracheal topography

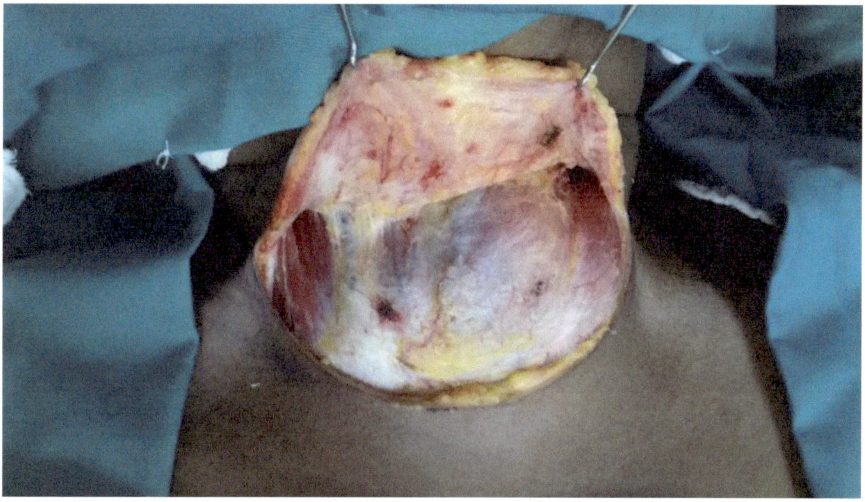

Fig. 10 Lifting of the subplatysmal patch

(Fig. 11). When it is not possible to fold these muscles because of tumor invasion, they should be sectioned (Fig. 12).

After removal of the prethyroid muscles, we reach the volume of the tumor mass that is causing the compression and obstruction of the airway. The thyroid cartilage is an important anatomical reference at this point, and the surgeon must be guided by it in search of a viable tracheal area (Fig. 13).

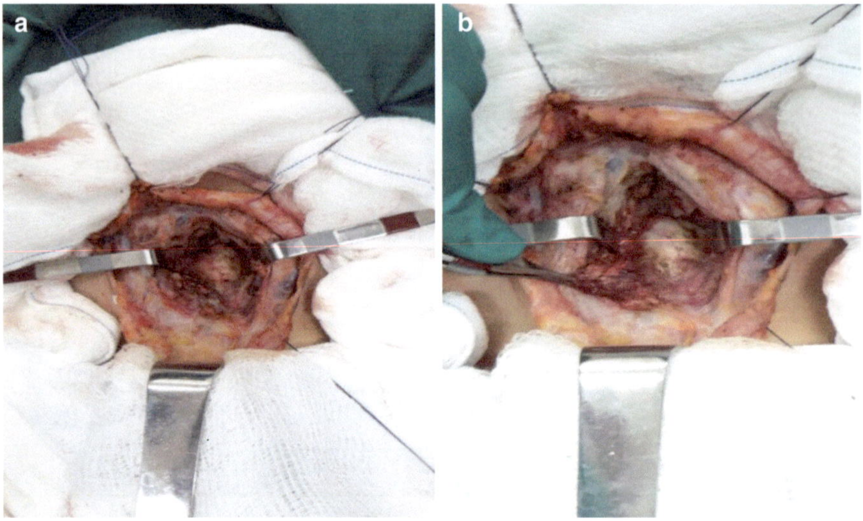

Fig. 11 The sternohyoid and sternothyroid muscles are retracted laterally or sectioned if there is a tumor invasion

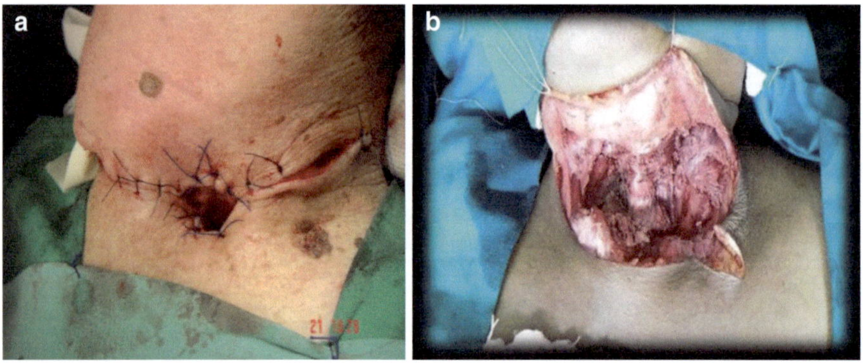

Fig. 12 (**a**) A large cervical incision is made for the safest possible approach to the already performed transtumoral tracheostomy. (**b**) Section of the musculature

At this point the surgeon should evaluate the resectability of the lesion that is anterior to the trachea. Whenever possible, it is important to remove the largest possible volume of the mass anteriorly for greater exposure of the airway, which should maintain the permeability of the access route and facilitate the fixation of the tracheostomy (Fig. 14).

When it is not possible to remove the anterior mass volume (Fig. 15), a tumor incision must be made, thinning it with electrocautery, until a viable trachea is achieved (Fig. 16).

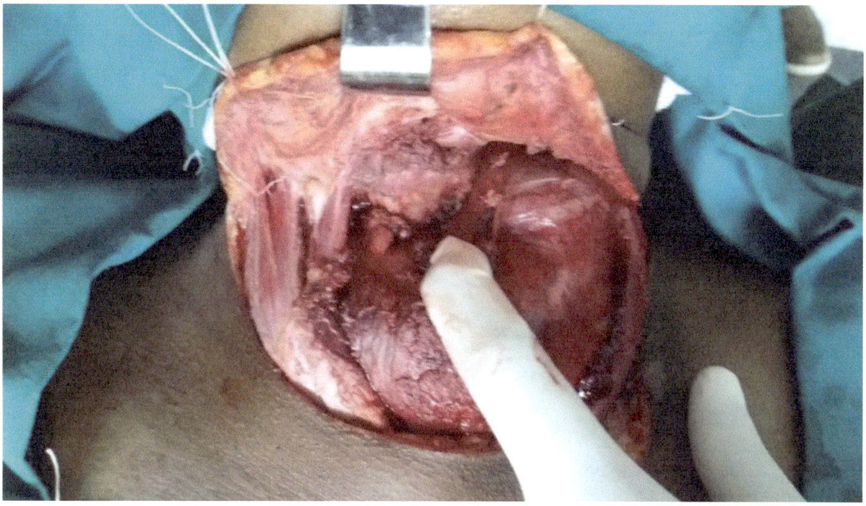

Fig. 13 During the procedure, with loss of the usual anatomy, in addition to the possibility of preoperative examinations to locate the trachea site, palpation to identify structures such as the carotid, cricoid, and thyroid cartilages is of great value

Fig. 14 Resection of as much of the neoplasm as possible, maintaining the safety of the procedure, with an emphasis on diagnosis, treatment, and improvement of the surgical condition

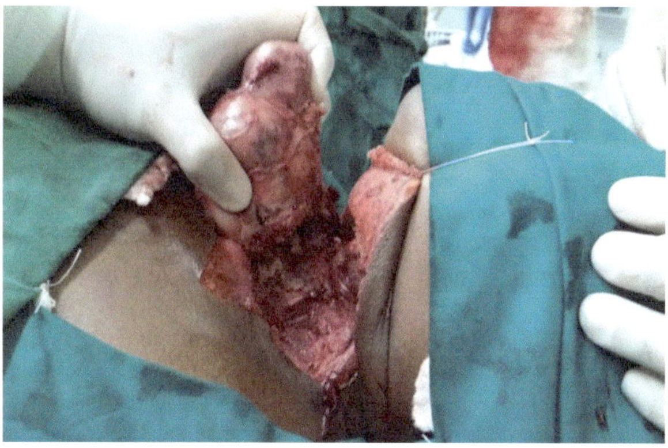

Once tumor debulking is performed, an inverted U-shaped incision (Bjork technique) is performed and a tracheal flap is made of about one half to two thirds the width of the trachea. The incision is performed in the intercartilaginous portion between the first and second tracheal rings and extends inferiorly, promoting the section of two rings. The fixation of the tracheal flaps is performed with non-absorbable thread with stitches surrounding the tracheal flap and the skin of the incised region, promoting fixation of the tracheal orifice to the skin [16, 17] (Fig. 17). Another possible technique is an H-shaped tracheal incision [18, 19, 20] (Fig. 18).

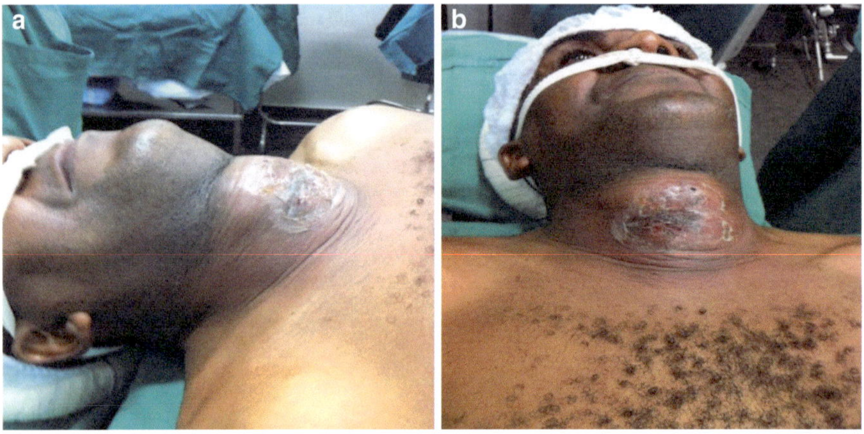

Fig. 15 Putting the surgical procedure at risk (of bleeding, infection, and complications such as a fistula), the removal of a large volume of the mass anterior to the tracheal tract during transtumoral tracheostomy is avoided

Fig. 16 Trachea with an endotracheal tube

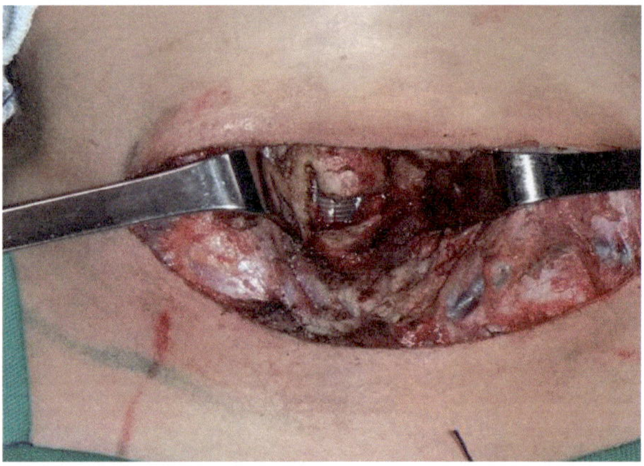

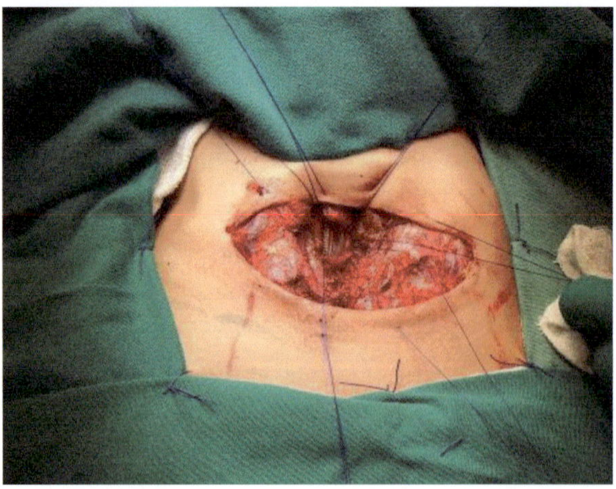

Fig. 17 Fixation of the tracheostoma on the skin after resection of the anterior wall of the trachea

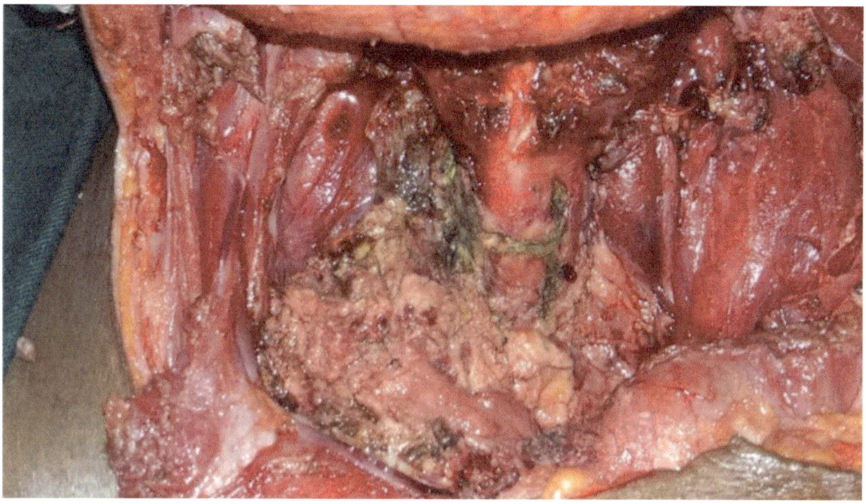

Fig. 18 H-shaped incision in the trachea

Cervical drainage may be required, depending on the debulking performed (Fig. 19), as well as cutaneous cannula fixation to avoid the risk of dislocation of the cannula outlet and exaggerated manipulation of the site (Fig. 20).

It is not always possible to follow the predetermined surgical plan. Depending on the degree of injury, destruction, and tracheal deviation, what happens depends on the status of the airway. This is consistent with important points: the new tracheal location (Fig. 21) and the location of the obstruction, structures that may be in the way, and the environment (the procedure site, anesthesia, and materials). The first two can be evidenced by physical examination when the patient has had a previous medical appointment and the history of the neoplastic lesion is known, or by complementary examination. The third one will depend on the hospital structure available to the head and neck surgery at the moment to perform the procedure and the surgeon should determine what he needs to do this procedure.

Technical Care

In addition to preparation of the patient and the family regarding the risk of the procedure and the prognosis of each case, sufficient time should be allowed for suitable preparation of the setting in which the procedure will be performed. The information given to the anesthesia team and the surgical room team is important for preparing the materials and avoiding distress and a sense of unpreparedness on the part of the patient, which could cause desperation during the procedure if general anesthesia is not feasible. Having surgical materials, a choice of cannulae, and materials for difficult anesthesia in place is essential to avoid prolonging the procedure.

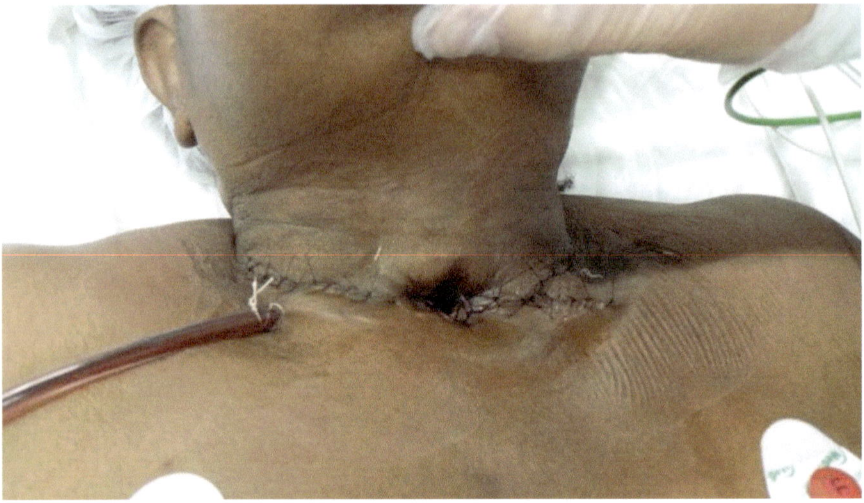

Fig. 19 Necessary cervical drainage after a large detachment, with significant removal of the lesion and risk of bleeding, reducing the chances of complication

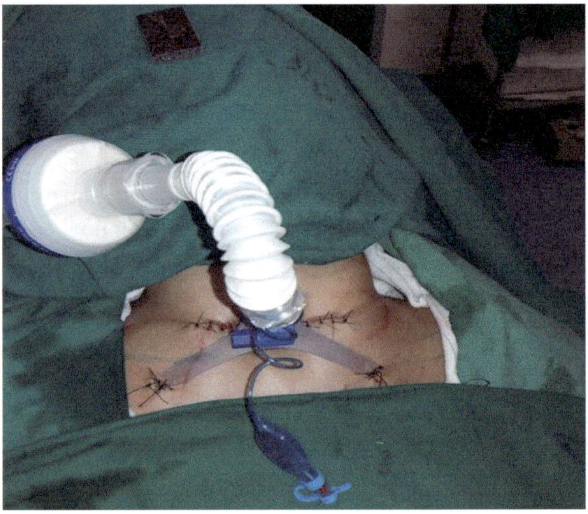

Fig. 20 Secure fixation of the Portex cannula, avoiding improper manipulation and risk of displacement of the cannula

In debulking, all removed material should be sent for histopathological study, even with a previous diagnosis. If this is the first approach to the patient, enough material should be collected and sent for histopathological and immunohistochemical study to optimize the chance of a conclusive diagnosis and suitable treatment for the patient.

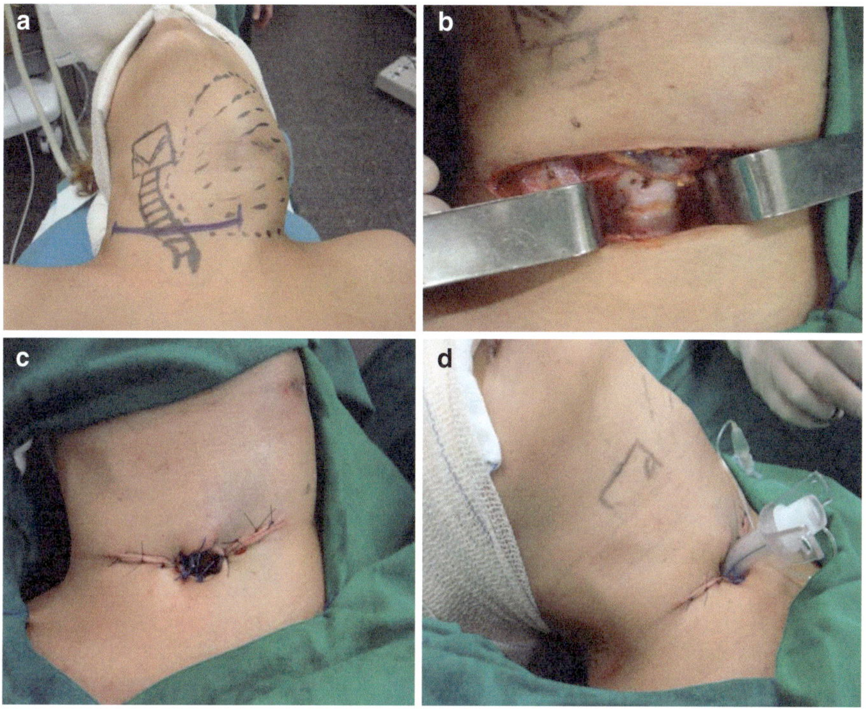

Fig. 21 (**a**) Anesthetized patient in the surgical room, with the team aware of the new cervical anatomy and the design of the tracheal topography. (**b**) Wide incision for safety in approaching the trachea. (**c**) Tracheostoma fixed to the skin. (**d**) Portex cannula

The most suitable preoperative examination for transtumoral tracheostomy, when there is doubt about a tracheal location, is one that will confirm the upper airway and obstruction site. It will depend on the availability of time and resources at the time of nomination. More accurate examinations are obviously more consistent and may facilitate the approach (Fig. 22), since they will also show the location of other significant structures to avoid complications during the procedure. Transcutaneous tracheostomies guided by ultrasonography have previously been described [13].

Performance of the procedure in an environment not suitable for use as an emergency room, in an emergency room, in a small surgery, or in another environment, can generate a desperate situation in an attempt to save the patient's life. Cricothyroidostomy can serve as a salvage option with the availability of suitable materials—preferably long- and short-caliber metal cannulae—where an attempt can be made to avert a worse outcome.

It is appropriate that after the cricothyroidostomy, tracheostomy is performed in an appropriate environment.

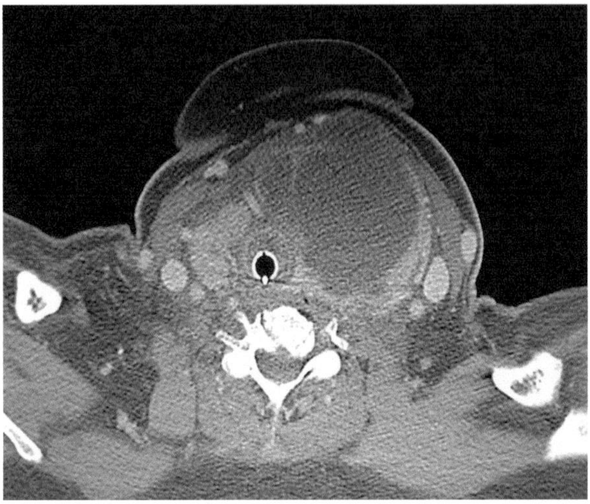

Fig. 22 Imaging greatly assists in tracheal identification and preparation for transtumoral tracheostomy

Complications

The possibility of complications in transtumoral tracheostomy is greater than in traditional tracheostomy, due to the distortion of the cervical anatomy, mainly. Subcutaneous emphysema, which is present in about 9% of patients in the postoperative period of tracheostomy [14], is not so frequent in transtumoral tracheostomies. Bleeding is the most frequent complication of the procedure, often occurring intraoperatively, and for this to happen, some reasons stand out: interposition of vessels in the altered path to the lumen, when not compressed by the injury, making it difficult to identify them; patients who are already receiving palliative treatment with worse anatomical circumstances; impossibility of general anesthesia, causing discomfort; need for optimization of the procedure, thus putting at risk visualization of the anatomical structures; and clotting disorders due to a paraneoplastic syndrome.

An esophageal fistula (cutaneous or due to the new route of the airway) can also happen during the procedure. This event should not be overlooked, even during ongoing palliative treatment. In the preoperative period, there is no investigation of the esophageal pathway; however, if there is any doubt, the patient should be investigated to see if there has been any injury after the end of the tracheostomy. If this yields a positive result, the appropriate repair should be performed, even in patients who are already gastrostomized.

In the event of a fistula already caused by the neoplasia, a cervical esophagostomy should be performed with cannula placement until a gastrostomy is performed, with the possibility of changing the cannula to a metallic one for hospital discharge.

The loss of a cannula after transtumoral tracheostomy can occur in cases in which there was no possibility of tracheal fixation in the skin. Replacement of the cannula by an insufficiently trained professional can lead to risks for the patient—not just a risk of malpositioning of the cannula but also risks of bleeding and destruction of important structures, with a further risk of obstruction. Therefore, the best thing to do is to allow a cervical positioning that allows the patency of the airway until a more qualified professional can perform the replacement of the cannula.

Conclusion

Prudent management is essential. Observing the natural history and the risk, depending on the treatment, from the evolution to the obstruction due to the development of the neoplasm, the head and neck surgeon should immediately inform the patient and relatives about the seriousness of the patient's condition, with proper orientation and indications to avoid increasing the risk of death. When the previous indication was not feasible or there was a negative outcome of the initial treatment, prompt action should be taken.

In the time available, the surgical center should be notified about the urgent requirement for immediate availability of an operating room, with preparation by the anesthesia team and the room staff to assemble the materials to be used, to avoid wasting time during the actual course of the procedure.

The hospital in which the head and neck surgery team is present should always have access to at least the minimum required emergency room equipment for tracheostomy, with surgical materials, cannulae, and surgical light or headlight.

Intraoperative care should be taken to avoid injury, including carotid artery disease, since in patients undergoing radiotherapy, a carotid lesion may develop with ligature of the carotid artery due to the friability of the vessel wall and the impossibility of suturing and maintaining viability. Consequently, in addition to cerebral sequelae, there is a risk of fatal evolution.

The postoperative course should involve care of the family or caregiver, informing them of the severity and the prognosis, with referral to another team if appropriate (clinical oncology, palliative care, radiotherapy), and follow-up of test results on tissue from the tracheostomy that is sent for histopathology analysis. In the latter case, it is always important to consider requesting immunohistochemistry analysis to optimize the diagnosis and treatment of the patient.

Consent for Publication Informed consent was obtained from all individual participants for whom identifying information is included in this article.

References

1. Alexander Patterson G, Pearson FG. Pearson's thoracic and esophageal surgery. 3rd ed. London: Churchill Livingstone; 2008.
2. Shaha AR. Airway management in anaplastic thyroid carcinoma. Laryngoscope. 2008;118(7):1195–8.
3. Pasieka J. Anaplastic thyroid cancer. Curr Opin Oncol. 2003;15:78–83.
4. Glaser SM, Mandish SF, Gill BS, Balasubramani GK, Clump DA, Beriwal S. Anaplastic thyroid cancer: prognostic factors, patterns of care, and overall survival. Head Neck. 2016;38(S1):E2083–90. Available from: http://doi.wiley.com/10.1002/hed.24384.

5. Nikiforov YE. Genetic alterations involved in the transition from well-differentiated to poorly differentiated and anaplastic thyroid carcinomas. Endocr Pathol. 2004;15(4):319–27. https://doi.org/10.1385/EP:15:4:319.
6. O'Neill JP, Shaha AR. Anaplastic thyroid cancer. Oral Oncol. 2017;49(7):702–6. https://doi.org/10.1016/j.oraloncology.2013.03.440.
7. Lu W, Lin J, Huang H, Chao T. Does surgery improve the survival of patients with advanced anaplastic thyroid carcinoma? Otolaryngol Head Neck Surg. 1998;118:728–31.
8. Wein RO, Weber RS. Anaplastic thyroid carcinoma: palliation or treatment? Curr Opin Otolaryngol Head Neck Surg. 2011;19(2):113–8.
9. Xu J, Liao Z, Li J, Wu X, Zhuang S. The role of tracheostomy in anaplastic thyroid carcinoma. World J Oncol. 2015;6(1):262–4.
10. Maipang T, Singha S, Panjapiyakul C, Totemchokchyakarn P. Mediastinal tracheostomy. Am J Surg. 1996;171(6):581–6.
11. Wang JC, Takashima S, Takayama F, Kawakami S, Saito A, Matsushita T, et al. Tracheal invasion by thyroid carcinoma: prediction using MR imaging. Am J Roentgenol. 2001;177(4):929–36. Available from: http://www.ncbi.nlm.nih.gov/pubmed/11566708.
12. Binelfa LF, García J. La traqueostomía en el cáncer anaplásico del tiroides: más vale temprano que nunca, vol. Vol. 145. Buenos Aires: Compumedicina.com; 2008. p. 1–7.
13. Honings J, Stephen AE, Marres HA, Gaissert HA. The management of thyroid carcinoma invading the larynx or trachea. Laryngoscope. 2010;120:682–9.
14. De Virgilio A, Greco A, Gallo A, Martellucci S, Conte M, de Vincentiis M. Tracheostomal stenosis clinical risk factors in patients who have undergone total laryngectomy and adjuvant radiotherapy. Eur Arch Otorhinolaryngol. 2013;270(12):3187–9. Available from: http://www.ncbi.nlm.nih.gov/pubmed/24057098.
15. de Figueiredo A. Tratado de oncologia. 1st ed. Rio de Janeiro: Revinter; 2013. p. 417–28.
16. Kinley CE. A technique of tracheostomy. Can Med Assoc J. 1965;92:79–81.
17. Dukes HM. Tracheostomy. Thorax. 1970;25:573–7.
18. Walts PA, Murthy SC, DeCamp MM. Techniques of surgical tracheostomy. Clin Chest Med. 2003;24:413–22.
19. Cheung NH, Napolitano LM. Tracheostomy: epidemiology, indications, timing, technique, and outcomes. Respir Care. 2014;59(6):895–915. https://doi.org/10.4187/respcare.02971.
20. Mani N, McNamara K, Lowe N, Lougrhran S, Yap B. Management of the compromised airway and role of tracheotomy in anaplastic thyroid carcinoma. Head Neck. 2016;38(1):85–8.

Tracheostomy and Radiotherapy

Célia Maria Pais Viégas, Diego Chaves Rezende Morais, and Carlos Manoel Mendonça de Araujo

Introduction

The overall annual incidence of head and neck tumors is more than 550,000 new cases with about 300,000 deaths [1]. The figures for 2016 in the USA [2] and in Brazil [3] are approximately 62,000 and 23,000 new cases and 13,000 and 10,000 deaths, respectively. In this context, radiotherapy appears to be an important therapeutic modality in the management of patients with head and neck cancer. It uses ionizing radiation and, through water radiolysis, produces free radicals that promote irreparable double breaks in tumor cell DNA molecules, leading to their deaths.

Specifically, in patients with head and neck cancer, radiotherapy can be employed in all subsets and clinical stages. In initial tumors, it is used as a single therapeutic modality, with results similar to those obtained with surgery. It may also be used as an adjuvant treatment to surgery in patients who present with predictors that indicate a high risk for locoregional recurrence (lymph node involvement, positive margins, locally advanced disease with adjacent extension, etc.). In addition, in recent years there has been increasing interest in the use of radiotherapy in combination with chemotherapy in organ preservation protocols, without detrimental effects on survival and providing organ preservation. Finally, radiotherapy can be used alone or in combination with chemotherapy in patients with unresectable or nonsurgical tumors due to comorbidities, and also has an important role as palliative treatment in the relief of local pain, bleeding, and/or imminent obstruction of the airway.

Conventional radiotherapy was traditionally used in the decades preceding the 1990s, and in this approach there was minimal conformation to the tumor, generating many treatment-related side effects, since there was exposure to radiation of large volumes of mucosa, the swallowing organs, skin, and salivary glands.

C.M.P. Viégas, M.D., Ph.D., M.Sc. (✉) • D.C.R. Morais, M.D. • C.M.M. de Araujo, M.D.
Department of Radiotherapy, Brazilian National Cancer Institute, Rio De Janeiro, Brazil
e-mail: cmpviegas@yahoo.com.br

T.P. de Farias (ed.), *Tracheostomy*, https://doi.org/10.1007/978-3-319-67867-2_13

With the emergence of three-dimensional (3D) techniques and imaging acquisition using computed tomography (CT) scans and magnetic resonance, as well as positron emission tomography (PET) CT, it was possible to specifically delineate the areas of interest to be treated, as well as adjacent healthy organs (salivary glands, medulla, spinal cord, healthy segments of the oral cavity, nontumoral larynx, swallowing musculature, among others) in order to report and constrain the dosage delivered to each of these volumes. This technique is called *conformational radiotherapy* and, with it, a better conformation of the treatment dose begins to occur. However, only with the advent of important radiotherapy accessories, such as the multileaf collimator and specific software, it has been possible to modulate the intensity of the treatment beam and, consequently, to intensify the dose designated for the tumor volume and to perform differentiated escalating dosages between tumor regions and potential healthy volumes, consequently increasing the protection of healthy tissues. This technique is called *intensity-modulated radiotherapy* (IMRT). Improvements in this technique have been made possible by rotational arcs, meaning that the radiation beam is delivered by a rotating arc performed by the head device and concurrent fluency energy, that allows beam modulation and results in a complex delivery system wich can provide IMRT dinamically, with the rotation of the entire device. This approach also allows to decrease the total time in active beam, so it's good for departmental expedience and improves device wear. This technique is called *radiotherapy with dynamic arc modulation*, or a *modulated dynamic arc*. It is important to note that regardless of the technique used (conventional, conformational, IMRT, or dynamic arc), radiotherapy offers good rates of local control and survival. What will actually vary will be the frequency and intensity of early and late side effects of treatment [4–8].

In view of these various indications, the use of radiotherapy in tracheostomized patients is not infrequent, nor is the need for tracheostomy during or after radiotherapy. Therefore, it is essential that the staff involved in radiotherapy treatment are accustomed to the presence of tracheostomy and have the necessary knowledge and expertise to deal with its presence.

The objective of this chapter will be to address some aspects considered relevant to tracheostomy and directly related to the approach with radiotherapy.

Radiotherapy and Tracheostomy: Important Care and Recommendations

Fundamentally, there are three situations in which patients with tracheostomy may undergo radiotherapy:

- Patients with imminent airway obstruction who undergo prophylactic tracheostomy before starting radiotherapy, leaving the tumor lesion intact;
- Patients undergoing total laryngectomy or definitive tracheostomy, resulting from surgery at other tumor sites (thyroid, pharynx, or trachea) and who have clinical, radiological, and/or pathological predictors that indicate a high risk of locoregional recurrence, with consequent indication of adjuvant radiotherapy;

- Patients undergoing procedures that may lead to risk of airway obstruction (examples are total glossectomy or tongue brachytherapy), with a need for tracheostomy to protect the airway.

In this context, it is imperative that the presence of tracheostomy be considered in the planning and process of treatment with ionizing radiation. In patients undergoing total laryngectomy and therefore with a permanent tracheostomy, it is recommended that at the time of planning and treatment, the tracheotomy tube (if it is in use) is removed in full and the patient undergoes such procedures without its presence. In patients without a definitive tracheostomy, the ideal is that at the time of planning and treatment, the metal tracheotomy tube is replaced by a plastic one (Fig. 1).

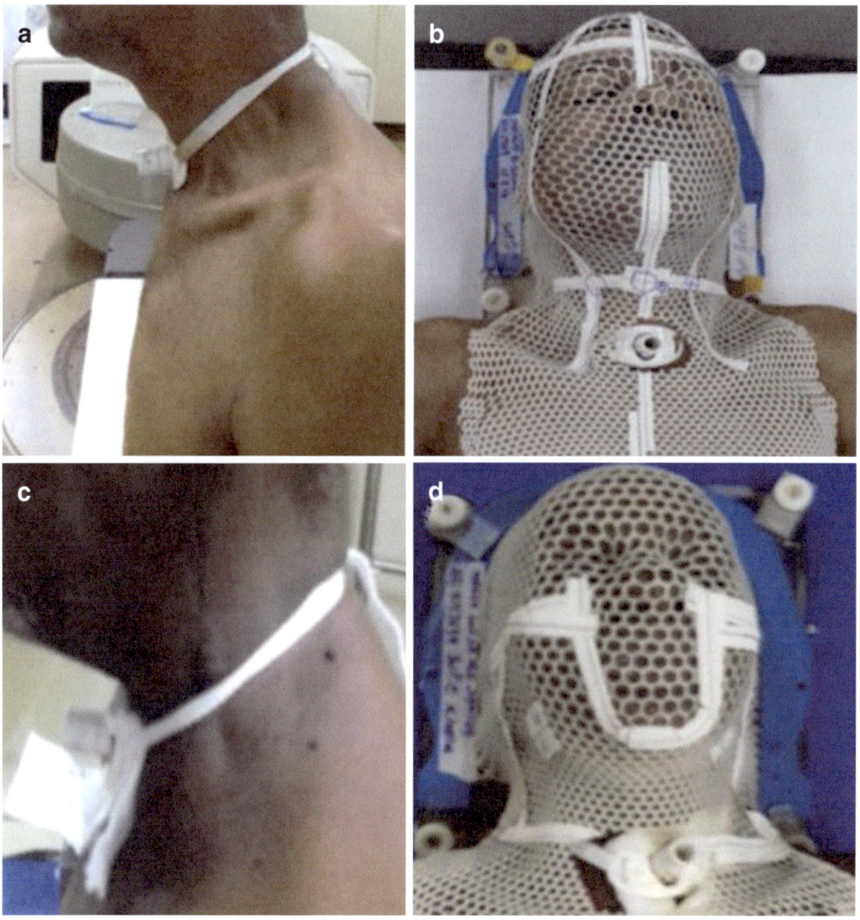

Fig. 1 Patients with a tracheostomy with plastic cannulae irradiated for similar periods (16th radiotherapy fraction). *Upper images* (**a**, **b**): treatment performed in a 6 MV linear accelerator, showing the lateral and frontal views, respectively. *Lower images* (**c**, **d**): treatment performed in a telecobalt therapy unit, showing the lateral and frontal views, respectively. Observe the increased skin reaction in the treatment performed with telecobalt therapy—an inherent characteristic of the treatment beam. It is important to emphasize that when using a thermoplastic mask, the tracheostomy must not be obstructed

The presence of a metallic tracheostomy tube could interfere with the radiation dose distribution, causing an increase in the dosage received by the underlying stoma and the surrounding skin, due to the production of secondary electrons. In addition, the posterior region of the beam trajectory could receive an underdosage due to the "shadow" produced by its path, increasing the risk of relapse in the stoma, which is estimated to occur in 3–15% of cases [9]. Likewise, if the patient makes use of some type of foam or any other preparation around the tracheostomy tube, it should, whenever possible, be removed prior to treatment, as the presence of such materials may increase the dose received by the underlying skin and cause a more intense acute reaction [10].

In addition, great care must be taken to ensure that the tube is handled by experienced and safe hands, mainly to ensure that accidental removal of the tube does not occur in patients with a temporary tracheostomy, avoiding more significant problems, besides ensuring that it is repositioned correctly rather than in a false trajectory.

Tracheotomy tube manipulation procedures during radiation should be performed preferably under nurse responsibility [11, 12]. At the Brazilian National Cancer Institute (INCA), a study was conducted with 153 patients with laryngeal tumors enrolled in the Head and Neck Surgery Department and undergoing exclusive surgery and radiotherapy, chemoradiotherapy, or exclusive radiotherapy. Almost 20,000 nursing procedures related to the tracheostomy were performed in the period, and each patient received nursing procedures 12 times, on average (6–37 times).

Among these procedures, there were some as simple as changing dressings, trichotomies and aspiration of secretions, and removal of surgical wound and tracheostomy stitches; and more complex procedures such as emergency tracheostomy for airway viability, definitive tracheostomy, training instructions for home dressing, or instrumental debridement. Among the almost 20,000 nursing procedures performed, the technical procedures related to dressings (TPRDs) were predominantly defined, and included oral cavity, tracheostoma and/or cervical region cleaning; application of topical healing medications; occlusion with sterile gauze over the operative wound; exchange of the endotracheal cannula; and application and fixation of a bandage with gentle compression. On average, 113 TPRDs per day were performed, which corresponded to approximately 17,000 nursing procedures performed in the period. The therapeutic combinations that most required nursing procedures, in increasing order of need, were chemoradiotherapy (11.1%), exclusive surgery (15.7%), surgery followed by radiotherapy (30.7%), and exclusive radiotherapy (36.6%) [11].

Tracheostomy Prior to or During Radiotherapy as a Predictor of Worse Prognosis

Eventually, patients with laryngeal and/or hypopharyngeal tumors present with significant airway involvement, requiring a tracheostomy prior to radiotherapy. In addition, laryngeal edema induced by radiotherapy may reduce the already compromised airway and could precipitate a surgical intervention with emergency tracheostomy. In this context, pretreatment tracheostomy has been associated with lower overall survival among patients undergoing surgery for transglottic tumors [13]. Such evidence also exists for patients treated with radiotherapy, since several studies have clearly demonstrated the prognostic importance of tracheostomy as a predictor of worse local control, worse disease-free survival, and worse overall survival in patients who are irradiated [14–16]. A prospective study conducted at INCA included 49 patients with locally advanced laryngeal tumors treated with radiochemotherapy. Of the 49 patients recruited, 12 patients (24.5%) underwent tracheostomy prior to initiation, and these patients had worse progression-free survival (hazard ratio [HR] 2.83, 95% confidence interval [CI] 1.61–4.89, $p < 0.001$), worse median survival (12 versus 56 months, HR 2.37, 95% CI 1.43–3.93, $p < 0.001$) and worse overall survival at 3 years (6% versus 61%, $p = 0.001$) than patients without tracheostomy [17].

In the Royal Marsden Hospital series, 21 of 150 patients (14%) with T3 or T4 laryngeal tumors underwent tracheostomy prior to initiation of treatment and also presented with significantly worse therapeutic results. Of these 21 patients, 16 died from the disease and only two patients survived for 5 years with an intact larynx [18].

Another study conducted by the Toronto Sunnybrook Regional Cancer Center [19], with 270 patients, demonstrated that patients without tracheostomy had 74% 2-year disease-free survival, while tracheostomized patients had a 2-year disease-free survival rate of 41%. Although more evident in glottic tumors (78% versus 32%), this difference was also found in supraglottic tumors (64% versus 47%). Regarding local control, there was also a difference: it was achieved in 94% and 81% of patients with glottic and supraglottic tumors without tracheostomy, respectively, and in 69% and 80% of those with glottic and supraglottic tumors with tracheostomy, respectively. A fundamental counterpoint to be made, however, is that the clearly worse results obtained in such patients leads to the misperception that radiochemotherapy is unlikely to be able to preserve the larynx in a patient with compromised airways. This has motivated some centers to even consider pretreatment tracheostomy as a formal indication for primary laryngectomy. The Canadian series published by the Toronto Sunnybrook Regional Cancer Center demystifies this issue. In this study, preservation of the larynx was feasible in more than 40% of patients treated with radiotherapy who underwent pretreatment tracheostomy, without compromising the cause-specific survival. The authors of the aforementioned study also emphasized that the need for tracheostomy should not be ruled out or considered a formal contraindication to conservative treatment with radiochemotherapy, but it makes a realistic and judicious assessment of the success of laryngeal preservation therapy mandatory and fundamental in these patients with unfavorable clinical presentation [19].

Chronic and/or Definitive Tracheostomy in Patients Undergoing Organ Preservation Protocols with Radiochemotherapy

In recent decades there has been increasing interest in organ preservation protocols for larynx and hypopharynx tumors with the use of radiotherapy with concomitant and/or neoadjuvant chemotherapy. These protocols were introduced in the 1990s as an alternative to total laryngectomy, with the objective of preserving a functional larynx, without compromising the final oncological outcome. Since then several randomized studies have been published showing equivalent results in terms of overall survival, when comparing such organ preservation protocols with immediate surgical treatment [20–22]. It is important to note that eventually such patients may remain free of the disease but with a nonfunctioning larynx and, as a result, they undergo a laryngectomy with a tracheostomy anyway.

However, such an outcome is extremely rare, and laryngectomies as a consequence of severe laryngeal dysfunction and/or laryngeal necrosis are infrequent following organ preservation protocols with radiochemotherapy. In a recent update of the Intergroup Radiation Therapy Oncology Group 91-11 (RTOG 91-11) study, only nine of the 547 patients included in the study presented with this complication, which represents an incidence lower than 1.65% of the patients [23]. A phase II study using a significantly more toxic chemotherapy regimen (docetaxel and cisplatin weekly) in conjunction with radiotherapy recruited 116 patients, and only one patient (0.86%) underwent tracheostomy after the end of radiochemotherapy, without showing signs of local recurrence. This patient presented with significant laryngeal edema after bilateral cervical dissection and retained his tracheostomy even after 2 years of radiochemotherapy treatment [24]. In summary, tracheostomy as a complication of conservative treatment with radiotherapy and chemotherapy is an *extremely rare* event described in the literature, occurring in a significantly small percentage (<2%) of patients when current radiotherapy techniques are used, even in conjunction with more aggressive chemotherapy.

Another situation described in the literature refers to patients who undergo tracheostomy before starting treatment with radiochemotherapy, and who remain with a chronic tracheostomy, even after the end of treatment; and also patients who present with locoregional recurrence after conservative treatment, who are surgically rescued with a consequent definitive tracheostomy. This evolution is not infrequent, especially in patients with bulky tumors. In a recent series published by the MD Anderson Cancer Center, including 60 patients with T4 laryngeal tumors treated with organ preservation strategies, the rates of locoregional control at 5 and 10 years were 63% and 58%, respectively, with a high rescue rate (63%) in patients with local recurrence, which resulted in final 5-year and 10-year locoregional control rates of 80% and 73%, respectively. However, the tracheostomy rate in these patients was 45%, indicating that this is a relatively frequent outcome in patients with T4 tumors treated with nonsurgical approaches.

It is worth noting, however, that in this study, 40% of the patients already presented with a tracheostomy before starting conservative treatment [25]. In another study conducted at Illinois University, 109 patients with locally advanced laryngeal and/or hypopharyngeal squamous cell carcinoma undergoing radiochemotherapy were evaluated for factors predictive of definitive tracheostomy dependence. The multivariate analysis showed that the need for definitive tracheostomy was associated with the following factors: presence of tracheostomy prior to irradiation, subglottic tumor extension, conformal radiotherapy instead of IMRT, and postradiotherapy lymphadenectomy. When the primary tumor site was considered, it was observed that for primary laryngeal tumors, the need for definitive tracheostomy was associated with all previously described factors and that for primary hypopharyngeal tumors, tracheostomy prior to radiotherapy and tube dependence were predictive factors. In this study, tracheostomy dependence did not influence local control, progression-free survival, or overall survival [26].

Tracheostomy Stenosis in Patients Undergoing Laryngectomy and Adjuvant Radiotherapy

Tracheostomy stenosis is an event with a variable incidence in the literature, and is reported in the main series available as occurring in 4–42% of laryngectomized patients [27]. Because total laryngectomy is indicated primarily for patients with locally advanced tumors, most of these patients will undergo adjuvant radiotherapy, and this may have some role in the genesis of future stenosis. In a series published by the University of Hong Kong, with 207 laryngectomized patients, tracheostomy stenosis was described in 13% of the cases and the only independent determinants for the development of tracheostomy stenosis were female sex and tracheostomy infection. Seventeen percent of patients irradiated postoperatively presented with tracheostomy stenosis, although the use of adjuvant radiotherapy was not considered a determining factor for this occurrence in the statistical analysis [28]. In another publication from West Virginia University Hospitals [29], 106 laryngectomized patients with a stenosis rate of 28.4% were included. Again, female sex was a determinant of its occurrence, being, in this study, the only predisposing factor with statistical significance. Infection at the stoma site, the presence of a fistula, use of steroids, neck dissection, use of a myocutaneous flap, and radiotherapy were not correlated with an increase in the incidence of stenosis [29]. A more recent publication from the University of Rome, with 85 patients, reported a 35% incidence of tracheostomy stenosis and identified, on univariate and multivariate analysis, diabetes mellitus and local infection as the only predictors in laryngectomized patients undergoing adjuvant radiotherapy [27].

In summary, tracheostomy stenosis is a possible outcome in laryngectomized patients with highly variable incidence; adjuvant radiation, when clinically indicated, has not been linked to it as a risk factor for its occurrence in any study, and the main predisposing factors described in the literature were female sex, tracheostomy infection, and associated diabetes mellitus.

Tracheostomy Stoma as a site Risk for Relapse: Implications for the Radio-oncologist

In the literature, the reported occurrence of stomal recurrence in laryngectomized patients varies between 2% and 15% [9, 30]. Several factors have been described as predictors of an increased risk of peritracheostomy recurrence, such as the presence of subglottic extension [31]. Emergency tracheostomy prior to surgery has also been clearly associated with an increased risk of recurrence in and/or around the stoma [32]. In a study published by Keim et al., peristomal recurrence was observed in nine (41%) of 22 patients undergoing pretreatment tracheostomy, compared with four (6%) of 65 patients undergoing surgery without prior tracheostomy [33]. Stell and Van Den Broek also identified tracheostomy as an adverse prognostic factor and reported peritracheostomy recurrence in four (21%) of 19 patients undergoing tracheostomy before laryngectomy [34].

Despite the use of aggressive treatments with surgery, radiotherapy, and chemotherapy, the rescue rates for stomal recurrence are poor, with the prognosis and overall survival data being quite discouraging. In view of this, prevention of peritracheostomy recurrence is extremely important and is the only means of reducing its incidence [35].

In this context, adjuvant radiotherapy plays an important role, and some care must be taken. Fundamentally, in patients undergoing emergency tracheostomy prior to definitive surgical treatment, and in other patients with an increased risk of peritracheostomy recurrence (such as patients with subglottic tumor extension and with metastases to paratracheal lymph nodes), special attention should be paid during radiotherapy and special consideration should be given to the peristomal dose. Eventually, dressings and/or materials considered tissue-equivalent (called *bolus*) may be deliberately placed around the stoma or a plastic tracheostomy tube may be inserted during treatment, with the intention of increasing the dose in this region, ensuring suitable dose coverage.

A study conducted by Montefiore Medical Center and the Memorial Sloan-Kettering Cancer Center evaluated the various options available to ensure adequate dosage of the surface and back wall of the tracheostoma. Dosimetric studies demonstrated that the various alternatives tested (1.0 cm thick bolus, plastic tracheostomy tube number 06, plastic tracheostomy tube number 08, 3 mm Aquaplast® plate, and 6 mm Aquaplast® plate) were suitable for a treatment radiation beam of 6 MV. The only exception was the use of bolus with only 0.5 cm of thickness, which resulted in significant underdosing. The authors of the study concluded that although most of the alternatives provided an acceptable dose for the surface and posterior wall of the tracheostoma, the best technique dosimetrically consisted of use of the 6 mm Aquaplast® plate, which also was associated with better patient positioning reproducibility and reduced trauma, did not interfere with the patient's breathing, and was compatible with vocalization [36].

What is most important to emphasize is that with relatively simple measures, it can be ensured that a suitable dose of radiotherapy is administered to peritracheostomy tissues in patients undergoing emergency tracheostomy prior to laryngectomy and/or with significant subglottic extension, thus minimizing the risk of future stomal recurrence (Figs. 2, 3, and 4).

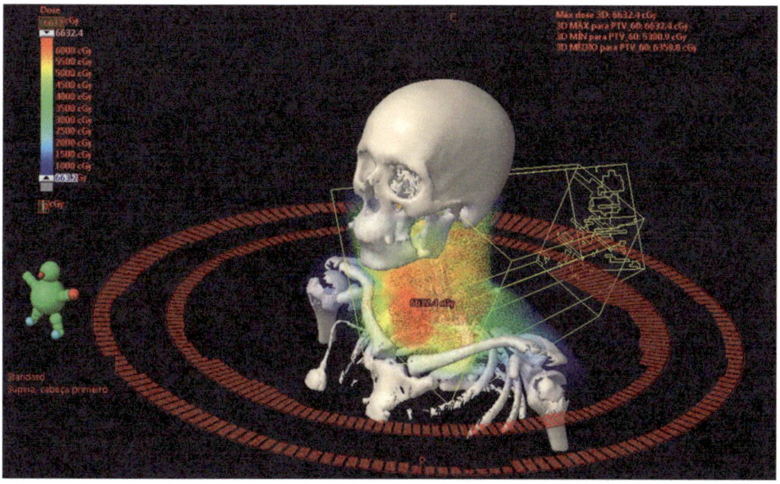

Fig. 2 Example of treatment with postoperative teletherapy using the volumetric arc technique with three-dimensional vision in a male patient aged 66 years old with a laryngeal tumor (pT4N1M0), operated on and treated with emergency tracheostomy. Observe the necessary areas of greater dosage in the ventral region of the neck, characterized by reddish coloration

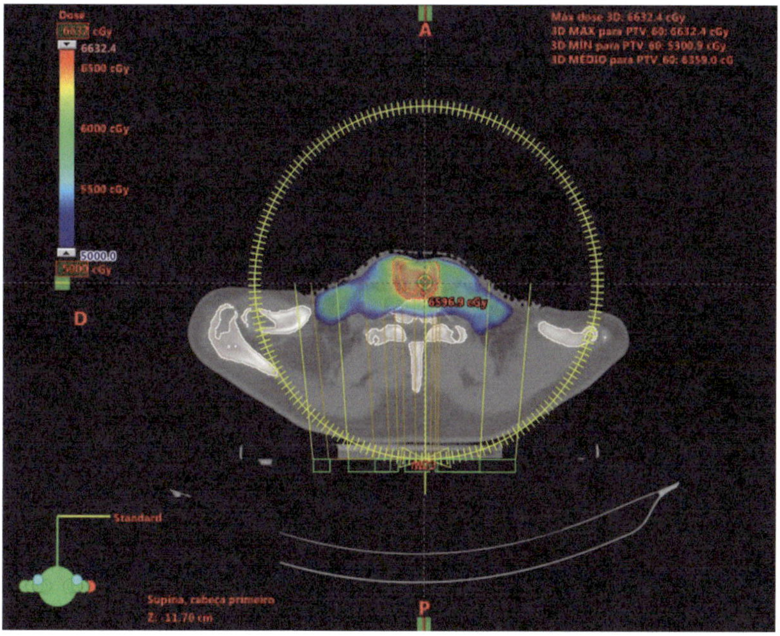

Fig. 3 Example of treatment with postoperative teletherapy using the volumetric arc technique, shown in cross-section, in a male patient aged 66 years old with a laryngeal tumor (pT4N1M0), operated on and treated with emergency tracheostomy. Observe the necessary areas of greater dosage in the ventral region of the neck, with special attention to the area of the tracheostomy, with reinforcement of the dose integrated into the treatment plan, represented by reddish coloration

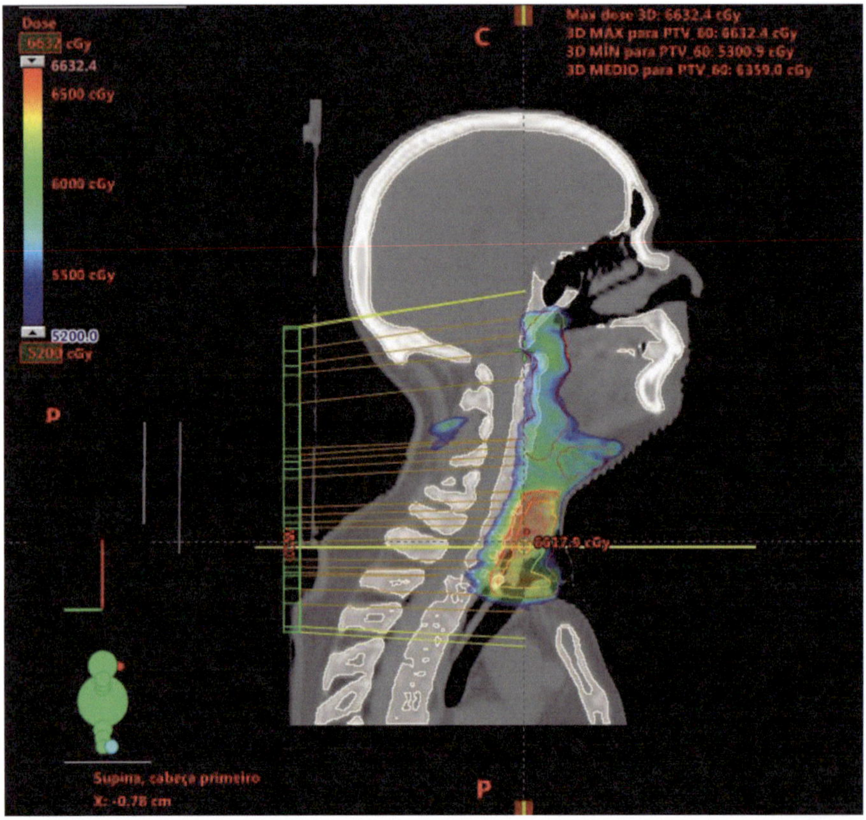

Fig. 4 Example of treatment with postoperative teletherapy using the volumetric arc technique, showing the sagittal cut, in a male patient aged 66 years old, with a laryngeal tumor (pT4N1M0), operated on and treated with emergency tracheostomy. Observe the necessary areas of greater dosage in the ventral region of the neck, with special attention to areas of the previous tumor bed (laryngeal bed with 66 Gy, reddish color) and the tracheostomy area, with dose reinforcement integrated into the treatment plan, represented by more orange coloration. Calculations were performed to ensure a minimum dose of 60 Gy in the tracheostomy area

Defensive Tracheostomy for Interstitial Brachytherapy of Head and Neck Tumors

Brachytherapy can be used in a significant proportion of patients with head and neck tumors, exclusively in patients with initial tumors, as consolidation for a dose boost after teletherapy, after the appearance of a second primary in a previously irradiated head and neck region, or in a rescue approach for locally recurrent tumors, including in patients with peritracheostomy recurrence [37]. This treatment offers the advantage of delivering a high radiation dosage in the tumor vicinity, with rapid dose reduction in healthy tissues contiguous with the area to be irradiated [38, 39].

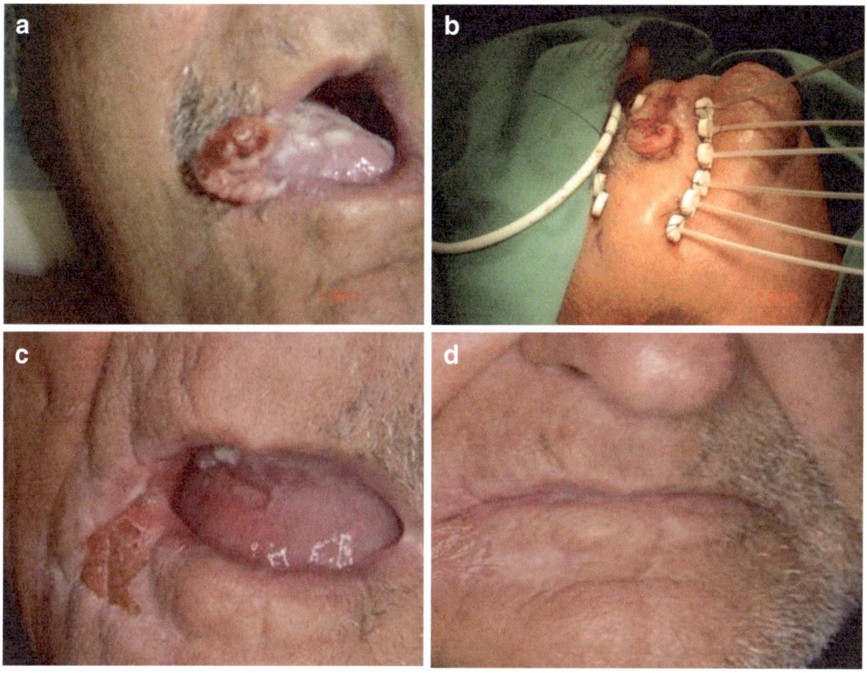

Fig. 5 Squamous carcinoma of the labial commissure treated with interstitial brachytherapy, in which it was possible to avoid a tracheostomy. Observe the evolution with regression of the ulcerous-fungating lesion: (**a**) at the time of diagnosis; (**b**) at the time of catheter insertion; (**c**) 28 days after stopping brachytherapy; and (**d**) 60 days after the end of treatment, with a complete response and functional preservation. 60 Gy/20 fractions were prescribed with two daily fractions

In addition, the vast majority of head and neck sites—such as the lip, oral cavity, oropharynx, and nasopharynx, as well as the cervical region—are accessible for the insertion of needles or brachytherapy catheters [38, 40]. However, manipulation for insertion of catheters can cause edema, bleeding, and increased production of local secretions, which can lead to a compromised airway. In addition, oral intubation procedures precede interstitial brachytherapy, and except in situations where nasal intubation occurs, the tracheostomy provides alternative access for intubation. Although it is possible to avoid tracheostomy in small anterior oral cavity lesions [40], we prefer to perform prophylactic tracheostomy routinely when treating patients with interstitial brachytherapy for tumors of the head and neck, except for lip tumors (Fig. 5).

The American Brachytherapy Society (ABS) recommends that prophylactic tracheostomy be performed in patients with oropharyngeal tumors, due to the risk of possible compromise of the airways (Figs. 6 and 7).

It is important to emphasize that intracavitary nasopharyngeal brachytherapy, on the other hand, dispenses with this care, since the oral cavity remains free for breathing.

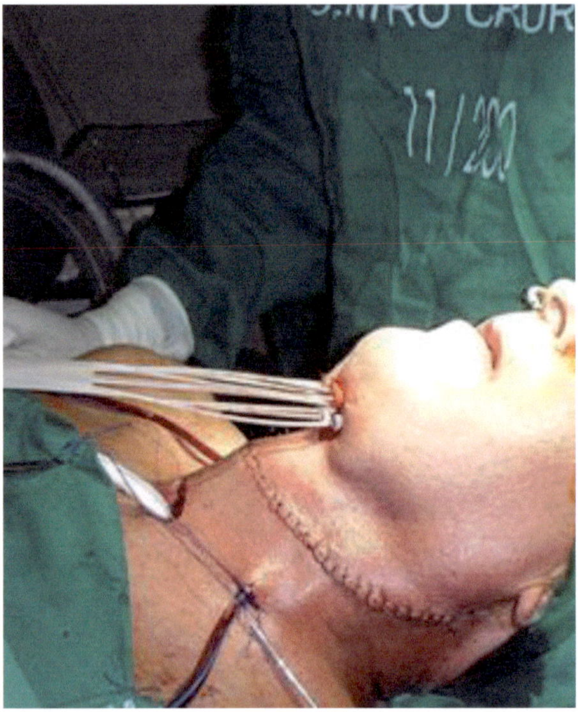

Fig. 6 Interstitial brachytherapy of the oropharynx. Observe the cervical dissection performed, the catheters inserted through the submental access, and the defensive tracheostomy, which also served to allow patient intubation during the procedure. The patient underwent a full treatment course with the tracheostomy until the catheters were definitively removed. 45Gy was prescribed in nine fractions with two fractions per day. The patient had previously received radiotherapy for a laryngeal tumor with a full dose (66 Gy/33 fractions)

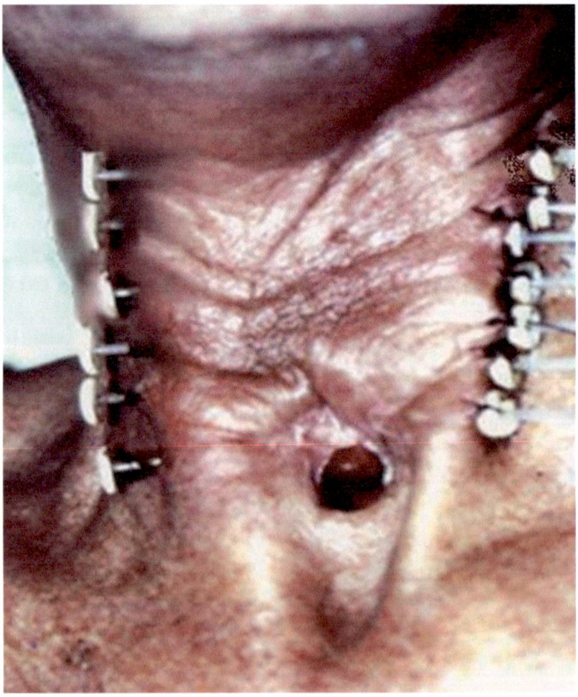

Fig. 7 Interstitial brachytherapy of the cervical region. Note the cervical dissection scar, transverse catheters, and tracheostomy also previously performed, due to advanced and recurrent carcinoma of the larynx. The patient had already been previously irradiated due to an advanced tumor of the larynx with full dose (70Gy/35fractions)

References

1. Locally Advanced Squamous Carcinoma of the Head Neck. Union for International Cancer Control. 2014 Review of Cancer Medicines on the WHO List of Essential Medicines. Available in: www.who.int/selection_medicines/committees/expert/20/applications/HeadNeck.pdf. Last access: 15/09/2016.
2. American Cancer Society. Cancer Facts and Figures 2016. Atlanta: American Cancer Society; 2016.
3. Brasil MS. Estimativa 2016: incidência de câncer no Brasil/Instituto Nacional de Câncer José Alencar Gomes da Silva—Rio de Janeiro: INCA, 2015.
4. Nutting CM, Morden JP, Harrington KJ, Urbano TG, Bhide SA, Clark C, Miles EA, Miah AB, Newbold K, Tanay M, Adab F, Jefferies SJ, Scrase C, Yap BK, A'Hern RP, Sydenham MA, Emson M, Hall E, PARSPORT Trial Management Group. Parotid-sparing intensity modulated versus conventional radiotherapy in head and neck cancer (PARSPORT): a phase 3 multicentre randomised controlled trial. Lancet Oncol. 2011;12(2):127–36.
5. Gupta T, Agarwal J, Jain S, Phurailatpam R, Kannan S, Ghosh-Laskar S, Murthy V, Budrukkar A, Dinshaw K, Prabhash K, Chaturvedi P, D'Cruz A. Three-dimensional conformal radiotherapy (3D-CRT) versus intensity modulated radiation therapy (IMRT) in squamous cell carcinoma of the head and neck: a randomized controlled trial. Radiother Oncol. 2012;104(3):343–8.
6. Kam MK, Leung SF, Zee B, Chau RM, Suen JJ, Mo F, Lai M, Ho R, Cheung KY, Yu BK, Chiu SK, Choi PH, Teo PM, Kwan WH, Chan AT. Prospective randomized study of intensity-modulated radiotherapy on salivary gland function in early-stage nasopharyngeal carcinoma patients. J Clin Oncol. 2007;25(31):4873–9.
7. Pow EH, Kwong DL, McMillan AS, Wong MC, Sham JS, Leung LH, Leung WK. Xerostomia and quality of life after intensity-modulated radiotherapy vs. conventional radiotherapy for early-stage nasopharyngeal carcinoma: initial report on a randomized controlled clinical trial. Int J Radiat Oncol Biol Phys. 2006;66(4):981–91.
8. Eisbruch A, Schwartz M, Rasch C, Vineberg K, Damen E, Van As CJ, Marsh R, Pameijer FA, Balm AJ. Dysphagia and aspiration after chemoradiotherapy for head-and-neck cancer: which anatomic structures are affected and can they be spared by IMRT? Int J Radiat Oncol Biol Phys. 2004;60(5):1425–39.
9. Breneman JC, Bradshaw A, Gluckman J, Aron BS. Prevention of stomal recurrence in patients requiring emergency tracheostomy for advanced laryngeal and pharyngeal tumors. Cancer. 1988;62(4):802–5.
10. Yorke ED, Kassaee A, Doyle T, et al. The dose distribution of medium energy electron boosts to the laryngectomy stoma. J Appl Clin Med Phys. 2001;2(1):9–20.
11. Alcantara LS, Oliveira ACAM, Guedes MTS, et al. Interdisciplinaridade e integralidade: a abordagem do assistente social e do enfermeiro no INCA. Revista Brasileira de Cancerologia. 2014;60(2):109–18.
12. Araujo CRG, Rosas AM. O papel da equipe de enfermagem no setor de radioterapia: uma contribuição para a equipe multidisciplinar. Revista Brasileira de Cancerologia. 2008;54(3):231–7.
13. Mittal B, Marks JE, Ogura JH. Transglottic carcinoma. Cancer. 1984;53:151–61.
14. Mendenhall WM, Parsons JT, Mancuso AA, Pameijer FJ, Stringer SP, Cassisi NJ. Definitive radiotherapy for T3 squamous cell carcinoma of the glottic larynx. Int J Radiat Oncol Biol Phys. 1997;15:2394–402.
15. Meredith AP, Randall CJ, Shaw HJ. Advanced laryngeal cancer: a management perspective. J Laryngol Otol. 1987;101:1046–54.
16. Mucha-Małecka A, Składowski K. High-dose radiotherapy alone for patients with T4-stage laryngeal cancer. Strahlenther Onkol. 2013 Aug;189(8):632–8.
17. Herchenhorn D, Dias FL, Ferreira CG, Araújo CM, Lima RA, Small IA, Kligerman J. Impact of previous tracheotomy as a prognostic factor in patients with locally advanced squamous cell carcinoma of the larynx submitted to concomitant chemotherapy and radiation. ORL J Otorhinolaryngol Relat Spec. 2008;70(6):381–8.

18. Tennant PA, Cash E, Bumpous JM, Potts KL. Persistent tracheostomy after primary chemoradiation for advanced laryngeal or hypopharyngeal cancer. Head Neck. 2014;36(11):1628–33.
19. MacKenzie R, Franssen E, Balogh J, Birt D, Gilbert R. The prognostic significance of tracheostomy in carcinoma of the larynx treated with radiotherapy and surgery for salvage. Int J Radiat Oncol Biol Phys. 1998;41(1):43–51.
20. Department of Veterans Affairs Laryngeal Cancer Study Group. Induction chemotherapy plus radiation compared with surgery plus radiation in patients with advanced laryngeal cancer. N Engl J Med. 1991;324:1685–90.
21. Richard JM, Sancho-Garnier H, Pessey JJ, Luboinski B, Lefebvre JL, Dehesdin D, et al. Randomized trial of induction chemotherapy in larynx carcinoma. Oral Oncol. 1998;34:224–8.
22. Forastiere AA, Goepfert H, Maor M, Pajak TF, Weber R, Morrison W, et al. Concurrent chemotherapy and radiotherapy for organ preservation in advanced laryngeal cancer. N Engl J Med. 2003;349:2091–8.
23. Forastiere AA, Zhang Q, Weber RS, Maor MH, Goepfert H, Pajak TF, Morrison W, Glisson B, Trotti A, Ridge JA, Thorstad W, Wagner H, Ensley JF, Cooper JS. Long-term results of RTOG 91-11: a comparison of three nonsurgical treatment strategies to preserve the larynx in patients with locally advanced larynx cancer. J Clin Oncol. 2013;31(7):845–52.
24. Inohara H, Takenaka Y, Yoshii T, Nakahara S, Yamamoto Y, Tomiyama Y, Seo Y, Isohashi F, Suzuki O, Yoshioka Y, Sumida I, Ogawa K. Phase 2 study of docetaxel, cisplatin, and concurrent radiation for technically resectable stage III–IV squamous cell carcinoma of the head and neck. Int J Radiat Oncol Biol Phys. 2015;91(5):934–41.
25. Rosenthal D, Mohamed AS, Weber RS, Garden AS, Sevak PR, Kies MS, Morrison WH, Lewin JS, El-Naggar AK, Ginsberg LE, Kocak-Uzel E, Ang KK, Fuller CD. Long-term outcomes after surgical or nonsurgical initial therapy for patients with T4 squamous cell carcinoma of the larynx: a 3-decade survey. Cancer. 2015;121(10):1608–19.
26. Jefferson GD, Wenig BL, Spiotto MT. Predictors and outcomes for chronic tracheostomy after chemoradiation for advanced laryngohypopharyngeal cancer. Laryngoscope. 2016;126(2):385–91.
27. De Virgilio A, Greco A, Gallo A, Martellucci S, Conte M, de Vincentiis M. Tracheostomal stenosis clinical risk factors in patients who have undergone total laryngectomy and adjuvant radiotherapy. Eur Arch Otorhinolaryngol. 2013;270(12):3187–9.
28. Kuo M, Ho CM, Wei WI, Lam KH. Tracheostomal stenosis after total laryngectomy: an analysis of predisposing clinical factors. Laryngoscope. 1994;104(1 Pt 1):59–63.
29. Wax MK, Touma BJ, Ramadan HH. Tracheostomal stenosis after laryngectomy: incidence and predisposing factors. Otolaryngol Head Neck Surg. 1995;113(3):242–7.
30. De Jong PC. Intubation and tumor implantation in laryngeal carcinoma. Practica Otorhinolaryngol. 1969;31:119–21.
31. León X, Quer M, Burgués J, Abelló P, Vega M, de Andrés L. Prevention of stomal recurrence. Head Neck. 1996;18(1):54–9.
32. Imauchi Y, Ito K, Takasago E, Nibu K, Sugasawa M, Ichimura K. Stomal recurrence after total laryngectomy for squamous cell carcinoma of the larynx. Otolaryngol Head Neck Surg. 2002;126(1):63–6.
33. Keim WF, Shapiro MJ, Rosin HD, Montclair NJ. The study of post laryngectomy stomal recurrence. Arch Otolaryngol. 1965;81:183–6.
34. Stell PM, Van Den Broek P. Stomal recurrence after laryngectomy: aetiology and management. J Laryngol Otol. 1971;85:131–40.
35. Reséndiz-Colosia JA, Gallegos-Hernández JF, Hernández-San Juan M, Barroso-Bravo S, Flores-Díaz R. Post total laryngectomy stomal recurrence. Case report and review of the literature. Cir Cir. 2003;71(5):387–90.
36. Beitler JJ, Yaparpalvi R, Della Biancia C, Fontenla DP. Methods of bolusing the tracheostomy stoma. Int J Radiat Oncol Biol Phys. 2001;50(1):69–74.

37. Doyle LA, Harrison AS, Cognetti D, Xiao Y, Yu Y, Liu H, Ahn PH, Anné PR, Showalter TN. Reirradiation of head and neck cancer with high-dose-rate brachytherapy: a customizable intraluminal solution for postoperative treatment of tracheal mucosa recurrence. Brachytherapy. 2011;10(2):154–8.
38. Nag S, Cano ER, Demanes DJ, Puthawala AA, Vikram B, American Brachytherapy Society. The American Brachytherapy Society recommendations for high-dose-rate brachytherapy for head-and-neck carcinoma. Int J Radiat Oncol Biol Phys. 2001;50(5):1190–8.
39. Hepel JT, Syed AM, Puthawala A, Sharma A, Frankel P. Salvage high-dose-rate (HDR) brachytherapy for recurrent head-and-neck cancer. Int J Radiat Oncol Biol Phys. 2005;62(5):1444–50.
40. Montemaggi P, Trombetta M, Brady L. Brachytherapy—an international perspective. 1st ed. Philadelphia; 2016. p. 98.

Tracheostomy in Orthognathic Surgery and Facial Trauma Surgery: Is There a Place?

Ricardo Lopes da Cruz, Fernando Cesar A. Lima, and Antônio Albuquerque de Brito

General Considerations

Dealing with the upper airways is an integral part of a maxillofacial surgeon's daily life, and understanding how to better deal with them is one of the aims of this practice, in collaboration with other specialists.

Indications for performing tracheostomy in maxillofacial trauma and orthognathic surgery, as well as some considerations about procedures in craniomaxillofacial anomalies, will be discussed in this chapter. Literature data and the authors' personal expertise are taken into account.

Other methods besides tracheostomy will also be briefly presented in this chapter, as there is a close relation between maxillofacial surgery and maintenance of the upper airway.

R.L. da Cruz, M.D. (✉)
Private Practice, Rio de Janeiro, RJ, Brazil

Department of Craniomaxillofacial Surgery, National Institute of Traumatology and Orthopedics, Rio de Janeiro, RJ, Brazil
e-mail: ricardolopescruz@gmail.com

A.A. de Brito, D.D.S., M.D., M.Sc.
Private Practice, Belo Horizonte, MG, Brazil

F.C.A. Lima, D.D.S., M.D.
Department of Oral and Maxillofacial Surgery, Hospital Federal dos Servidores, Rio de Janeiro, RJ, Brazil

Private Practice, Rio de Janeiro, RJ, Brazil

T.P. de Farias (ed.), *Tracheostomy*, https://doi.org/10.1007/978-3-319-67867-2_14

Craniomaxillofacial Trauma and Tracheostomy

Indications for Use of Tracheostomy in Craniomaxillofacial Trauma

Although tracheostomy is a common procedure, the decision to perform it in craniomaxillofacial trauma patients can be complex [1]. Not a lot has been researched or written regarding the objectives of tracheostomy in the management of these fractures [2].

Airway management in trauma patients should take multiple factors into consideration, such as trauma etiology, extent of the injuries, existence of comorbidities, and surgeon experience and preference. Tracheostomy is usually performed in multisystem trauma and is considered a safe method for airway stabilization in craniomaxillofacial trauma patients (Fig. 1) [2–4].

During the Second World War, the roles of hemostatic control and airway maintenance became widely recognized, and these procedures were established as immediate screening in campaign hospitals. At the time, most patients had a need for prolonged intermaxillary fixation, and tracheostomy was seen as a way to protect airway function as well as facilitating a surgical approach. Subsequent technological advances at the end of the twentieth century imposed changes on the routine use of tracheostomy for airway maintenance during trauma surgery [5, 6]. Monitoring

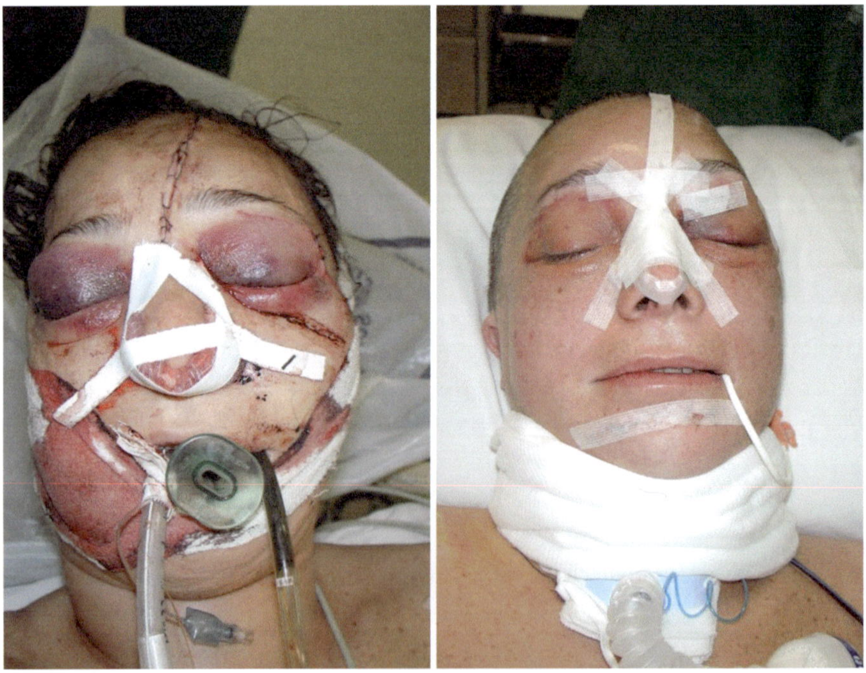

Fig. 1 Panfacial trauma before and after tracheostomy and treatment

techniques and equipment allowed more accurate assessment of vital functions, diagnostic resources became more precise, and the use of internal rigid fixation (Figs. 2 and 3) eliminated the need for long periods of intermaxillary fixation. As a result of these innovations, many surgeons oppose routine use of tracheostomy in complex facial trauma [4, 7].

Tracheostomy is one of the most common procedures performed in intensive care units, having many benefits for patients under mechanical ventilation, such as maintaining unobstructed upper airways, achieving better control of mechanical support ventilation, protection of direct laryngeal lesions, facilitating basic nursing care, enabling aspiration of tracheobronchial mucus, and making it more

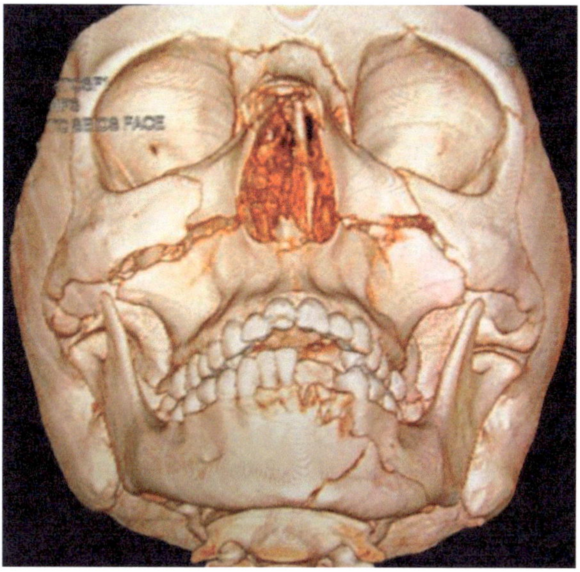

Fig. 2 Panfacial fractures

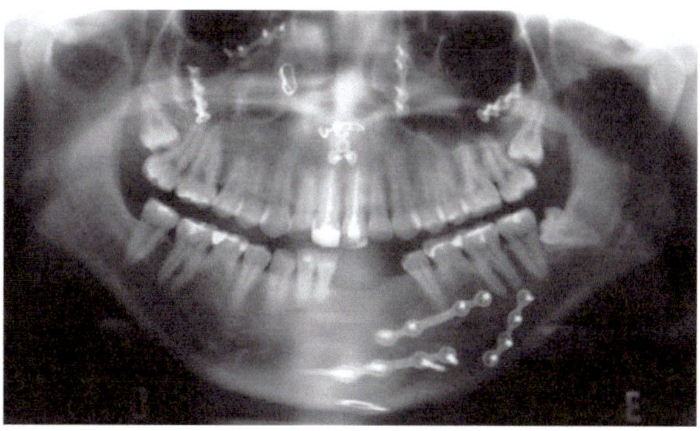

Fig. 3 The same patient from Fig. 2 after rigid internal fixation of the fractures

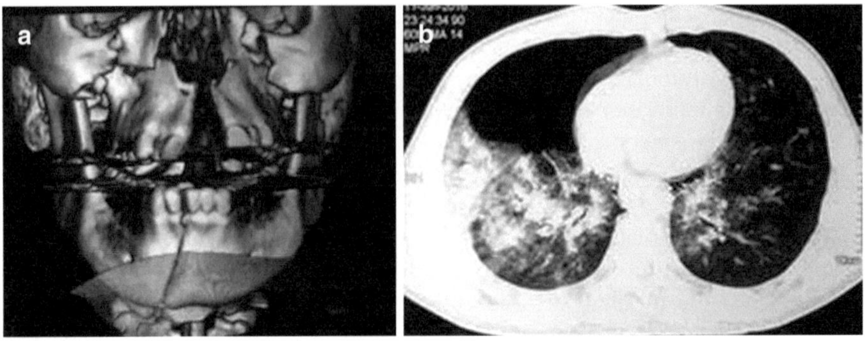

Fig. 4 (**a**) Computed tomography (CT) scan of facial trauma. (**b**) Chest CT scan of the same patient, showing chest trauma. (Courtesy of Roger Lanes, MD, DDS, PhD, FHEMIG)

comfortable for the patients [8, 9]. In general, the best indications for performing tracheostomy are upper airway obstruction, facial swelling, whenever oral or naso-tracheal intubation are deemed unsafe, airway deviation during or after facial fracture repair, frequent need for tracheobronchial hygiene, prolonged mechanical ventilation, and associated trauma (Fig. 4) [10–12].

Some specific patient variables are predictive of long-term need for mechanical ventilation, including cranial lesions, a low Glasgow Coma Scale score, the mechanism of injury, and patient comorbidities [13]. For instance, oral or nasotracheal intubation that lasts longer than 2–3 weeks increases the risk of complications for the patient, including tracheal stenosis, vocal cord dysfunction, gastric hemorrhage, vascular lesions, pneumothorax, and tracheoesophageal fistula [14]. However, some studies have suggested that glottic and subglottic stenosis, pneumonia, and death are no more frequent in patients who remain intubated for over 2 weeks than in those who have early tracheostomy performed (Fig. 5) [15].

Other studies have demonstrated a decrease in the amount of time spent in the intensive care unit, a lower incidence of pneumonia, decreased mortality rates, and facilitation of basic nursing care when tracheostomy is performed at the beginning of the hospital stay [16].

Aside from the indications for tracheostomy intended for better clinical stabilization of the craniomaxillofacial trauma patient, one must consider airway maintenance during the surgical procedure for the treatment of the fractures. In cases of simultaneous inferior and medial third facial fractures, oral and nasotracheal intubation may incur limitations for performing the necessary surgical procedures. In this context, tracheostomy may be useful. With regard solely to the surgical procedure, submental intubation is also possible, providing satisfactory airway access [8]. It consists of orotracheal intubation, followed by submental access to the buccal cavity and transposition of the extremity of the intubation tube through this access, with its exteriorization through the skin incision in the submental region. The benefits of this technique are discussed below (Fig. 6).

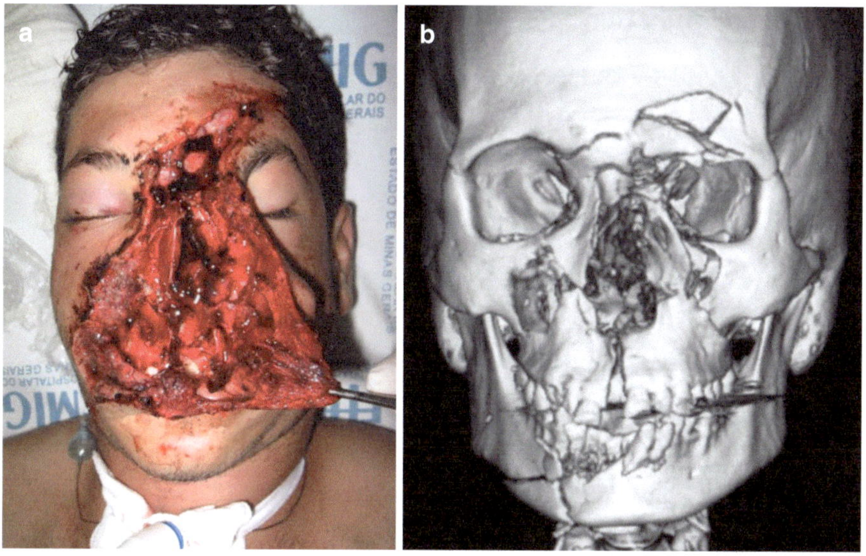

Fig. 5 (**a**) Multiple-trauma patient with severe facial airway-compromising trauma and tracheostomy. (**b**) Computed tomography (CT) scan of the same patient's facial fractures. (Courtesy of Davidson Rodarte, DDS, MSc, FHEMIG)

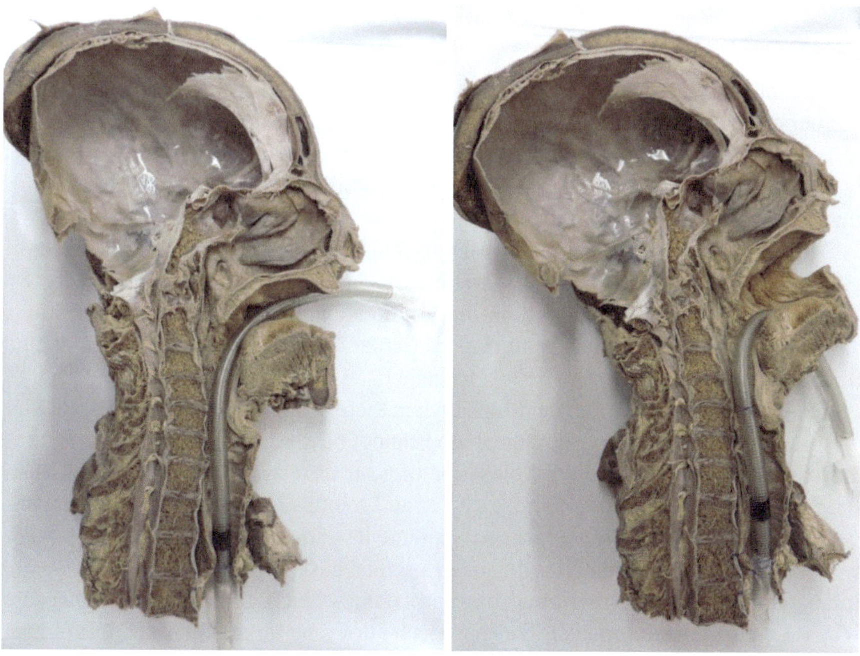

Fig. 6 Sagittal view of submental intubation on a cadaver specimen

Submental Intubation

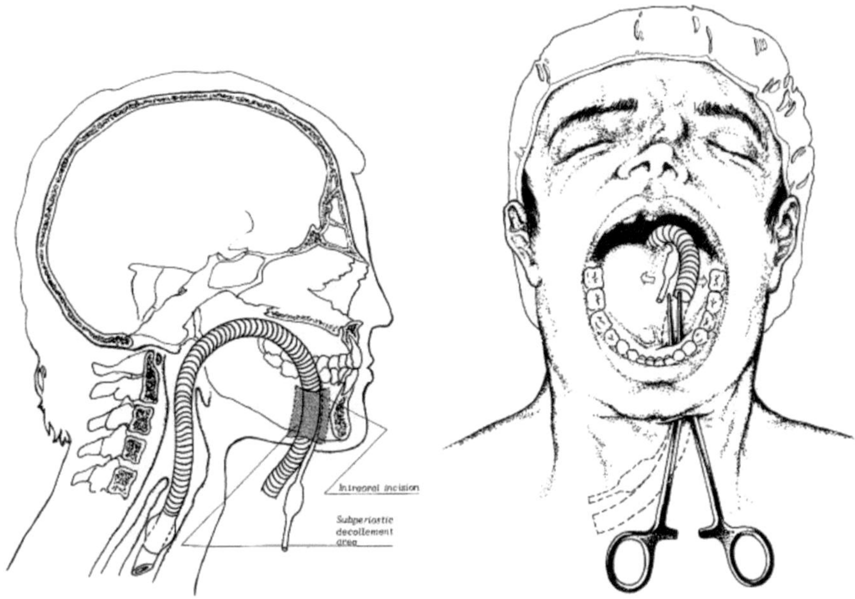

Fig. 7 Submental intubation [8]

Submental intubation is regarded as a less invasive technique than tracheostomy, although it has a more limited set of indications. The technique was first described in 1986 (Fig. 7) for acute airway management of craniomaxillofacial trauma patients where nasotracheal intubation was not a viable choice due to the need for maxillomandibular blockage during the surgical procedure [8].

More frequently used in trauma patients, submental intubation can also be indicated during orthognathic surgery and cranial base surgical procedures [17, 18]. Maxillofacial trauma remains its primary indication [19, 20]. It is described as a safe and efficient technique, requiring participation of both anesthesiologists and maxillofacial surgeons for its performance [1].

Submental intubation can be utilized when there is a need for maxillomandibular fixation in cases where a nasotracheal tube cannot be used, such as in nasal fractures and naso-orbital-ethmoidal complex fractures. It also avoids tracheostomy when long-term intubation is not mandatory. It can be indicated when orthognathic surgery is associated with rhinoplasty and in patients undergoing orthognathic surgery who have anatomical anomalies that make use of a nasal tube impossible. Submental intubation can be used in cranial base procedures, such as transmaxillary access with o Le Fort I osteotomy [2]. This approach allows better maxillary exposure than orotracheal intubation.

Submental intubation is not indicated when a long period of intubation is likely. In any patient with severe brain lesions—a condition frequently seen in facial trauma patients—this procedure should not be chosen.

The advantages of submental intubation, as compared with tracheostomy, are avoidance of morbidity such as infection, hemorrhage, laryngeal nerve lesions, tracheal stenosis, pneumothorax, pneumomediastinum, subcutaneous emphysema, and tracheoesophageal fistula. Simplicity of postoperative care and ease of reversibility are also benefits to be considered [19].

One of the few described disadvantages of submental intubation is the skin scar; this can be minimized with a small incision and meticulous suturing (Fig. 8). There have been cases of superficial wound infections due to the passage of the tube from orotracheal to submental placement. Less frequent are orocutaneous fistulae, temporary lingual nerve palsy, venous bleeding, and mucocele formation [1, 3].

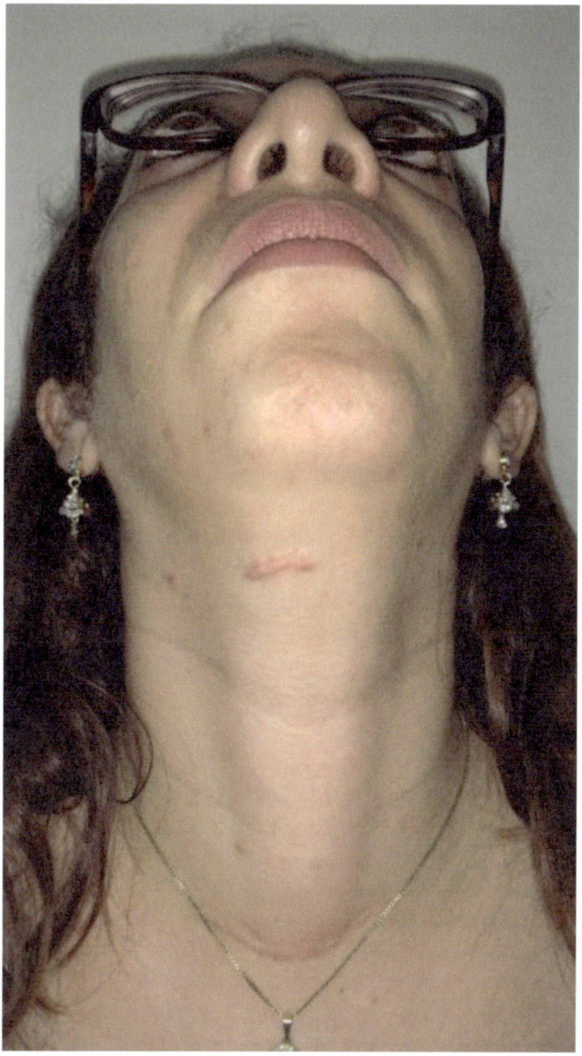

Fig. 8 Submental intubation scar

Airway Management in Pediatric Patients

Severe craniofacial and laryngeal traumas are not common in pediatric patients. When they do happen, these lesions present specific challenges in airway management because of the smaller size of the oropharynx, laryngeal swelling, displacement of soft tissue, and excessive bleeding. These can rapidly compromise airway permeability in children. Also seen, though less frequently, are foreign bodies in the aerodigestive tract and laryngotracheal rupture. Both can lead to devastating consequences in pediatric patients. Brain hypoxia can quickly ensue, and death is imminent if proper ventilation and oxygenation are not promptly re-established [4].

The anatomy and location of the tongue, larynx, and trachea are different in children compared with adults. In children, the tongue's size is bigger compared with the size of the oral cavity and oropharynx. The same applies to the epiglottis, which occupies more space in the laryngeal segment of the airways, impairing a proper view of the glottis during orotracheal intubation. On top of that, the pediatric larynx is more cephalically placed (at the C3–C4 level, compared with the C4–C5 level in adults), with subsequent superior placement of the tongue [5].

Craniomaxillofacial trauma in pediatric patients requires rapid assessment and management of the airways. The small lumen and unique development characteristics of the aerodigestive tract in children make it difficult to ensure the safety of airway permeability, even in a nonemergency setting. There are options for managing the airways in children affected by craniofacial trauma, but the best approach depends on evaluation of each individual patient [6].

In general, orotracheal intubation is a fast and efficient way to stabilize the airways in children, though it can lead to hoarseness, coughing, and a sore throat, which resolve spontaneously 2–3 days after extubation. Rarely seen are complications such as massive barotrauma and misguided esophageal intubation [18]. Nasotracheal intubation is an alternative and can be useful in repairing craniofacial fractures with maxillomandibular fixation. But there are drawbacks in its use. In patients with extensive nasoethmoidal frontal trauma, it may result in intracranial misguided intubation through a basilar cranial fracture, especially if done by inexperienced professionals [7].

Cricothyroidostomy is not an option in pediatric patients, as mentioned in Chap.15. This procedure has a high level of complications in this group of patients. In cases of laryngeal trauma, tracheostomy can be used to surpass the injured site, thus avoiding potential complications of orotracheal intubation [6].

Other than the specific conditions mentioned above, the indications for tracheostomy in pediatric patients follow the same principles as those for adult patients.

Orthognathic Surgery and Tracheostomy

Orthognathic surgery consists of maxilla and/or mandible osteotomies in order to correct dentofacial discrepancies (Figs. 9 and 10). The indications to perform this surgery are for treatment of dentofacial deformities (DFD), and the etiology can be

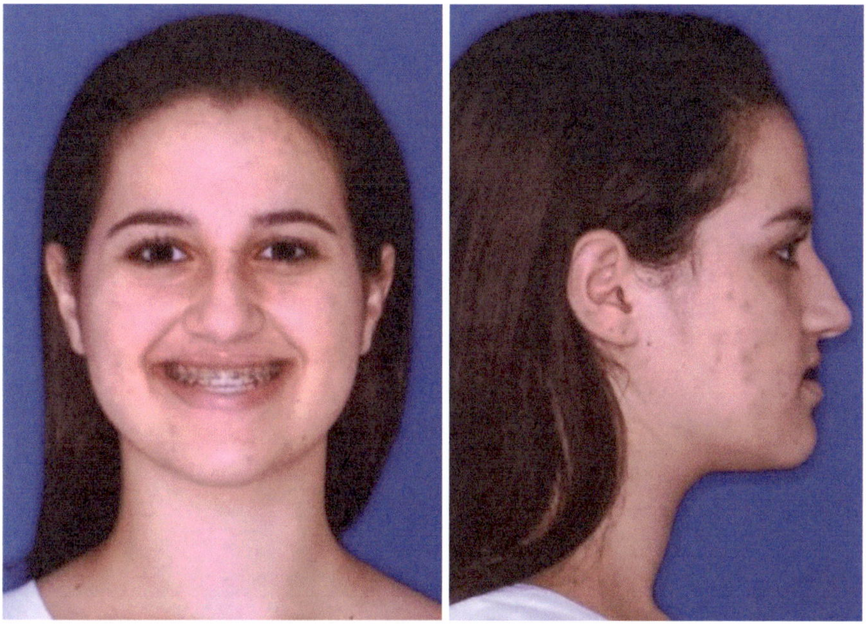

Fig. 9 Patient with dentofacial discrepancy on preoperative view

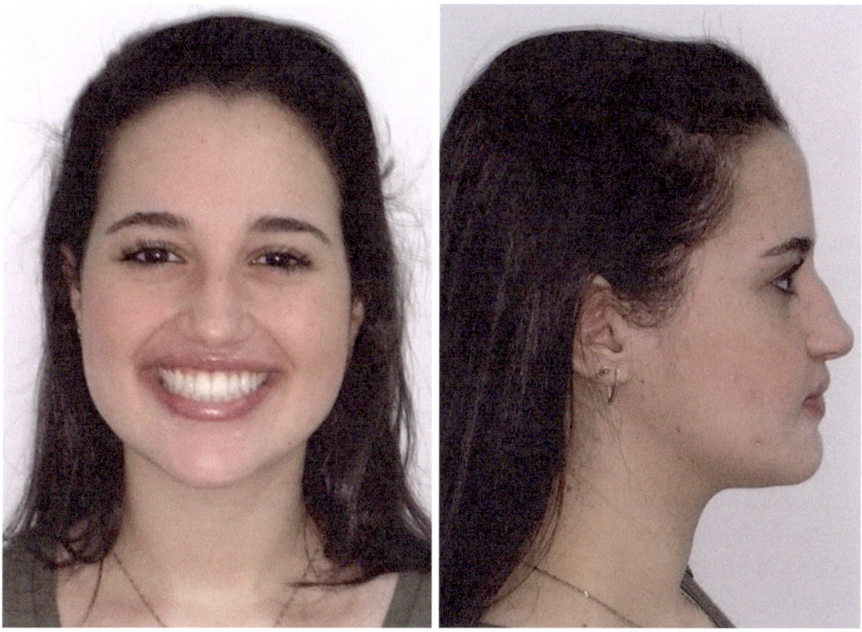

Fig. 10 The same patient from Fig. 9, 1 year postoperatively (orthodontist: Bernardo Quiroga, DDS, PhD)

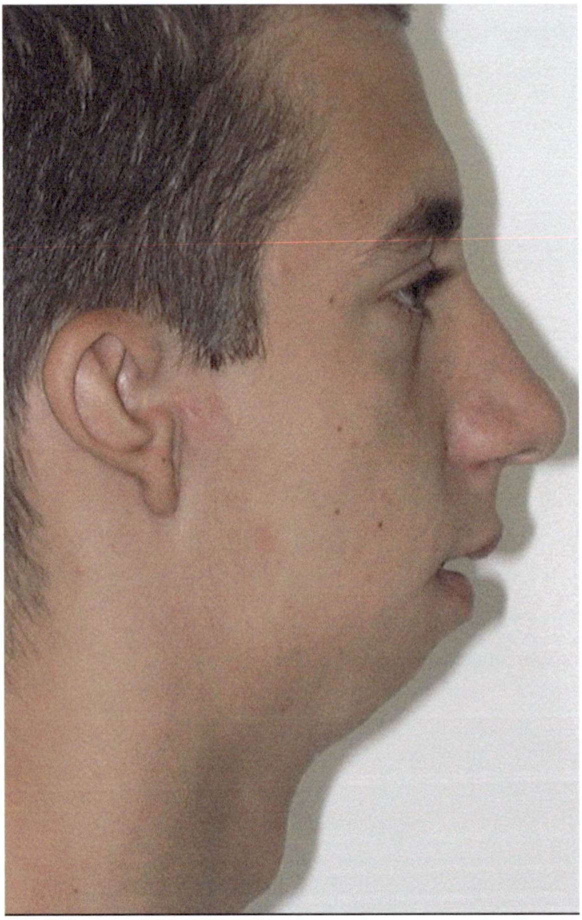

Fig. 11 Severe dentofacial discrepancy with probable difficult airway

facial development derangements, craniofacial congenital anomalies, facial fracture sequelae, inheritance deformities, and others. Other types of surgery in the head and neck area and considerations regarding the upper airway are also important for orthognathic patients, especially because of some etiologic factors, the surgery itself, and/or the anesthesiological procedure (Fig. 11).

Despite these first considerations, ventilatory complications due to orthognathic surgery are uncommon, although not impossible. Some of them have been experienced during the practice of the authors, and certainly by some other surgeons. Posnick states that a patient with DFD should be considered to have difficulties in the upper airway, unless proved otherwise [8].

The purpose of this chapter is to present the indications to perform tracheostomy (after previous cricothyroidostomy or not), as well as submental intubation, establishing the relationships with the biotype or physical characteristics of the patient, the type of DFD, and treatment planning [10, 11]. Considerations regarding preoperative, perioperative, and postoperative evaluation and care are also presented.

Biotype or Physical Characteristics of the Patient

Orthognathic surgery is applied to a great number of patients and to treat a large variety of facial diseases. In some cases, due to some physical characteristics of the patient, a tracheostomy may become a necessity.

Obese patients with DFD, mainly where a mandibular setback is to be done, may have respiratory difficulties during the postoperative period, which might require a tracheostomy.

For those with craniofacial syndromes that require orthognathic surgery as part of the treatment—such as hemifacial microsomia, Treacher Collins syndrome (Fig. 12), cleft palate, or craniosynostosis (Fig. 13)—a preoperatively defined tracheostomy may be a standard procedure in order to make the orthognathic surgery possible and also to promote better postoperative care and safety, especially when external appliances such as external distracters (Fig. 14) are used.

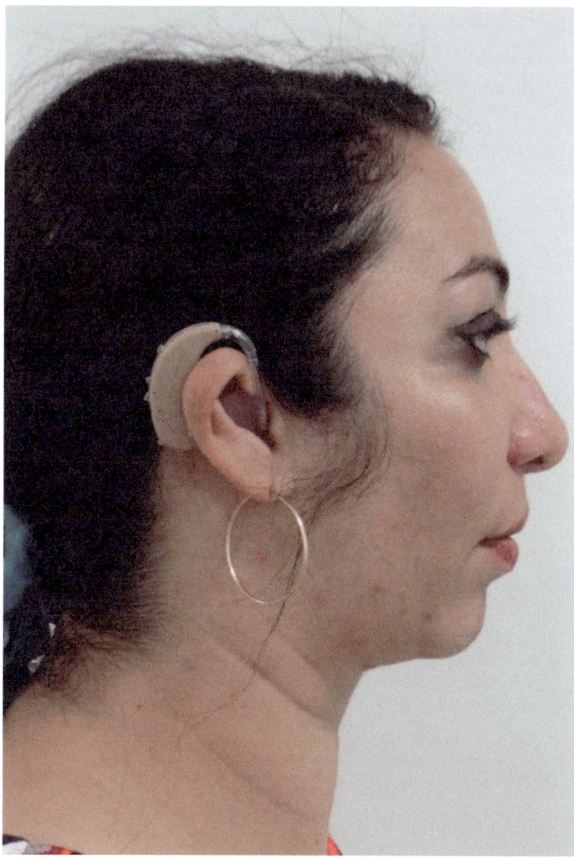

Fig. 12 Lateral view after orthognathic surgery and rhinoplasty for Treacher Collins syndrome (rhinoplasty: Paulo Henrique Rodrigues, MD; orthodontist: Silvia Reis, DDS, PhD)

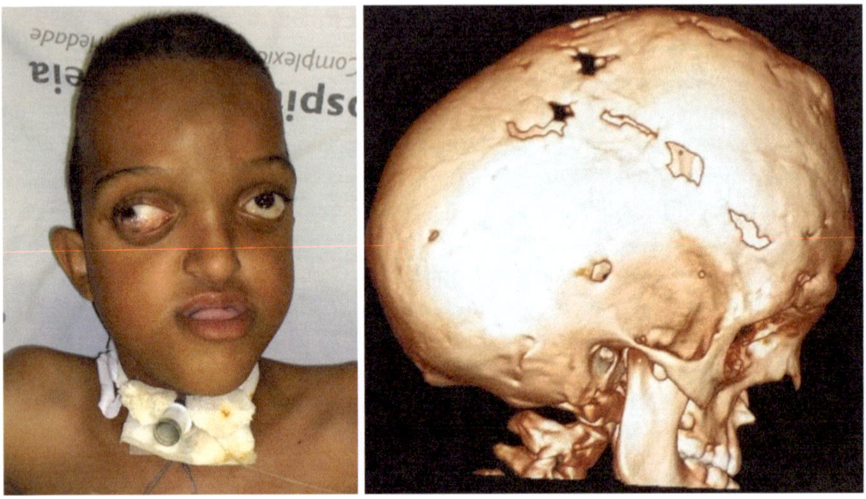

Fig. 13 Child with Crouzon syndrome electively tracheostomized before facial middle third distraction (neurosurgeon: Sandro Lemos, MD)

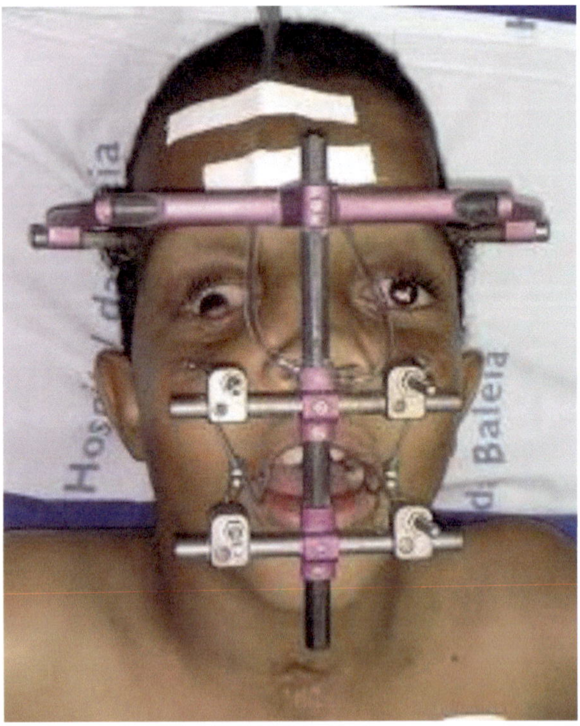

Fig. 14 The same patient from Fig. 13 with a facial middle third distractor

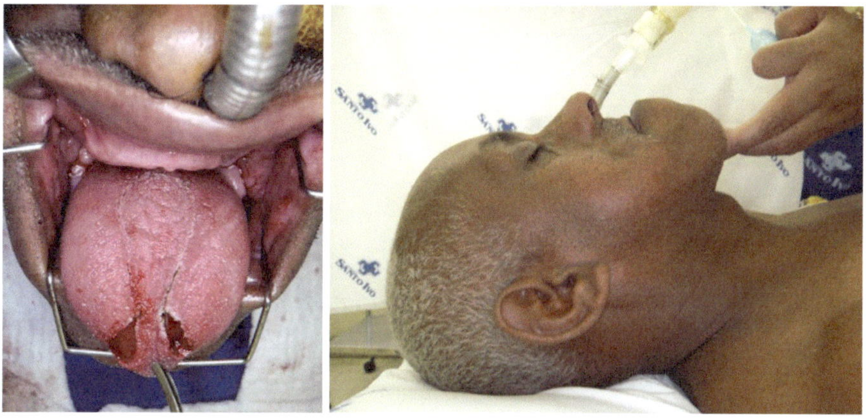

Fig. 15 Macroglossia in a patient with mandibular prognathism

Whenever macroglossia is presented and a glossectomy is to be performed (Fig. 15), tongue swelling may pose a risk of upper air way obstruction and/or dysphagia and a higher risk of aspiration. Special care should be taken in patients with a wide and short neck who are to have a mandible setback, and for those who—even when they do not present with sleep obstructive apnea syndrome (SOAS)—complain of snoring. In these cases, tracheostomy may be necessary to prevent airway collapse during the postoperative period. An intensive care unit stay is recommended for these patients during the initial postoperative period due to the risk of respiratory obstruction when tracheostomy is not the first option.

Finally, some comments are needed on the choice of the tracheostomy cannula. Since it is common to have some blood coming from the nose and mouth, together with saliva, after orthognathic surgery, and considering some dysphagia on the first days, the cannula must have a cuff. In patients who require a long period of tracheostomy, a cannula with a cuff and an inner cannula is the best choice.

Dentofacial Deformity Characteristics and Their Relationship with the Airway

Normally, patients who are to be treated by orthognathic surgery are classified according to the deformity presented. As an example, deformities such as a long or short face, asymmetries, anterior/posterior excess or deficiency, or transverse deficiencies of the maxilla or the mandible can present in isolation or together in a patient (Fig. 16).

Deformities with a deficiency, such as retrognathia or maxillary atresia, can be associated with a narrow upper airway, and the best method to maintain it during and after the surgery should be defined preoperatively. For some cases, bronchofibroscopy may be indicated for the intubation procedure (Fig. 17).

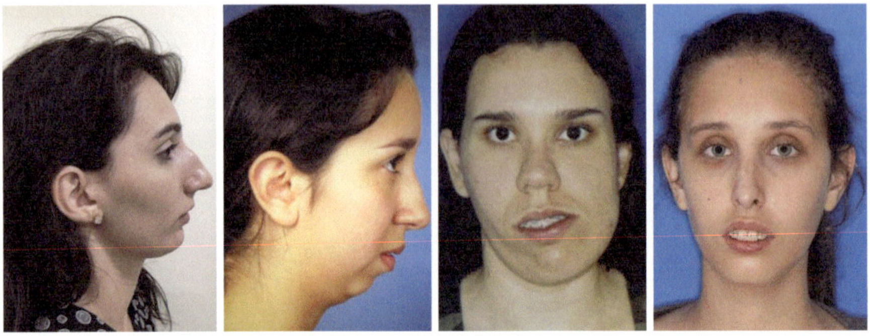

Fig. 16 Examples of dentofacial discrepancies

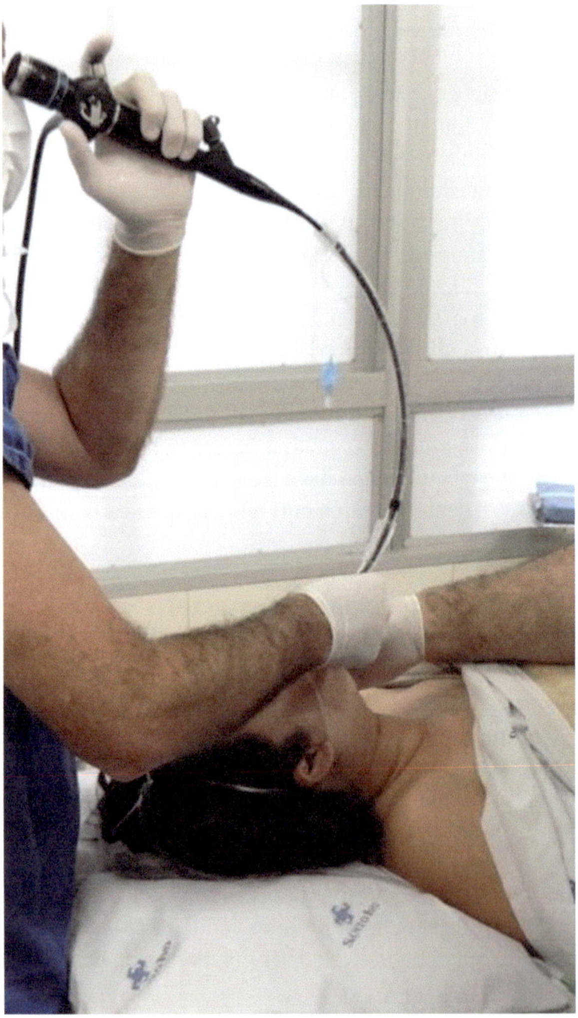

Fig. 17 Orotracheal intubation with a fibrobronchoscope in a patient with Treacher Collins syndrome (chest surgeon: Agnaldo Eisenberg, MD)

In cases in which a narrow nasal cavity is presented, the choice of submental intubation should be considered [8, 21]. The necessity for maintaining maxillomandibular immobilization during orthognathic surgery prevents the possibility of performing oral intubation. For these cases, oral intubation followed by submental intubation, as previously described in this chapter, are highly recommended [13].

In order to surgically treat these patients, tracheostomy is rarely employed, since the main concern is to provide an airway for surgical and anesthesiological purposes. In case of a restricted bone anatomy and constricted airway, the outcome of the surgical treatment normally improves the airway volume, leading to a better breathing pattern, even during the immediate postoperative period.

In contrast to this, DFD with excess in the sagittal, coronal, and/or axial planes may acquire a more constricted condition postoperatively. It may also imply a more constricted airway. Naturally, the treatment planning must consider these possibilities, and the patient might need a longer period of intubation or a tracheostomy. In fact, only in very rare situations will an orthognathic patient undergo these procedures.

Although unlikely to happen, some special conditions should be mentioned due to the high risk of complications arising from them. Whenever it is necessary to employ any kind of positive pressure ventilator system, such as continuous positive airway pressure (CPAP) or bilevel positive airway pressure (BiPAP), during the postoperative period (especially in the first month), an elective tracheostomy is indicated as the first step of the surgery. This avoids the risk of subcutaneous emphysema or further complications such as pneumomediastinum [14, 15]. These are conditions that would probable compromise the airway, and under these circumstances, a tracheostomy or even a cricothyroidostomy would be very difficult to perform.

As a clinical example, a case of DFD and myasthenia gravis depending on BiPAP is presented (Fig. 18). An elective tracheostomy was performed and orthognathic surgery, together with rhinoplasty, was done. Ventilatory assistance was applied and, after a couple of months, the patient was decannulated without any concern.

Dentofacial Deformity Treatment Planning

Orthognathic treatment planning involves measurement of dentofacial discrepancies and makes a prediction regarding the surgical movements of the maxilla and/or the mandible. With the possibility of doing this procedure virtually, with computer-aided design and manufacturing (CAD/CAM) resources, additional information concerning the airway evaluation can be obtained. However, some bias can be noted when this planning is based on a computed tomography (CT) scan and not on a dynamic evaluation of the upper airways. These methods can partially predict the airway volume after surgery, acting as a warning about the risk of airway compromise. Nevertheless, they cannot be taken as a secure predictable method for this purpose (Fig. 19).

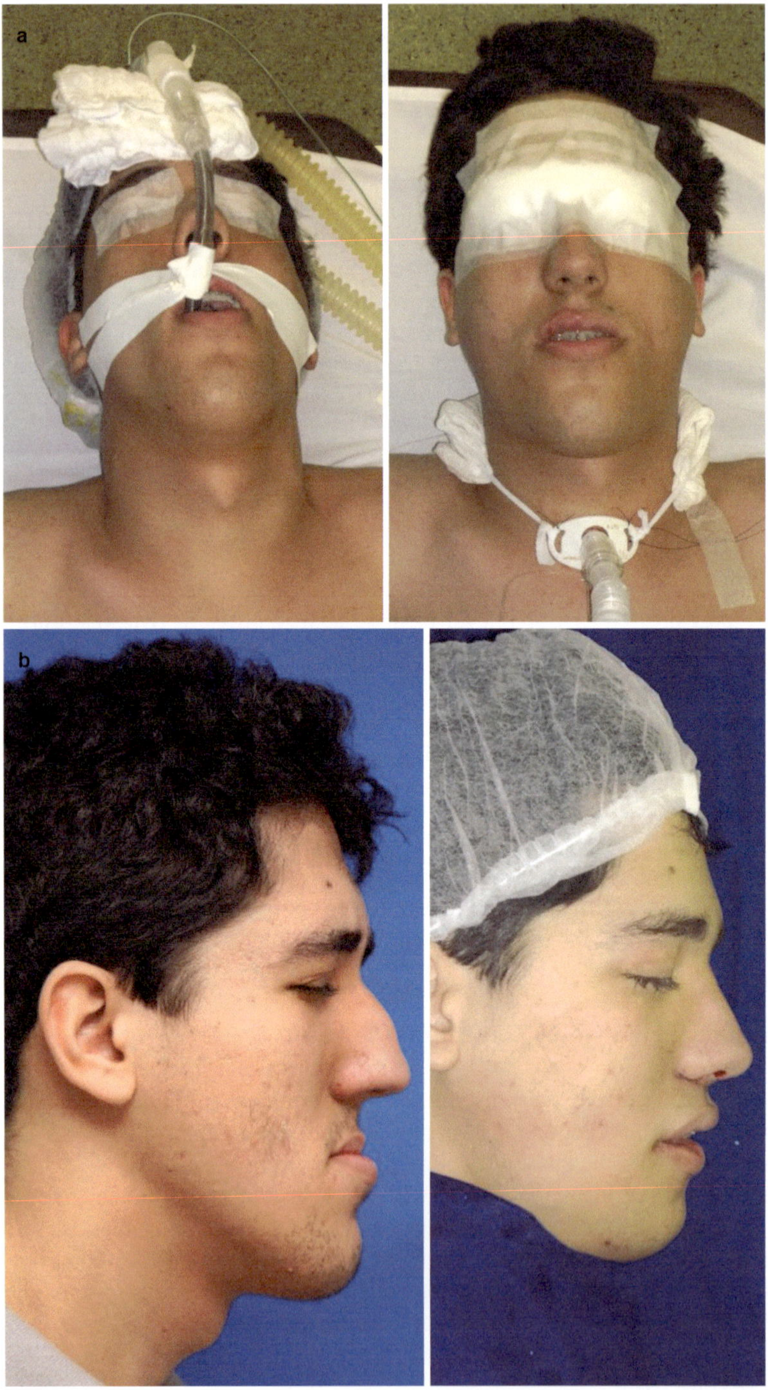

Fig. 18 (**a**) Patient with myasthenia gravis and dentofacial discrepancy using bilevel positive airway pressure (BiPAP). Elective tracheostomy was performed. (**b**) Pre- and immediate postoperative views after tracheostomy, orthognathic surgery, and rhinoplasty (rhinoplasty: Paulo Henrique Rodrigues, MD)

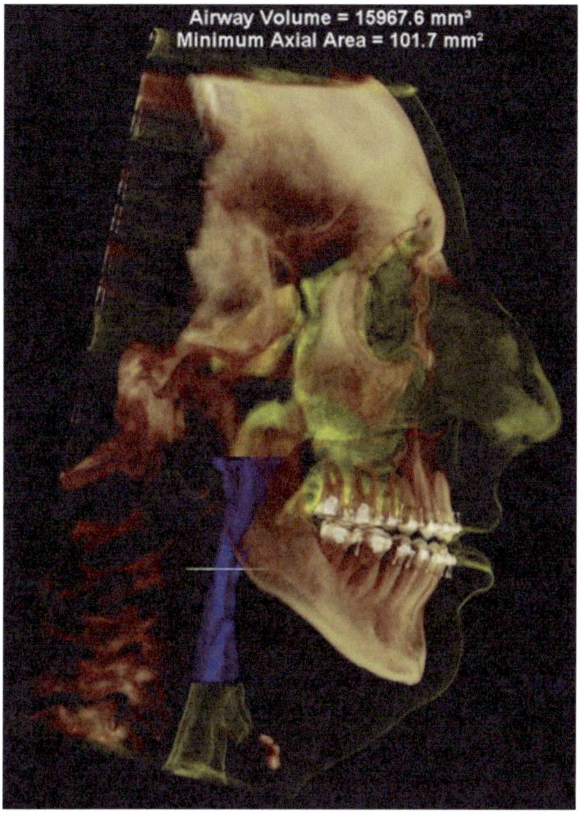

Fig. 19 Airway evaluation with a cone beam computed tomography (CT) scan. (Courtesy of Eduardo Januzzi, DDS, PhD)

Still, treatment planning can consider the necessity of surgical procedures for the osteotomies, such as glossectomy, rhinoplasty, septoplasty, or turbinectomy [16, 22].

With the increasing indication of orthognathic surgery as a treatment method for SOAS, uvulopalatoplasty and other pharyngeal procedures can be put together with the previously described surgeries [17, 18]. Although these are procedures normally performed separately from orthognathic surgery, elective tracheostomy should be an available choice if they are done together.

Endonasal surgeries, such as septoplasty and/or turbinectomy, are often done together with orthognathic surgery without worsening the risk of airway obstruction. When performed, glossectomy of the anterior two thirds of the tongue can compromise the airway and cause an obstruction [16, 19]. In cases such as this, effort in breathing can be the etiology of subcutaneous emphysema and pneumothorax. There are literature data presenting cases of pneumothorax and pneumomediastinum due to the effort to breathe after orthognathic surgery [14, 15, 20]. A tracheostomy may be indicated in these cases, but not electively.

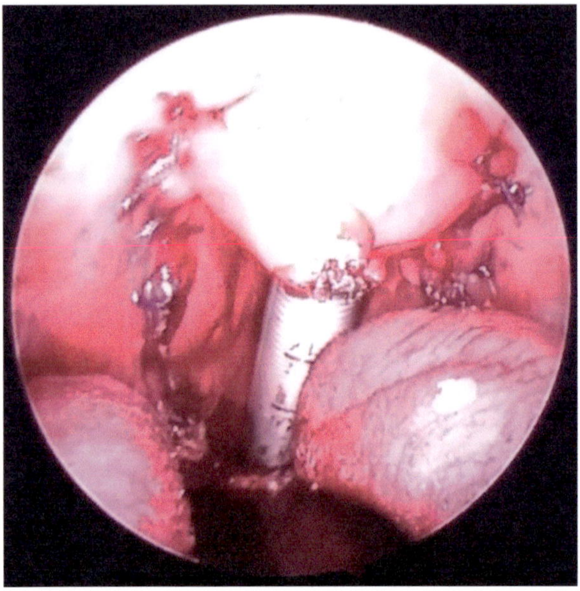

Fig. 20 Screen view of uvulopalatoplasty and posterior glossectomy. Note the nasotracheal tube in the oropharynx (Surgeon: Arturo Carpes, MD, PhD)

Uvulopalatoplasty and/or glossectomy of the base of the tongue are presented as possible treatments for SOAS (Fig. 20). Whenever they are planned to be performed together with orthognathic surgery, special care should be taken related to the risk of postoperative airway obstruction due to the increased swelling expected with these procedures, although smaller soft tissue pharyngeal surgeries may be done along with the orthognathic surgery with minor risk [8]. Elective tracheostomy may also be considered in these cases.

Rhinoplasty can be done together with orthognathic surgery whenever it appears to be necessary, or according to the wishes of the patient [22]. Since the orthognathic surgery is performed first, nasotracheal intubation is used because it is mandatory to immobilize the maxilla and the mandible together while establishing and fixing them. To perform rhinoplasty, a change from naso- to orotracheal intubation is needed. Care should be taken for this procedure; the anesthesiologist must be confident in doing it, and the use of a bronchofiberscope or a bougie may be necessary. When changing the endotracheal tube is not an option, submental intubation is the best choice (Figs. 21 and 22). A tracheostomy would be indicated only if a complication is presented.

Finally, an accurate preoperative evaluation related to the upper airways such as maximum mouth opening, temporomandibular joint (TMJ) mobility, a Mallampati test, and other data can classify the degree of difficulty in accessing the airway [32].

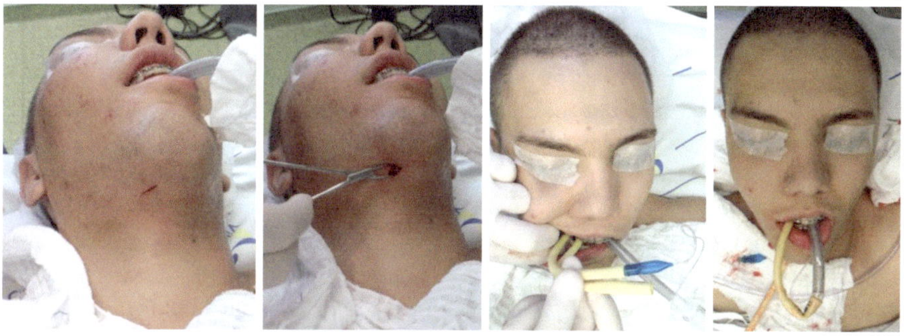

Fig. 21 Sequence for submental intubation in a patient with dentofacial discrepancy and fibrous dysplasia of the right maxilla, undergoing orthognathic surgery with ostectomy to treat the fibrous dysplasia, and rhinoplasty (rhinoplasty: Paulo Henrique Rodrigues, MD; orthodontist: Heloísio Leite, DDS, MSc)

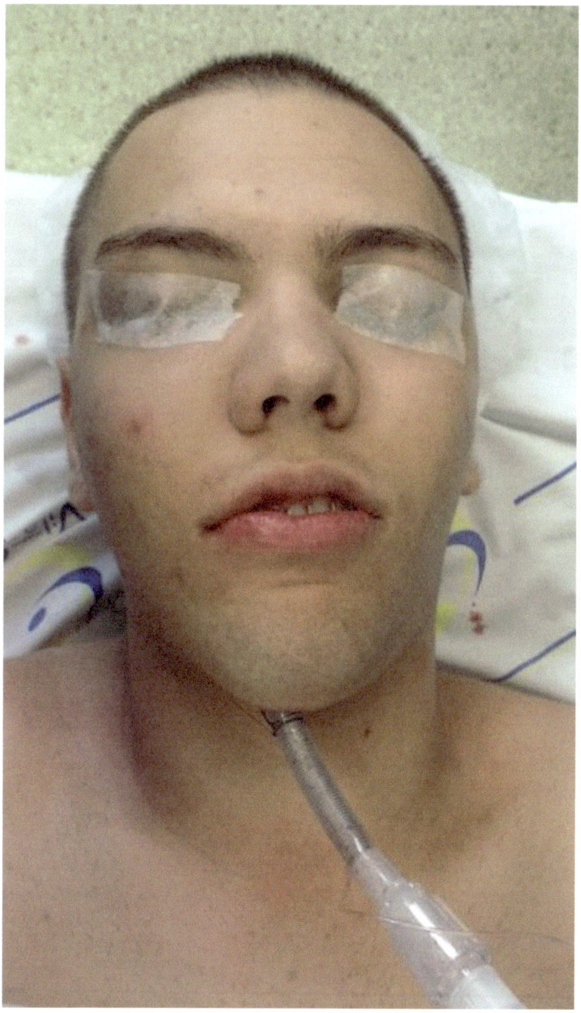

Fig. 22 View of the submental intubation of the patient from Fig. 19

Final Considerations

Tracheostomy has a relevant role in cranial and maxillofacial surgery, and its use should be considered whenever any procedures of this surgical modality are being planned [2, 6, 15, 23–26]. Although it is rare, patients undergoing orthognathic surgery, patients with trauma or trauma sequelae, patients with craniomaxillofacial congenital anomalies, and those about to undergo reconstruction procedures in this field may need a tracheostomy in order to make an airway viable, in either an emergency or elective manner. All of these clinical conditions have received attention from the authors concerning whether to perform a tracheostomy or not. The literature also presents data on this subject.

Nasotracheal intubation is the first option for orthognathic surgery, such as mandible fractures and fractures of the lower middle third of the facial skeleton. Upper middle third and superior facial third fractures will require orotracheal intubation. In cases of combined fractures, such as panfacial fractures, submental intubation or tracheostomy should be chosen, unless it is feasible not to do it. If necessary, perioperative maxillomandibular immobilization, nasotracheal intubation, or submental intubation is the first choice.

Whenever a long period of intubation is expected—for instance, in a patient with facial fractures, brain injuries, and chest trauma—there is an indication to perform a tracheostomy, if it has not yet been done [27].

References

1. Mittal G, Mittal R, Katyal S, Uppal S, Mittal V. Airway management in maxillofacial trauma: do we really need tracheostomy/submental intubation. J Clin Diagn Res. 2014;8:77–9.
2. Holmgren EP, Bagheri S, Bobek S. Utilization of tracheostomy in craniomaxillofacial trauma at a level-1 trauma center. J Oral Maxillofac Surg. 2007;65:2005–10.
3. Watkins TA, Opie NJ, Norman A. Airway choices in maxillofacial trauma. Trends in Anaest Crit Care. 2011;1:179–90.
4. Perry M, Morris C. Advanced trauma life support (ATLS) and facial trauma: can one size fit all? Part 2: ATLS, maxillofacial injuries and airway management dilemmas. Int J Oral Maxillofac Surg. 2008;37:309–20.
5. Taicher S, Givol N, Peleg M, Ardekian L. Changing indications for tracheostomy in maxillofacial trauma. J Oral Maxillofac Surg. 1996;54:292–5.
6. Demas PN, Soteranos GC. The use of tracheotomy in oral and maxillofacial surgery. J Oral Maxillofac Surg. 1988;46:483–6.
7. Kim KF, Doriot R, Morse MA, Al-Attar A, Dufresne CR. Alternative totracheostomy: submental intubation in craniomaxillofacial trauma. J Craniofac Surg. 2005;16:498–500.
8. Hernández AF. The submental route for endotracheal intubation. A new technique. J Maxillofac Surg. 1986;14:64–5.
9. Plummer AL, Gracey DR. Consensus conference on artificial airways in patients receiving mechanical ventilation. Chest. 1989;96:178–80.
10. Boffano P, Gallesio C, Roccia F, Bvd B, Forouzanfar T. Clinical outcomes of surgical management of anterior bilateral mandibular fractures. J Craniofac Surg. 2013;24:e387–90.
11. Keller MW, Han PP, Galarneau MR, Brigger MT. Airway management in severe combat maxillofacial trauma. Otolaryngol Head Neck Surg. 2015;153:532–7.

12. Branco BC, Plurad D, Green DJ, Inaba K, Lam L, Cestero R, Bukur M, Demetriades D. Incidence and clinical predictors for tracheostomy after cervical spinal cord injury: a national trauma databank review. J Trauma. 2011;70:111–5.
13. Lanza DC, Koltai PJ, Parnes SM, Decker JW, Wing P, Fortune JB. Predictive value of the Glascow Coma Scale for tracheostomy in head-injured patients. Ann Otol Rhinol Laryngol. 1990;99:38–41.
14. Barquist ES, Amortegui J, Hallal A, Giannotti G, Whinney R, Alzamel H, MacLeod J. Tracheostomy in ventilator dependent trauma patients: a prospective, randomized intention-to-treat study. J Trauma. 2006;60:91–7.
15. Zachariades N, Rapidis AD, Papademetriou J, et al. The significance of tracheostomy in the management of fractures of the facial skeleton. J Maxillofac Surg. 1983;11:180–6.
16. Lanza DC, Parnes SM, Koltai PJ, Fortune JB. Early complications of airway management in head-injured patients. Laryngoscope. 1990;100:958–61.
17. Schütz P, Hamed HH. Submental intubation versus tracheostomy in maxillofacial trauma patients. J Oral Maxillofac Surg. 2008;66:1404–9.
18. McNiece WL, Dierdorf SF. The pediatric airway. Semin Pediatr Surg. 2004;13:152Y–165.
19. Jundt JS, Cattano D, Hagberg CA, Wilson JW. Submental intubation: a literature review. Int J Oral Maxillofac Surg. 2012;41:46.
20. Das S, Das TP, Ghosh PS. Submental intubation: a journey over the last 25 years. J Anaesthesiol Clin Pharmacol. 2012;28:291–303.
21. Mak PHK, Ooi RGB. Submental intubation in a patient with beta-thalassaemia major undergoing elective maxillary and mandibular oeteotomies. Br J Anaesth. 2002;88:288–91.
22. Lima SM Jr, Asprino L, Moreira RWF, de Moraes M. A retrospective analysis of submental intubation in maxillofacial trauma patients. J Oral Maxillofac Surg. 2011;69:2001–5.
23. Imahara SD, Hopper RA, Wang J, Rivara FP, Klein MB. Patterns and outcomes of pediatric facial fractures in the United States: a survey of the National Trauma Data Bank. J Am Coll Surg. 2008;207:710–6.
24. Manley L. Essentials of airway management for the injured child. Int J Trauma Nurs. 1997;3:27–30.
25. Jackson C. Tracheostomy. Laryngoscope. 1909;19:285–90.
26. Galloway TC. Tracheostomy in bulbar poliomyelitis. JAMA. 1943;128:1096–7.
27. Stranc MF, Skoracki R. A complication of submandibular intubation in a panfacial fracture patient. J Craniomaxillofac Surg. 2001;29:174–6.
28. Eisemann B, Eisemann M, Rizvi M, Urata MM, Lypka MA. Defining the role for submental intubation. J Clin Anesth. 2014;26:238–42.
29. Biglioli F, Mortini P, Goisis M, Bardazzi A, Boari N. Submental orotracheal intubation: an alternative to tracheotomy in transfacial cranial base surgery. Skull Base. 2003;13:189–95.
30. Avarello JT, Cantor RM. Pediatric major trauma: an approach to evaluation and management. Emerg Med Clin North Am. 2007;25:803–36.
31. Castilla DM, Dinh CT, Younis R. Pediatric airway management in craniofacial trauma. J Craniofac Surg. 2011;22:1175–8.
32. Posnick JC. Anesthesia techniques, blood loss/fluid replacement, airway management and convalescence in the treatment of dentofacial deformities. In: Posnick JC, editor. Orthognathic surgery—principles and practice. Amsterdam: Elsevier; 2014. p. 308–36.
33. Haspel AC, Coviello VF, Stevens M. Retrospective study of tracheostomy indications and perioperative complications on oral and maxillofacial surgery service. J Oral Maxillofac Surg. 2012;70:890–5.
34. Badjate SJ, Shenoi SR, Budhraja NJ, Ingole P. Transmylohyoid orotracheal intubation: case series and review. J Clin Anest. 2012;24:460–4.
35. Gadre KS, Waknis PP. Transmylohyoid/submental intubation: review, analysis, and refinaments. J Craniofac Surg. 2010;21:516–9.
36. Chandu A, Witherow H, Stewart A. Submental intubation in orthognathic surgery: initial experience. Br J Oral Maxillofac Surg. 2008;46:561–3.

37. Corega C, Vaida L, Festila D, Bertossi D. Bilateral pneumothorax and pneumomediastinum after orthognathic surgery. Chirurgia. 2014;109:271–4.
38. Chebel NA, Ziade D, Achkouty R. Bilateral pneumothorax and pneumomediastinum after treatment with continuous positive airway pressure after orthognathic surgery. Br J Oral Maxillofac Surg. 2010;48:e14–5.
39. Wolford LM, Cottrell DA. Diagnosis of macroglossia and indications for reduction glossectomy. Am J Orthod Dentofac Orthop. 1996;110:170–7.
40. Seah TE, Bellis H, Ilankovan V. Orthognathic patients with nasal deformities: case for simultaneous orthognathic surgery and rhinoplasty. Br J Oral Maxillofac Surg. 2012;50:55–9.
41. Knudsen TB, Laulund AS, Ingerslev J, Homoe P, Pinholt EM. Improved apnea–hypopnea index and lowest oxygen saturation after maxillomandibular advancement with or without counterclockwise rotation in patients with obstructive sleep apnea: a meta-analysis. J Oral Maxillofac Surg. 2015;73:719–26.
42. Andrews BT, Lakin GE, Bradley JP, Kawamoto HK. Orthognathic surgery for obstructive sleep apnea: applying the principles to new horizons in craniofacial surgery. J Craniofac Surg. 2012;23:2038–41.
43. Jones LC, Waite PD. Orthognathic surgery and partial glossectomy in a patient with merosin-deficient congenital muscular dystrophy. J Oral Maxillofac Surg. 2012;70:e141–6.
44. Goodson ML, Manemi R, Paterson AW. Pneumothorax after orthognathic surgery. Br J Oral Maxillofac Surg. 2010;48:180–1.
45. Heffner JE, Miller S, Sahn SA. Tracheostomy in the intensive care unit. Part 1: indications, technique, management. Chest. 1986;90:269–74.

Cricothyroidostomy

Adriana Eliza Brasil Moreira, Rodrigo Gonçalves, João Lisboa de Sousa Filho, José Francisco de Sales Chagas, Maria Beatriz Nogueira Pascoal, and Ricardo Alexander Marinho da Silva

Cricothyroidostomy or cricothyrotomy, is surgical access to the airways through the cricothyroid membrane, a procedure that promotes access to the airways by means of an incision in the cricothyroid membrane with placement of a tube for oxygenation and ventilation.

According to Mori, the procedure was first described by the French surgeon Vicq d'Azyr in the seventeenth century and later detailed by Tandler in 1916 and disseminated in the USA by Sicher in 1949 [1]. In 1909, Chevalier Jackson [2] described the surgical techniques and factors necessary to perform cricothyroidostomy, called

A.E.B. Moreira, M.D. (✉) • R.A.M. da Silva, D.D.S. •
Department of Oral and Maxillofacial Surgery, Hospital Santa Casa de Piracicaba, Piracicaba, SP, Brazil
e-mail: adrisolaris@hotmail.com

R. Gonçalves, D.D.S. • J.L. de Sousa Filho, D.D.S.
Department of Bucco-Maxillo-Facial Surgery and Traumatology, Hospital Santa Casa de Piracicaba, Piracicaba, SP, Brazil

J.F. de Sales Chagas, M.D., Ph.D.
Federal University, São Paulo, Brazil

Department of Head and Neck Surgery, São Leopoldo Mandic Medical School, Campus of Campinas, Campinas, Brazil

São Leopoldo Mandic Medical School, Campus of Araras, Araras, Brazil

M.B.N. Pascoal, M.D., Ph.D.
Department of Head and Neck Surgery, São Leopoldo Mandic Medical School, Campus of Campinas, Campinas, Brazil

University of São Paulo, São Paulo, Brazil

Department of Head and Neck Surgery, Dr. Mário Gatti Municipal Hospital, Campinas, SP, Brazil

Department of Integrated Clinical Meeting, São Leopoldo Mandic Medical School, Campus of Campinas, Campinas, Brazil

T.P. de Farias (ed.), *Tracheostomy*, https://doi.org/10.1007/978-3-319-67867-2_15

high tracheostomy. After hundreds of references to patients with tracheal stenosis, this author reviewed 200 of these cases, condemning the procedure [3]. In the decade of 1970, Brantigan and Grow reported on 655 patients undergoing the procedure, with a complication rate of 6.1%. Consequently, the use of cricothyroidostomy was resumed and became the surgical rescue technique of choice for a difficult airway in adults [4].

Cricothyroidostomy is a rapid and temporary alternative for maintenance of the airway, especially in emergency situations, and should be replaced by a tracheostomy within 24–72 h [5]. Its use is rare, with a 1% rate among all intubations in the emergency sector and 10.9% among prehospital intubations [6]. According to Chang et al., there has been a decline in the performance of cricothyroidostomy in cases of trauma in the last 10 years due to the establishment of emergency medical residency programs, with rates of 1.8% before these programs and 0.2% thereafter [7].

Indications

Cricothyroidostomy is indicated when there is an inability to perform orotracheal intubation due to a difficult airway or when an emergency airway is necessary.

Conditions associated with a difficult airway that may require cricothyroidostomy include severe facial trauma, including burns; severe hemorrhage of upper aerodigestive pathways; anatomical distortion due to neck trauma; inability to visualize the vocal cords due to accumulation of blood and secretions, airway edema, or trismus; pre-existing diseases of the larynx or trachea, such as tumors and infections; and abscesses of the cervical region [5]. Of all clinical conditions requiring cricothyroidostomy, 32% reportedly involved facial fractures, 32% were due to blood or vomiting in the airways, 7% were due to traumatic airway obstruction, and 11% were due to intubation failure in the absence of other specific problems [7].

When deciding whether to perform cricothyroidostomy, the patient's age; size and physical maturity in children; clinical conditions (presence of coexisting morbidities); cervical anatomy (palpability of the cricothyroid membrane); and the presence of trauma, masses, or previous surgeries should be considered.

Contraindications

There are no absolute contraindications to cricothyroidostomy in adults. Relative contraindications are trauma with transection of the trachea and extensive fracturing of the larynx. In these cases, tracheostomy is the best approach.

Cricothyroidostomy is relatively contraindicated in children due to cartilage fragility and airway conformation in the form of a funnel, which increases the risk of developing subglottic stenosis after the procedure. The preferred technique for accessing the airway in children is transtracheal ventilation using a 14-gauge needle. The age at which cricothyroidostomy can be safely performed in children is not well established, and recommendations range from 5 to 12 years of age.

Cricothyroidostomy is usually also contraindicated in patients with hemorrhagic diastasis, but in a life-threatening situation the need to establish an airway overcomes this concern [8].

How to Predict a Difficult Airway

In order to predict procedural difficulty, it is important to evaluate the airway before attempting intubation. Factors that may predict difficulties with airway maneuvers include cervical spine injuries, advanced cervical spine arthritis, significant mandibular or maxillomandibular trauma, limiting mouth opening, and anatomical variations such as micrognathism, prognathism, short neck, and muscle hypertrophy. The LEMON method (for difficult intubation evaluation) serves as a reminder to assess the potential airway difficulty [9] and is described below:

L = *Look Externally:* Look externally for features that are related to difficult intubation or ventilation.

E = *Evaluate:* Evaluate the 3–3–2 rule. To align the pharynx, larynx, and mouth axis and then intubate, the following relationships must be observed: (a) the distance between the incisor teeth must be at least three (3) fingers; (b) the distance between the hyoid bone and the mandible should be at least three (3) fingers; and (c) the distance between the thyroid protrusion and the mouth floor should be at least two (2) fingers.

M = *Mallampati:* The hypopharynx should be properly visualized. Traditionally, this has been done by evaluating the Mallampati classification (Fig. 1).

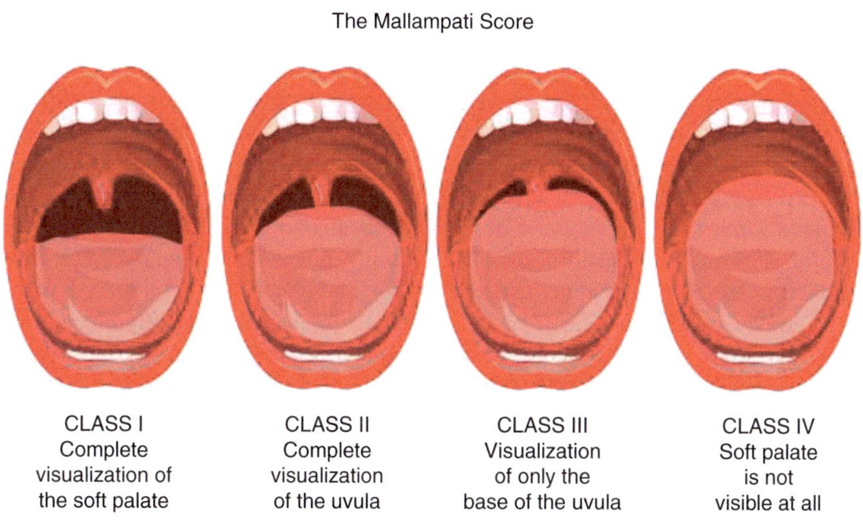

Fig. 1 Mallampati classification

O = *Obstruction:* Any condition that causes airway obstruction makes laryngoscopy and ventilation difficult. These conditions include epiglottis in omega, hypertrophy, tonsillar abscesses, and trauma.
N = *Neck Mobility:* This is of vital importance for successful intubation. It can be easily assessed by asking the patient to flex the chin to the chest and then extend the neck in such a way as to look up. Patients using a cervical collar obviously cannot move their neck and are more difficult to intubate.

The Advanced Trauma Life Support (ATLS) airway algorithm provides an overview of airway treatment in trauma. Many health centers have their own algorithms. Figure 2 shows the decision framework to approach the airway recommended by ATLS [10].

Ethical Aspects

The Regional and Federal Councils of Medicine of Brazil guide—through opinions, resolutions, and consultations—the standardization of procedures, best practice, competence, and responsibilities.

Orotracheal intubation is the passage of a tube through the oral or nasal cavity, aiming to maintain the airway, either in cases of airway obstruction or in cases of maintenance of the airways in anesthetic procedures. Impossibility of tracheal intubation in emergency situations is a clear indication for creation of a surgical airway. When the airways are obstructed by edema, severe facial trauma with significant anatomy alteration, or the presence of severe oral bleeding, surgical cricothyroidostomy should be performed. Tracheostomy is a surgical procedure, often performed in patients requiring prolonged mechanical ventilation. The incision is made between the second and third tracheal rings. Cricothyroidostomy consists of opening of the cricothyroid membrane on its midline, creating communication with the external environment and providing the patient with a respiratory alternative. In this way, both are medical procedures [5].

The Federal Council of Medicine published, on its website, the resolution of the Regional Council of Medicine of the State of Paraná no. 54/1995, which regulates the "normalization of medical activity in the urgency–emergency area in its prehospital phase of trauma care," establishing that "lifeguards are forbidden to practice invasive acts such as: vascular access, intubation, cricothyroidostomy, thoracocentesis, pericardiocentesis, prescription and administration of medications, etc.". Resolution no. 1718/2004 of the Federal Council of Medicine states that "it is prohibited [to teach] private medical acts or procedures, in any form of transmission of knowledge, to non-medical professionals, including those relevant to advanced life support, except emergency care at distance, through telemedicine, under medical supervision until ideal resources are achieved" [11].

Article 4 of law no. 12.842/2013 provides, among others, that the indication for the execution and the execution of invasive procedures—whether diagnostic,

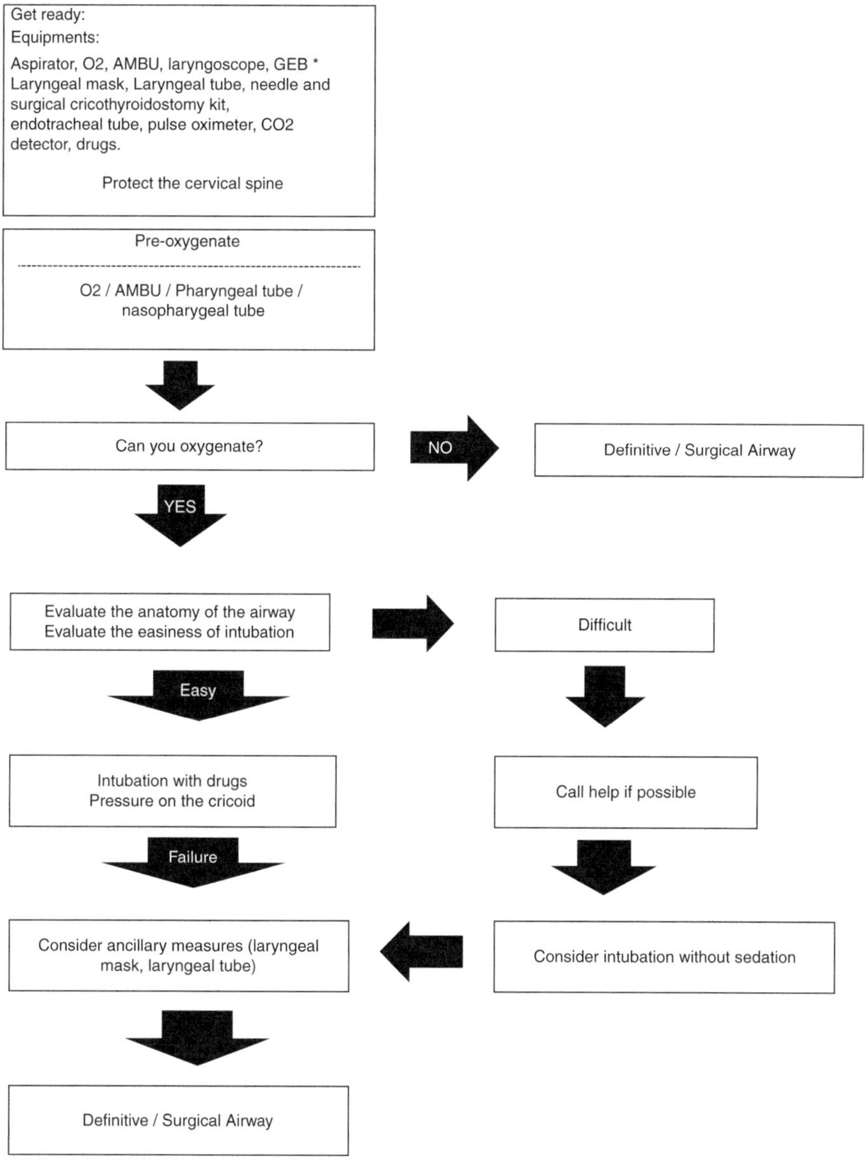

Fig. 2 Decision-making framework to approach the airway, recommended by the Advanced Trauma Life Support (ATLS) Program

therapeutic, or aesthetic, including deep vascular accesses, biopsies, and endoscopies, as well as tracheal intubation—are exclusive activities of the physician [12].

Thus, from May 2004, medical teaching by physicians of invasive procedures—for example, naso- or orotracheal intubation, venous dissection, thoracocentesis, puncture cricothyroidostomy, or surgical cricothyroidostomy—to those who are not physicians or medical students is prohibited.

Anatomical Considerations

The median structures anterior to the neck are easily palpable most of the time, and comprise (from top to bottom) the mandible, mouth floor, hyoid bone, thyroid membrane, thyroid cartilage, cricothyroid membrane, and cricoid cartilage.

One way to improve familiarity with the anatomy of the cervical region is to regularly palpate the neck structures when examining patients (Fig. 1). Begin by palpating the prominence of the larynx, which forms the upper border of the thyroid cartilage. There is often a V-shaped prominence with a palpable groove on the midline, and this is always more evident in men. The hyoid bone is in a position superior to the thyroid cartilage. In patients where the thyroid cartilage is not prominent, the hyoid bone may be confused with the laryngeal prominence [13].

The laryngeal prominence can be easily palpated in most patients; the index finger must slide down through the keel of the thyroid cartilage to find a depression that corresponds to the cricothyroid membrane just below the cartilage (Fig. 3).

The cricothyroid membrane is a trapezoidal membrane of dense, elastic, fibrous tissue, laterally bordered by the cricothyroid muscles. The medial portion of the membrane is specifically known as the *medial cricothyroid ligament* [13]. Its blood supply comes from the cricothyroid arteries—branches of the upper thyroid artery, which anastomose on the midline at the lower border of the thyroid cartilage. Therefore, incision of this membrane should be performed near the upper edge of the cricoid cartilage in order to avoid injury to these blood vessels and bleeding. The size of the membrane varies in adults from 22 to 33 mm in width and from 9 to 10 mm in height. The external diameter of the endotracheal tube should therefore not exceed 8 mm, and an internal diameter of at least 5 mm is recommended to provide good air flow [14].

Identification of the cricothyroid membrane is relatively easy and direct due to its superficial position in the neck. However, lack of familiarity may hinder rapid identification of the cricothyroid membrane, particularly in emergency situations or in patients with obesity, trauma, or previous surgeries in the cervical region. Ultrasonography has been proposed to identify the cricothyroid membrane, and observational studies on corpses suggest that it provides a rapid and accurate means of identification [15].

Surface Anatomy of the Cervical Region with the Corresponding Structures of the Respiratory Tract

The vocal cords are located superiorly, at least 1 cm above the incision site. The tube should be directed downward in order not to injure them. The subglottic space begins below the vocal cords and extends up to the inferior margin of the cricoid

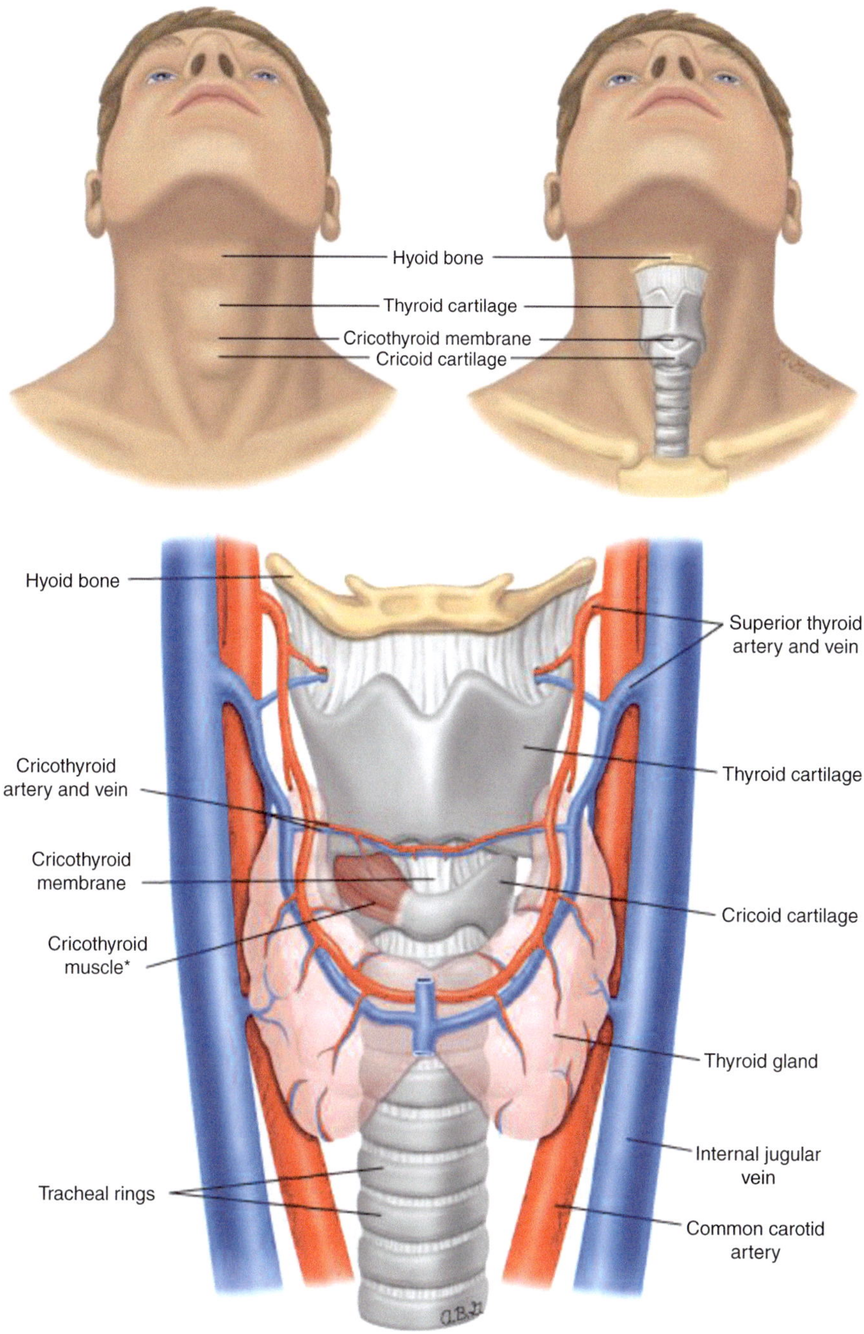

Fig. 3 Anatomy of the cervical region in relation to the thyroid gland, with its vascularization and laryngeal structures

cartilage. It is the site of the smallest internal diameter and is surrounded by the cricoid cartilage, which is the only complete cartilaginous ring of the airways—a characteristic that predisposes this space to numerous complications, with stenosis being the main one. This cartilage consists of an anterior arch and a posterior lamina, and is situated at the height of the sixth cervical vertebra. It serves as a support structure and is responsible for airway permeability [14].

Procedure

Assuming that anoxia can lead to death within 4–5 min, an emergency cricothyroidostomy should be performed within 2–3 min [16].

Precautions

As in all surgical procedures, some standardizations need to be followed:

(a) Take standard precautions for protection against exposure to blood and body fluids, which include wearing of gloves, a surgical mask, goggles, and adequate clothing.
(b) Keep the patient on the stretcher and, unless there is known or suspected cervical trauma, extend the cervical region to help identify the anatomical landmarks (the laryngeal prominence, thyroid and cricoid cartilages, and cricothyroid membrane), thus obtaining extensive exposure of the cricothyroid membrane, but it is important to keep in mind that the cricothyroidostomy will be guided mainly by palpation and not by direct visualization (Fig. 4).
(c) Monitor the heart rate, blood pressure, and respiratory rate.
(d) Prepare the skin with antiseptic solution.
(e) Use local anesthesia if the patient is conscious, involving the skin, subcutaneous tissue, and cricothyroid membrane.

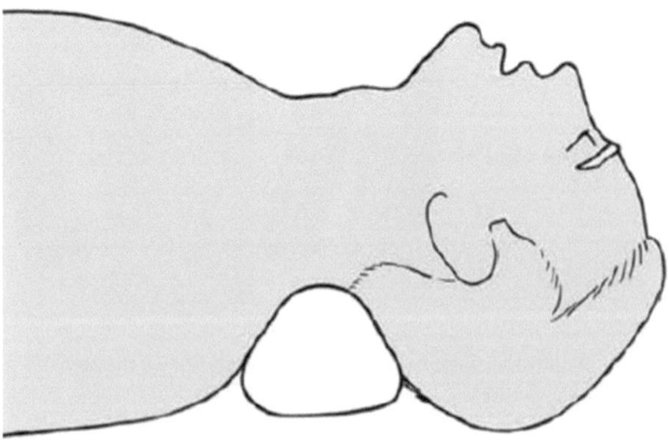

Fig. 4 Extension of the cervical region with a cushion, facilitating exposure of the cricothyroid membrane

During assembly of the equipment, perform preoxygenation of the patient by administration of high oxygen flow, using a mask.

Under certain emergency circumstances, there is no time to administer sedative or analgesic medications, since the main objective is maintenance of the airway, and in cases of respiratory depression, the use of sedatives may aggravate the condition. However, if the patient is agitated and this behavior is hampering the progress of the procedure, a sedative or analgesic may be given to help control the patient.

Cricothyroidostomy guarantees the airway for a given time, and it must be substituted with a tracheostomy within 24–72 h. Cricothyroidostomy is a short-term alternative because prolonged use of this airway access may be associated with an important risk of subglottic stenosis [12].

Types of Cricothyroidostomy

Surgical Cricothyroidostomy

Surgical cricothyroidostomy consists of making a transverse incision in the skin over the cricothyroid membrane and carefully deepening the incision until it reaches the tracheal lumen.

It can be performed by a standard technique or by a rapid procedure called the *rapid 4-step technique*.

The standard technique consists of immobilization of the larynx by the middle finger and thumb of the nondominant hand on the borders of the thyroid cartilage and identification of the cricothyroid membrane with the index finger of the same hand (Fig. 5). Proper immobilization of the larynx is essential for the procedure because it

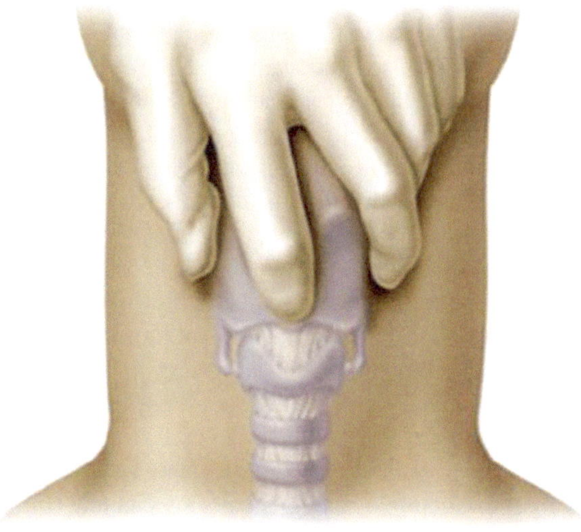

Fig. 5 Laryngeal immobilization with the nondominant hand

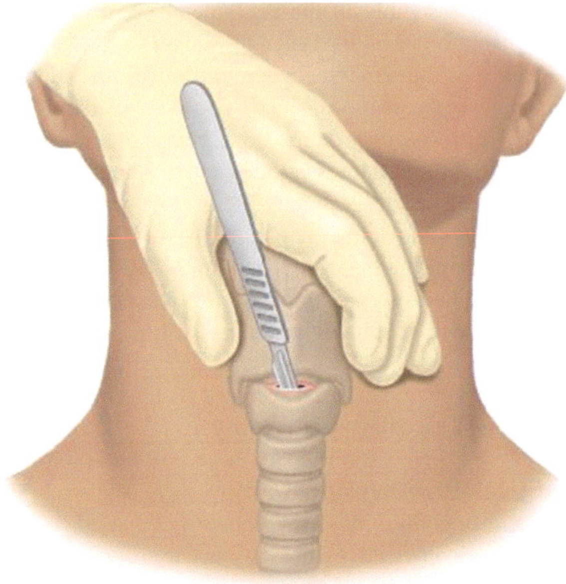

Fig. 6 Horizontal cutaneous incision

maintains its anatomical functions, and identification of the cricothyroid membrane indicates the site of the cutaneous incision. The incision is made in the vertical direction, extending about 3–5 cm on the midline, thus avoiding vascular structures located laterally (Fig. 6). The cricothyroid membrane is sectioned for 1 cm horizontally because its extension is greater than its height, allowing adequate separation of the thyroid and cricoid cartilages, which should be done without excessive force to avoid risk of injury to the vocal cords, located 1–2 cm above. The index fingertip of the nondominant hand should be kept within the cricothyroid membrane incision in order not to lose it. If it is difficult to maintain laryngeal immobilization due to obesity, trauma, edema, or other causes, the scalpel can be held in position until a hook or a claw is positioned to pull the thyroid cartilage so there is no loss of the membrane opening. Insert a dilator or Kelly tweezers into the opening of the membrane to facilitate the introduction of the tracheostomy cannula. Remove the dilator or Kelly tweezers and hook or claw carefully to avoid damaging the cuff of the tracheostomy cannula. Inflate the cuff of the tracheostomy cannula and fix it with a lace. Make a dressing with gauzes below the cannula flaps to protect the skin.

The rapid 4-step technique can be performed in a short time and requires only a scalpel with a number 11 or 15 blade, a traction hook or claw, and a tracheostomy cannula. It begins with palpation and identification of the cricothyroid membrane, followed by a horizontal incision extending about 2 cm, involving the skin, subcutaneous cellular tissue, and cricothyroid membrane. Before removal of the scalpel, insert the hook or the claw to pull the thyroid cartilage, which will help immobilize the larynx, allowing introduction of the tracheostomy cannula (Fig. 7). This can be assisted with an intubation cannula introducer (called a "bougie"), which will serve as a guide. This technique greatly reduces the surgical time, and its procedure is simpler than the standard technique [17] (Fig. 8).

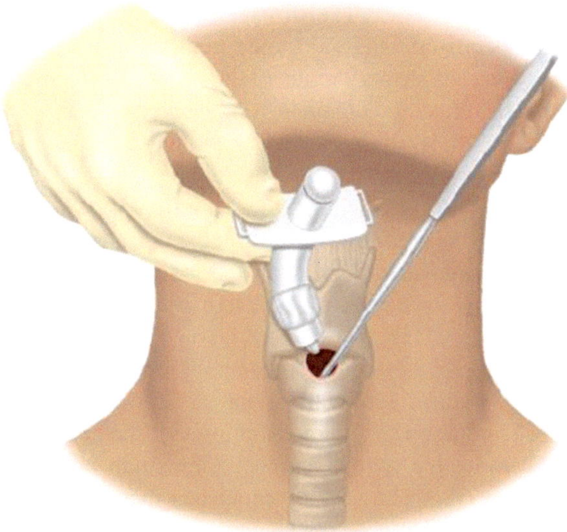

Fig. 7 Hook to facilitate insertion of the tracheostomy cannula

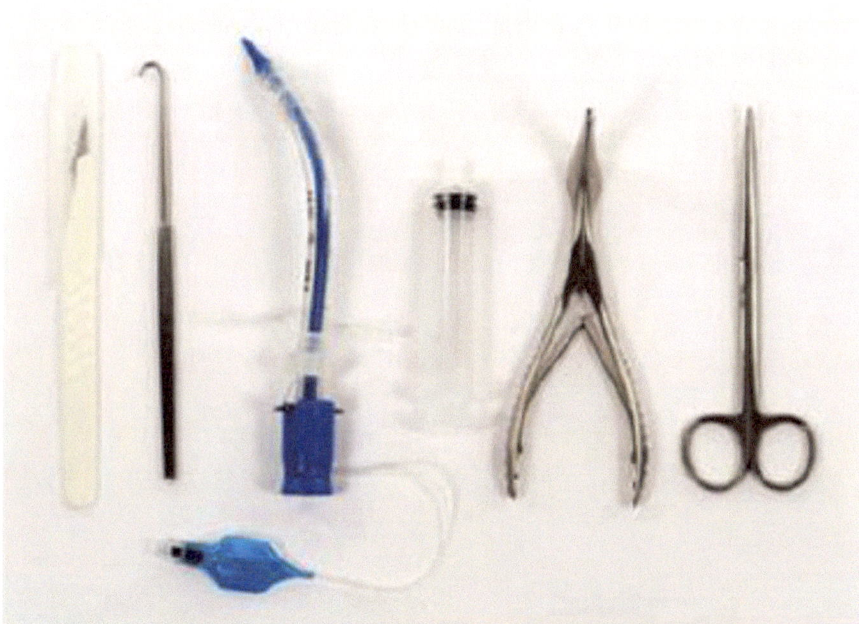

Fig. 8 Instruments needed for surgical cricothyroidostomy

Puncture Cricothyroidostomy (Seldinger Technique)

Puncture or percutaneous cricothyroidostomy consists of a rapid and emergency access to the airways by simple perforation of the cricothyroid membrane by a large-caliber needle catheter, creating communicating between the airway lumen and the external environment [18]. It requires specific instruments, usually in kits offered by the industry, which include a 6 to 10 ml syringe, large-caliber needle, guide wire, soft tissue dilator, and tracheostomy cannula (Fig. 9). Alternatively, an intubation cannula introducer (bougie) may be used, as described in the rapid 4-step technique.

Palpate the cricothyroid membrane with the index finger of the nondominant hand while immobilizing the larynx with the thumb and middle finger of this hand (Fig. 5).

Puncture in the region of the cricothyroid membrane with the needle and syringe, aspirating the syringe plunger until bubbles appear (if there is a physiological solution in the syringe) or air appears, demonstrating that the needle is in the tracheal lumen (Fig. 10). Remove the syringe and insert the guide wire through the needle lumen, then remove it (Fig. 11). Make a cutaneous incision of about 2 cm at the location of the guide wire entrance with a number 11 or 15 scalpel blade, including the cricothyroid membrane. Insert the tissue dilator into the tracheostomy cannula with the guide wire in the dilator until it reaches the tracheal lumen (Fig. 12). Remove the dilator and guide wire, leaving the cannula in position (Fig. 13). Fix the cannula with a lace. Make a dressing with gauze under the cannula flaps to protect the skin [18, 19].

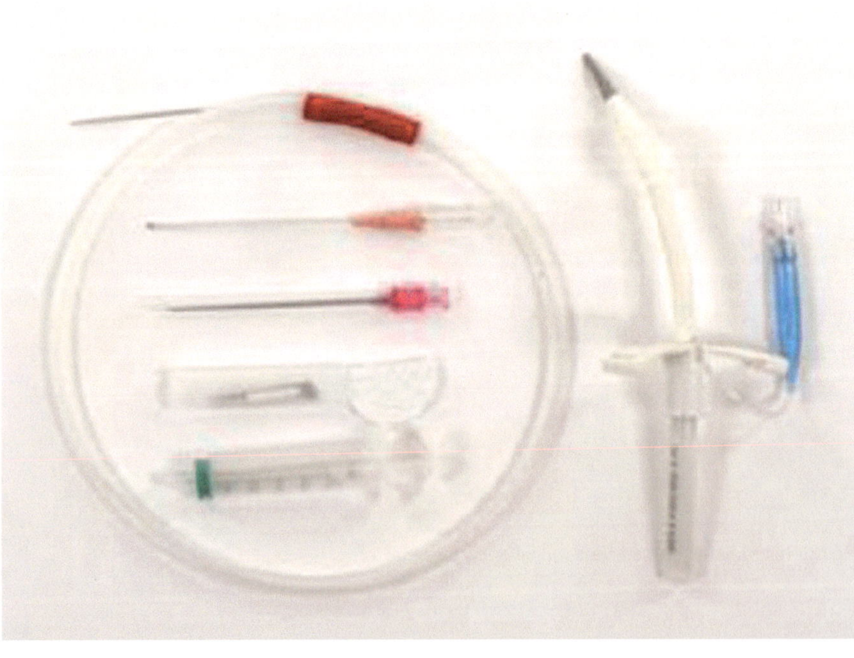

Fig. 9 Instruments needed for puncture cricothyroidostomy

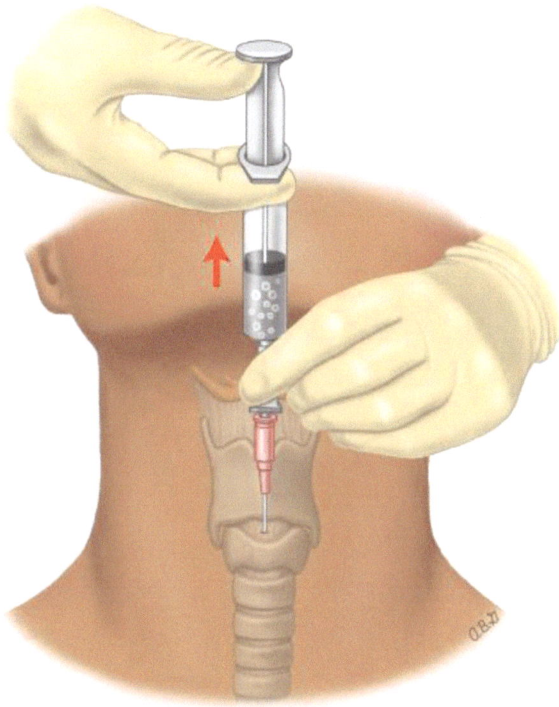

Fig. 10 Puncture with a syringe with saline solution and aspiration with bubbles, demonstrating that the lumen of the trachea has been reached

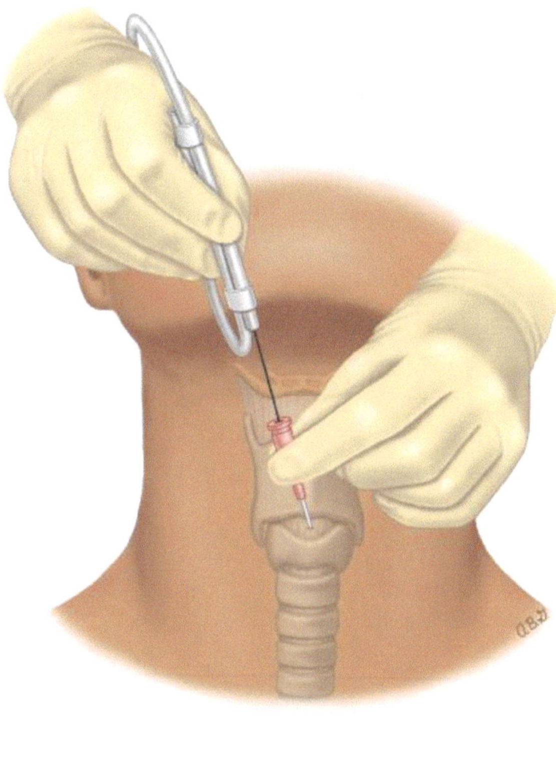

Fig. 11 Introduction of a guide wire after removal of the syringe

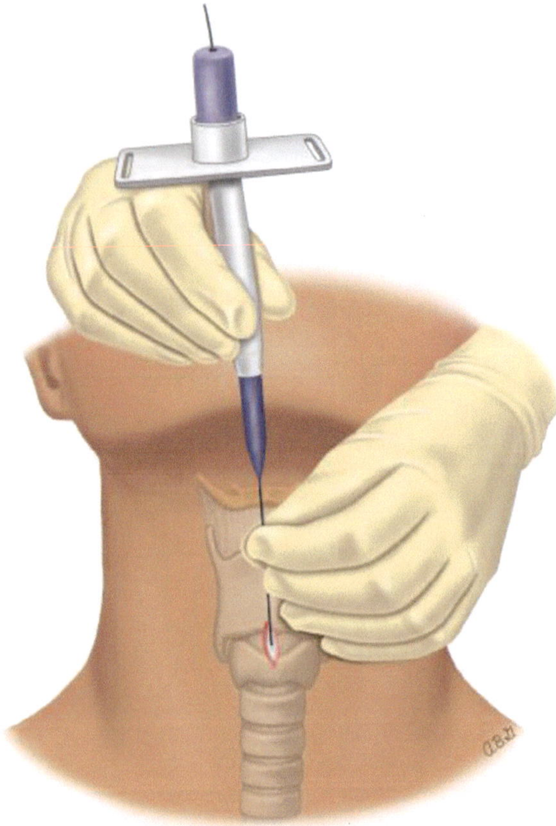

Fig. 12 Introduction of a soft tissue dilator together with the tracheostomy cannula

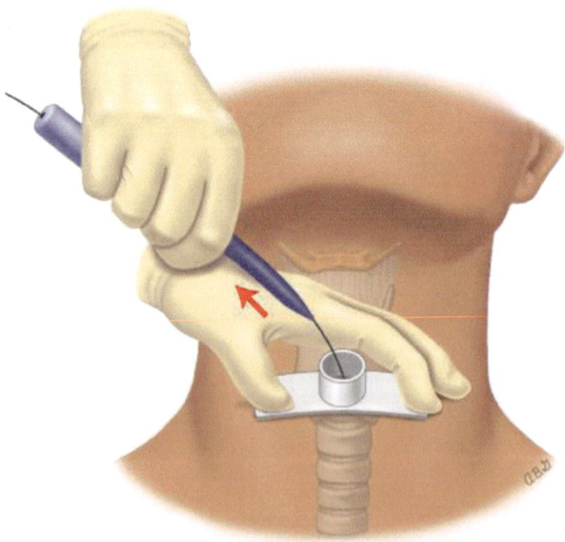

Fig. 13 Tracheostomy cannula in position and removal of the dilator together with the guide wire

Situations for Performing Cricothyroidostomy

Prehospital Care

Cricothyroidostomy should be used as a last resort for control of the airways in the prehospital environment. When performed by trained professionals, this procedure can resolve cases of airway obstruction with difficult intubation.

Urgent tracheostomy is indicated for specific cases, since the risks of complications are two to five times higher than in elective situations; therefore, it is not a method to be used in urgency situations [19].

Hospital Care

Cricothyroidostomy in the hospital environment should also be used as a last resort. Considering that the hospital offers an adequate infrastructure for performing a surgical procedure, and has a trained team to perform tracheostomy, cricothyroidostomy is reserved for isolated cases.

Tracheostomy should be performed in the surgery center with all necessary support, and its performance at the bedside should be avoided. The exception is in an intensive care setting, when removal of the patient from that location can create risks [18].

The time and success of a cricothyroidostomy procedure depend on the technique used, the patient, and the experience of the physician. Studies on cricothyroidostomy techniques are limited due to the absence of randomized clinical protocols, and the current literature is based on reports of cadaver or animal studies, with conflicting findings. Thus, the best technique and the best clinical circumstances are still unknown. An observational study reported that experienced physicians needed an average of 73 s (ranging from 53 to 255 s), while inexperienced ones required an average of 180 s to complete cricothyroidostomy with the standard technique in unfixed corpses. Studies using unfixed corpses have demonstrated an 88% success rate in performing cricothyroidostomy with the standard technique and with the rapid 4-step technique, but the latter was faster, taking an average time of 43.2 s versus 133 s with the standard technique [18, 20].

Complications

Complication rates vary, depending on the type of patient, the clinical aspects, the physician's training level, and the setting for the procedure (i.e., the hospital or prehospital environment). Studies have reported complication rates ranging from 0% to 54%. Emergency cricothyroidostomy has a higher complication rate than the elective procedure, as expected, because it is indicated for critically ill patients with a difficult airway in conjunction with emergency conditions.

Bleeding usually occurs early and usually is not intense, being resolved with dressings. Other early complications include laceration of the cricoid cartilage or thyroid cartilage, perforation of the posterior trachea wall, esophageal laceration, aspiration of blood or secretions, hematoma, subcutaneous and mediastinal emphysema, and laceration of the thyroid gland [18, 21, 22].

Concluding Remarks

Cricothyroidostomy is a surgical approach classically indicated in cases of acute upper airway obstruction, when urgent or emergency care is required, or when other techniques of access to such routes are not possible or not indicated. However, in order to perform such a procedure, it is essential to know the cervical topographic anatomy and the surgical steps involved in order to avoid complications inherent in the technique.

Thorough knowledge of the anatomy involved in cricothyroidostomy can reduce the anxiety of doctors when performing the procedure. Anxiety exists due to the precipitous and potentially fatal nature of the situation where an emergency airway needs to be established. Cricothyroidostomy continues to be a safe and rapid means of ensuring emergency access to the airways in the absence of contraindications.

References

1. Mori ND. Cricotireoidostomia e trauma. In: Clínica cirúrgica e fundamentos yeóricos e práticos, vol. Vol. 1. New York: Atheneu; 2002. p. 376–9.
2. Jackson C. Tracheotomy. Laryngoscope. 1909;18:285.
3. Jackson C. High tracheotomy and other errors the chief cause of chronic laryngeal stenosis. Surg Gyneco Obstet. 1921;32:392.
4. Brantigan CO, Grow JB. Cricothyroidotomy: elective use in respiratory problems requiring tracheotomy. J Thorac Cardiovasc Surg. 1976;71(1):72–81.
5. Goon SSH, Stephens RCM, Smith H. The emergency airway. Br J Hosp Med. 2009;70(12):186–8.
6. Fortune JB, Judkins DG, Scanzaroli D, Mc Leod KB, Johnson SB. Efficacy of prehospital surgical cricothyrotomy in trauma patients. J Trauma. 1997;42(5):832–6.
7. Chang RS, Hamilton RJ, Carter WA. Declining rate of cricothyrotomy in trauma patients with an emergency residency: implications for skills training. Acad Emerg Med. 1998;5(3):247–51.
8. Schroeder AA. Cricothyroidotomy: when, why, and why not? Grand Rounds. 2000;21(3):195–201.
9. Norskov AK, Rosenstock CV, Wetterslev J, Astrup G, Afshari A, Lundstrom LH. Diagnostic accuracy of anaesthesiologists prediction of difficult airway management in daily clinical practice: a cohort study of 188 064 patients registered in the Danish Anaesthesia Database. Anaesthesia. 2015;70:272–81.
10. American College of Surgeons Committee on Trauma. Advanced Trauma Life Suport – ATLS. 8 ED., 2009.
11. Conselho Federal de Medicina, www.portal.cfm.org.br, visited on November 14, 2017 at 10:00 p.m.
12. Presidência da República, Casa Civil, Subchefia para Assuntos Jurídicos, http://www.planalto.gov.br/ccivil_03/_Ato2011-2014/2013/Lei/L12842.htm, visited on November 14, 2017 at 10:00 p.m.
13. Aslani A, Ng SC, Hurley M, Mc Carthy KF, Mc Nicholas M, Mc Caul CL. Accuracy of identification of the cricothyroid membrane in female subjects using palpation: an observational study. Anesth Analg. 2012;114(5):987–92.
14. Fernanda S'A, de Souza FAC, Arlei C, Alvarez RM. Cricotireotomia no manejo de obstrução aguda das vias aéreas. Rev cir traumatol buco-maxilo-fac. 2010;10(2):35–41.
15. Curtis K, Ahern M, Dawson M, Mallin M. Ultrasound-guided,bougie-assisted cricothyroidotomy: a description of a novel technique in cadaveric models. Acad Emerg Med. 2012;19(7):876.

16. James H, Victor P-F. Videos in clinical medicine: cricothyroidotomy. N Engl J Med. 2008;358(22):e25.
17. Salvino CK, Dries D, Gamelli R, Murphy-Macabobby M, Marshall W. Emergency cricothyroidotomy in trauma victims. J Trauma. 1993;34(4):503.
18. Schaumann N, Lorenz V, Schellongowski P, Staudinger T, Locker GJ, Burgmann H, Pikula B, Hofbauer R, Schuster E, Frass M. Evaluation of Seldinger technique emergency cricothyroidotomy versus standard surgical cricothyroidotomy in 200 cadavers. Anesthesiology. 2005;102(1):7.
19. Hill C, Reardon R, Joing S, Falvey D, Miner J. Cricothyrotomy technique using gum elastic bougie is faster than standard technique: a study of emergency medicine residents and medical students in an animal lab. Acad Emerg Med. 2010;17(6):666.
20. Holmes JF, Panacek EA, Sakles JC, Brofeldt BT. Comparison of 2 cricothyrotomy techniques: standard method versus rapid 4-step technique. Ann Emerg Med. 1998;32(4):442.
21. Bair AE, Panacek EA, Wisner DH, Bales R, Sakles JC. Cricothyrotomy: a 5-year experience at one institution. J Emerg Med. 2003;24(2):151.
22. Erlandson MJ, Clinton JE, Ruiz E, Cohen J. Cricothyrotomy in the emergency department revisited. J Emerg Med. 1989;7(2):115.

Indications for Performing Tracheostomy in the Intensive Care Unit: When and Why?

Carlos Eduardo Ferraz Freitas, Gustavo Trindade Henriques-Filho, Marcos Antonio Cavalcanti Gallindo, Maria Eduarda Gurgel da Trindade Meira Henriques, Maria Alice Gurgel da Trindade Meira Henriques, and Maria Eduarda Lima de Moura

C.E.F. Freitas, M.D.
Intensive Care Specialist by the Brazilian Intensive Care Medicine Association (AMIB) and Brazilian Medical Association (AMB), Recife, Pernambuco, Brazil

Santa Joana Recife Hospital, Recife, Pernambuco, Brazil

Esperança Recife Hospital, Recife, Pernambuco, Brazil

Esperança Olinda Hospital, Olinda, Pernambuco, Brazil

G.T. Henriques-Filho, M.D. (✉)
Intensive Care Specialist by the Brazilian Intensive Care Medicine Association (AMIB) and Brazilian Medical Association (AMB), Recife, Pernambuco, Brazil

Santa Joana Recife Hospital, Recife, Pernambuco, Brazil

Oswaldo Cruz University Hospital, Universidade de Pernambuco (HUOC/UPE), Recife, Pernambuco, Brazil
e-mail: gustavotrindadefilho@gmail.com

M.A.C. Gallindo, M.D.
Intensive Care Specialist by the Brazilian Intensive Care Medicine Association (AMIB) and Brazilian Medical Association (AMB), Recife, Pernambuco, Brazil

Santa Joana Recife Hospital, Recife, Pernambuco, Brazil

Agamenon Magalhães Hospital, Recife, Pernambuco, Brazil

Royal Portuguese Hospital, Recife, Pernambuco, Brazil

M.E.G. da Trindade Meira Henriques, M.S., (Medical Student).
Faculdade Pernambucana de Saúde (FPS), Recife, Pernambuco, Brazil

M.A.G. da Trindade Meira Henriques, M.S., (Medical Student).
Centro Universitário Maurício de Nassau (UNINASSAU), Recife, Pernambuco, Brazil

M.E.L. de Moura, M.S., (Medical Student).
Faculdade de Medicina Nova Esperança (FAMENE), João Pessoa, PB, Brazil

T.P. de Farias (ed.), *Tracheostomy*, https://doi.org/10.1007/978-3-319-67867-2_16

Introduction

The need for invasive mechanical ventilation is a major cause of admission to intensive care units [1–6]. The maintenance of an artificial airway for advanced support in several acute and chronic pathologies is the reality of services that deal with critical patients. Such a profile is found at various levels of care, from low-complexity units to intermediate support units to intensive care units with patients that demands 100% of human resources and specialized materials for critical care.

For these reasons, 10% of patients requiring at least 3 days of mechanical ventilation may need a definitive airway. In this case, the alternative is the tracheostomy [1–6].

Tracheostomy is usually an elective procedure in the intensive care context. Although several techniques have been developed in recent years (conventional or percutaneous techniques), the lack of appropriately designed studies to evaluate short- and long-term complications—such as major bleeding, infections, and tracheal stenosis—makes it difficult to choose the most appropriate method in the intensive care unit. Concerning the complications, the risk seems to be the same, with slight superiority of percutaneous techniques related to infections and cosmetic changes, and, depending on the technique, a lower risk of major bleeding [1–6].

Furthermore, although there is extensive experience with the procedure, with known indications and presumed benefits, many of the suggested benefits are based on uncontrolled studies, observational studies, expert opinion, and controversial data [1–3, 7]. Regarding the timing of the tracheostomy, there is no consensus on the best time to perform it, whether early (at 4–10 days), at 10–14 days, or at up to 21 days of translaryngeal cannula use. The need for individualization of each patient's situation by the intensivist for effective prediction of the ideal time to execute the procedure, using clinical judgment, is well known though [1–3, 7–9].

This chapter has the main objective of delineating the main indications for tracheostomy in intensive care, with a description of techniques, complications, and the most appropriate time for performing tracheostomy in general and specific situations.

Indications, Advantages, and Disadvantages of Tracheostomy

Indications

In the intensive care environment, there are five main indications for tracheostomy [1, 4, 5, 10, 11]:

(a) Obstructed airway, either by a foreign body, tumor, laryngeal stenosis, burns, trauma, or infection
(b) To provide continued invasive mechanical ventilation to patients who have difficulty in weaning off artificial ventilation or patients who have chronic neuromuscular diseases or degenerative diseases

(c) To prevent damage to the airway with prolonged translaryngeal cannulation
(d) To prevent aspiration in high-risk patients
(e) To optimize clearance of pulmonary secretions, improving airway patency

It should be emphasized that tracheostomy is not performed due to a disease itself, but due to complications generated by the pathology. In addition, tracheostomy has been used in airway management, but today it is used only in specific cases, except for the aforementioned indications leading to supraglottic direct trauma, preventing oral intubation [2, 3, 6, 8, 9].

Benefits and Disadvantages

As already mentioned, there are several presumed benefits provided by tracheostomy for eligible patients: to protect the larynx from lesions such as tracheal stenosis; reduction in the incidence of ventilator-associated pneumonia; greater comfort for the patient; less need for sedation and mechanical ventilation; shorter intensive care length of stay and shorter hospital stay; possibility of returning to oral nutrition; return of phonation; more secure ventilatory support; and easier nursing care [1–6].

On the other hand, while many of these benefits are supported by scientific data, some of these gains that the procedure can supposedly provide are theoretical and based on observational studies and clinical experience [1, 8, 10] , except for lower use of sedatives, (reported in several randomized controlled trials and one multicenter study), fewer days of mechanical ventilation, and shorter intensive care and hospital stays [2, 3, 6, 8, 9].

The presumed tracheal protection against stenosis or long-term complications, despite being observed in patients in daily practice, should not be taken as irrefutable truth. There is also a shortage of large studies following tracheostomized patients for more than 6 months. Moreover, according to a systematic review published in 2015 in *Critical Care Medicine*, comparing long-term outcomes in critically ill patients, most analyzed studies have been unable to demonstrate a relationship between the procedure and reduced rates of these complications, especially regarding tracheal stenosis. Such complications are underdiagnosed and lack structured criteria [12].

Likewise, there is controversial evidence concerning the reduction in ventilator-associated pneumonia; from the point of view of evidence-based medicine, it cannot be proven that such a strategy—although it can reduce the use of sedatives and may lead to more days free of mechanical ventilation—can effectively minimize the risk of developing this complication [6, 9].

In relation to the patient's quality of life and safety, even if there is a practical hypothesis that the tracheostomized patient would be less subject to events related to airway cannulation, manifold observational and controlled studies have shown increases in the number of endotracheal cannula replacements and severe events such as hypoxia, subcutaneous emphysema, false pathway, and even cardiorespiratory arrest being related to endotracheal cannula obstruction. However, these events are more related to patient discharge to units with a patient-to-nurse ratio of >2:1 and lack of continuous monitoring. In addition, there is flexibility in monitoring and surveillance, even in closed units. In fact, it is believed that there is a relationship between decannulation and increased mortality [1, 6, 8, 9, 12, 13, 14] when that occurs in lower-complexity care units.

There is also the fact that patients report self-image changes, especially in relation to aesthetic factors; they present with fewer painful events and complaints of discomfort [1, 8, 12, 13].

The disadvantages of the procedure are related to the procedure itself, which will be discussed later, and to the permanence of the tracheal cannula, such as:

(a) Tracheal complications such as tracheal stenosis, tracheomalacia, tracheoesophageal fistula, tracheal granuloma, soft tissue infection, and tracheobronchitis
(b) Risk of a false pathway in the replacement of the cannula, lumen obstruction, hypoxemia due to obstruction, subcutaneous emphysema, and cardiorespiratory arrest
(c) Increased mortality after discharge from the intensive care unit, as discussed above
(d) Failure in the cicatrization process, with the need for tracheoplasty

Patients also report a high incidence of anxiety attacks and panic syndrome after decannulation, in addition to the aforementioned changes in the way the patients see themselves [1, 3, 4, 11, 12].

When to Perform Tracheostomy

Initially, it is important to make clear that we have not yet been able to define the ideal time for performing tracheostomy. Some authors in the 1990s and early 2000s suggested that early tracheostomy would be beneficial, both from the point of view of weaning off mechanical ventilation and in preventing ventilator-associated pneumonia, with a shorter intensive care unit length of stay. However, these advantages have not been replicated in major studies and systematic reviews [1, 11, 13].

The last major randomized controlled trial that was published—the *TRACMAN* study, performed in different centers of intensive care in the UK—failed to demonstrate superiority of early tracheostomy (after 4 days of intubation) in comparison with tracheostomy at between 10 and 14 days. There were no significant differences in mortality at 90 days, hospitalization times, or infection rates, i.e., there was no difference in outcome. However, it was demonstrated that in the early tracheostomy group the use of sedatives was lower, leading to shorter mechanical ventilation time. An important finding was that the physicians involved in direct patient care failed to predict the optimal timing of tracheostomy. Despite this, the authors recognized flaws in the design of the study. First, it was impossible for a blinded study to be conducted. A second point was that the study was discontinued by suspension of research funding, making it impossible to achieve the sample size originally calculated to prove the hypothesis. Another problem was the absence of patient subtypes that presumably would benefit from the early strategy, such as neurocritical and postoperative cardiovascular surgery patients [10].

In 2015, after a meta-analysis, *Cochrane* concluded that the early strategy would be the most beneficial for shorter mechanical ventilation and early discharge from the intensive care unit. However, in this review, only four studies were considered adequate for evaluation [7].

Therefore, in general, we do not have enough data to recommend an early strategy for all patients, thus further research is required. Individualization is always important, and there seems to be a consensus based on expert opinion and clinical experience that an indication for tracheostomy at between 12 and 14 days of orotracheal intubation is more adequate [1, 4, 7, 10].

Analyzing the data from clinical experience and the available literature, we recommend that tracheostomy in critical care patients be generally performed between the 10th and the 14th days of intubation.

Important Exceptions

There are some exceptions that warrant discussion: patients with moderate and severe traumatic brain injury predicted to require more than 4 days of mechanical ventilation; postoperative cardiovascular surgery patients who have failed weaning off mechanical ventilation; and patients with amyotrophic lateral sclerosis of the bulbar type.

Moderate and Severe Traumatic Brain Injury

In patients with moderate to severe traumatic brain injury who are expected to need more than 4 days of mechanical ventilation, early choice of tracheostomy, according to literature data, appears to reduce infectious complications, especially ventilator-related pneumonia, and the durations of mechanical ventilation and hospitalization. The Brazilian guideline for mechanical ventilation, in its latest (2013) edition, recommends that in these patients the procedure should be performed after the first 4 days if there is no possibility of mechanical ventilation withdrawal [15–18].

It should be noted that in unstable patients with uncontrolled intracranial hypertension, the approach should be delayed until stabilization, as manipulation of the trachea increases intracranial pressure, leaving the patient at risk [15, 16, 18, 19].

In neurocritical patients, for different reasons, there is no such strong recommendation, and we must use an individual approach. A study published in *Stroke* showed that tracheostomy at 4 days had a relative benefit, although it was a small study and had some measurement bias, thus this study was not sufficient to change paradigms [15–19].

After Cardiac Surgery

Some authors suggest that performing early tracheostomy in cardiovascular surgery patients who have failed mechanical ventilation weaning at the fourth postoperative day may reduce the rate of ventilator-associated pneumonia, use of sedatives, the duration of mechanical ventilation, and the incidence of delirium. A randomized trial from a French group, published in 2011 in the *Annals of Internal Medicine*, also suggested such advantages, although it was a single-center study [20].

Amyotrophic Lateral Sclerosis

In patients with amyotrophic lateral sclerosis who present with respiratory insufficiency and quite compromised muscular force—mainly patients with bulbar involvement—the best option is tracheostomy. In this case, the recommendation is that tracheostomy is the first choice when an artificial airway is needed, avoiding tracheal intubation [17, 21, 22].

Tracheostomy Techniques, Complications Related to the Procedure, and Contraindications

Conventional (Open) Tracheostomy

There is a consensus opinion among the authors of this chapter that the best place in which to perform the tracheostomy, whether conventional or percutaneous, is the intensive care unit itself because this avoids unnecessary transportation of the patient. Moreover, experience shows that a well-trained intensive care physician can replace the surgeon, even for performing the conventional technique [1, 4].

Preparation of the Patient

In order to perform the open technique, it is necessary to position the patient with neck extension (if there are no contraindications) and to identify anatomical marks. The points of anatomical reference, which are easily identifiable, are the lower border of the cricoid cartilage, cricothyroid membrane, cricoid cartilage, and sternal notch. Adequate preparation of the aseptic technique with placement of sterile fields and anesthetic induction should be performed [1, 4, 5, 11, 23].

Incision and Access to the Trachea

A vertical or horizontal incision can be performed; however, the latter gives the best aesthetic results.

From the incision, which must have adequate depth to surpass the platysma, hemostasis with an electric scalpel is performed. The anatomical sequence begins with the sternohyoid muscle, the anterior jugular veins, the sternothyroid muscle, and the thyrohyoid muscle. After stretching the muscles with retractors, we can easily reach the area that contains the isthmus of the thyroid, at which time special care must be taken. In most situations, with cranial displacement of the isthmus, we can easily reach the third tracheal ring; in some cases it may be necessary to dissect the isthmus or even perform isthmectomy [1, 4, 10, 11, 24–26].

Tracheal Incision and Cannula Insertion

The incision is made from the second to the fourth tracheal ring. Most authors recommend performing suturing at the lateral edges of the tracheal incision to better identify the structures, although this may vary among surgeons, then the appropriate tracheal cannula is inserted through the incision [1, 4, 11, 24–26].

Percutaneous Techniques

Percutaneous tracheal dilatation is currently the most commonly used percutaneous method for performing tracheostomies in intensive care units. Here, again, a trained intensivist can replace the surgeon. There are several forms of training. There are courses recognized by the international societies of intensive care medicine, thoracic surgery, otorhinolaryngology, and head and neck surgery; and there is the possibility of the training intensive care physician to accompany an experienced surgeon or intensivist to become familiar with the technique. It is recommended that in both cases the professional is able to perform the procedure without supervision only after at least 20 supervised procedures [23, 24, 27–31].

Some studies postulate that if the professional does not have the necessary experience to perform the percutaneous technique, it is safer to perform the conventional surgical technique. Even though the percutaneous technique is apparently simpler to perform, it requires adequate identification of anatomical landmarks and some other aspects, which will be discussed below [27, 29–31].

Percutaneous techniques are similar; only the commercially available kits for carrying them out differ. They are based on the Seldinger technique with the use of a guide wire, which can be blinded or assisted by bronchoscopy (more recommended) and, more currently, with the use of ultrasonography. The use of ultrasonography involves a shorter learning time and involves materials less fragile than the optical fiber of the bronchoscope [4, 27, 29–31].

Technique, Preparation, and Access to the Trachea

The patient should be in a supine position, with neck extension, and needs to be ventilated continuously with a 100% inspiratory oxygen fraction. The orotracheal tube is then withdrawn with direct visualization after deflation of the cuff, identifying the third and fourth tracheal rings. Adequate skin disinfection is performed with placement of surgical fields. The visualization of the natural anatomical landmarks in this case is more important than in the surgical technique [4, 23, 29–31].

We use a 14-gauge needle attached to a syringe filled with distilled water or saline solution, puncturing from the second to the fourth tracheal ring until there is a decrease in resistance, air aspiration, and evidence of bubble formation in the solution. We confirm the placement of the cannula under direct visualization with a bronchoscope, insert the guide wire through the needle, fit the dilator through the guide wire, and, with a little pressure, dilate the tracheal ring and remove and mount the dilator. The cannula is then positioned in the trachea. The patient is then ventilated, observing the resistance in the airway and confirming the position of the cannula with the bronchoscope [4, 27, 29–31].

Performing a simple chest X-ray to rule out immediate complications of the procedure is necessary. A major advantage of using ultrasonography is the ability to waive this test [4, 23, 29–31].

There are several commercial kits available on the market, and dilatation can be performed with curved, straight, or tapered dilators, or even using a balloon.

Conventional Versus Percutaneous Techniques

Although researchers have failed to demonstrate clear superiority (from the point of view of long-term structural complications) of either percutaneous or conventional tracheostomy, and although the studies have been mostly observational and nonrandomized, a meta-analysis performed by Dempsey et al., published in *Critical Care Medicine* in 2015, suggested that the majority of events such as major bleeding, infection, and tracheal stenosis are less frequent with the percutaneous technique [12].

Complications Related to the Procedure

The following complications can occur, related to the procedure [1, 3–5, 11, 12, 25, 26, 32, 33]:

(a) Pneumothorax (1–5%)
(b) Vascular lesions with major bleeding (up to 5%)
(c) Injury of the thyroid isthmus (<1%)
(d) Recurrent laryngeal nerve injury (<1%)
(e) False pathway (<1%)
(f) Subcutaneous emphysema (<1%)
(g) Esophageal lesion with tracheoesophageal fistula (<1%)
(h) Tracheal laceration (<1%)
(i) Tracheal stenosis (<1%)
(j) Hypoxia and cardiorespiratory arrest (<1%)

The following complications can occur, related to the presence of the cannula [1, 3–5, 11, 12, 25, 26, 32, 33]:

(a) Cannula obstruction
(b) Surgical wound infection
(c) Tracheobronchitis
(d) Tracheomalacia
(e) Formation of granuloma
(f) Stoma necrosis
(g) Esophagotracheal fistula and tracheal stenosis

Contraindications

The following are contraindications to the procedure [1, 3–5, 11, 12, 25, 26, 32, 33]:

(a) Platelet count <50,000 or coagulopathy (with both techniques). In this case it is recommended to perform a platelet transfusion before the procedure: 1 unit for each 10 kg of patient weight until a target above 50,000 platelets is reached [33].
(b) Active bleeding in the cervical region, cervical trauma, thyroid goiter (with both techniques).
(c) Cervical instability (with both techniques).
(d) Abnormal anatomy/tumors (with the percutaneous technique).

Conclusions

Tracheostomy is one of the most common procedures performed in the intensive care unit. The indications for the procedure in patients who require intensive care are due not to their diagnosis per se but to the inherent complications of caring for patients with severe acute or chronic disease [1–6].

Continuous use of mechanical ventilation is one of the main indications. Advances in education and training of professionals, and the development and evolution of critical care medicine as an internationally recognized medical specialty, make the intensive care physician the most appropriate professional, with suitable training, to perform the procedure in the context of critical patient care [1–6].

However, with the aging population and the increases in chronic degenerative diseases, urban violence, and accidental injuries, more patients will require this strategy. We still require appropriate studies to assess the long-term complications of the procedure, the best time to perform it, and the issues of whether it provides real benefits or comfort to patients, whether the benefits exceed the aesthetic disadvantages, and the quality of life of patients undergoing tracheostomy [1–12, 32, 34–37].

Finally, perhaps the greatest challenge for professionals dealing with this population is to individualize the management of patients more and more, to make families aware of the importance and safety of tracheostomy, and to demystify the idea that the procedure is an eternal sentence for patients, since this airway path is nothing more than a bridge to facilitate withdrawal of the ventilatory strategy and resumption of the functional potential of each patient. With improvements in rehabilitation strategies, physical therapy, speech therapy, and occupational therapy, cannula withdrawal can then be performed safely in a controlled environment [1–5, 7–11].

References

1. Durbin Charles G Jr. Tracheostomy: why, when, and how? Respir Care. 2010;55(8):1056–68.
2. Huang CT, Lin JW, Ruan SY, Chen CY, Yu CJ. Preadmission tracheostomy is associated with better outcomes in patients withprolonged mechanical ventilation in the postintensive care respiratory care setting. J Formos Med Assoc. 2016;9:1–8.

3. Frutos-Vivar F, Esteban A, Apezteguía C, International Mechanical Ventilation Study Group, et al. Outcome of mechanically ventilated patients who require a tracheostomy. Crit Care Med. 2005;33:290–8.
4. Friedman Y, Sobeck S. Tracheostomy. In: Parrillo JE, Phillip Dellinger R, editors. Critical care medicine: principles of diagnosis and management in the adult. 4th ed. Amsterdam: Elsevier Inc; 2008. p. 202–13.
5. Tobin M, Stauffer Jonh L. Chapter 39: Complications of translaryngeal intubation. In: Tobin M, editor. Principles and practice of mechanical ventilation. 3rd ed. New York: McGraw-Hill; 1991. p. 895–940.
6. Terragni PP, Antonelli M, Fumagalli R, et al. Early vs late tracheotomy for prevention of pneumonia in mechanically ventilated adult ICU patients: a randomized controlled trial. JAMA. 2010;303:1483–9.
7. Andriolo BNG, Andriolo RB, Saconato H, Atallah ÁN, Valente O. Early versus late tracheostomy for critically ill patients. Cochrane Database Syst Rev. 2015;52(1):1–66.
8. Young D, Harrison DA, Cuthbertson BH, TracMan Collaborators, et al. Effect of early vs late tracheostomy placement on survival in patients receiving mechanical ventilation: the TracMan randomized trial. JAMA. 2013;309:2121–9.
9. Moeller MG, Slaikeu JD, Bonelli P, et al. Early vs late tracheostomy in the surgical intensive care unit. Am J Surg. 2005;189:293–6.
10. Durbin CG Jr. Indications for and timing of tracheostomy. Respir Care. 2005;50(4):483–7.
11. Tobin M, Heffner JE. Chapter 40: Care of the mechanically ventilated. In: Principles and practice of mechanical patient with a tracheotomy in principles and practice of mechanical ventilation. 3rd ed. New York: McGraw-Hill; 2015. p. 941–71.
12. Dempsey GA, Morton B, Hammell C, et al. Long-term outcome following tracheostomy in critical care: a systematic review. Crit Care Med. 2016;44:617–28.
13. Boynton JH, Hawkins K, Eastridge BJ, et al. Tracheostomy timing and the duration of weaning in patients with acute respiratory failure. Crit Care. 2004;8:R261–7.
14. Freeman-Sanderson AL, Togher L, Elkins MR, Phipps PR. Quality of life improves with return of voice in tracheostomy patients in intensive care: an observational study. J Crit Care. 2016;33:186–91.
15. Baron DM, Hochrieser H, Metnitz PGH, Mauritz W. Tracheostomy is associated with decreased hospital mortality after moderate or severe isolated traumatic brain injury. Wien Klin Wochenschr. 2016;128:397–403.
16. Julian Bösel MD, et al. Stroke-Related Early Tracheostomy Versus Prolonged Orotracheal Intubation in Neurocritical Care Trial (SETPOINT): a randomized pilot trial. Stroke. 2013;44:21–8; originally published online November 29, 2012.
17. Diretrizes Brasileiras de ventilação mecânica. AMIB-SBPT;2013, p.13–16; p. 93–100.
18. Longworth A, Veitch D, Gudibande S, Whitehouse T, Snelson C, Veenith T. Tracheostomy in special groups of critically ill patients: who, when, and where? Indian J Crit Care Med. 2016 May;20(5):280–4.
19. Arabi Y, Haddad S, Shirawi N, et al. Early tracheostomy in intensive care trauma patients improves resource utilization: a cohort study and literature review. Crit Care. 2004;8:R347–52.
20. Trouillet JL, Luyt CE, Guiguet M, et al. Early percutaneous tracheotomy versus prolonged intubation of mechanically ventilated patients after cardiac surgery: a randomized trial. Ann Intern Med. 2011;154:373–83.
21. Tandan R, Bradley WG. Amyotrophic lateral sclerosis: part 1. Clinical features, pathology, and ethical issues in management. Ann Neurol. 1985;18:271–80.
22. Braun SR. Respiratory system in amyotrophic lateral sclerosis. Neurol Clin. 1987;5:9–31.
23. Rumbak MJ, Newton M, Truncale T, et al. A prospective, randomized, study comparing early percutaneous tracheotomy to prolonged translaryngeal intubation (delayed tracheotomy) in critically ill medical patients. Crit Care Med. 2004;32:1689–94.
24. Fattahi T, Vega L, Fernandes R, et al. Our experience with 171 open tracheostomies. J Oral Maxillofac Surg. 2012;70(7):1699–702. Epub 2011 Oct 22.

25. Straemans J, Schloendorff G, Herzhoff G, et al. Complications of midline-open tracheotomy in adults. Laryngoscope. 2010;120:84–92.
26. Halum SL, Ting JY, Plowman EK, et al. A multi-institutional analysis of tracheostomy complications. Laryngoscope. 2012;122:38–45.
27. Pilarczyk K, Carstens H, Heckmann J, Lubarski J, Marggraf G, Jakob H, Pizanis N, Kamler M. Safety and efficiency of percutaneous dilatational tracheostomy with direct bronchoscopic guidance for thoracic transplant recipients. Respir Care. 2016;61(2):235–42.
28. Blot F, Similowski T, Trouillet JL, et al. Early tracheostomy versus prolonged intubation in unselected severely ill ICU patients. Intensive Care Med. 2008;34:1779–89.
29. Jackson LM, Davis JW, Kaups KL, et al. Percutaneous tracheostomy: to bronch or not to bronch—that is the question. J Trauma. 2011;71:1553–6.
30. Beltrame F, Zussino M, Martinez B, et al. Percutaneous versus surgical bedside tracheostomy in the intensive care unit: a cohort study. Minerva Anesthesiol. 2008;74:529–35.
31. Pappas S, Maragoudakis P, Vlastarakos P, et al. Surgical versus percutaneous tracheostomy: an evidence-based approach. Eur Arch Otorhinolaryngol. 2011;266:323–30.
32. Hess DR. Chapter 33: airway management. In: Essentials of mechanical ventilation. New York: McGraw-Hill Education; 2014. p. 335–43.
33. Kaufman RM, et al. Platelet transfusion: a clinical practice guideline from the AABB. Ann Intern Med. 2015;162(3):205–13.
34. Hsu CL, Chen KY, Chang CH, et al. Timing of tracheostomy as a determinant of weaning success in critically ill patients: a retrospective study. Crit Care. 2005;9:R46–52.
35. Freeman BD, Stwalley D, Lambert D, et al. High resource utilization does not affect mortality in acute respiratory failure patients managed with tracheostomy. Respir Care. 2013;58:1863–72.
36. Anón JM, Araujo JB, Escuela MP. González-Higueras E, por el Grupo de Trabajo de Insuficiencia Respiratoria Aguda de la SEMICYUC. Traqueotomía percutánea en el paciente ventilado Med Intensiva. 2014;38:181–93.
37. Brass P, Hellmich M, Ladra A, Ladra J, Wrzosek A. Percutaneous techniques versus surgical techniques for tracheostomy. Cochrane Database Syst Rev. 2016;20:7.

Considering the best place to do a Tracheostomy: At the Bedside or in the Operating Room?

Jose Gabriel Miranda da Paixão, Jorge Pinho Filho, Fernando Luiz Dias, Adilis Stepple da Fonte Neto, Juliana Fernandes de Oliveira, and Terence Pires de Farias

Patients with nasal or orotracheal tubes requiring ventilatory support for long periods usually undergo tracheostomy at some time during their hospitalization [1]. More than 100,000 tracheostomies are performed annually in the USA, and about 20,000 are performed in England [2, 3], most commonly in intensive care unit (ICU) patients. It is a procedure that, historically, has had high rates of complications [4], but under controlled conditions it can be performed safely in critically ill patients [5].

J.G.M. da Paixão, M.D. (✉) • J.F. de Oliveira, M.D.
Department of Head and Neck Surgery, National Cancer Institute – INCA, Rio de Janeiro, RJ, Brazil
e-mail: jgmp.gabriel@gmail.com

J.P. Filho, M.D., F.A.C.S.
Memorial Hospital São José, Recife, PE, Brazil

F.L. Dias, M.D., Ph.D., M.Sc., F.A.C.S.
Head and Neck Surgery Department, Brazilian National Cancer Institute – INCA, Rio de Janeiro, RJ, Brazil

Head and Neck Department, Pontifical Catholic University of Rio de Janeiro, Rio de Janeiro, RJ, Brazil

A.S. da Fonte Neto, M.D.
Department of Head and Neck Surgery, Integral Medicine Institute of Pernambuco (Instituto de Medicina Integral de Pernambuco-IMIP), Recife, PE, Brazil

Pernambuco Cancer Hospital (Hospital de Câncer de Pernambuco), Recife, PE, Brazil

Department of Head and Neck Surgery, Brazilian Head and Neck Surgery Society (Sociedade Brasileira de Cirurgia de Cabeça e Pescoço), São Paulo, SP, Brazil

T.P. de Farias, M.D., Ph.D., M.Sc., Researcher.
Department of Head and Neck Surgery, Brazilian National Cancer Institute—INCA, Rio de Janeiro, RJ, Brazil

Department of Head and Neck Surgery, Pontifical Catholic University, Rio de Janeiro, RJ, Brazil

T.P. de Farias (ed.), *Tracheostomy*, https://doi.org/10.1007/978-3-319-67867-2_17

Although there is a well-established technique for performing a tracheostomy, its management still provokes discussion. There are several variables affecting the tracheostomy patient's clinical course, such as the issue of early or late tracheostomy, and the issue of appropriate steps for decannulation [2]. Even though it is one of the most frequently performed procedures in ICUs, underreporting and a lack of information on records makes it difficult to discuss these variables [3].

As one of the oldest surgical procedures, tracheostomy is currently undergoing a "rationalization period" in which it has been established as a safe method for controlling and managing airways, together with orotracheal intubation, but tends to be used only in selected cases [6–8]. In addition, development of percutaneous tracheostomy [9] and its variants, which can be performed at the bedside [10, 11], have allowed for a shorter learning curve and less surgical trauma.

All efforts to refine the practice of tracheostomy have potential to affect both the quality of care for critically ill patients and its costs [12].

The costs associated with tracheostomized patient are related to longer hospitalization, a higher mortality risk, and several other requirements due to the complexity of care that this type of patient requires (mechanical ventilation weaning, respiratory physiotherapy, and speech therapy, among others). A study by Baylor College of Medicine [13] estimated a average cost of US$155,469 per case of tracheostomy (not including medical services), and this cost varies according to the institution [13, 14], concluding that each patient who needs a tracheostomy causes a financial impact on the hospital or health care system. Therefore, there is an effort to reduce the expenses associated with the procedure, either by reviewing its indication time in patients on mechanical ventilation [14] or by avoiding it when possible [7].

This fact led to the attempt to create several algorithms for the indication and management of tracheostomies, related to the duration of orotracheal intubation that indicates tracheostomy, criteria for early procedure performance, and care with the cannula and aspiration, for example [13]. The diversity of established protocols is linked to the multidisciplinary care that this type of patient requires and often reflects a lack of coordination among the involved professionals, since there are no formal and universally accepted clinical guidelines regarding the issues raised.

Considering that tracheostomy is associated with morbidity in 8–45% of cases [7], there is also a tendency to avoid it. A study by Coyle et al. (2012) [7] discussed a series of 55 cases of mouth tumor resection followed by reconstruction with a microsurgical free flap in which no patient received a tracheostomy postoperatively, showing that corticosteroid therapy in anesthetic induction and early extubation may result in less invasive management of the patient's airway.

Within this context, deciding when to perform tracheostomy is already widely discussed in the literature [14, 15]. However, the place where the procedure is to be performed has an impact on its cost and presents caveats that must be known so that doctor can choose, on a case-by-case basis, the best environment in which to perform it. Whether performed electively or due to urgency, three types of procedures are the most studied regarding cost effectiveness: surgical tracheostomy in the operating room (STOR), surgical tracheostomy at the bedside (STBS), and percutaneous tracheostomy (PT).

Costs

Regarding costs, PT is generally considered more cost effective than STOR or STBS [16, 17]. The costs analyzed by Levin and Trivikram (2001) [16] took into account the expenses of the surgeon, anesthesiologist (when necessary), equipment, and operating room time. In PT, the cost is around US$1700 [16, 18, 19] without considering bronchoscopy use, which increases this cost by about US$700 to US$1000 [18]. The average costs of a procedure such as this are difficult to estimate, because of variables that can affect them, such as in the same study by Levin and Trivikram (2001), where the authors themselves developed a list of medical materials and services based on medical records to estimate how much would be charged for a PT, STBS, or STOR. Retrospective data collection also occurred in the review by Cools-Lartigue et al. (2013) [17], who compiled data from several other studies to conclude that PT is less costly than STOR.

Comparing STOR and STBS, there is a small cost difference considering the value per procedure, the former costing an estimated US$2071.70 and the latter US$1997.90 [16]. It is difficult to calculate the exact procedure costs because most studies have analyzed billing codes in a retrospective fashion, as well as equipment rental time, surgery room time, and professional services based on hospital charts records. Yoo et al. (2011) [20] reported a much greater discrepancy between STBS and STOR expenditures (US$511 and US$5086, respectively) because in this series, the complication costs and length of ICU stay were excluded from the calculations since they did not present a statistically significant difference between the two types of procedure and the costs were prospectively counted [20]. Massick et al. (2001) [21] reported similar results using strict patient selection criteria (for clinical and anatomical conditions), randomized individuals who would undergo PT/STBS/STOR, and studied a single surgical team performing the procedures, showing a significant cost reduction with any of the bedside procedures, with each STBS costing US$436 less than one PT. Considering only bedside procedures, STBS has the potential to be much more cost effective than PT [20, 21].

It is important to note that this cost may vary according to different institutional protocols. For example, the STBS cost can be reduced to a value lower than the PT cost if there is no need for an anesthesiologist routinely at the time of the procedure and if there is standardization of the procedure's logistics (organization and availability of materials similar to what would happen in an operating room). A team comprising a surgeon, intensive care physician, and respiratory therapist exclusively dedicated to a single procedure can guarantee adequate anesthesia and greater ease in performing a bedside tracheostomy [16, 20]. There is a trend to not use bronchoscopy in order to lessen expenditure on PT, with series showing similar results between bronchoscopy-assisted PT and non-bronchoscopy-assisted PT [18], but there is no sufficient scientific evidence to not use it [15].

Complications

There are proposals for standardization of tracheostomy-related complications, although there are still different ways to define them, and there is no homogeneity between studies. Generally speaking, there is a generalization in which major complications are those that require significant surgical or clinical intervention, such as closed chest tube insertion or antibiotic therapy, and minor complications are those that do not require any intervention [16, 20]. There is another one that distinguishes early complications (happening within the first 7 days) and late complications (after 7 days) [11].

In the ICU or operating room, there are comparable complication rates [22].

Considering bedside procedure complications, most studies have focused on PT. There are complications that are more common in PT, such as obstruction and problems in decannulation [23]. This happens because the cannula used in this procedure hinders nursing care, requiring continuous attention to avoid mucus plug formation and/or clots that cause obstruction. Decannulation is difficult in a subset of patients who develop subglottic stenosis due to cartilage and mucosal trauma caused at the time of tracheostoma tube insertion [24], which occurs to a lesser extent with the open technique [25].

When it comes to complications such as hemorrhage and infection, PT and STOR have similar complication rates, the same being true for long-term effects (such as the resulting scar or related to quality of life) [26, 27]. PT has low rates of hemorrhage ranging from 0% to 5.7% in some series [18, 26, 27] and infection rates ranging from 4% to 10% [12]. STOR, on the other hand, presents hemorrhage rates between 0% and 33% and infection ranging from 0% to 63% [28–32]. The lower rates of bleeding and infection with PT in most studies can be justified by the smaller amount of dissected tissue and the lesser amount of dead space, allowing better compression of small bleeding points and making it difficult for microorganisms that would cause infections to become established [12].

Considering all of the complications of tracheostomy performed in the ICU or in the operating room, there is no statistical difference based on the place where the procedure is performed, according to some series [12, 22]. Kilic et al. (2011) [22], performing a prospective study of 121 patients who underwent STOR and 85 who underwent PT by the Griggs technique, found that bleeding was the main complication in both groups, but surgical revision was necessary only in PT cases; they concluded, however, that for the sample studied there was no statistically significant difference in complications between the two groups. Freeman and Morris (2012) [12], in a review of the literature, highlighted the lower rate of blood loss and infection with PT compared with STOR, but there were similar rates of late complications (for example, clinically significant tracheal stenosis) on long-term follow-up.

There is no association between the specialty of the physician who performs the tracheostomy and the rate of complications [19], and a physician trained in surgery can perform either STBS or PT without a significant difference in complication rates [28]. PT is perhaps the most commonly used method in the ICU due to its technical simplicity, which does not demand advanced surgical training; for example, it can be performed by anesthesiologists, intensive care physicians, and pulmonologists, without this influencing the rate of complications, as concluded by Bowen et al. (2001) [19]. Porter and Ivatury, in 1999 [28], studying ICU patients with the same indication for tracheostomy in groups undergoing PT or STBS performed by experienced intensivist physicians, and with a control group undergoing STOR performed by surgeons, found similar complication rates between the groups.

Caveats and Pitfalls of Operating Room Versus Intensive Care Unit Tracheostomy

The indications, optimal timing, and definition of the ideal technique for tracheostomy are a major controversy in the literature [15]. Therefore, deciding where to do it can be an arduous task, taking into account only the available case reviews and series, most often comparing PT (in the vast majority of cases carried out at the bedside) and STOR, with only a few authors including STBS in the discussion [16, 20, 28].

In the operating room, tracheostomy allows better positioning of the patient with adequate cervical hyperextension and sufficient space between the surgeon and the operative field (Fig. 1). A table suitable for surgical procedures avoids complications that may result from poor patient positioning, such as a pulmonary apex lesion followed by subcutaneous emphysema and stoma positioning below the third tracheal ring (which increases the risk of erosion of the innominate artery by the cannula) [33].

In addition, the presence of an anesthesiologist and a nursing team as support for a single procedure ensures adequate tracheostomy progress. The anesthesiologist observes vital sign monitoring, analgesia, and sedation, giving comfort to the patient, whether he or she is intubated or not (Fig. 2). The nursing staff performs the preoperative checklist and provides all necessary surgical materials for the procedure, with enough space for the movement of personnel and equipment, as well as providing an instrument table ready for use (Figs. 3 and 4). An operating room has

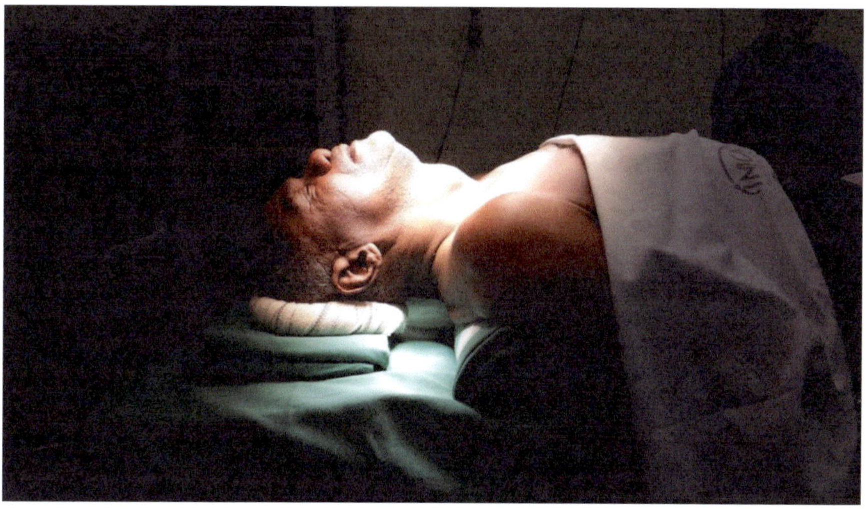

Fig. 1 Patient positioning in the operating room, with hyperextension for proper tracheal exposure and a proper surgery table with sufficient space between the surgeon and the operative field

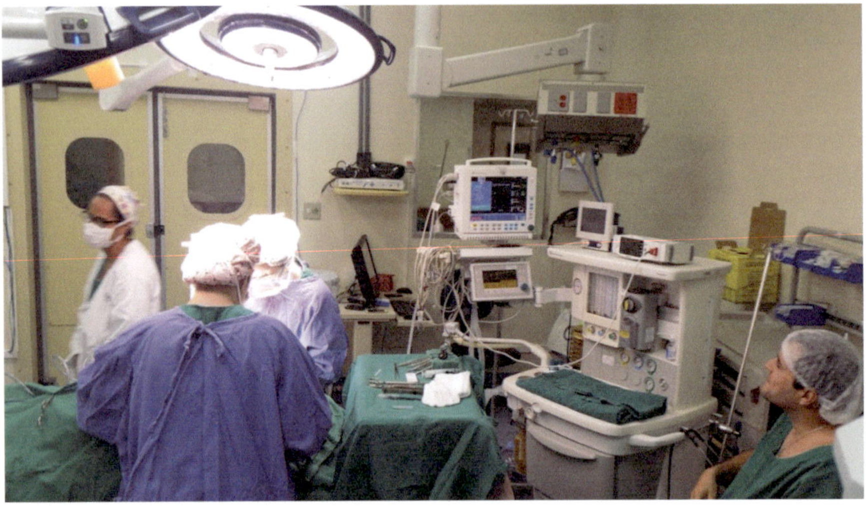

Fig. 2 The anesthesiologist helps in monitoring vital signs and supports analgesia and sedation

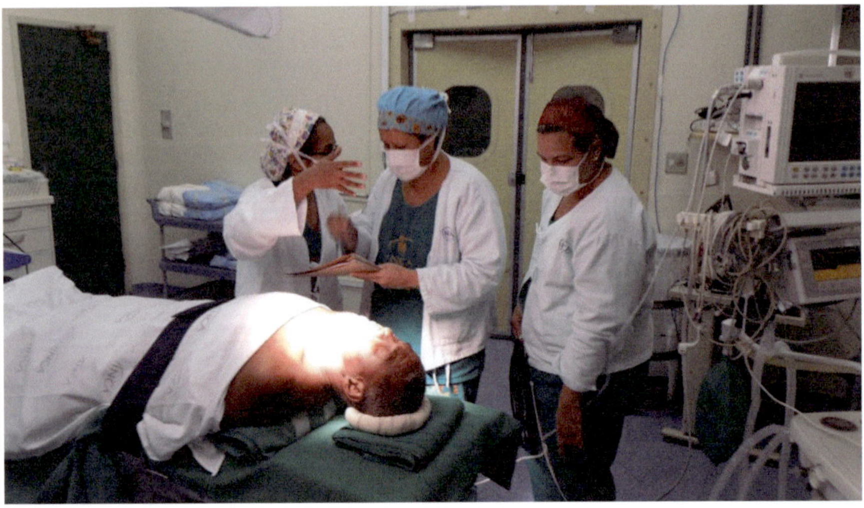

Fig. 3 Nursing team performing the preoperative checklist and organizing necessary materials for the procedure

an adequate structure and space for surgical procedures, such as overhead operating lights, electrocautery, a proper operating table, and suction, all of which are mobile for different setups according to the procedure (Fig. 5).

Adequate light allows accurate identification of structures such as blood vessels, the thyroid gland, and the apical pleura, which may be the site of intra- and postoperative complications. The surgical table and operating room provide the surgeon and the assistant with better ergonomics in performing the procedure (Fig. 6).

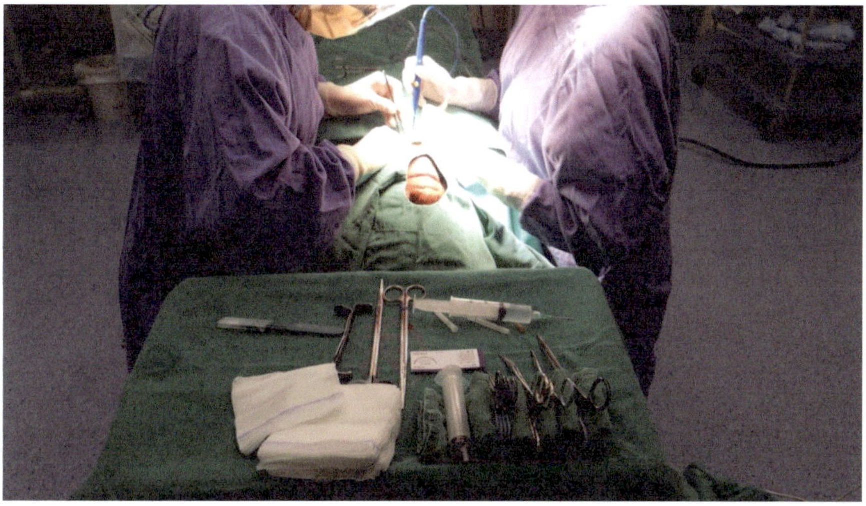

Fig. 4 Instrument table routinely organized by the nursing team with all necessary instruments. Note the position of the Mayo table in a place that allows easy access for the surgeon and the assistant

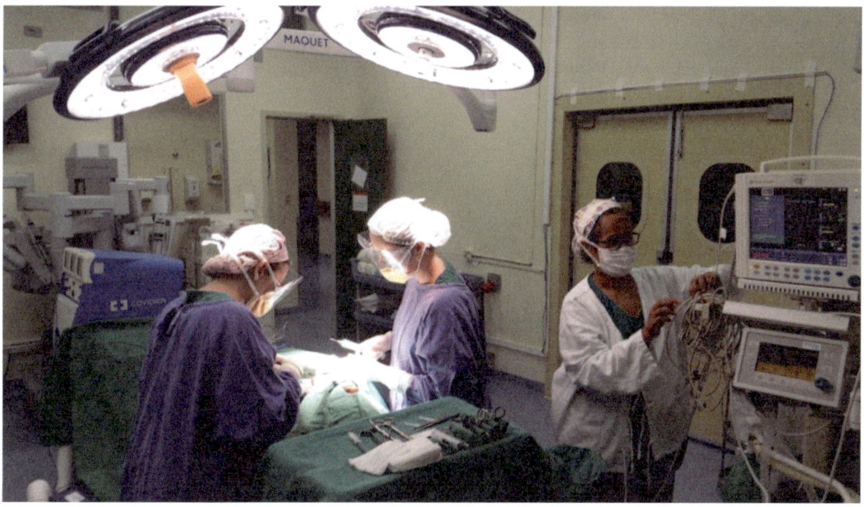

Fig. 5 Space in the operating room, with overhead operating lights, electrocautery, instrument table, and anesthesia cart in a convenient arrangement

According to the protocol of the hospital where the procedure is performed, there may be the possibility of providing a postprocedural observation bed for clinical patient surveillance, which allows better control of analgesia and immediate complications such as minor bleeding or subcutaneous emphysema, and dedicated nursing care (Fig. 7).

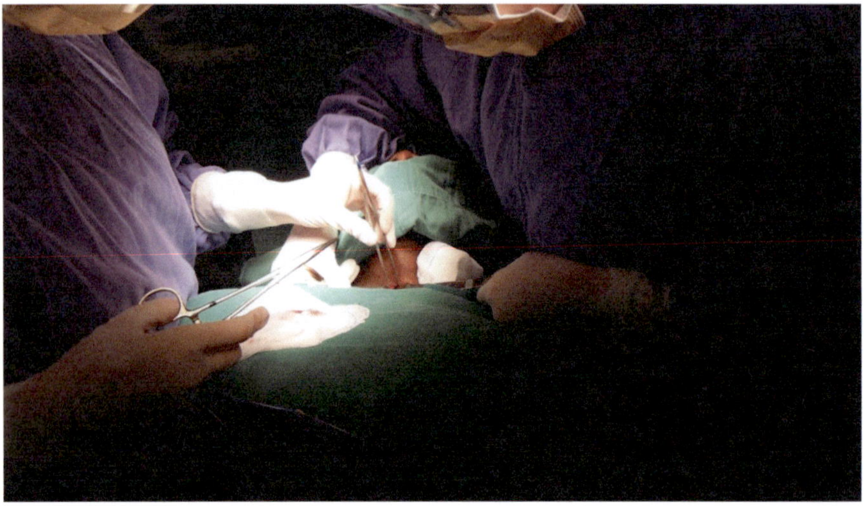

Fig. 6 Surgical table positioning, patient positioning, and adequate arrangement of instruments ensure good ergonomics for the surgeon and the assistant

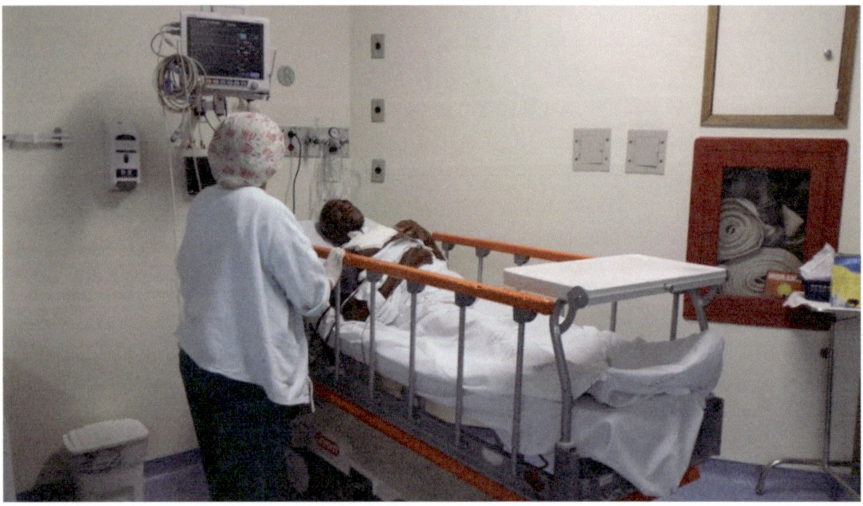

Fig. 7 Postprocedure bed recovery, in which the patient remains monitored and under clinical surveillance and nursing care

With the patient controlled by an anesthesiologist, and with the surgeon and the assistant properly supplied and able to work in an ergonomic posture, there is more secure access to the patient's airways.

However, there are disadvantages as inherent difficulties in the transportation of the patient to the surgical center, the costs that operating room time can generate for the hospital or health system, and related to the time prior to performance of the procedure.

Transporting ICU or urgent patients to the operating room can cause potentially life-threatening complications [33, 34]. There are risks of poor monitoring of vital parameters, cardiovascular or respiratory instability, inadequate administration of medications, and numerous mechanical difficulties regarding limb positioning and transfer of stretchers. It is estimated that one third of patient transported for a therapeutic procedure will incur at least one of these complications [33]. Minimizing the risks of such transportation can add an indirect value to the cost of an elective tracheostomy in a surgical center, as it requires experienced staff for transportation of critical patients, use of pretransport checklists, use of drug administration guidelines, and contingency plans [35].

The operating room time cost is associated with an increase in the STOR cost compared with PT at the bedside [22]. This is due to what is spent on staff time, use of surgical materials (a tracheotomy tray and disposable materials), and considering the time spent on the procedure, which can vary from 3 to 39 min [16, 36, 37]. When the use of an operating room is avoided, it is estimated that expenses are reduced by between US$851 and US$1645 [38].

The time prior to performance of the procedure takes into account the difficulty in obtaining time in the surgical center routine to schedule an elective tracheostomy. This fact often leads to a delay in performing it and delays the treatment of the patient [20], which may cause tube compression injury in upper airways and greater difficulty in ventilatory weaning. However, previous studies have not stated that this delay increases the length of the ICU stay.

In the ICU, depending on the institutional protocol, bedside tracheostomy can be a cost-effective, quick, and easy procedure, with a complication rate comparable to that of STOR [20, 39]. It may be performed using one of the various percutaneous techniques in a traditional open manner. The tracheostomy can be performed more quickly after the request of the intensivist physician, since the surgeon only needs to make time available in his own schedule and inform the ICU to provide the necessary materials in a convenient arrangement near the bed in which the procedure will be performed (Fig. 8).

A checklist with all of these materials can be standardized as a protocol for the nursing team, who can set it up upon request, including a spotlight, electrocautery unit, sterile drapes, instrument tray, and all other requirements—such as gauzes, tracheostomy cannulas, and surgical sutures—that would be available in the operating room. Another option is the PT that can be performed by different techniques [17], requiring a specific kit for each technique, and may require bronchoscopy support or not [18].

The availability of a circulating nurse, a respiratory physiotherapist, and an intensive care physician to attend to the patient's analgesia and sedation make the procedure more comfortable for the patient and safe for the surgeon [16, 20] (Figs. 9 and 10).

There is the possibility of an anesthesiologist supporting the procedure, although this may increase the final cost of the procedure [16].

The greatest difficulties in performing a tracheostomy in the ICU are related to patients' particular conditions and to the physical space and restricted infrastructure

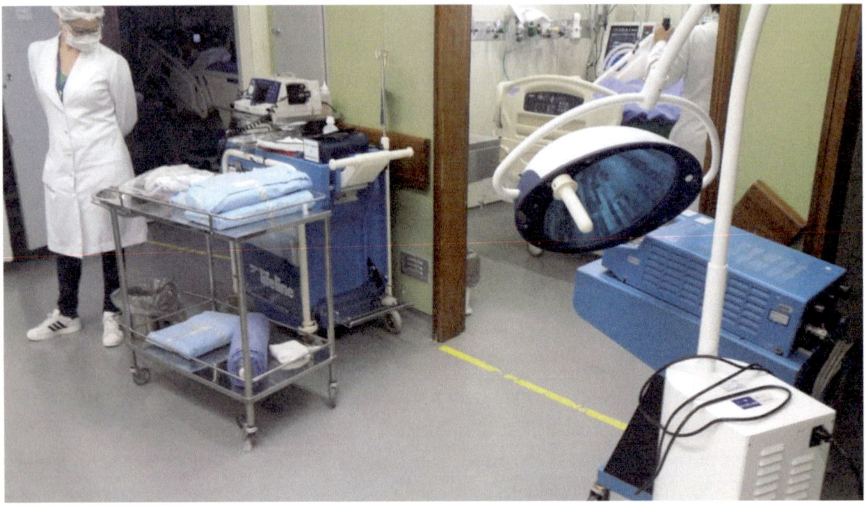

Fig. 8 Materials needed to perform open tracheostomy at the bedside in the intensive care unit: instrument tray, disposable materials, shoulder roll, sterile drapes and scrubs, electrocautery unit, and spotlight

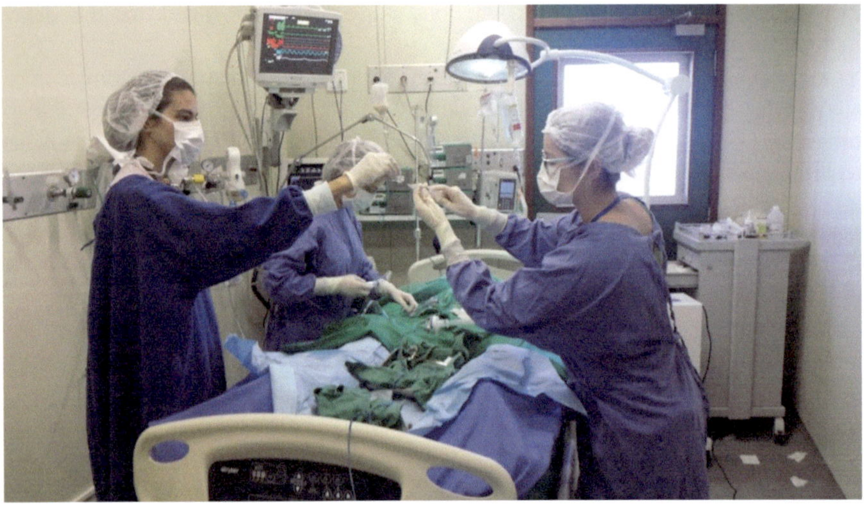

Fig. 9 Nursing team assistance in preparation for the procedure

of ICU beds. The major disadvantage of bedside tracheostomy, either PT or STBS, is that it cannot be done safely in patients who present with factors that restrict proper neck positioning (such as morbid obesity and cervical vertebral arthrodesis), patients who present with access pitfalls for surgical manipulation of the airway (such as a bulky goiter or tracheomalacia), or cases involving the delicate structures and anatomy of a child's trachea [16, 22]. In these specific cases it is imperative to use the infrastructure and staff of the surgical center.

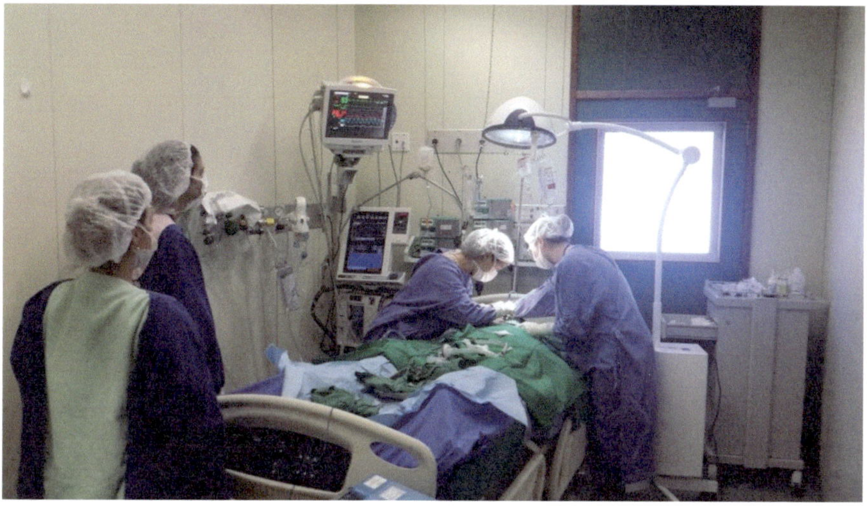

Fig. 10 Intensive care physician and nurse supporting the bedside procedure. A team is specifically assigned to the procedure, stopping other activities until the tracheostomy is finished. This ensures greater safety and speed of the procedure

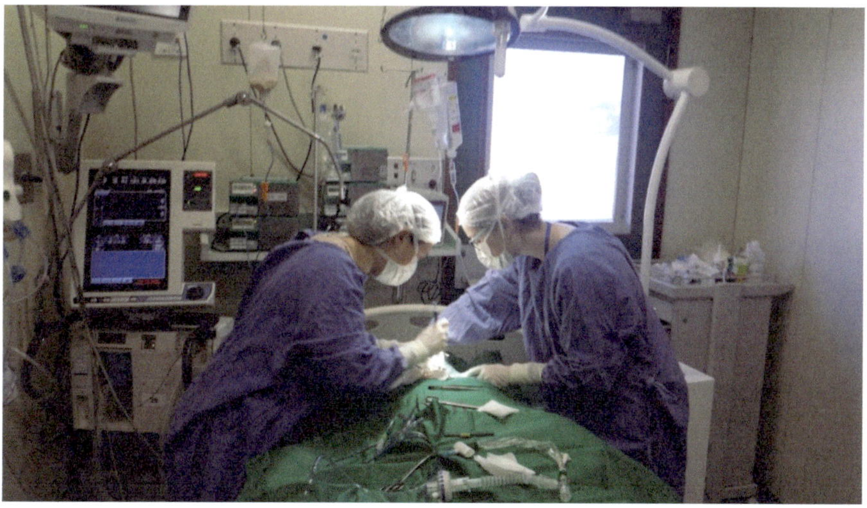

Fig. 11 Unergonomic positioning of the surgeon and the assistant for bedside open tracheostomy. Mechanical ventilation and infusion pumps divide the space with the spotlight and sterile drapes. Note that there is no instrument table for the sterile materials to be organized on

The positioning of the surgeon in bedside tracheostomy may be hampered by the width of the stretcher, which may force the surgeon and the assistant to assume unergonomic positions and make operative field exposure more difficult [39] (Fig. 11). The position may become more uncomfortable if the procedure is prolonged and muscle fatigue increases. Adding to this, there may be no suitable place to organize the surgical

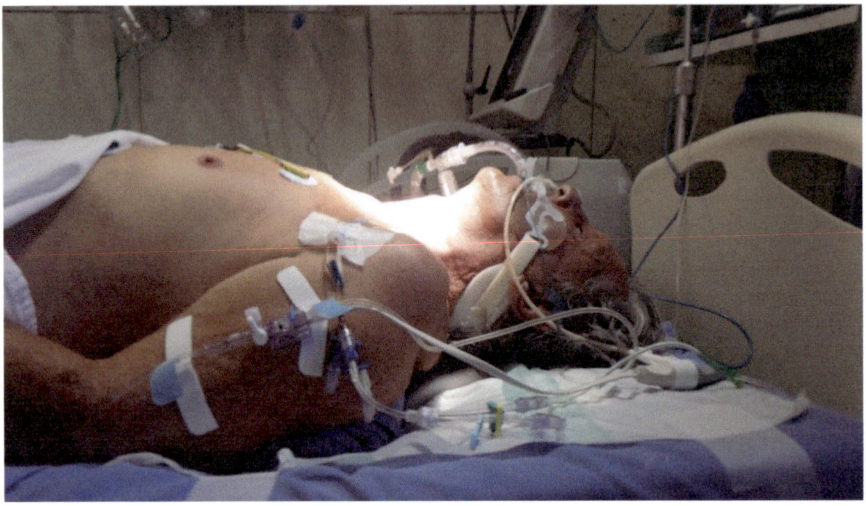

Fig. 12 Patient positioning can be hampered by venous access and cardiac monitor electrodes. Notice the deformity that the shoulder roll causes on the mattress. It may increase as the procedure lengthens and jeopardize the procedure

instruments and disposable materials that will be used in the procedure, making it difficult to access them. Another challenge is patient positioning (Fig. 12), which can change throughout the procedure by deformation of the mattress on the ICU bed, which is made to avoid areas of high pressure—a fact that may jeopardize the procedure.

Bedside or Operating Room Tracheostomy?

Deciding where to do a tracheostomy depends fundamentally on two factors: available resources and patient conditions.

It should be assessed if there is a trained professional available to use the desired technique, and if there is availability of resources to perform it (operation room time, safe transport for a ICU patient, a well-established bedside procedure protocol, an intensive care team experienced in organizing the appropriate materials and assisting a tracheostomy, a PT kit, etc.). Finally, the patient's clinical condition must be assessed with regard to laboratory tests, cardiorespiratory stability, possibility of cervical hyperextension, and access to the airway.

Considering these points, the surgeon is then able to decide, on a case-by-case basis, where is the best place to do the tracheostomy.

"Informed consent was obtained from any individual participant for whom identifying information is included in this article."

References

1. Pogue MD, Pecaro BC. Safety and efficiency of elective tracheostomy performed in the intensive care unit. J Oral Maxillofac Surg. 1995;53(8):895–7.

2. Yu M. Tracheostomy patients on the ward: multiple benefits from a multidisciplinary team? Crit Care. 2010;14(1):109.
3. Straffon G. The use of a multidisciplinary team in the management of tracheostomy patients, with specific attention to the hole of a physiotherapist [fellowship report]. London: Winston Churchill Memorial Trust Fellowship; 2015.
4. Upadhyay A, Maurer J, Turner J, Tiszenkel H, Rosengart T. Elective bedside tracheostomy in the intensive care unit. J Am Coll Surg. 1996;183(1):51–5.
5. Stock MC, Woodward CG, Shapiro BA, Cane RD, Lewis V, Pecaro B. Perioperative complications of elective tracheostomy in critically ill patients. Crit Care Med. 1986;14(10):861–3.
6. McClelland RMA. Tracheostomy: its management and alternatives. Proc R Soc Med. 1972;65:401–4.
7. Coyle MJ, Shrimpton A, Perkins C, Fasanmade A, Godden D. First do no harm: should routine tracheostomy after oral and maxillofacial oncological operations be abandoned? Br. J Oral Maxillofac Surg. 2012;50(8):732–5.
8. Clec'h C, Alberti C, Vincent F, Garrouste-Orgeas M, De Lassence A, Toledano D, et al. Tracheostomy does not improve the outcome of patients requiring prolonged mechanical ventilation: a propensity analysis. Crit Care Med. 2007;35(1):132–8.
9. Ciaglia P, Firsching R, Syniec C. Elective percutaneous dilatational tracheostomy: a new simple bedside procedure; preliminary report. Chest. 1985;87(6):715–9.
10. Molardi A, Benassi F, Manca T, Ramelli A, Vezzani A, Nicolini F, et al. Parma tracheostomy technique: a hybrid approach to tracheostomy between classical surgical and percutaneous tracheostomies. J Thorac Dis. 2016;8(12):3633–8.
11. Karimpour HA, Vafaii K, Chalechale M, Mohammadi S, Kaviannezhad R. Percutaneous dilatational tracheostomy via Griggs technique. Arch Iran Med. 2017;20(1):49–54.
12. Freeman BD, Morris PE. Tracheostomy practice in adults with acute respiratory failure. Crit Care Med. 2012;40(10):2890–6.
13. Altman KW, Banoff KM, Tong CC. Medical economic impact of tracheotomy patients on a hospital system. J Med Econ. 2015;18(4):258–62.
14. Tong CC, Kleinberger AJ, Paolino J, Altman KW. Tracheotomy timing and outcomes in the critically ill. Otolaryngol Head Neck Surg. 2012;147(1):44–51.
15. Raimondi N, Vidal MR, Calleja J, Quintero A, Cortés A, Celis E, et al. Evidence-based guidelines for the use of tracheostomy in critically ill patients. J Crit Care. 2017;38:304–18.
16. Levin R, Trivikram L. Cost/benefit analysis of open tracheotomy, in the or and at the bedside, with percutaneous tracheotomy. Laryngoscope. 2001;111(7):1169–73.
17. Cools-Lartigue J, Aboalsaud A, Gill H, Ferri L. Evolution of percutaneous dilatational tracheostomy—a review of current techniques and their pitfalls. World J Surg. 2013;37(7):1633–46.
18. Gadkaree SK, Schwartz D, Gerold K, Kim Y. Use of bronchoscopy in percutaneous dilational tracheostomy. JAMA Otolaryngol Head Neck Surg. 2016;142(2):143–9.
19. Bowen CP, Whitney LR, Truwit JD, Durbin CG, Moore MM. Comparison of safety and cost of percutaneous versus surgical tracheostomy. Am Surg. 2001;67(1):54–60.
20. Yoo DB, Schiff BA, Martz S, Fraioli RE, Smith RV, Kvetan V, et al. Open bedside tracheotomy: impact on patient care and patient safety. Laryngoscope. 2011;121(3):515–20.
21. Massick DD, Yao S, Powell DM, Griesen D, Hobgood T, Allen JN, et al. Bedside tracheostomy in the intensive care unit: a prospective randomized trial comparing open surgical tracheostomy with endoscopically guided percutaneous dilational tracheotomy. Laryngoscope. 2001;111(3):494–500.
22. Kilic D, Fındıkcıoglu A, Akin S, Korun O, Aribogan A, Hatiboglu A. When is surgical tracheostomy indicated? Surgical "U-shaped" versus percutaneous tracheostomy. Ann Thorac Cardiovasc Surg. 2011;17(1):29–32.
23. Higgins KM, Punthakee X. Meta-analysis comparison of open versus percutaneous tracheostomy. Laryngoscope. 2011;117(3):447–54.

24. Khalid AQ, Adamis J, Tse J, Harris J, Islam T, Seikaly H. Ultra percutaneous dilation tracheotomy vs mini open tracheotomy. A comparison of tracheal damage in fresh cadaver specimens. BMC Res Notes. 2015;8(1):237.
25. Stoeckli SJ, Breitbach T, Schmid SA. clinical and histologic comparison of percutaneous dilational versus conventional surgical tracheostomy. Laryngoscope. 1997;107(12):1643–6.
26. Antonelli M, Michetti V, Di Palma A, Cont G, Pennisi MA, Arcangeli A, et al. Percutaneous translaryngeal versus surgical tracheostomy: a randomized trial with 1-yr double-blind follow-up. Crit Care Med. 2005;33(5):1015–20.
27. Delaney A, Bagshaw SM, Nalos M. Percutaneous dilatational tracheostomy versus surgical tracheostomy in critically ill patients: a systematic review and meta-analysis. Crit Care. 2006;10(2):R55.
28. Porter JM, Ivatury RR. Preferred route of tracheostomy—percutaneous versus open at the bedside: a randomized, prospective study in the surgical intensive care unit. Am Surg. 1999;65(2):142–6.
29. Hazard P, Jones C, Benitone J. Comparative clinical trial of standard operative tracheostomy with percutaneous tracheostomy. Crit Care Med. 1991;19(8):1018–24.
30. Crofts SL, Alzeer A, McGuire GP, Wong DT, Charles D. A comparison of percutaneous and operative tracheostomies in intensive care patients. Can J Anaesth. 1995;42(9):775–9.
31. Holdgaard HO, Pedersen J, Jensen RH, Outzen KE, Midtgaard T, Johansen LV, et al. Percutaneous dilatational tracheostomy versus conventional surgical tracheostomy. Acta Anaesthesiol Scand. 1998;42(5):545–50.
32. Friedman Y, Fildes J, Mizock B, Samuel J, Patel S, Appavu S, et al. Comparison of percutaneous and surgical tracheostomies. Chest. 1996;110(2):480–5.
33. Papson JP, Russell KL, Taylor DM. Unexpected events during the intrahospital transport of critically ill patients. Acad Emerg Med. 2007;14(6):574–7.
34. Smith IRA, Fleming S, Cernaianu A. Mishaps during transport from the intensive care unit. Crit Care Med. 1990;18(3):278–81.
35. Hurst JM, Davis K Jr, Johnson DJ, Branson RD, Campbell RS, Branson PS. Cost and complications during in-hospital transport of critically ill patients: a prospective cohort study. J Trauma. 1992;33(4):582–5.
36. Heikkinen M, Aarnio P, Hannukainen J. Percutaneous dilational tracheostomy or conventional surgical tracheostomy? Crit Care Med. 2000;28(5):1399–402.
37. Muhl E, Franke C, Hansen M. Costs and time savings by dilatation tracheotomy with bronchoscopic control. Langenbecks Archiv für Chirurgie. Supplement. Kongressband. Deutsche Gesellschaft für Chirurgie. Kongress. 1993;113:353–5.
38. Hsia DW, Ghori UK, Musani AI. Percutaneous dilational tracheostomy. Clin Chest Med. 2013;34(3):515–26.
39. Terra RM, Fernandez A, Bammann RH, Castro ACP, Ishy A, Junqueira JJM. Open bedside tracheostomy: routine procedure for patients under prolonged mechanical ventilation. Clinic. 2007;62(4):427–32.

Tracheostomy Complications

Gabriel Manfro, Fernando Luiz Dias,
and Terence Pires de Farias

Tracheostomy is a frequently performed procedure. The variety of indications and different characteristics of the patients makes attention necessary to avoid complications The decision regarding the performance of tracheostomy should consider the risks and benefits of this procedure [1].

More important than knowing the possible complications of the tracheostomy, making the diagnosis early, and treating them, is to identify in advance possible characteristics of the procedure that increase the chances of events, such as tracheostomies in obese patients or pediatric patients, and retracheostomy [2].

G. Manfro, M.D., Ph.D. (✉)
Department of Head and Neck Surgery, Santa Teresinha University Hospital, Universidade do Oeste de Santa Catarina, UNOESC, Joaçaba, Santa Catarina, Brazil
e-mail: manfro1976@gmail.com

F.L. Dias, M.D., Ph.D., M.Sc., F.A.C.S.
Head and Neck Surgery Department, Brazilian National Cancer Institute—INCA, Rio de Janeiro, RJ, Brazil

Head and Neck Department, Pontifical Catholic University of Rio de Janeiro, Rio de Janeiro, RJ, Brazil

T.P. de Farias, M.D., Ph.D., M.Sc., Researcher
Department of Head and Neck Surgery, Brazilian National Cancer Institute—INCA, Rio de Janeiro, RJ, Brazil

Department of Head and Neck Surgery, Pontifical Catholic University, Rio de Janeiro, RJ, Brazil

T.P. de Farias (ed.), *Tracheostomy*, https://doi.org/10.1007/978-3-319-67867-2_18

Transoperative Complications

Bleeding

This is the most frequent complication, affecting between 1% and 37% of cases [3]. Most of the time the bleeding is minor, without hemodynamic repercussions for the patient (Fig. 1). it usually occurs due to failure of vessel exposure and exacerbated traction on these structures, especially the anterior jugular veins and inferior thyroid veins (Fig. 2).

The treatment of this kind of bleeding normally is done with hemostatic maneuvers with suturing or electrocauterization.

Pneumothorax

This occurs by inadvertent injury of the apical pleura (Fig. 3), which is more easily exposed in patients who are on mechanical ventilation. In addition, this pleural segment is more exposed in children, which increases the risk of this complication from 4% in adults to up to 17% in children [3, 4].

To diagnose this complication, it is necessary to perform a chest X-ray after the tracheostomy [3, 4].

Another cause of pneumothorax is the placement of the cannula on a false path anteriorly and laterally to the trachea (Fig. 4).

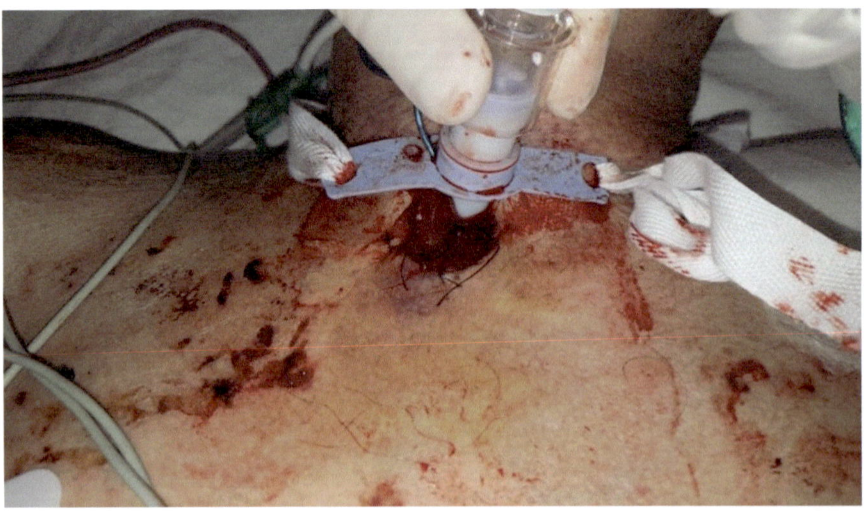

Fig. 1 A small bleeding posttracheostomy treated with surgical re-exploration and bleeding suture

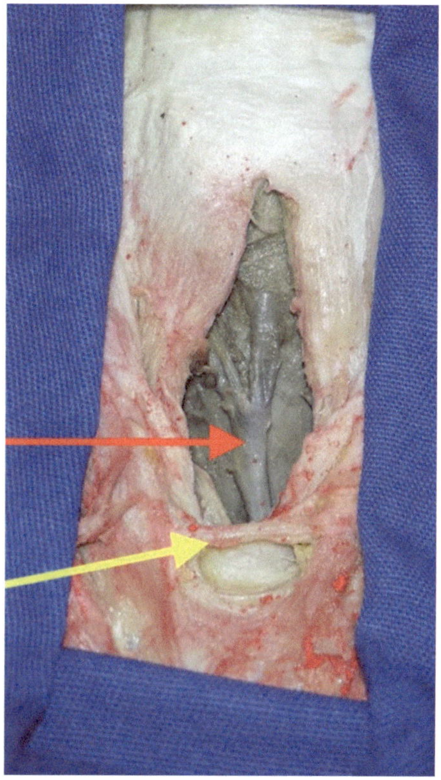

Fig. 2 *Red arrow:* inferior thyroid vein; *yellow arrow:* anterior jugular vein (anterior jugular arch)

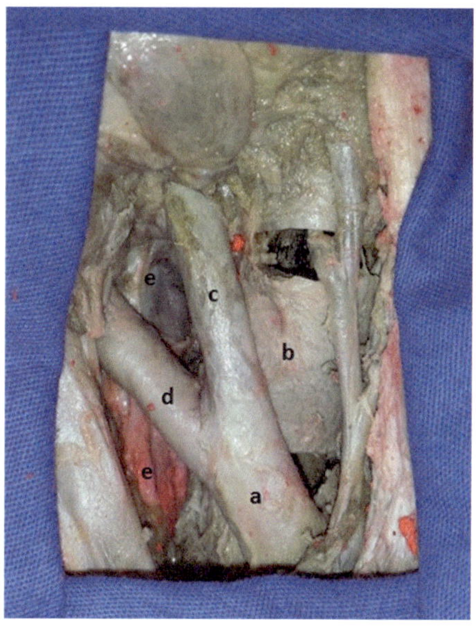

Fig. 3 (**a**) Brachiocephalic trunk. (**b**) Trachea. (**c**) Right carotid common artery. (**d**) Right subclavian artery. (**e**) Right apical pleura

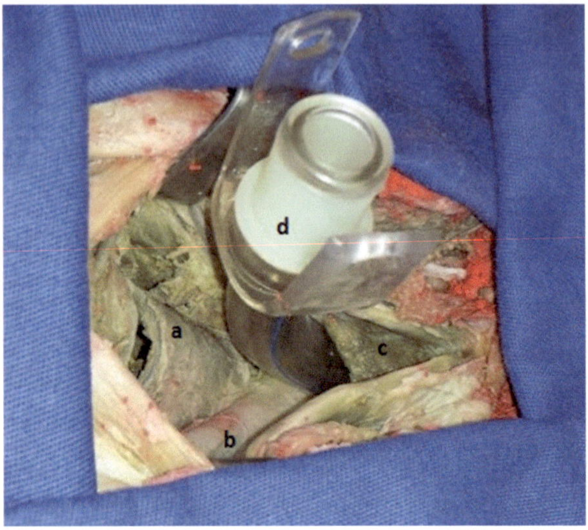

Fig. 4 (**a**) Trachea. (**b**) Brachiocephalic trunk. (**c**) Brachiocephalic vein. (**d**) Tracheal cannula (false path between brachiocephalic trunk and brachiocephalic vein)

Esophageal Perforation

This iatrogenic lesion is rare, occurring in fewer than 1% of cases, and should be treated immediately, with suturing in two planes, in addition to diversion of food intake with nasoenteric feeding. Late diagnosis of this complication significantly worsens the prognosis, based on the risk of mediastinitis [3, 4].

Normally it happens with lateral traction of the trachea, exposing the anterior wall of the esophagus, confusing the muscular esophagus wall with the strap muscles, which could resulting in a surgical esophagus injury (Figs. 5 and 6).

Recurrent Laryngeal Nerve Injury

This occurs during lateral dissection of the trachea, and happens more easily when it is deviated. This complication usually is diagnosed after decannulation, with significant dysphonia and changes in swallowing with aspiration of varied intensity, and is confirmed by laryngoscopy examination. This neural deficit may be definitive or temporary [5, 6].

Cardiopulmonary Resuscitation

Several factors can result in cardiorespiratory arrest during the performance of a tracheostomy: delay in airway clearance, cardiac arrhythmia, vagal stimulation, hypertensive pneumothorax, postobstruction pulmonary edema, and excessive inhalation of oxygen in patients with chronic hypercarbia [3, 7].

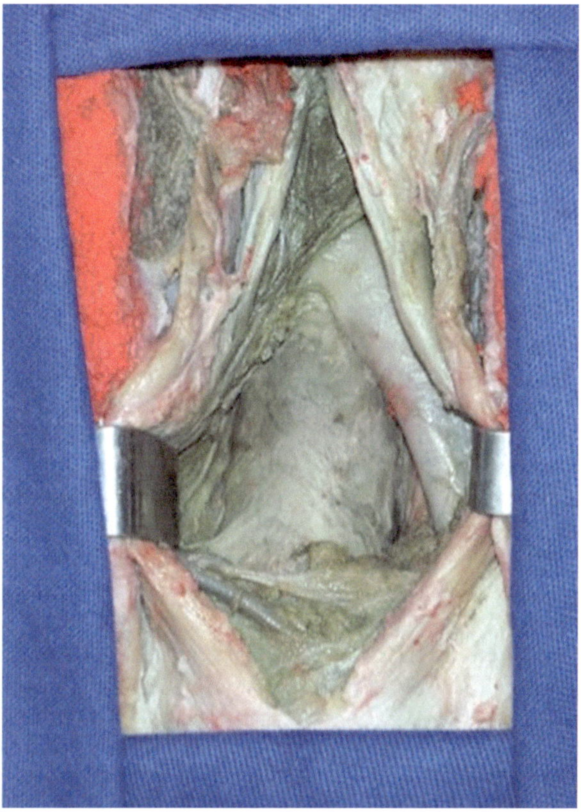

Fig. 5 Normal exposure during a tracheostomy. The trachea is in a central position

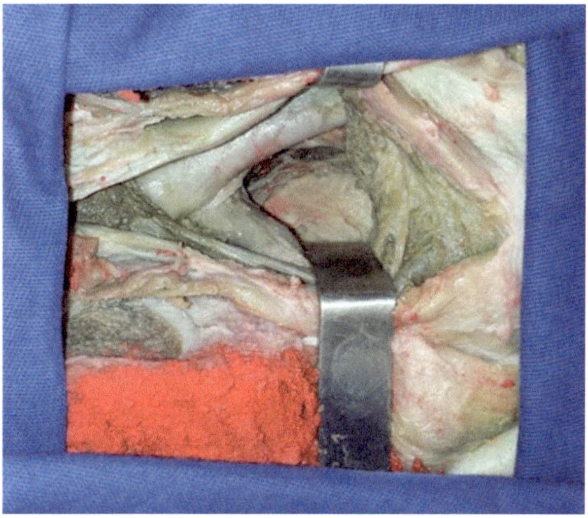

Fig. 6 Lateral tracheal retraction with anterior esophagus wall exposure

Pneumomediastinum

This occurs more often in children and is usually diagnosed on routine chest X-rays. This complication can be caused by dissection of the paratracheal soft tissues, especially in cases of excessive respiratory effort and also when accompanied by cough.

In most cases, pneumomediastinum is asymptomatic and does not require treatment [8].

Combustion

This rare complication can be a catastrophic event. The use of electrocautery on a surface that has received an alcoholic solution, in the presence of oxygen in a high concentration, may result in ideal conditions for the occurrence of severe burns.

Care should be taken to avoid this complication; however, if it occurs, treatment should be instituted to minimize the complications of airway burns, such as antibiotics, intravenous fluids, and corticosteroids [8].

Late debridement will be necessary in the following days to avoid secondary infection of the burned tissue.

Early Complications

Cannula Obstruction

The presence of mucous secretions or blood clots can occur frequently and immediately after performing the tracheostomy. This can be avoided by using proper humidification and frequent aspiration of the tracheostomy. To avoid complete obstruction of the cannula, the use of a prosthesis with an inner cannula is essential, otherwise replacement is indicated [8].

Displacement of the Tracheostomy Tube

The earlier this occurrence happens, the more serious a complication it can be. In the immediate postoperative period, the peritracheal soft tissue does not present fibrosis. Then there is no defined path between the skin and the trachea, and immediate recannulation could be difficult to perform. Decannulation more frequently occurs in patients without favorable anatomy such as obesity, agitated patients, or those with a severe cough. Incorrect cannula fixation and inappropriate dressing may also facilitate the occurrence of this complication.

One of the clear signs of cannula displacement is the possibility of the patient speaking even with a tracheostomy.

For the repositioning of the cannula, a suture in the tracheal ring can help in the exposure of the tracheal orifice. In cases where repositioning of the cannula is not possible, the orotracheal tube should be replaced, following by posterior repositioning of the tracheostomy cannula [8].

Bleeding

In the early postoperative period the source of bleeding would be the same as that in the transoperative period (see Sect. 1.1). Cases of major bleeding should be surgically re-explored [8].

Surgical Wound Infection

Colonization of the tracheal wound occurs within the first 48 h after surgery. The main colonizing germs are Gram positive bacteria, *Pseudomonas,* and *Escherichia coli*. Because it is an open operative wound, colonization is inevitable, but some maneuvers are important for reducing the risks of major infectious complications, such as frequent cannula replacement, removal of the tracheal ring suture, and minimal devascularization of peritracheostoma and tracheal tissue, avoiding lateral tracheal dissection.

Necrotizing stoma infection is an uncommon complication; however, it presents a high rate of serious complications such as exposure of large vessel ruptures (Fig. 7). Treatment should be performed with antibiotic therapy whenever possible, guided by cultures and debridement of devitalized tissue [8].

Subcutaneous Emphysema

Accumulation of air in the subcutaneous space usually is not very serious, requiring no treatment at all. The cause of this complication may be excessive cough, a cannula without a cuff, or near-total obstruction of the skin around the cannula. Usually the treatment is cannula replacement with a cuffed cannula or correct cuff inflation [8].

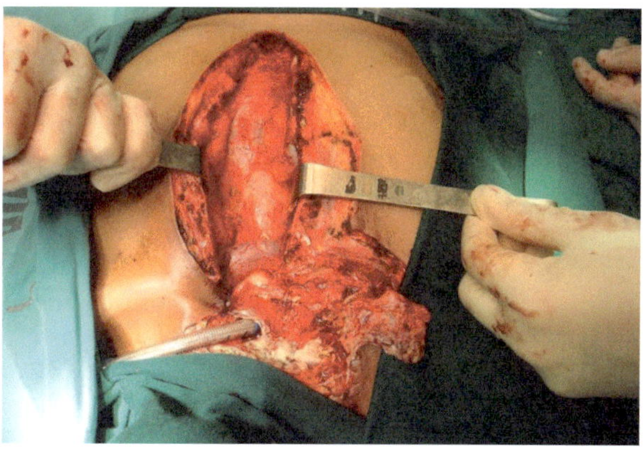

Fig. 7 Sternotomy approach for a brachiocephalic trunk rupture due to tracheostomy infection

Late Complications

Tracheal Stenosis

After tracheostomy, tracheal narrowing occurs more frequently at the stomal level, but this also can occur in a lower incidence in the suprastomal region [9, 10, 11], in the region of contact with the cuff, and in the contact region between the tip of the cannula and the tracheal wall [12]. Some factors such as local infection favor weakening of the tracheal walls, facilitating the occurrence of this stenosis.

Although a large number of patients show a certain degree of tracheal caliber reduction after a tracheostomy, only 3–12% of patients present with stenosis symptoms that require treatment [11].

At first, granulation tissue formation occurs, which can lead to decannulation difficulties. Later, fibrous tissue formation begins at the site of granulation, followed by epithelization of this tissue and stenosis.

Some factors are indicated as risk factors for developing tracheal stenosis, such as sepsis, stoma infection, hypotension, elderly patients, steroids, cannula size, excessive cannula mobility, prolonged cannulation, or disproportionate excision of the anterior wall of the trachea during the surgical procedure [9].

The risk of this complication occurs equally with the surgical and percutaneous procedures [13, 14, 15].

One third of tracheal stenoses are located in the cuff region due to a pressure higher than the capillary perfusion, resulting in an ischemic lesion of the tracheal wall. These types of lesions decrease by ten times after standard cuffs, prioritizing high-volume and low-pressure cuffs [16, 17].

The position and contact of the distal cannula tip are important and can result in posterior tracheal wall trauma, especially in obese patients with a large distance between the skin and the tracheal orifice, allowing contact between its extremity and the posterior wall of the trachea [12].

For diagnosis of tracheal stenosis, a lot of signs and symptoms should be observed. The most frequent symptom is dyspnea, beginning weeks to months after decannulation. Half of the patients start experiencing symptoms before 6 weeks and two thirds before 2 months after decannulation [18]. Usually the symptoms start with a reduction in the tracheal lumen of greater than 50%.

A computed tomography (CT) scan and tracheoscopy are the most useful examinations to define the exact level and the extension of the stenosis, and help to define the treatment [12] (Fig. 8).

Laser resection of the granulation tissue (Fig. 9) formed in the tracheostomy is the treatment of choice [19]. Bronchoscopy dilation may also be an appropriate approach for this type of complication [20]. When stenosis of a short segment of the trachea occurs, resection with laser therapy achieves up to 60% success. When the laser approach does not achieve an adequate outcome, surgical segmental resection of the trachea and reanastomosis is the treatment of choice [11, 18, 21, 22].

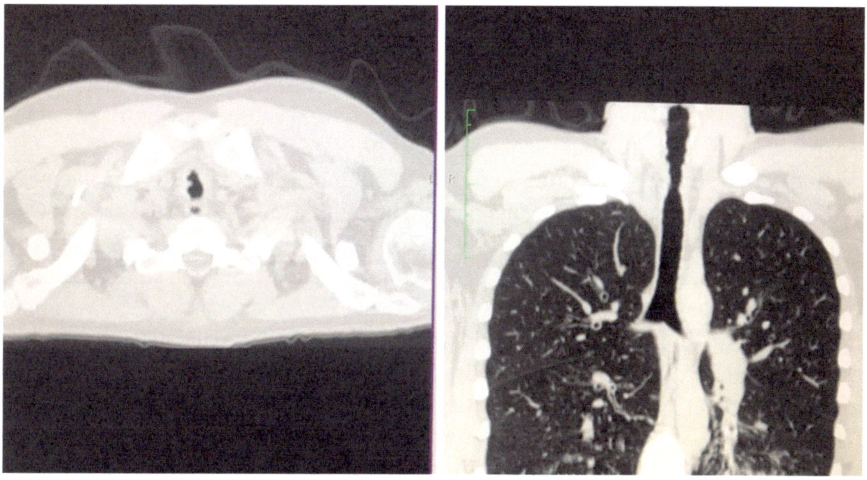

Fig. 8 Transversal and coronal section showing extensive tracheal stenosis due to cuff hyperinflation

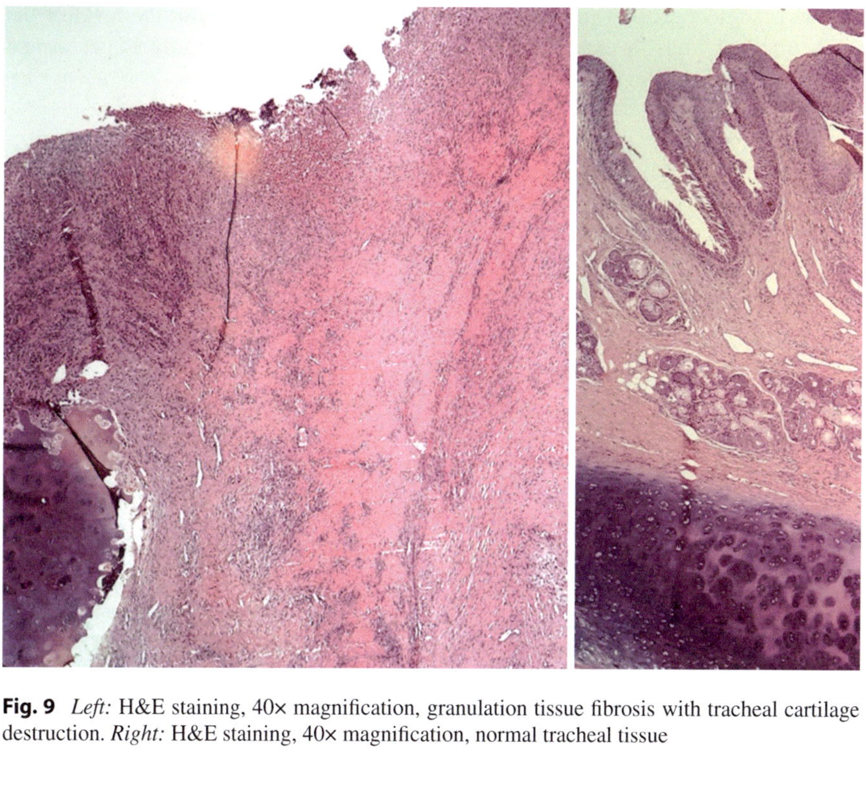

Fig. 9 *Left:* H&E staining, 40× magnification, granulation tissue fibrosis with tracheal cartilage destruction. *Right:* H&E staining, 40× magnification, normal tracheal tissue

Tracheomalacia

This is weakening of the walls of the trachea, which results in a decrease in caliber during expiration. It occurs secondary to chondritis and subsequent cartilage necrosis, resulting in loss of airway caliber support [9, 23].

It may arise acutely, resulting in failure to attempt withdrawal from mechanical ventilation, or in a more chronic manner, manifesting itself with dyspnea associated with a previous history of tracheostomy [12].

A high degree of suspicion is also required for diagnosis. Several complementary examinations may aid in diagnosis, such as tracheoscopy showing a decrease in the tracheal caliber during expiration, and spirometry with characteristics of intrathoracic flow obstruction, in addition to dynamic tracheal tomography [24].

The treatment depends on the severity of the symptom [25]. The options include retracheostomy, stent placement, and tracheal resection [12].

Tracheoinnominate Fistula

This is one of the most feared complications of tracheostomy [9]. The risk factors for the occurrence of this fistula are similar to those of other late complications and are related to local trauma secondary to excessive movement of the tracheal cannula, hyperinflation of the cuff, and inferior placement of the cannula [12].

The brachiocephalic trunk crosses the trachea approximately at the level of the ninth tracheal ring—a region easily reachable if the tracheostomy is performed below the third cartilaginous ring (Fig. 10).

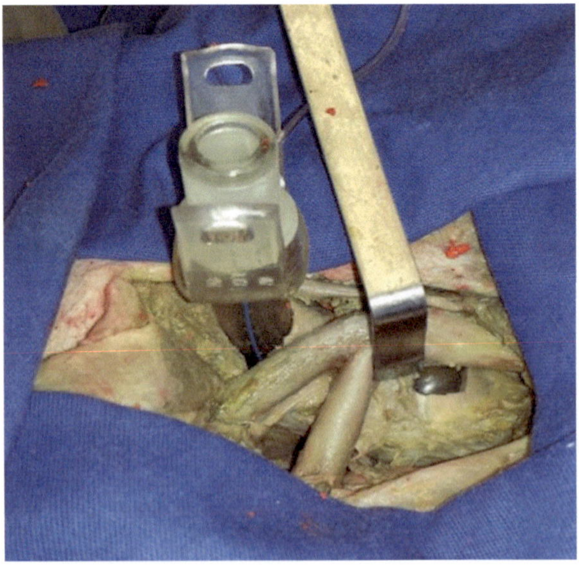

Fig. 10 Relationship between the posterior wall of the brachiocephalic trunk, the anterior tracheal wall, and the cuff pressure

This complication occurs in fewer than 1% of tracheostomized patients, and approximately 75% of these occur between the third and fourth week of tracheostomy. Mortality is close to 100%, even in cases where surgical exploration is possible.

Clinically it presents with a bleeding prodrome by the tracheostomy, evolving to massive hemoptysis [12]. Immediate surgical exploration is mandatory to attempt to correct the fistula [26].

Tracheoesophageal Fistula

This is a rare complication, which occurs in fewer than 1% of cases [27]. This iatrogenic complication occurs due to trauma to the posterior wall of the trachea, which may occur acutely during a percutaneous tracheostomy procedure, or it may be due to chronic trauma causing ischemia of the posterior tracheal wall [12]. The presence of a nasoenteric catheter may also cause trauma to the esophagus, facilitating the formation of the fistula [24, 28].

The clinical manifestation of this complication occurs with aspiration pneumonia, increased dyspnea, and gastric distension [9]. The diagnosis is made with esophagography and a thoracic CT scan. The treatment is surgical, and, depending on the level of the fistula, a thoracic approach beyond the cervical one could be necessary [29].

Pneumonia

Old studies have reported that tracheostomy reduced the occurrence of pneumonia [30]. However, a study analyzing more than 3000 intensive care patients reported that tracheostomy increased the incidence of pneumonia by 6.7 times [31].

Aspiration

Placement of the tracheostomy alters the swallowing movement, predisposing the patient to aspiration, in addition to compression of the esophagus by the cuff of the cannula. Aspiration can occur in up to 50% of patients on mechanical ventilation and with an inflated cuff. Based on this high incidence, a swallowing study is recommended in all patients who remain tracheostomized for a long time before starting oral intake of food.

References

1. Durbin CG Jr. Early complications of tracheostomy. Respir Care. 2005;50(4):511–5.
2. Taylor CB, Otto RA. Open tracheostomy procedure. Atlas Oral Maxillofac Surg Clin North Am. 2015;23(2):117–24.

3. Myers EM, Stool SE, Thonson JT. Complications of tracheostomy. In: Myers EM, Stool SE, Thonson JT, editors. Tracheotomy. New York: Churchill Livingstone; 1985. p. 147–69.
4. Barlow DW, Weymuller EA Jr, Wood DE. Tracheotomy and the role of postoperative chest radiography in adult patients. Ann Otol Rhinol Laryngol. 1994;103(9):665–8.
5. Pereira KD, MacGregor AR, Mitchell RB. Complications of neonatal tracheostomy: a 5-year review. Otolaryngol Head Neck Surg. 2004;131(6):810–3.
6. Kremer B, Botos-Kremer AI, Eckel HE, Schlöndorff G. Indications, complications, and surgical techniques for pediatric tracheostomies—an update. J Pediatr Surg. 2002;37(11):1556–62.
7. Christopher KL. Tracheostomy decannulation. Respir Care. 2005;50(4):538–41.
8. Kost KM, Myers EM. Traqueostomia. In: Myers EM, editor. Otorrinolaringologia Cirúrgica; 2008. p. 609–27.
9. Sue RD, Susanto I. Long-term complications of artificial airways. Clin Chest Med. 2003;24(3): 457–71.
10. Stauffer JL, Olson DE, Petty TL. Complications and consequences of endotracheal intubation and tracheotomy. A prospective study of 150 critically ill adult patients. Am J Med. 1981;70(1):65–76.
11. Streitz JM Jr, Shapshay SM. Airway injury after tracheotomy and endotracheal intubation. Surg Clin North Am. 1991;71(6):1211–30.
12. Epstein SK. Late complications of tracheostomy. Respir Care. 2005;50(4):542–9.
13. Benjamin B, Kertesz T. Obstructive suprastomal granulation tissue following percutaneous tracheostomy. Anaesth Intensive Care. 1999;27(6):596–600.
14. Koitschev A, Graumueller S, Zenner HP, Dommerich S, Simon C. Tracheal stenosis and obliteration above the tracheostoma after percutaneous dilational tracheostomy. Crit Care Med. 2003;31(5):1574–6.
15. Briche T, Le Manach Y, Pats B. Complications of percutaneous tracheostomy. Chest. 2001;119(4):1282–3.
16. Lewis FR Jr, Schiobohm RM, Thomas AN. Prevention of complications from prolonged tracheal intubation. Am J Surg. 1978;135(3):452–7.
17. Leigh JM, Maynard JP. Pressure on the tracheal mucosa from cuffed tubes. Br Med J. 1979;1(6172):1173–4.
18. Brichet A, Verkindre C, Dupont J, Carlier ML, Darras J, Wurtz A, Ramon P, Marquette CH. Multidisciplinary approach to management of postintubation tracheal stenoses. Eur Respir J. 1999;13(4):888–93.
19. Shapshay SM, Beamis JF Jr, Hybels RL, Bohigian RK. Endoscopic treatment of subglottic and tracheal stenosis by radial laser incision and dilation. Ann Otol Rhinol Laryngol. 1987;96(6):661–4.
20. Reilly JS, Myer CM. Excision of suprastomal granulation tissue. Laryngoscope. 1985;95(12): 1545–6.
21. Mehta AC, Lee FY, Cordasco EM, Kirby T, Eliachar I, De Boer G. Concentric tracheal and subglottic stenosis. Management using the Nd-YAG laser for mucosal sparing followed by gentle dilatation. Chest. 1993;104(3):673–7.
22. Laccourreye O, Naudo P, Brasnu D, Jouffre V, Cauchois R, Laccourreye H. Tracheal resection with end-to-end anastomosis for isolated postintubation cervical tracheastenosis: long-term results. Ann Otol Rhinol Laryngol. 1996;105(12):944–8.
23. Wood DE, Mathisen DJ. Late complications of tracheotomy. Clin Chest Med. 1991;12(3): 597–609.
24. Aquino SL, Shepard JA, Ginns LC, Moore RH, Halpern E, Grillo HC, McLoud TC. Acquired tracheomalacia: detection by expiratory CT scan. J Comput Assist Tomogr. 2001;25(3):394–9.
25. Feist JH, Johnson TH, Wilson RJ. Acquired tracheomalacia: etiology and differential diagnosis. Chest. 1975;68(3):340–5.
26. Cooper JD. Trachea-innominate artery fistula: successful management of 3 consecutive patients. Ann Thorac Surg. 1977;24(5):439–47.
27. Reed MF, Mathisen DJ. Tracheoesophageal fistula. Chest Surg Clin N Am. 2003;13(2):271–89.

28. Dartevelle P, Macchiarini P. Management of acquired tracheoesophageal fistula. Chest Surg Clin N Am. 1996;6(4):819–36.
29. Macchiarini P, Verhoye JP, Chapelier A, Fadel E, Dartevelle P. Evaluation and outcome of different surgical techniques for postintubation tracheoesophageal fistulas. J Thorac Cardiovasc Surg. 2000;119(2):268–76.
30. Dunham CM, LaMonica C. Prolonged tracheal intubation in the trauma patient. J Trauma. 1984;24(2):120–4.
31. Ibrahim EH, Tracy L, Hill C, Fraser VJ, Kollef MH. The occurrence of ventilator-associated pneumonia in a community hospital: risk factors and clinical outcomes. Chest. 2001;120(2):555–61.

Predicting Factors for Tracheal Stenosis

Paulo Soltoski, Paola Andrea Galbiatti Pedruzzi, and Monique Pierosan Cardoso

Introduction

A new disease named *tracheal stenosis* was created when modern society became capable of keeping critically ill patients alive under mechanical ventilation.

The reported incidence of stenosis associated with endotracheal intubation was nearly 26% in the 1970s, and it remains elevated in most institutions that still do not measure the endotracheal tube cuff pressure routinely [1].

As observed by Pearson et al., tracheal and subglottic stenosis are usually acquired and in most cases caused by intubation or tracheostomy. The reported incidence rates of tracheal stenosis following laryngotracheal intubation and tracheostomy range from 6% to 21% and from 0.6% to 21%, respectively [1]. With the introduction of endotracheal tubes with a large area of contact (high-volume, low-pressure cuffs) the incidence of postintubation tracheal stenosis in intensive care units (ICUs) has decreased [1–3].

Despite technological improvements and more skillful patient care in ICUs, tracheal and laryngotracheal stenoses still constitute an important group of iatrogenic sequelae after intubation in tracheostomy [2–4].

P. Soltoski, M.D., M.Sc.
Assistant Professor of Surgery, Universidade Federal do Parana, Curitiba, PR, Brazil
e-mail: psoltoski@gmail.com

P.A.G. Pedruzzi, M.D., M.Sc. (✉)
Hospital Erasto Gaertner de Curitiba — Paraná, Curitiba, PR, Brazil
e-mail: paolapedruzzi@yahoo.com.br

M.P. Cardoso, M.D.
Hospital Universitário Evangélico de Curitiba – Paraná, Curitiba, PR, Brazil

T.P. de Farias (ed.), *Tracheostomy*, https://doi.org/10.1007/978-3-319-67867-2_19

Discussion

The trachea extends from the larynx, at the inferior margin of the cricoid cartilage on the fifth or sixth cervical vertebrae to the right and left main bronchi at the carina, near the fourth thoracic vertebral body level. It measures 12–15 cm in length and 1.5–2.0 cm in width. The stenosis is typically 1.5–2.5 cm in length [5].

As Epstein stated, diagnosing tracheal stenosis is not easy and very often the diagnosis is delayed. A high index of suspicion is important, especially when a patient has a history of previous intubation or tracheostomy. Tracheal stenosis may be present very early while the patient is still undergoing mechanical ventilation, and can be clinically manifested as difficulty in weaning from the ventilator or attempts at removal of the endotracheal tube [6].

Some degree of tracheal stenosis is present in almost all patients with a tracheostomy tube, but only 3–12% of patients have clinically significant stenosis requiring intervention [7].

Dyspnea, stridor, and respiratory failure may be present after extubation. In addition, clinical manifestations of stenosis may present weeks to years after development, but they are typically evident within 2 months following removal of the endotracheal tube. Tracheal stenosis may produce no symptoms until the lumen has been reduced by 50–75%. The initial manifestations may be increased cough and difficulty in clearing secretions. Once the tracheal lumen has been reduced to 10 mm, exertional dyspnea occurs. When the lumen is narrowed to 5 mm, dyspnea at rest or a stridor is noted [6].

Stauffer et al., in 1981, considered tracheal stenosis as a reduction of more than 10% in the tracheal lumen [4], but in our experience clinically evident symptoms do not occur until approximately 75% of the airway is compromised. Tracheal stenosis symptoms occur in the first month in the majority of patients, but may occur as late as several years afterward [8].

Patients who present subacutely are often incorrectly diagnosed as having asthma, chronic obstructive pulmonary disease, or pneumonia, and frequently have a history of multiple prior visits to the emergency department with unclear respiratory symptoms. Some patients may develop difficulty in expectoration and dyspnea on exertion and can progress to airway obstruction with the development of a stridor. Postintubation tracheal stenosis is often misdiagnosed as asthma in as many as 44% of patients [9, 10].

Rumbak et al. conducted a retrospective study of 756 patients at a long-term care facility who had been ventilated for at least 15 weeks (3 weeks with an endotracheal tube followed by 12 weeks with a tracheostomy tube). Thirty-seven patients (5%) developed failure to wean secondary to tracheal stenosis or obstruction from granulation tissue, often manifested as higher peak airway pressures or difficulty in passing a suction catheter. Intervention (a longer tube in 34 patients and airway stenting in 3) led to successful weaning in 34 of 37 patients within 1 week. This study raised the question of whether all patients should undergo bronchoscopic investigation of the trachea prior to tracheal tube capping or decannulation [11].

Flexible bronchoscopy remains the gold standard for diagnosis and planning of tracheal stenosis treatment. Computed tomography (CT) scans with three-dimensional reconstruction can predict the size and location of the stenosis, but these imaging studies are only necessary in complete tracheal obstructions, since in most cases, bronchoscopy provides all of the information we require for treatment.

One personal experience has deeply marked our practice. A young man presented to the emergency department in severe respiratory distress, requiring endotracheal intubation. A heavy guide wire was necessary to overcome a stenotic lesion with a number four cuffless endotracheal tube. His only past medical history was a gallbladder resection 30 days before this admission, with a short period of general anesthesia involving endotracheal intubation. There was no prior history of endotracheal intubation. This otherwise healthy male, with no other medical problems besides gallstones, was now facing tracheal reconstruction because of less than 2 h of mechanical ventilation.

This case alone is the cornerstone of our chapter. The major predictive factor for laryngeal and tracheal stenosis is elevated cuff pressure during mechanical ventilation. All other causes combined account for just a few of the patients we currently treat at our institution.

Pathophysiology

Considering that excessive cuff pressure is the key element in the spectrum of tracheal and laryngeal stenosis, most lesions will be located at the transition between these structures, but some complications may be related to the tip of the tube, especially when it impinges upon the posterior tracheal wall [12].

Intracuff pressure is transmitted laterally against the wall of the trachea. Overinflation of the cuff can cause tissue ischemia, ulceration, and necrosis. When the endotracheal tube cuff pressure exceeds the mucosal perfusion pressure (15–20 mmHg) in the trachea, the mucosa that lies between the cuff and the underlying cartilage develops ischemia [2, 13].

Different levels of pressure will result in different degrees of tracheal lesion. Normal to mildly elevated cuff pressures will result in mucosal lesions, which may readily heal upon removal of the tube. A deeper lesion is expected when higher cuff pressures are utilized. Since cartilaginous tracheal rings are poorly vascularized, moderate pressures may cause cartilaginous ischemia and degeneration, in addition to the mucosal lesion.

Necrosis of the tracheal mucosa leads to sloughing and ulceration of the mucosal membrane, exposing the tracheal cartilage. This reaction stimulates the formation of scar tissue, which obstructs the airway; this process may lead to a tight fibrous stricture, resulting in tracheal stenosis [6, 14, 15].

Immediately upon endotracheal tube placement, the mucosa underlying the tube cuff will suffer an ischemic process, which lasts for the entire period of endotracheal intubation, but only a small percentage of patients will develop tracheal stenosis.

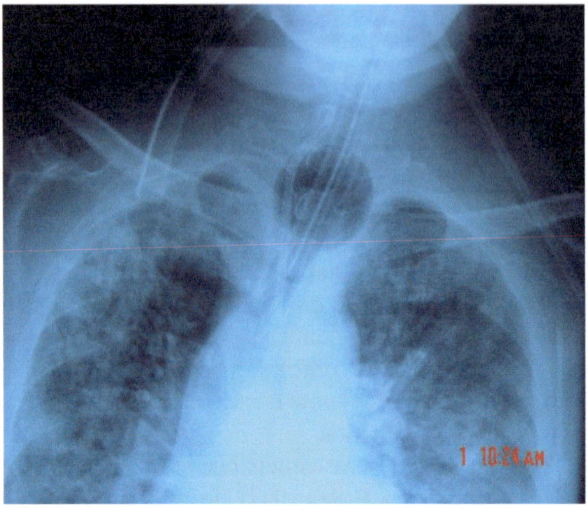

Fig. 1 A bedside chest X-ray demonstrates diffusely infiltrated lungs and an overinflated endotracheal tube cuff. Note the nasogastric tube deviated to the right. (Author's files with permission)

This explains why it is inappropriate pressure of the cuff, not its presence inside the trachea, that is the cause of stenosis. Worsening respiratory function demands increasing ventilatory pressure, and air leakage is controlled with increasing volume of the cuff. At very high pressures, and consequently high volumes, such as in (Fig. 1), transmural ischemia occurs, which may progress to complete occlusion of the trachea approximately 30 days after the injury (Fig. 1).

Causes

Gelbard et al. evaluated 150 patients, demonstrating that the most common etiology was iatrogenic (54.7%), followed by idiopathic (18.5%), autoimmune (18.5%), and traumatic (8%). They divided, in a very practical way, the most common causes of adult subglottic and tracheal stenosis [16].

The idiopathic causes, presenting as 18.5% of the total, involved no significant laryngotracheal injury and no history of endotracheal intubation or tracheotomy within 2 years of the presentation, no thyroid or major anterior neck surgery, no neck irradiation, no caustic or thermal injuries to the laryngotracheal complex, no history of vasculitis, and negative titers for angiotensin-converting enzyme and antinuclear cytoplasmic antibody. The lesion had to involve the subglottis.

The autoimmune subgroup, also presenting as 18.5% of the total, corresponded to patients with documented clinical and serologic and/or histologic diagnosis of granulomatosis with polyangiitis (Wegener's granulomatosis), relapsing polychondritis, systemic lupus erythematosus, rheumatoid arthritis, epidermolysis bullosa, sarcoidosis, or amyloidosis.

The polytrauma subgroup, corresponding to 8% of the patients, included patients presenting with laryngotracheal stenosis following documented traumatic injuries involving multiple organ systems.

The iatrogenic subgroup, accounting for 54.7% of the patients, included those who developed subglottic or tracheal stenosis following tracheostomy or within 2 years after intubation. Overall, 59% of iatrogenic injuries occurred within the subglottis and, therefore, were attributable to intubation. 83% of healthy patients with iatrogenic stenosis were women, suggesting that endotracheal tube size may contribute to tracheal injury and should be carefully considered in the smaller female trachea [16].

Our experience in Brazil is very similar, since nearly 90% of our patients present with iatrogenic stenosis of the larynx and trachea, and many of them develop this lesion secondary to mechanical ventilation due to multiple trauma. We have observed, particularly in the trauma setting, that tracheal intubation at the scene, often under severely adverse conditions, contributes to initially elevated cuff pressures [17].

Upon arrival at the hospital, trauma patients are not infrequently taken to the operating room immediately after the initial trauma evaluation, and many hours will pass before the first cuff pressure measurement can be performed, much later, in the ICU. Attempts at correcting the pressure at this stage often result in significant air leakage, and this appears to be one of the primary signs of laryngotracheal complications [17].

Risk Factors

There are many predisposing factors for complications after endotracheal intubation, and these may be classified as patient-, physician-, or equipment-related factors [13, 18].

The elevated cuff pressure of endotracheal tubes is the most important factor in the development of tracheal damage. Endotracheal tube cuffs can be high-volume, low-pressure cuffs or low-volume, low-pressure cuffs. High-volume, low-pressure cuffs markedly reduce the occurrence of cuff-related injury [2, 19].

With regard to patient factors, the incidence is high in infants, children, and adult women, as they have a relatively small larynx and trachea and are more prone to airway edema. Patients who have a difficult airway are more prone to injury as well as hypoxic events. Also, those with congenital or chronic acquired disease may experience difficult intubation or may be more prone to physiological trauma during intubation. Another significant patient factor to be considered is the hemodynamic status. Patients with sepsis who require inotropic agents have a higher chance of developing mucosal ischemia, since the tracheal perfusion pressure is greatly affected by these drugs [13].

Complications are more likely to occur during emergency situations. It seems to be extremely important to establish an adequate cuff pressure from the very beginning of the tracheal intubation. We have demonstrated that it is impossible to subjectively estimate the cuff pressure by simple digital palpation of the external balloon of the endotracheal or tracheostomy tube; therefore, the pressure of the endotracheal cuff should be routinely, promptly, and frequently measured, even in the trauma scenario, during the transfer of the patient to the hospital [13, 17].

The usual shape of the standard endotracheal tube results in maximal pressure being exerted on the posterior aspect of the larynx. The degree of damage to this area depends on the size of the tube, and a frequently identified lesion is erosion of the posterior commissure of the true vocal cords. Inadequate use of stylets and bougies also predisposes the patient to trauma and tracheal lesions. Another important factor, frequently related to limited medical resources in developing countries, is use of sturdier ventilator tubing, since it needs to be utilized several times for cost containment reasons [13].

This heavy tubing occasionally hangs at the bedside, causing standing traction on the tracheostomy or on the endotracheal tube, which results in additional pressure against the tracheal wall or the cricoid cartilage, respectively. The excessive pressure of the cuff, followed by its inappropriate location inside the trachea, are the two most important determinants of intubation-related tracheal stenosis, accounting for approximately 90% of all lesions, in our personal experience [17].

Considering that the blood supply to the trachea originates from various sources and different levels, entering the tracheal wall from both sides, any radial pressure inside the trachea that exceeds the capillary perfusion pressure can result in ischemic changes at that particular site, and a spectrum of tracheal lesions, ranging from mild and reversible tracheal mucosal lesions to complete transmural necrosis, followed by stenosis, will be observed in the treatment of this disease.

These lesions include granulomas, ulcers, membranous stenotic lesions, and dense fibrotic rings. This also explains why not all patients develop tracheal stenosis, since multiple factors are involved in this disease, including the hemodynamic status of the patient.

Sarper et al., studying 45 patients under mechanical ventilation who subsequently developed laryngotracheal stenosis, observed that trauma, hypotension, infection at the tracheostomy site, technical errors during the construction of the tracheostomy, acute attacks of chronic respiratory disease, and cardiopulmonary disorders were some of the most frequent causes of stenosis [20].

When secondary to endotracheal intubation, tracheal laceration may occur due to overinflation of the cuff, traumatic intubation with multiple intubation attempts, use of stylets, misplacement of the tube tip, tube repositioning without cuff deflation, inadequate tube size (large tubes; >8 mm in men and >7 mm in women), vigorous coughing, and nitrous oxide in the cuff. But these lesions generally heal without problems if no ischemia is involved. The risk is also greater in patients with tracheal distortion caused by a neoplasm or large lymph nodes, chronic obstructive lung disease, and corticosteroid therapy [2]. Our opinion regarding the diameter of the tube is a little different, since we rarely use a tube smaller than a number 9 in men and a number 8 in women [17].

Sasaki and associates believe that tracheal stenosis may be more common when tracheostomy follows prolonged intubation—possibly a result of tracheostomy introducing bacteria and thereby aggravating chondritis with mucosal and submucosal necrosis and mucosal ulceration [21, 22].

We attribute this higher incidence of tracheal complications following tracheostomies after prolonged tracheal intubation to the fact that the tracheal stoma will be created in an already severely diseased segment of the trachea. Once airway injury occurs, other exacerbating factors can coexist, such as chemical injury from either gastroesophageal reflux or laryngopharyngeal reflux, and pooling of inflammatory secretions above the tracheostomy cuff can further injure the airway [23, 24]. The extent of airway injury may be greatest in patients with multiple organ failure [25].

The presence of shock may compromise the mucosal blood flow and lead to airway mucosal ischemia. Wound sepsis and previous cervical or tracheal trauma negatively affect healing of the stoma [20].

Sites of Larynx and Tracheal Lesions

The majority of laryngeal and tracheal lesions occur between the true vocal cords superiorly and the upper third of the trachea distally, since this is the area most commonly affected by the endotracheal tube. The vocal cords are often spared by cuff lesions, but they are often less than 2 cm from the suture line in tracheal reconstructions.

Tracheal lesions are often divided, according to their anatomical location in relation to the stoma, as suprastomal, stomal, and infrastomal (Fig. 2).

Most tracheal stenoses commonly occur at the level of the stoma or above it (suprastomal) but below the vocal cords (subglottic). Tracheal stenosis may also

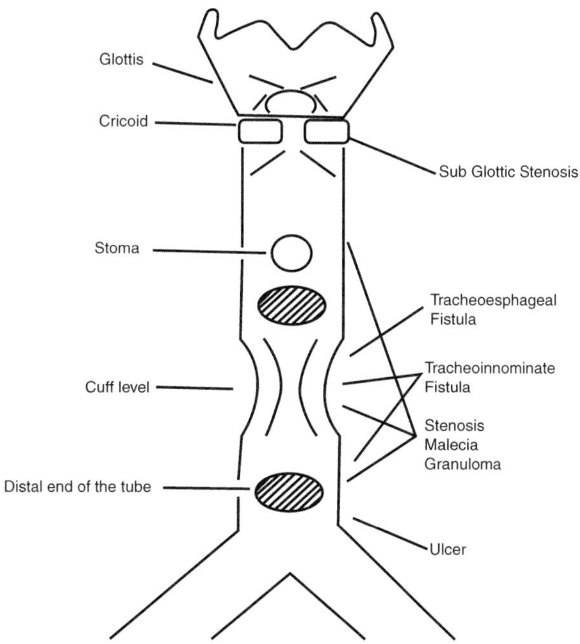

Fig. 2 Anatomical locations of tracheostomy complications. (Reproduced from Lanza et al. [26], with permission)

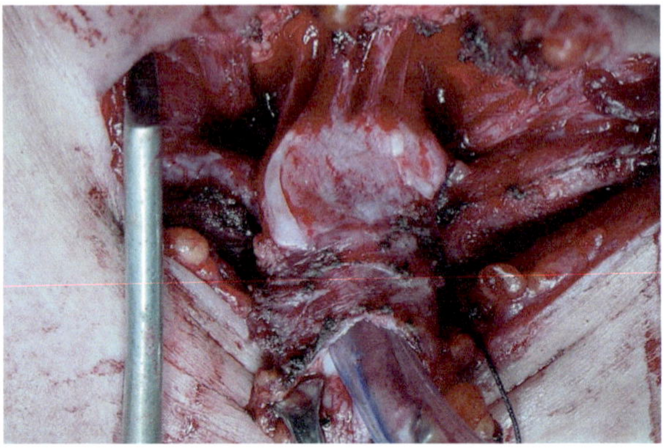

Fig. 3 Total stenosis at the cricoid cartilage. The tracheal tube was inserted through the tracheostomy stoma for ventilation

occur at the site of the tracheostomy tube cuff or at the site of the tube's distal tip [6]. Tracheal stenosis occurs most frequently at the level of the cuff.

The most important reason for stenoses at the stoma site is damaged cartilage, probably due to excessive pressure [4, 27]. Although infraglottic stenosis most commonly results from endotracheal tube damage, it may occur after damage of the first tracheal ring or the cricoid cartilage during tracheostomy (Fig. 3). High tracheostomy should be avoided as far as possible [20]. Suprastomal lesions are often a result of cricothyroidotomy, high tracheostomy tube placement, or friction of the proximal aspect of an overinflated balloon against the tracheal wall or the cricoid. These lesions include subglottic stenosis, tracheal stenosis, and granulation tissue formation [26, 28, 29].

Infrastomal complications include tracheal stenosis, tracheomalacia, and tracheoesophageal and tracheoinnominate fistulas. Infrastomal lesions typically result from ischemia of the tracheal mucosa due to endotracheal tube cuff balloon pressure exceeding the perfusion pressure [6].

Risk factors for infrastomal lesions include female sex, older age, and excessive endotracheal tube cuff pressures. Malacia may also complicate the stenotic segment. The mechanism of malacia formation is not fully understood but may be related to concomitant chronic airway inflammation secondary to bacterial colonization or acid reflux, as stated by Scott K. Epstein, and it certainly is related to ischemic changes secondary to elevated cuff pressures. Finally, stenosis may occur near the distal tip of the tracheostomy tube. The latter may occur because standard tracheostomy tubes may be too short in patients with abundant soft tissue in the anterior neck. The resulting injury to the posterior membranous wall may lead to stenosis or to tracheoesophageal fistula [6].

Sarper et al. reviewed postintubation tracheal stenoses in 45 patients, after intubation or tracheostomy for ventilation support, with special regard to the etiology of the stenoses. There were 38 tracheal and seven subglottic stenoses. The cuffs of tubes accounted for 12 lesions and in 29 patients, the stenoses were located at the stoma site only. Twenty-two patients underwent open tracheostomy, and seven patients had a percutaneous procedure. In five of these patients, high tracheostomy was performed by mistake, resulting in subglottic stenosis. In another patient, a

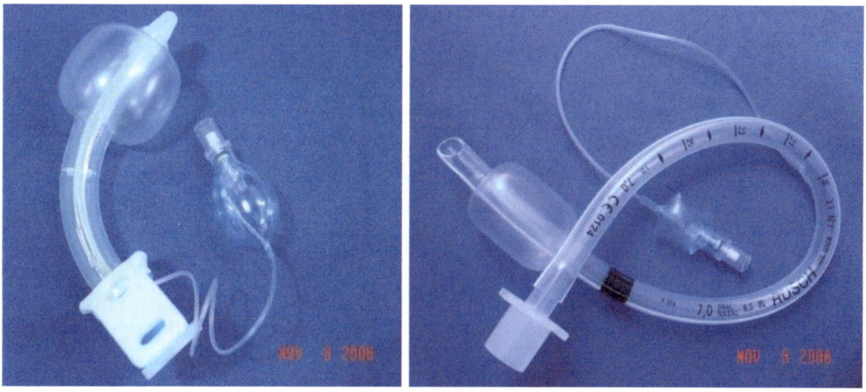

Fig. 4 Cuff balloon and external balloon on a tracheostomy tube (*left*) and an orotracheal tube (*right*). (Author's files, with permission)

large tube was used, and tracheal stenosis developed as a result of tracheal cartilage damage. Two patients had double stenoses, at both the stoma and cuff sites [30].

Recent studies have demonstrated there is no significant difference between tracheostomies or oral intubation in terms of stenosis, but we believe this only holds true when the cuff pressure in both situations is kept within acceptable limits (Fig. 4). We believe, considering adequate cuff pressure maintenance, that the only advantage of a tracheostomy over an endotracheal tube will be that the tracheal lesion, if it occurs, will hopefully be away from the cricoid cartilage—a fact that greatly simplifies treatment [17].

Tracheostomy Techniques and Stenosis

If we compare the incidence rates of tracheal stenosis with different tracheostomy techniques, we observe that stenosis is not related to the type of incision in the trachea but to additional damage to an already injured tracheal wall.

There still is much controversy about the influence exerted by the type of tracheostomy on tracheal stenosis post–tracheostomy. Coelho studied 117 patients, 86 male (73.5%) and 31 female (26.5%), with an average age of 33 years. The author compared two techniques (resection tracheostomy and longitudinal tracheostomy) in relation to their predisposing, triggering, and aggravating factors, as well as the predisposing, triggering, and aggravating factors that influence tracheal stenosis or are influenced by it. The patients underwent fibrolaryngotracheobronchoscopy on days 7, 14, 21, and 28, and every 30 days until the end of the first year if they still had the tube in place, and on the 30th and 180th days after having had the tube taken out. The conclusion was that the stenosis rate was not influenced by the tracheostomy type [31].

Tracheostomy tube placement can be performed surgically via open surgical tracheostomy, or percutaneously via percutaneous dilational tracheostomy. Either open tracheostomy or percutaneous tracheostomy should be performed by experienced physicians [32, 33].

When we compare the percutaneous and surgical approaches, in general, most studies have demonstrated a low incidence of long-term complications with the percutaneous approach [34, 35]. Similarly, a meta-analysis of trials (in 1985–1996) comparing surgical and percutaneous tracheostomy found more frequent perioperative complications with the percutaneous approach but more postoperative complications with surgery [36].

The main perioperative complications of percutaneous tracheostomy include bleeding, pneumothorax, and posterior tracheal injury. Posterior tracheal injury may be confined to the mucosa or may involve the entire posterior wall and, more seriously, may result in a tracheoesophageal fistula or tracheal stenosis. It has been suggested that visualization by fiberoptic bronchoscopy of the tracheal puncture and dilatation can substantially reduce the incidence of such complications [37, 38].

Excessive force must not be applied to the trachea, to prevent cartilage damage particularly during percutaneous tracheostomy. Stoma lesions may result from fracture of the anterior tracheal wall following percutaneous tracheostomy. As a result, the anterior tracheal wall is invaginated and protrudes into the tracheal lumen, resulting in a fixed obstruction [29, 39]. During percutaneous tracheostomy, placement of the stoma must be done carefully, with bronchoscopic guidance [40, 41].

Prevention of Stenosis

There is only one method for prevention of tracheal stenosis, which is careful monitoring of the pressure of the cuff. Although this may seem quite obvious, we have frequently observed patients who are not connected to ventilation and still have their endotracheal tube cuffs fully inflated.

Daily endotracheal tube care should be provided to avoid complications, and includes monitoring of cuff pressure, oral and endotracheal suctioning of secretions, inspection of the tube position, and rotation [42]. Endotracheal tube cuffs can be high-volume, low-pressure cuffs or low-volume, low-pressure cuffs. High-volume, low-pressure cuffs markedly reduce the occurrence of cuff injury [19].

The incidence of stomal stenosis can be reduced by not making a large stoma and by use of lightweight, mobile, swivel connectors to minimize mechanical trauma. The stoma must not have been made too large, and a large-sized tube must not have been inserted into a small stoma by force [8, 43].

Our reality demands studies on ventilation tubing, since it needs to be utilized several times. This heavy tubing occasionally hangs at the bedside, causing traction on the tracheostomy or endotracheal tube, and the cricoid cartilage will act as a ring to prevent extubation. This explains why most subglottic stenosis involve the cricoid cartilage.

It is therefore essential to inflate the cuff with only as much air as is required to just seal the air leak (a minimal inflation technique), and to check the intracuff pressure with a cuff pressure manometer (Fig. 5) [13]. Cuff pressures should be monitored; the frequency depends on the routine of the institution, but it is usually performed daily. The cuff pressure differs from one patient to

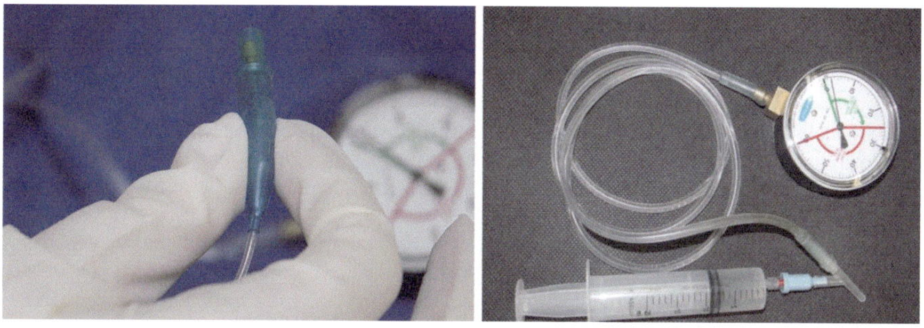

Fig. 5 Digital palpation of the cuff (*left*) and cuff pressure manometer (*right*). (Author's files with permission)

another because there are many factors that can affect cuff pressure, including the endotracheal tube size, tracheal size, ventilatory pressure, and patient position. As a guideline, the cuff pressure should be maintained between 20 and 30 mmHg [2, 13].

Considering that, we have demonstrated that it is impossible to subjectively estimate the cuff pressure by simple digital palpation (Fig. 5) of the external balloon of the endotracheal or tracheostomy tube. Our suggestion is the addition of the cuff pressure parameter to the routine measurement parameters in the ICU, to be verified and documented on the patient's flow sheet every 2 h.

Conclusion

The most important aspect of tracheal stenosis prevention is careful management of the endotracheal cuff. Maintaining adequate position of the endotracheal tube or tracheostomy and appropriate pressure of the cuff are crucial to minimize airway complications related to mechanical ventilation.

References

1. Pearson FG, Andrews MJ. Detection and management of tracheal stenosis following cuffed tube tracheostomy. Ann Thoracic Surg. 1971;12:359–74.
2. Sajal D, Sarmishtha D. Post intubation tracheal stenosis. Indian J Crit Care Med. 2008;12(4):194–7.
3. Grillo HC, Donahue DM, Mathisen DJ, Wain JC, Wright CD. Postintubation tracheal stenosis: treatment and results. J Thorac Cardiovasc Surg. 1995;109:486–93.
4. Stauffer JL, Olson DE, Petty TL. Complications and consequences of endotracheal intubation and tracheotomy: a prospective study of 150 critically ill adult patients. Am J Med. 1981;70(1):65–76.
5. Brand-Saberi BE, Schafer T. Trachea: anatomy and physiology. Thorac Surg Clin. 2014;24(1):1–5.
6. Epstein SK. Late complications of tracheostomy. Respir Care. 2005;50:542–9.
7. Streitz JM, Shapshay SM. Airway injury after tracheostomy and endotracheal intubation. Sur Clin North Am. 1991;6:1211–29.
8. Brichet A, Verkindre C, Dupont J, Carlier ML, Darras J, Wurtz A, et al. Multidisciplinary approach to management of posintubation tracheal stenoses. Eur Respir J. 1999;13(4):888–93.

9. Spittle N, McCluskey A. Tracheal stenosis afer intubation. BMJ. 2000;321:1000–2.
10. Herth FJF. Clinical presentation, diagnostic evaluation, and management of central airway. Ed. UpToDate. Waltham, MA: UpToDate Inc. http://www.uptodate.com. Accessed Feb 2017.
11. Rumbak MJ, Walsh FW, Anderson WM, Rolfe MW, Solomon DA. Significant tracheal obstruction causing failure to wean in patients requiring prolonged mechanical ventilation: a forgotten complication of long-term mechanical ventilation. Chest. 1999;115(4):1092–5.
12. Sue RD, Susanto I. Long-term complications of artificial airways. Clin Chest Med. 2003;24(3): 457–71.
13. Divatia JV, Bhowmick K. Complications of endotracheal intubation and other airway management procedures. Indian J Anaesth. 2005;49(4):308–18.
14. Leigh JM, Maynard JP. Pressure on the tracheal mucosa from cuffed tubes. Br Med J. 1979;1:1173–4.
15. Majid A, Fernandez L, Fernandez-Bussy S, et al. Tracheobronchomalacia. Arch Bronconeumol. 2010;46:196–202.
16. Gelbard A, Francis DO, Sandulache VC, Simmons JC, Donovan D, Ongkasuwan J. Causes and consequences of adult laryngotracheal stenosis. Laryngoscope. 2015;125(5):1137–43.
17. Soltoski PR. Estenose laringitraqueal: doença ou descaso. Aferição da pressão do balão endotraqueal por palpação digital comparada à verificação da pressão com manômetro. 49f. Dissertação (Mestrado em Clínica Cirúrgica)—Setor de Ciências da Saúde. Universidade Federal do Paraná; 2008.
18. Flemming DC. Hazards of tracheal intubation. In: Orkin FK, Cooperman LH, editors. Complications in anaesthesiology. Philadelphia: JB Lippincott; 1983.
19. Grillo HC. Management of nonneoplastic diseases of the trachea. In: Shields TW, Cicero JL, Ponn RB, editors. General thoracic surgery. 5th ed. Philadelphia: Lippincott Williams and Wilkins; 2000. p. 885–97.
20. Sarper A, Ayten A, Eser I, Ozbudak O, Demircan A. Tracheal stenosis after tracheostomy or intubation: review with special regard to cause and management. Heart Inst J. 2005;32:154–8.
21. Sasaki CT, Horiuchi M, Koss N. Tracheostomy-related subglottic stenosis: bacteriologic pathogenesis. Laryngoscope. 1979;89:857–65.
22. Santos PM, Afrassiabi A, Weymuller EA Jr. Risk factors associated with prolonged intubation and laryngeal injury. Otolaryngol Head Neck Surg. 1994;111(4):453–9.
23. Maronian NC, Azadeh H, Waugh P, Hillel A. Association of laryngopharyngeal reflux disease and subglottic stenosis. Ann Otol Rhinol Laryngol. 2001;110:606–12.
24. Havas TE, Priestley J, Lowinger DS. A management strategy for vocal process granulomas. Laryngoscope. 1999;109(2 Pt 1):301–6.
25. Lanza DC, Parnes SM, Koltai PJ, Fortune JB. Early complications of airway management in head-injured patients. Laryngoscope. 1990;100(9):958–61.
26. Fernandez-Bussy S, Mahajan B, Folch E, Caviedes I, Guerrero J, Majid A. Tracheostomy tube placement early and late complications. J Bronchol Interv Pulmonol. 2015;22:357–64.
27. Mathias DB, Wedley JR. The effects of cuffed endotracheal tubes on the tracheal wall. Br J Anaesth. 1974;46:849–52.
28. Benjamin B, Kertesz T. Obstructive suprastomal granulation tissue following percutaneous tracheostomy. Anaesth Intensive Care. 1999;27:596–600.
29. Koitschev A, Graumueller S, Zenner HP, et al. Tracheal stenosis and obliteration above the tracheostoma after percutaneous dilational tracheostomy. Crit Care Med. 2003;31:1574–6.
30. Sarper A, Ayten A, Eser I, Demircan A, Isin E. Review of posttracheostomy and postintubation tracheal stenosis with special regard to etiology and treatment. Internet Journal of Thoracic and Cardiovascular Surgery. 2002;6(1).
31. Coelho MS. Influência da traqueostomia longitudinal e da traquestomia de ressecção sobre a estenose traqueal. 155f. Dissertação (Mestrado em Clínica Cirúrgica)—Setor de Ciências da Saúde. Universidade Federal do Paraná; 2001.
32. Westphal K, Byhahn C, Rinne T, Wilke HJ, Greinecker GW, Lischke V. Tracheostomy in cardiosurgical patients: surgical tracheostomy versus Ciaglia and Fantoni methods. Ann Thorac Surg. 1999;68:486–92.

33. Leinhardt DJ, Mughal M, Bowles B, Glew R, Kishen R, MacBeath J, Irving M. Appraisal of percutaneous tracheostomy. Br J Surg. 1992;79:255–8.
34. Hazard P, Jones C, Benitone J. Comparative clinical trial of standard operative tracheostomy with percutaneous tracheostomy. Crit Care Med. 1991;19(8):1018–24.
35. Wagner F, Nasseri R, Laucke U, Hetzer R. Percutaneous dilatational tracheostomy: results and long-term outcome of critically ill patients following cardiac surgery. Thorac Cardiovasc Surg. 1998;46(6):352–6.
36. Dulguerov P, Gysin C, Perneger TV, Chevrolet JC. Percutaneous or surgical tracheostomy: a meta-analysis. Crit Care Med. 1999;27(8):1617–25.
37. Paul A, Marelli D, Chiu RCJ, et al. Percutaneous endoscopic tracheostomy. Ann Thorac Surg. 1989;47:314–5.
38. Winkler WB, Karnik IR, Seelman O, et al. Bedside percutaneous dilational tracheostomy with endoscopic guidance: experience with 71 patients. Intensive Care Med. 1994;20:476–9.
39. Walz MK, Schmidt U. Tracheal lesion caused by percutaneous dilatational tracheostomy—a clinico-pathological study. Intensive Care Med. 1999;25:102–5.
40. Toursarkissian B, Zweng TN, Kearney PA, Pofahl WE, Johnson SB, Barker DE. Percutaneous dilational tracheostomy: report of 141 cases. Ann Thorac Surg. 1994;57:862–7.
41. Leonard RC, Lewis RH, Singh B, Heerden PV. Late outcome from percutaneous tracheostomy using the Portex kit. Chest. 1999;115:1070–5.
42. Choi YS, Chae YR. Effects of rotated endotracheal tube fixation method on unplanned extubation, oral mucosa and facial skin integrity in ICU patients. J Korean Acad Nurs. 2012;42:116–24.
43. Hyzy RC. Complications of the endotracheal tube following initial placement. Ed. UpToDate. Waltham, MA: UpToDate Inc. http://www.uptodate.com. Accessed Feb 2017.

Difficult Intubation: How to Avoid a Tracheostomy

Ronald Lima, Leonardo Vianna Salomão, and Pedro Rotava

Abbreviations

BURP	Backward, upward, rightward pressure
CPAP	Continuous positive airway pressure
LMA	Laryngeal mask airway

Introduction

A pair of small mirrors and sunlight were the only equipment used to perform the first laryngoscopy in 1848. Remarkably, this procedure was actually done not by a physician, but by a speech therapist. Another 30 years elapsed before the first endotracheal intubation [1]. Numerous devices have since been developed to improve airway management, from traditional laryngoscopes to fiberoptic bronchoscopes, laryngeal masks and, more recently, videolaryngoscopes.

Difficulty in airway management is a clinically important complication, which can lead to considerable morbidity and mortality. A significant proportion of airway complications occur in intensive care units and emergency departments, and are associated with suboptimal care [2]. To reduce the risk, knowledge, careful assessment, good planning, and judgment, as well as the use of a wide range of techniques and devices, are required. Randomized, controlled trials are unsuited for studying many aspects of difficult-airway management, and in many areas where such studies might be possible, they have not been done; consequently, practices vary according to local expertise [2].

R. Lima, M.D., Ph.D. • L.V. Salomão, M.D. (✉) • P. Rotava, M.D., M.Sc.
National Cancer Institute-INCA, Rio de Janeiro, RJ, Brazil
e-mail: ronielima1@gmail.com; leonardo.vianna@terra.com.br; pedrorotava@hotmail.com

T.P. de Farias (ed.), *Tracheostomy*, https://doi.org/10.1007/978-3-319-67867-2_20

Creating an emergency surgical airway is a rescue technique which, despite being a rare event, is often associated with a poor outcome. It results from failure to recognize airway red flags during assessment, or failure of bag mask ventilation at some point. It is a situation to be addressed immediately, and there are reports of attempts to create a surgical airway even before applying a rescue device such as a laryngeal mask airway. It is critical to bear in mind that, when other techniques fail and an emergency surgical airway is required, the procedure itself is not as harmful as the delay in performing it.

History

In the 19th century, diphtheria led to the death of many patients due to the pseudomembrane formed in the airway. Mortality reached 70% even when tracheostomies were performed. In 1858, Eugène Bouchut developed a small metal tube that passed through the characteristic laryngeal obstruction. The results were unsatisfactory but created an opportunity to develop a nonsurgical airway access. In 1878 the first elective endotracheal oral intubation was performed, by William Macewan. It was used in a patient with glottal edema that led to severe respiratory distress.

Two years later, Joseph P. O'Dwyer developed a thinner tube than that of Bouchut. It had rounded edges, which allowed gentler and less traumatic placement and increased the rate of successful intubations. In 1889, a rubber tube, developed by Thomas Annandale, replaced the metal tubes. One of the hallmarks of a modern endotracheal tube, the inflatable cuff—designed to prevent air leakage and protect the lower from the upper airway and gastric secretions—was created in 1893 by Vitor Eisenmenger. Despite these improvements in endotracheal tubes, the placement was still done blindly. Another device needed to be added to the airway management arsenal, in order to allow direct visualization: the laryngoscope.

In 1895, Alfred Kirstein developed the first precursor of the modern laryngoscope. His apparatus was designed to create a straight pathway between the mouth and the trachea, where direct visualization and surgical treatment of the airway could be performed. After a few years, Chevalier Jackson developed a new laryngoscope, with a light source added to the blade, facilitating the procedure. Several other blades were developed, and in the early 1940s, Robert Miller developed the straight blade and Robert Macintosh developed the classic and very popular curved blade. Both are currently and widely used, with minor variations [3, 4]. Endotracheal oral intubation using direct laryngoscopy has evolved and been aided by innumerable technological improvements through the years. To this day, it remains the method that is most often used to place an advanced airway.

The next outstanding device to be developed for airway management was the laryngeal mask airway, invented in the 1980s by Archie Brain. Although it does not provide as complete a seal of the lower from the upper airway and gastric secretions as the endotracheal tube, it is very practical and has become widely used. By 1995, it was included in the American Society of Anesthesiologists' Difficult-Airway Algorithm, due to its simple and rapid placement technique. The laryngeal mask can definitely be a life-saving device in some situations. It is an ever present part of the airway management arsenal.

Recent years have seen exceptional developments of optical devices and videolaryngoscopes. They can not only provide better visualization of the larynx, but also increase the success rate of endotracheal intubations in patients with a difficult airway.

Airway Assessment

The purpose of airway assessment is to identify personal features that can lead to failed direct laryngoscopy and/or bag mask ventilation. This consists of taking a history and performing a careful physical examination. Imaging is valuable but may not be feasible for routine assessment. A correct assessment helps to anticipate a difficult airway, whether in an elective or urgent situation, thus considerably decreasing the possibility of needing an emergency surgical airway.

Medical History

The medical history may reveal important information such as snoring, use of a continuous positive airway pressure (CPAP) machine for sleep, or even a formal diagnosis of obstructive sleep apnea, which are all part of the same spectrum and require particular caution. A history of previous airway difficulty, whether in a verbal or written report, should lead to a high degree of suspicion of true airway difficulty.

The presence and nature of any difficult airway should be well documented and notified to the patient. The documentation must include a description of the difficulty, how it was managed, and the number and duration of attempts. Patients, especially the elderly, can use a difficult-airway bracelet, indicating the need for an expert in the event of an emergency situation.

Physical Examination

There are no clinical tests or signals that lead to a high degree of sensitivity and specificity in the detection of a difficult airway, so a combination of anatomical features and tests is used. Mouth opening must be assessed and the interincisor distance measured. Then, the Mallampati classification is commonly applied. This consists of the visibility of the pharyngeal structures while the patient is sitting up with the head in a neutral position, the mouth open, and the tongue fully protracted (Fig. 1). Prognathic inability of the mandible has also been associated with difficult intubation, and an upper lip bite test has been proposed (prognathic inability evidenced by the inability of the lower incisors to touch the upper lip). Measuring the thyromental distance, or the distance between the chin and the

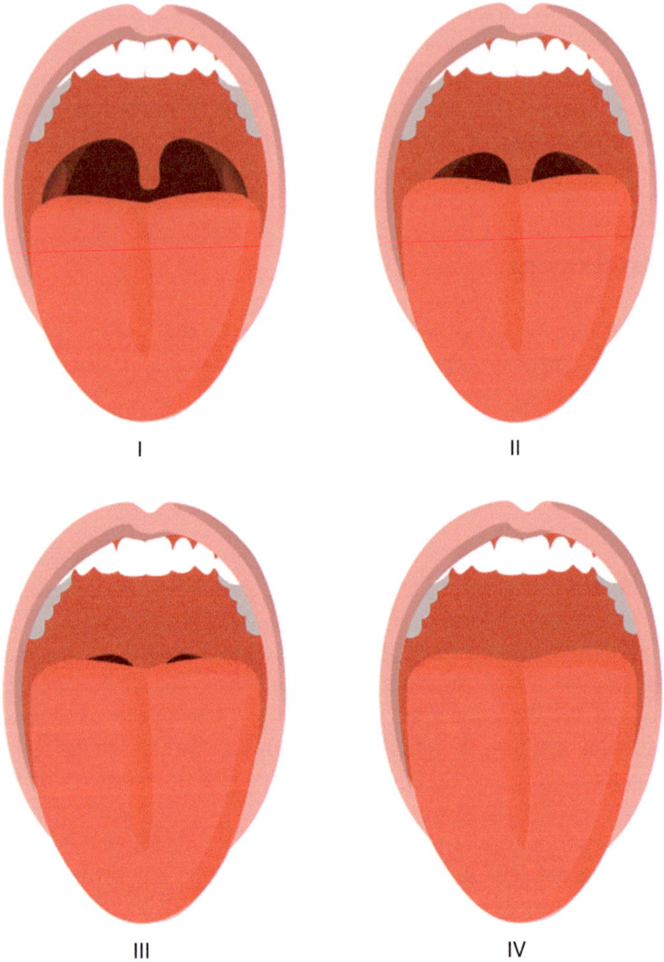

Fig. 1 Mallampati classification. Class I: soft palate, uvula, fauces, and tonsillar pillars visible; Class II: soft palate, uvula, and fauces visible; Class III: only base of the uvula visible; Class IV: uvula not visible [6]

thyroid cartilage, is also useful. Short distances can indicate possible difficulties in direct laryngeal visualization. The neck range of motion is also an indicator to be assessed. The capacity for hyperextending the head is critical for direct laryngoscopy. A mouth opening of less than 3 cm, low Mallampati classification score, thyromental distances less than three fingerbreadths, and restricted neck motion are all associated with difficult intubations. Of note, the circumference of the neck should be measured in obese patients. A value above 43 cm also indicates difficulty in airway management [5]. Special care should be taken if anatomical changes are present, such as macroglossia, acromegaly, or head and neck neoplasms. All of these have the potential to distort the airway and impair visualization of the larynx.

Table 1 Recommended set of devices to manage a difficult airway

Device	Comments
Facial mask	Three different sizes
Oropharyngeal airway	Three different sizes
Nasopharyngeal airway	Three different sizes
Laryngeal mask	Three different sizes each of two different types
Endotracheal tube	Two of each size
Laryngoscope	Sizes 3, 4, and 5 of Macintosh and Miller blades Hinged-tip blades, sizes 3 and 4
Endotracheal tube introducers	Malleable stylet and bougie
Magill forceps	–
Videolaryngoscope	Two different sizes of blades
Percutaneous cricothyrotomy kit	Two kits
Fiberoptic bronchoscope	–

It is of the utmost importance not only to evaluate the probability of a difficult endotracheal intubation but also to anticipate difficult bag mask ventilation. Endotracheal intubation can be postponed until a more advanced device or another expert is available; however, impossibility of ventilation can precipitate the need for a surgical airway. Predictors of difficult face mask ventilation are the presence of a beard, absence of teeth, a Mallampati classification score of III or IV, high body mass index, prognathic inability, and history of obstructive sleep apnea [7, 8].

Devices for Airway Management

A set of devices is recommended to be available wherever there is the possibility of difficult-airway management (Table 1). These devices should be of good quality, checked regularly, stored in an easily accessed location, and easily identifiable. An inadequate laryngoscope blade, as well as the absence of other accessories, can make the difference between successful endotracheal intubation and the need for a surgical airway.

Preoxygenation

In a patient breathing room air, hemoglobin saturation will fall below 90% after 45–60 s of apnea. Maximizing oxygen stores in advance of the onset of apnea prolongs the period before hypoxia sets in and increases the safety of airway management. Preoxygenation increases the oxygen reserve in the lungs and is achieved by having the patient breathe 100% oxygen from a close-fitting face mask. The term denitrogenation may also be used, as nitrogen in the lungs is replaced by oxygen with the maneuver [9].

Various preoxygenation techniques have been advocated, such as tidal breathing of 100% oxygen for 35 min, or eight deep vital capacity breaths of 100% oxygen within 60 s. A sufficient fresh gas flow (10–12 L/min) of oxygen must be provided to prevent rebreathing [10].

Patients with reduced functional residual capacity and with pulmonary shunt disorder have reduced oxygen storage in the lungs and consequently a shorter apnea interval before hypoxia. Some maneuvers, such as a head-up position (about 30 degrees), and application of positive end-expiratory pressure may further improve oxygenation in these clinical situations [11]. Adequate preoxygenation is recommended before any attempt at airway management, especially when bag mask ventilation is contraindicated or predicted to be difficult [9].

Bag Mask Ventilation

Bag mask ventilation is the least invasive type of airway management and can be done in any emergency situation. It appears to be simple but actually requires some previous training and skill acquisition. Face masks are designed to seal the mouth and nose area, while the provider must constantly check for air leakage and airway obstruction. The mask must be an appropriate size for the patient and have a low-pressure cushion around the edge to facilitate the seal. A transparent mask is ideal for prompt identification of any secretions in the upper airway and observation of the humidified gas exhaled with an unobstructed airway. The correct way to hold the mask in place is to support the mask with the thumb and index finger, while stabilizing the mandible with the other fingers (Fig. 2). Care must be taken not to press the soft tissue under the mandible, which may cause obstruction of the upper airway.

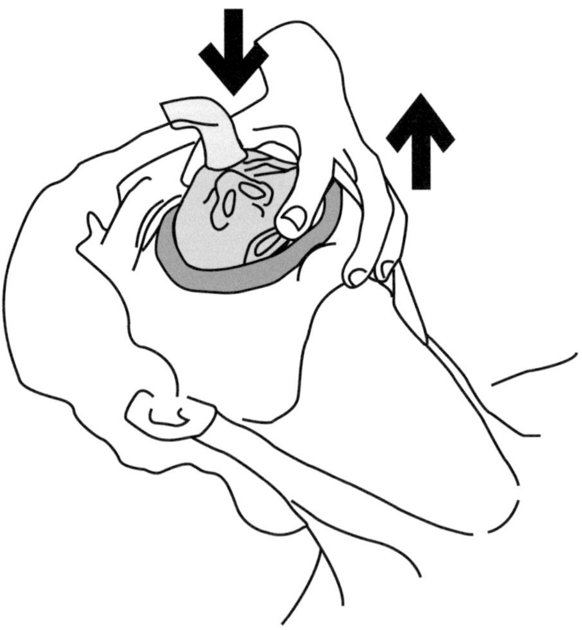

Fig. 2 Correct holding position for bag mask ventilation

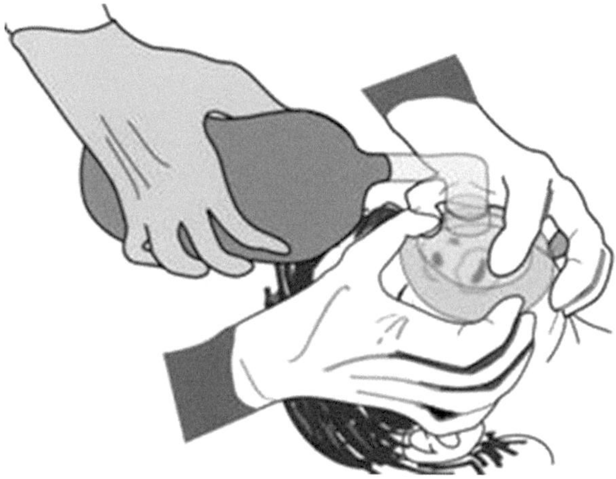

Fig. 3 Two-person technique for bag mask ventilation

Airway obstruction with spontaneous ventilation is characterized by noisy respiration, with inward movement of the upper chest and outward movement of the lower chest and abdomen. In controlled ventilation, airway obstruction will prevent chest movements as the reservoir bag is compressed, and much of the air will leak out by the face mask. Head extension and jaw thrust are maneuvers that open the pharyngeal soft tissues and can maintain adequate ventilation. An extra pair of hands can be especially helpful. A two-person technique is of proven value in patients for whom the conventional technique is proving to be less effective. Using this technique, the more experienced person should maintain the head extension, bimanual jaw thrust, and mask seal, while an assistant squeezes the bag (Fig. 3).

An oropharyngeal or nasopharyngeal airway can be used if the airway obstruction is not improved with head extension and jaw thrust. These devices displace the tongue from the soft tissues of the pharynx, creating a passage for the air. It is critical to use the correct size, since the device must be well positioned to be effective. The oropharyngeal airway is normally the first choice, and it should only be inserted when pharyngeal and laryngeal reflexes are depressed, to minimize the risk of coughing, vomiting, or laryngospasm. To ensure proper size selection, the airway should be placed against the side of the patient's face; with the flange of the airway at the corner of the mouth, the tip should reach the angle of the patient's mandible (Fig. 4). Lesions in the mouth or a cleft palate are contraindications to the oropharyngeal airway.

The nasopharyngeal airway can be used in awake patients or in those with upper airway reflexes present. Safe placement of the nasopharyngeal airway requires the device to be well lubricated with a water-soluble gel. Contraindications to the nasopharyngeal airway include facial traumas, skull base fractures, and coagulopathy (due to increased risk of epistaxis).

Fig. 4 Procedure for measuring the proper size of the oropharyngeal airway

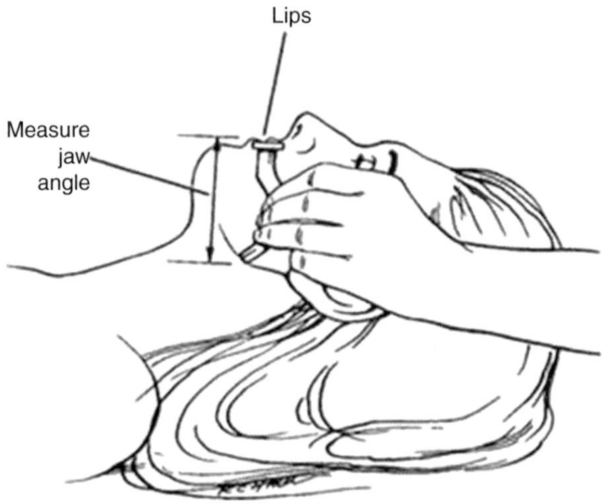

Direct Laryngoscopy

Laringoscopy Technique

The principle behind direct laryngoscopy is to manipulate the head, the neck, and the mandible, positioning a laryngoscope in the oral cavity and thus creating a direct visualization line between the larynx and the operator. For many decades, the classical theory has been that there are three axes (the first in the mouth, the second in the pharynx, and the third in the larynx), which need to be aligned in order to obtain an adequate view (Fig. 5). A pillow or roll underneath the occipital bone and hyperextension of the head (the sniffing position) would help to align the three axes [3]. This was challenged in 2001 by Adnet et al. Magnetic resonance images showed that the sniffing position does not align these axes. In fact, it is anatomically impossible to do so in healthy nonanesthetized subjects [12]. In 2011, Greenland et al. described another anatomical theory—the two-curve theory—that explains the observation of the vocal cord visualization in direct laryngoscopy: the first curve arcs along the tongue, while the second curve arcs along the larynx into the trachea, with the confluence point being the laryngeal vestibule. Rectification of these curves would allow observation of the vocal cords [13].

The technique requires a proper sniffing position. The laryngoscope blade is inserted into the right side of the mouth, displacing the tongue to the left, thus creating a pathway on the right. The blade is advanced until it is adequately placed into the vallecula or below the epiglottis (according to the type of blade chosen). The operator then pulls the blade in the direction of the laryngoscope handle, exposing the glottic aperture. The endotracheal tube is inserted using the right hand, by the right side of the mouth (Fig. 6).

Although it sounds straightforward, direct laryngoscopy requires practice in order to acquire the appropriate skills. The evidence is conflicting on how long it takes for the health care provider to master it. The vast majority of endotracheal

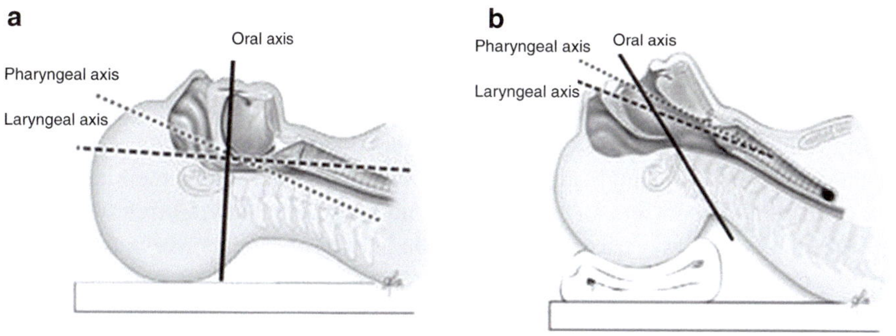

Fig. 5 Airway axes (oral, pharyngeal and laryngeal) and alignment during (**a**) normal and (**b**) sniffing position

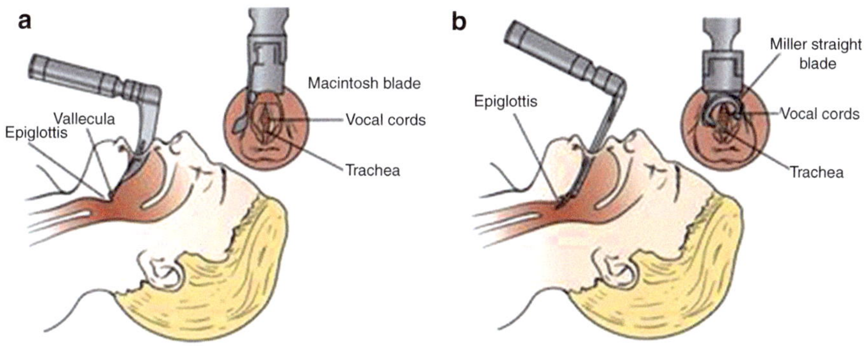

Fig. 6 Laryngoscope positioning in the airway according to blade selection (**a**) McIntosh or (**b**) Miller

intubations are performed electively in operating rooms; however, the most complex cases where skills are crucial occur in emergency situations. These are usually more challenging and harder to assess, and the time to perform the intubation is usually very short. In elective cases, probably more than 50 endotracheal intubations are necessary to eventually achieve a success rate above 90% [14]. Success rates during emergency situations will probably be higher if providers have performed at least this number of intubations in elective cases.

Laryngoscope Design

Since the earliest laryngoscope was invented, several designs have been proposed, some of which are commercially available. Older-generation laryngoscopes had a light bulb at the tip of the blade, whereas the newer generations have the light source at the handle and a fiberoptic bundle on the blade to transmit the light to its tip. The laryngoscope handle contains the batteries to power the light source, and they differ in size, diameter, and the type of batteries used (rechargeable or nonrechargeable). Small-diameter laryngoscopes require more delicate manipulation and are indicated for pediatric patients. Short handles can be more appropriate for morbidly obese patients, where there is little room for maneuvering. Personal preferences also play a role.

Although many different designs of blades are available, those most often used are the curved Macintosh blade and the straight Miller blade. Both are commercially available in different sizes. The main functional difference between them is that the Miller is a straight blade, placed below the epiglottis, while the McIntosh is a curved blade that fits into the vallecula, just above the epiglottis. Currently, straight blades are not routinely used, but they can be helpful in patients with a floppy epiglottis, especially small children. The different sizes of blades range from size 0, designed for neonates, to size 5, designed for large adults (Fig. 7). A variation of the traditional curved blade is the McCoy blade with a hinged tip. This blade allows additional lifting of the epiglottis, which can provide extra help, improving the laryngeal view in the case of a difficult airway (Fig. 8).

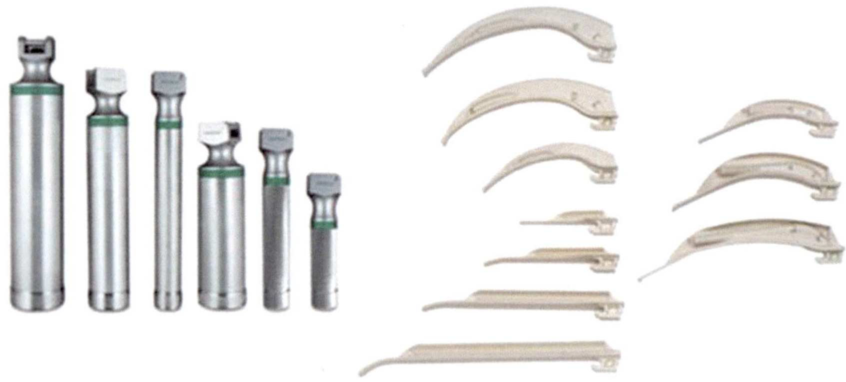

Fig. 7 Laryngoscope handle and blades. Straight blades (Miller) and curved blades (Macintosh) are shown in different sizes

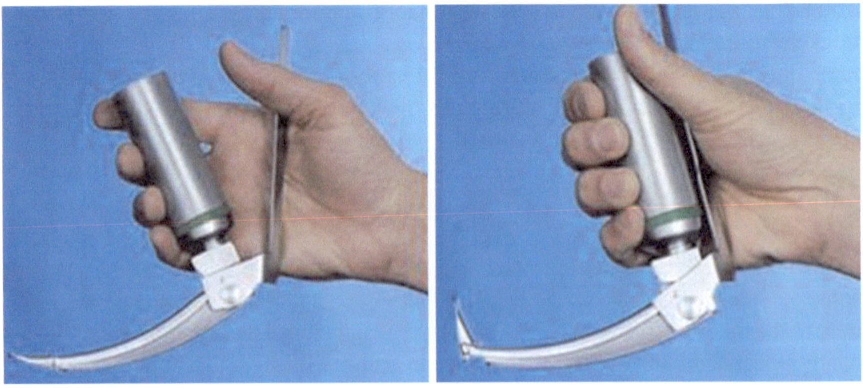

Fig. 8 Curved blade with hinged tip (McCoy)

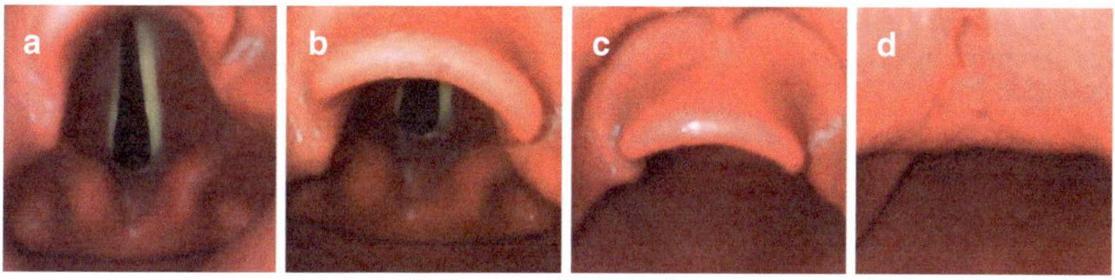

Fig. 9 Cormack–Lehane grade view. (**a**) Cormack I, (**b**) Cormack II, (**c**) Cormack III, (**d**) Cormack IV. Reproduced with permission from Daedalus Enterprises, Inc. [15]

The Cormack–Lehane Grade View

In order to classify the actual view of the larynx obtained by the operator, Cormack and Lehane described a scoring system with four grades [16]. Grade 1 is a visualization of the entire glottic aperture, grade 2 is a visualization only of the posterior part of the glottic aperture, grade 3 is a visualization of the epiglottis only, and grade 4 is a visualization of the soft palate only. This classification is important not only to help the operator in the decision-making process in the management of a difficult airway, but also for documentation (Fig. 9).

Adjuncts to Direct Laryngoscopy

In the event of an unanticipated difficult airway, different procedures and devices have been described that can lead to a successful endotracheal intubation. The backward, upward, rightward pressure (BURP) maneuver, initially described only as backward pressure, was reported to decrease the incidence of failed intubation from 9.6 to 1.3%. Later, Knill et al. added the other directions [17]. Commonly, the operator executes the maneuver with the right hand while performing the laryngoscopy with the left hand, to check the final Cormack view. Next, an assistant executes the maneuver, freeing the right hand of the operator. This procedure has been validated, improving Cormack–Lehane views and causing no complications, when performed in 630 patients [18].

The bougie is a device that can help in direct laryngoscopy. It was created by Robert Macintosh, the inventor of the curved blades, and was designed to overcome a common issue in difficult intubations: that the tube can sometimes block the laryngeal view. Since the bougie is slender, flexible, and easily manipulated, it can be placed into the trachea first and used as a guide to thread the tube (Fig. 10). Evidence comparing bougie-assisted intubations with stylet-loaded tubes is controversial. There may be a marginal advantage in using it when analyzing a large group of patients. It can be useful in properly selected cases [19].

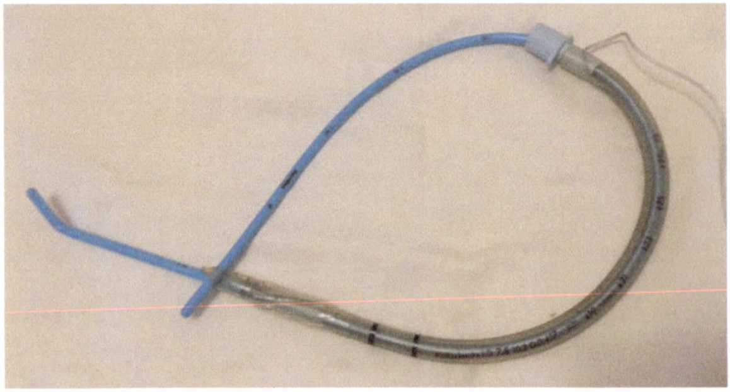

Fig. 10 Bougie loaded tube, prepared for intubation

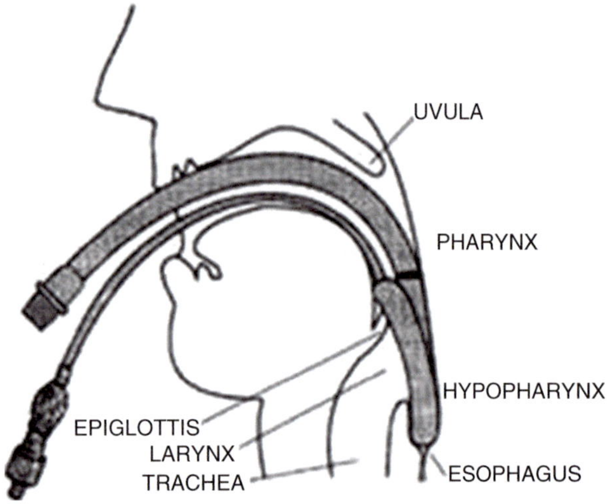

Fig. 11 Laryngeal mask in place

Laryngeal Mask

The laryngeal mask airway (LMA) was initially designed as a method to allow more effective ventilation and reduce the morbidity related to tracheal intubation. However, it had an important clinical impact and since 1995 has been included in difficult-airway algorithms. LMAs consist of a tube attached to a pneumatic cushion, which adapts to the supraglottic structures (Fig. 11). It is inserted blindly, and the quality of the ventilation is tested afterward. The provider needs to bag and carefully seek air leaks that will compromise ventilation.

Several models are available (Fig. 12). Second-generation devices incorporate recent improvements such as a gastric aspiration channel, an integrated bite block, and the ability to tolerate increased ventilatory pressure. Some studies suggest abandoning the use of first-generation models and adoption of second-generation versions as the first-choice LMAs [20].

Compared with endotracheal intubation, the LMA allows greater hemodynamic stability, less alteration of intracranial and intraocular pressure, and lower incidence of cough and pharyngeal pain. The basic skills for insertion of the laryngeal mask are acquired more rapidly than those of face mask ventilation or direct laryngoscopy [21–23].

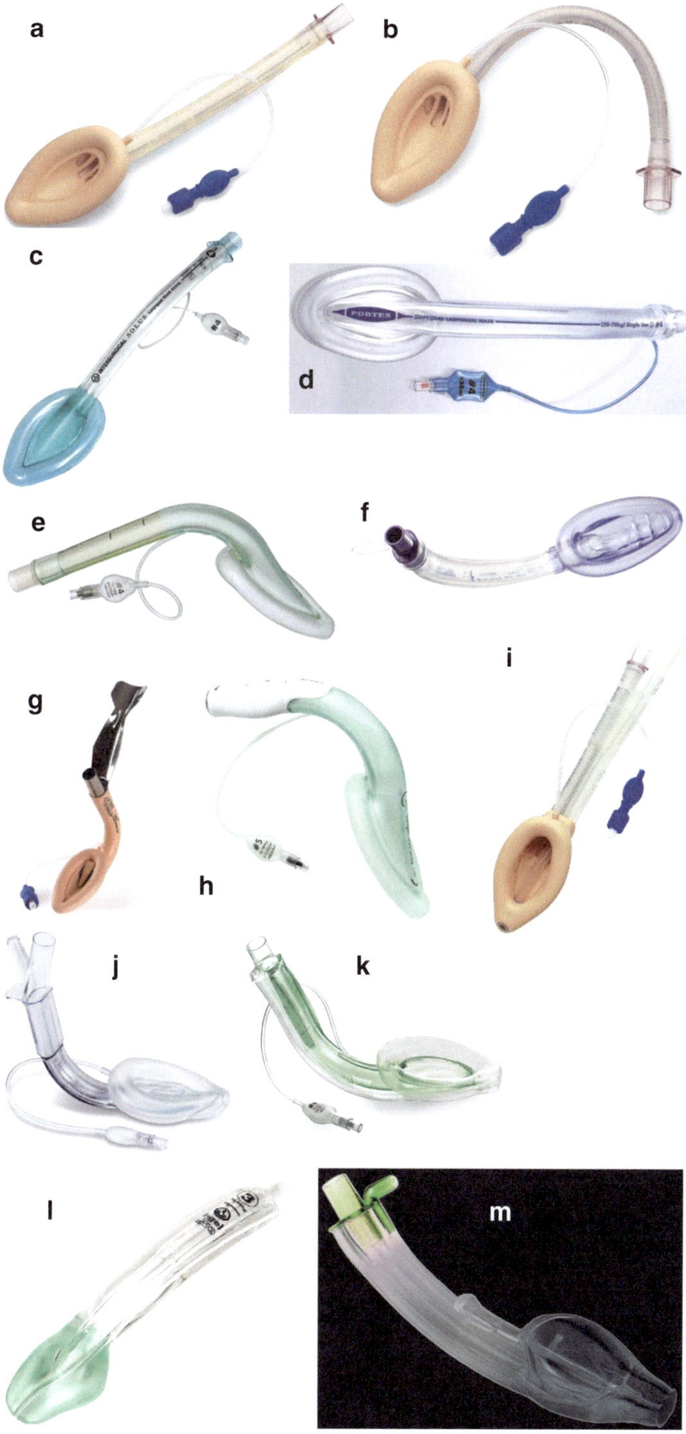

Fig. 12 Main commercially available laryngeal masks. First-generation: (**a**) LMA Classic, (**b**) LMA Flexible, (**c**) LM Solus, (**d**) LM Portex Soft Seal, (**e**) LM AuraOnce, (**f**) Air-Q intubating laryngeal airway, (**g**) LMA Fastrach, (**h**) LM Aura-i. Second-generation: (**i**) ProSeal LMA, (**j**) Supreme LMA, (**k**) AuraGain LM, (**l**) i-gel, (**m**) Baska mask

Insertion Technique

Several techniques for insertion of the laryngeal mask have been described; the most popular was described by its inventor, Archie Brain (Fig. 13). The size of the mask should be chosen according to the patient's weight (Table 2).

When correctly positioned, the mask surrounds the larynx and its distal tip is located in the upper esophageal sphincter. An adequate anesthetic depth should be obtained before attempting insertion, to avoid reflexes such as coughing, choking, laryngospasm, or even biting the finger of the provider. The technique is to slide the device along the soft palate and posterior wall of the pharynx, guiding with the finger, until an increase in resistance is observed. At this time, the mask is inflated, with a pressure of not more than 60 cm H_2O, and is coupled to the ventilation circuit. There may be a slight retrocession of the mask with insufflation, which indicates correct positioning. The adaptation of the mask is initially tested with light

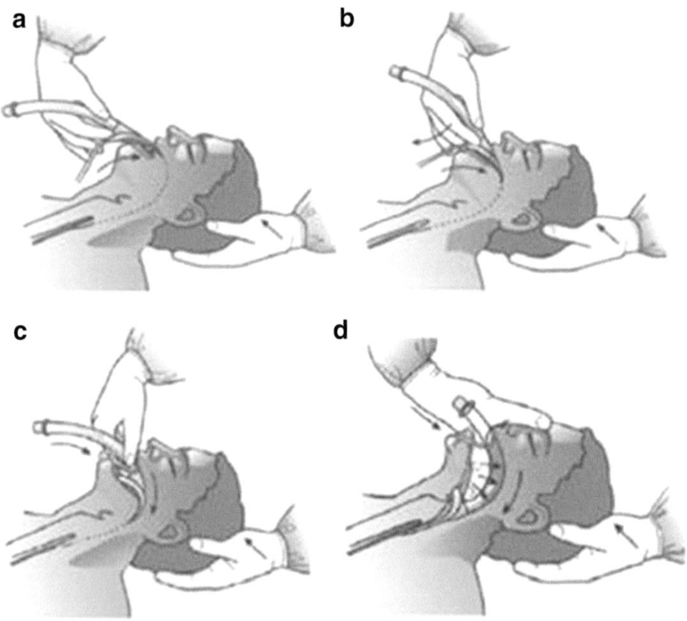

Fig. 13 Classic technique for insertion of a laryngeal mask device. With the neck flexed and the head extended by pushing the head from behind with one hand, the laryngeal mask airway (LMA) is inserted into the mouth with the other hand (**a**). The inserting hand is positioned like a pen, with the index finger placed at the junction of the cuff and the tube. The LMA tip is pushed up against the hard palate after verification that it is lying flat against the palate and that the tip is not folded over. Using the index finger, the mask is pushed into the patient's mouth, still maintaining pressure against the palate (**b**). As the mask moves in, the index finger maintains pressure against the posterior pharyngeal wall to avoid the epiglottis (**c**). The index finger is fully inside the mouth at the end of insertion (**d**). The other hand holds the LMA while the inserting finger is removed from the mouth. The cuff is inflated without holding the tube, permitting the device to position itself correctly

Table 2 Laryngeal mask size according to patient weight

Laryngeal mask size	Patient	Weight (kg)
1	Infants	<5
1.5	Infants	5–10
2	Children	10–20
2.5	Children	20–30
3	Children and young adults	30–50
4	Adults	50–70
5	Adults	>70

manual ventilation by observing the thoracic expansion, in addition to hearing sounds that indicate a leak or obstruction to the passage of air. Second-generation masks support airway pressures up to 37 cm H_2O [24].

Difficulties of insertion occur in up to 4.5% of cases. Head extension, protrusion of the mandible, and tongue traction may help. Factors that impair the efficiency of laryngeal mask ventilation include inadequate positioning, increased airway resistance, and reduced lung compliance. In the event of ineffective ventilation, one can attempt to reinsert the same mask or one of a different size. Small leaks that do not compromise ventilation can be tolerated, especially in emergency situations.

Role of the Laryngeal Mask Airway in Airway Management

The LMA is used in several clinical situations and has proved very useful in airway management. It has played an important role in difficult-airway algorithms, especially in "cannot intubate, cannot ventilate" situations. The main issues are that, even when well fitted, it does not provide a reliable airway seal and it is not recommended for long-term mechanical ventilation. In these cases, it acts as a rescue device until the patient can be awakened and intubated or, if necessary, a surgical airway can be obtained.

LMAs may be used to facilitate tracheal intubation, and the typical scenario in which this technique is useful is when an LMA has been placed as a rescue device due to failed direct laryngoscopy or failed intubation. It may be used for blind or fiberoptic bronchoscope-guided methods to aid intubation. A specific advantage of this technique is the ability to continue ventilating and anesthetizing the patient through the LMA until a conventional endotracheal intubation is performed. It is advisable to use fiberoptic bronchoscope-guided techniques to ensure greater success of tracheal intubation through an LMA.

Complications and Contraindications

The LMA offers less protection than the endotracheal tube against gastric aspiration. These devices are not recommended for patients at greater risk for

Fig. 14 Combitube in place

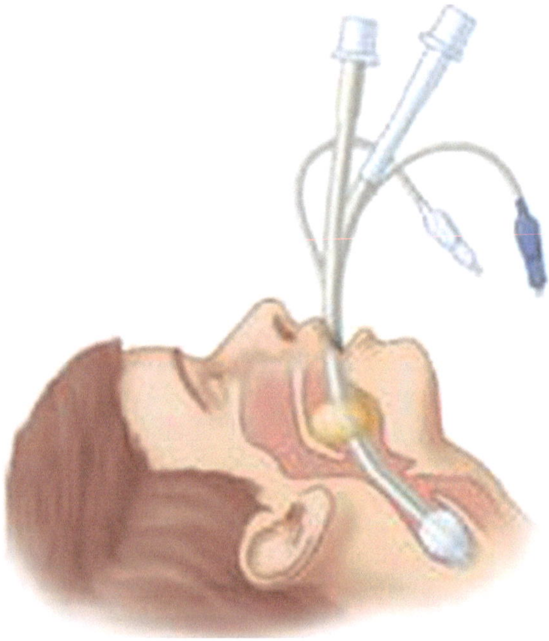

regurgitation or vomiting. Device failure related to inadequate ventilation is more likely to occur in patients with increased intrathoracic pressures, such as those with obesity or obstructive airway disease. Traumatic injuries can happen if positioning proves to be challenging, and upper airway bleeding and swelling can degenerate into a "cannot intubate, cannot ventilate" situation. In fact, a sore throat is a common complication after multiple placement attempts or if high cuff pressure is used.

Other Supraglottic Devices

Other less used supraglottic devices are available, including the Combitube and the laryngeal tube. The Combitube consists of a double-lumen tube with two cuffs. The insufflation of the distal cuff seals the esophagus while the proximal cuff closes the oropharynx. Its insertion is performed blindly, allowing adequate ventilation whether it is positioned in the esophagus or in the larynx (Fig. 14). It has been used in prehospital care.

The laryngeal tube is a single-lumen device in which both cuffs are insufflated from a single inflation line. Holes in the tube between the proximal seal and the distal cuffs deliver the fresh gas mixture to the laryngopharynx. Placement is rapid and it has been successfully used in "cannot intubate, cannot ventilate" situations and in LMA failure.

Videolaryngoscopes

Advances in fiberoptic and video technologies have led to the development of devices that facilitate the indirect visualization of the larynx, with minimal mouth opening and head extension. The indirect image of the larynx by these devices can be obtained in two ways: (1) through a fiberoptic bundle or a system of prisms to a lens or a video system; or (2) through a video camera that transmits a digital image to a display. The display can be integrated into the device or used as a stand-alone monitor.

The various models have different blade designs: (1) a traditional blade; (2) a nonchanneled angulated blade; or (3) a channeled angulated blade. The traditional blade devices are inserted using the direct laryngoscopy technique, while the other two designs require a slightly different technique. The blade is introduced on the midline of the oral cavity until its tip reaches the vallecula. The tongue can be pulled to facilitate the insertion of the blade. There is no need for the sniffing position, which is advantageous in patients with cervical spine injuries or limited neck extension. When in place, the blade can be pulled up for further view improvement. The nonchanneled blades require a stylet with a "hockey stick" curvature to be used to guide the tube. Once the blade is positioned, the next step is placing the tip of the tube in the oropharynx under direct visualization. Failure to do so can lead to accidental tearing or perforation of the tonsil pillars, causing profuse bleeding. The channeled blades have a more bulky structure which can hinder their insertion into small-opening mouths. In a simulated difficult-airway scenario (patients with a cervical collar), nonchanneled devices had a higher rate of successful airway management in the first attempt [25]. Glottic visualization does not always equate to successful endotracheal intubation.

Videolaryngoscopes have not been used only in emergency difficult-airway situations but also in routine airway management [26], as they allow a higher probability of successful intubations in unexpectedly difficult airways. This probability can range from 94% to 99% [27, 28]. Some authors have advocated the use of videolaryngoscopes as the new standard of care [29]. We do not suggest routine use of videolaryngoscopes, since it may lead to loss of the skills required for direct laryngoscopy. Videolaryngoscopes are not fail proof. The presence of secretion or blood in the upper airway may hinder the use of these devices. Failure to perform an optimal direct laryngoscopy prevents correct evaluation of patients, increasing the frequency of unsuccessful intubations. Insisting on direct laryngoscopy, however, can be harmful, since multiple attempts can lead to airway trauma and edema, making ventilation impossible. In these cases, videolaryngoscopy is highly recommended. We comment below on some of the commonly used devices.

Truview

The Truview (Truphatek, Netanya, Israel) can be considered a first-generation videolaryngoscope. It resembles a common laryngoscope with a handle and a Macintosh-design blade. The blade, however, contains a lens that allows a 45-degree view at its

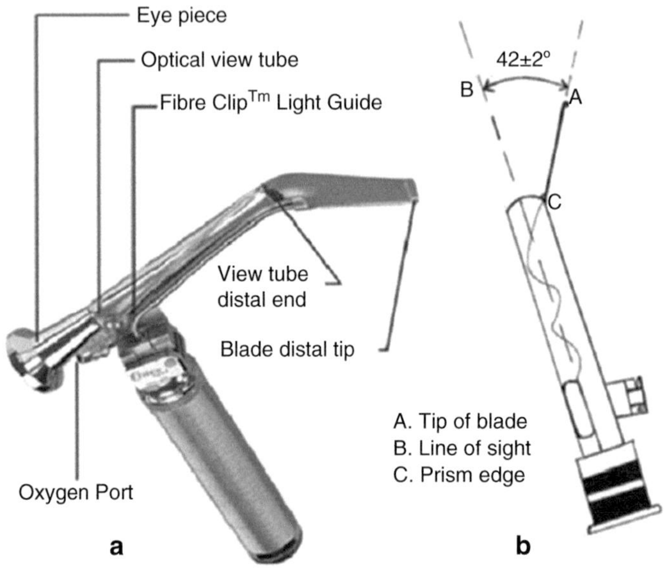

Fig. 15 Truview videolaryngoscope. (**a**) Truview handle and blades. (**b**) True view angle of view. Reproduced under Creative Commons Attribution License from [30]

tip (Fig. 15). The eyepiece of the lens can be connected to a video camera, but it can also be used without electronic equipment. It has the advantage of being more robust, with less chance of trouble because of electronic malfunction. The Truview can be used in patients with very small mouth openings. A bougie or a tube stylet is needed to guide the tube [30].

GlideScope

The GlideScope (Verathon, Seattle, WA, USA) is a flexible camera that is introduced into a plastic nonchanneled blade (Fig. 16). It has a high-resolution display, which can record the procedure. It is recommended to load the tube with a stylet matching the angulated profile of the blade.

C-MAC

The C-MAC (Karl Stortz, Tuttlingen, Germany) has a traditional blade design. A more angulated blade (D-blade) has been released recently, for more difficult intubation situations (Fig. 17). It has a display that is connected to the handle by a cable. The newer models have an integrated display at the handle, which facilitates operator use.

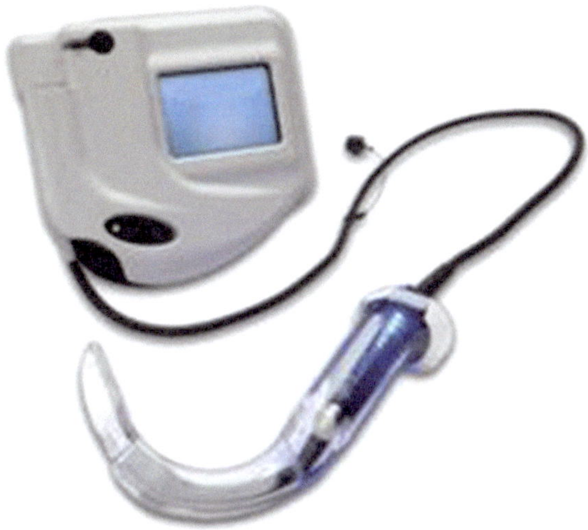

Fig. 16 GlideScope videolaryngoscope

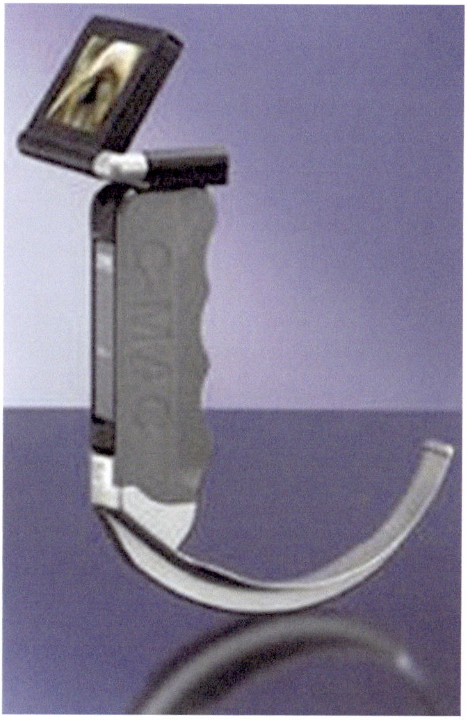

Fig. 17 C-MAC videolaryngoscope

McGrath

The McGrath (Aircraft Medical, Edinburgh, UK) has a traditional blade design, which allows direct or indirect laryngoscopy, by an integrated display. It has a narrower and more delicate blade, which facilitates intubation in patients with small mouths (Fig. 18).

King Vision

The King Vision (King Systems, Noblesville, IN, USA) has the advantage of offering two styles of blades: it can be used with nonchanneled or channeled angled blades. It has an integrated display (Fig. 19). The nonchanneled blade is easier to insert but requires the use of a stylet or bougie.

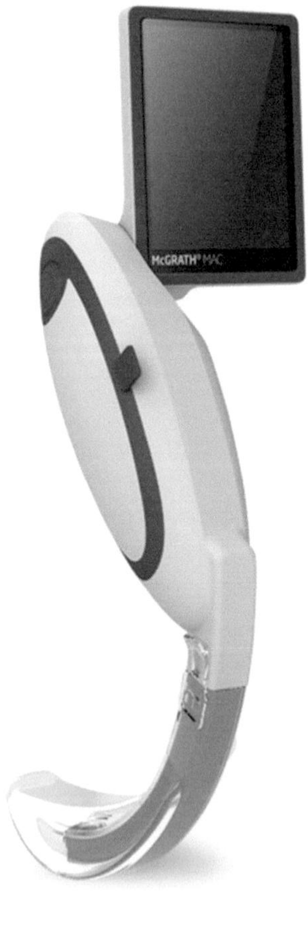

Fig. 18 McGrath videolaryngoscope

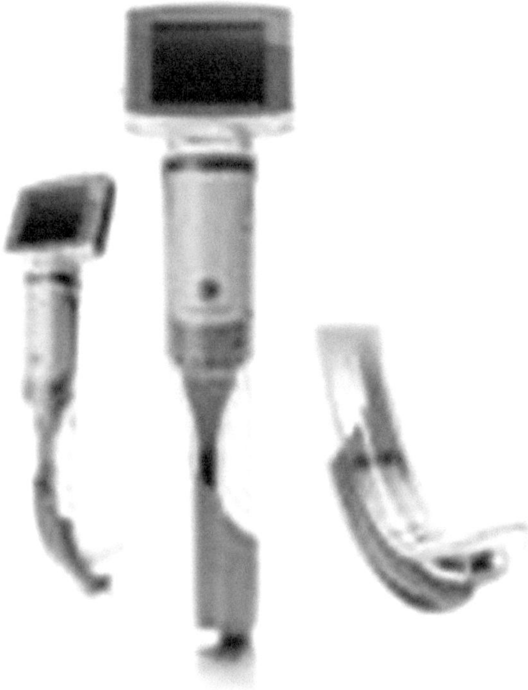

Fig. 19 King Vision videolaryngoscope

VividTrac

The VividTrac (Vivid Medical, Palo Alto, CA, USA) is a channeled angled-blade device. It has a USB cable, which plugs into a mobile or tablet device (Fig. 20). It has a low price compared to other videolaryngoscopes. It offers great visualisualization because it uses the full HD screen of the device (cellphone, tablet or computer).

Airtraq

The Airtraq SP (Prodol Meditec SA, Gueco, Spain) is a channeled angled-blade device, which has an integrated display (Fig. 21). It can also be used through direct visualization, which avoids the need for electronic components and can even be used in magnetic resonance rooms. It has a rapid learning curve and greater chance of successful airway management than direct laryngoscopy [31].

Fiberoptic Bronchoscope

The fiberoptic bronchoscope is the last-resort device for management of difficult airways but has some limitations. It consists of a flexible insertion cord with a working channel built in, fibers that conduct the light to the tip, and fibers that provide

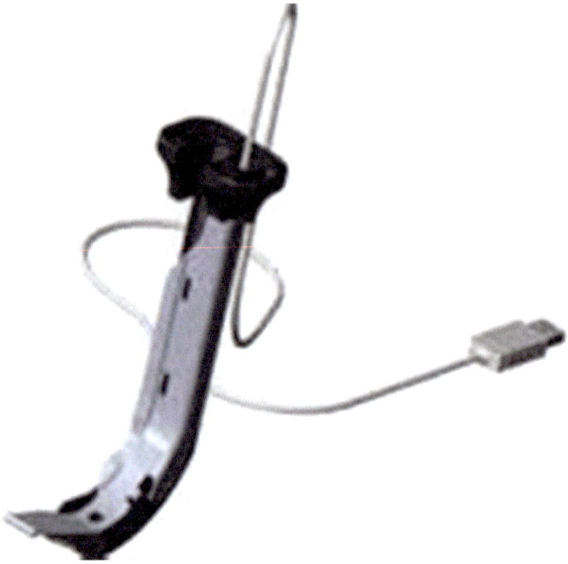

Fig. 20 VividTrac videolaryngoscope

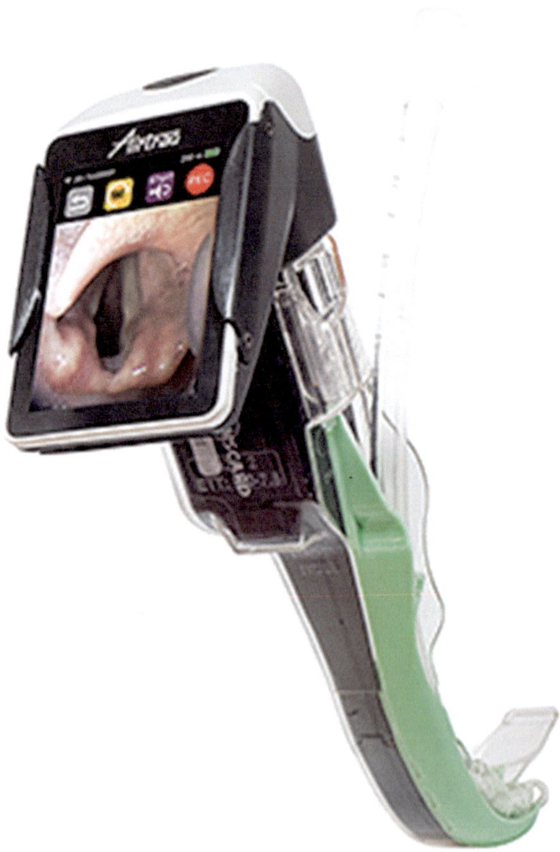

Fig. 21 Airtraq videolaryngoscope

Fig. 22 Ambu aScope 3

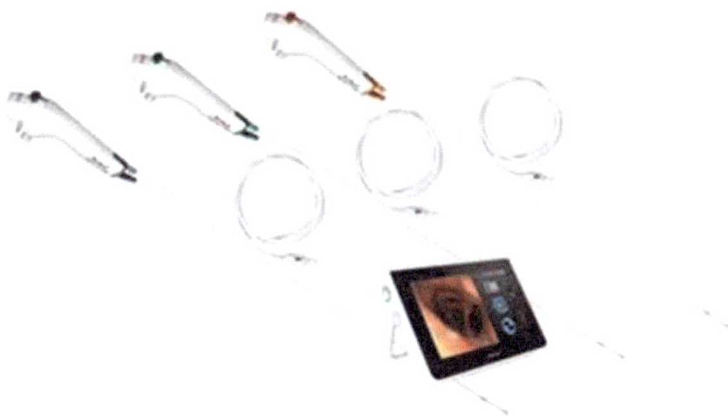

the image. It has a high cost of purchase and maintenance, and the fragile glass fibers require care. A bite block must be used when it is introduced orally. Due to its small diameter, it is possible to perform endotracheal intubations in patients with spontaneous ventilation, with minimal discomfort after topical anesthesia. It is not recommended to be used in patients under general anesthesia, because loss of tone in pharyngeal muscles makes it more difficult to visualize the larynx. The presence of excessive secretion or blood in the upper airway is also a difficulty with the use of the fiberoptic bronchoscope.

The Ambu aScope 3 (Ambu, Copenhagen, Denmark) is a device with the same functionality as the fiberoptic bronchoscope (Fig. 22). The lighting and visualization are electronically generated, which allows the device to be more resistant, portable, and affordable, since there are no fiberoptics. It is a disposable device.

Difficult-Airway Algorithms

A difficult airway can be caused by any clinical factor that complicates bag mask ventilation or endotracheal intubation, preventing proper endotracheal tube placement by experienced professionals. Difficult bag mask ventilation can be defined as impossible, inadequate, unstable, or requiring two providers to be effective. Difficult intubation is the need for more than three attempts at intubation, or a procedure that lasts longer than 10 min. The need for more than one specialist, or the need for blade changing or use of accessories, can also define a difficult intubation.

A difficult airway is not always predicted, so a strategy for the management of unanticipated difficulty is important. Several algorithms have been developed to provide a structured response to this life-threatening situation. The most widely used are the algorithms issued by the Difficult Airway Society [33] and by the American Society of Anesthesiologists [34]. Implementation of a standardized protocol has proved to significantly reduce the need for emergency surgical airway [32].

Difficult-Airway Algorithm from the Difficult Airway Society

This algorithm [33] has a simpler and more straightforward strategy for management of the airway. It does not go into details of different clinical situations such as an uncooperative patient or one with a full stomach. It is of great help in an emergency situation, when an unexpected difficulty is encountered (Fig. 23).

Plan A: It is of fundamental importance to correctly position the patient for endotracheal intubation. The appropriate equipment, such as a bougie and an oral airway or a nasopharyngeal airway, must be readily available. A videolaryngoscope must also be available and used if the attempts with a regular laryngoscope fail (the maximum number of attempts recommended is three). Adequate neuromuscular blockade must be done.

Plan B: If attempts at endotracheal intubation fail, it is recommended to place a supraglottic airway device. The guideline recommends second-generation devices and a maximum of three attempts (changing devices or size at each attempt). Different devices of different sizes must be available.

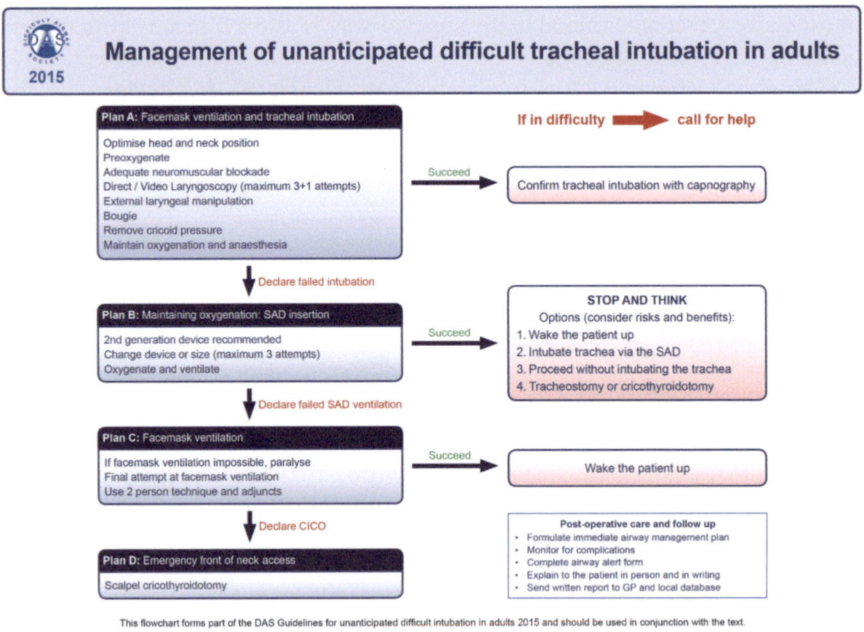

Fig. 23 Algorithm for unanticipated difficult tracheal intubation flowchart from the Difficult Airway Society (it includes all the information of the difficult airway algorithm of DAS) Reproduced from [33]

Plan C: If endotracheal intubation and ventilation through a supraglottic airway device fails, face mask ventilation must be attempted. The guideline recommends optimal positioning of the patient, the use of accessories (oral or nasopharyngeal airway), and a two-person technique.

Plan D: This envisions a situation of difficult endotracheal intubation and difficult face mask ventilation—a life-threatening scenario. No further attempts with the previous plans should be made. A cricothyroidotomy must be performed without delay.

Difficult-Airway Algorithm from the American Society of Anesthesiologists

The difficult-airway algorithm issued by the American Society of Anesthesiologists [34] includes more details and clinical scenarios, which may not be optimal for use by inexperienced professionals in an emergency situation. However, it must be studied by anyone who might possibly have to manage a difficult airway (Fig. 24).

The algorithm emphasizes that oxygenation is more important than intubation. Adequate preoxygenation must be offered to allow a longer apnea time before hemoglobin desaturation. The use of noninvasive positive-pressure ventilation prior to any attempt at airway management and a 20-degree upright position in obese patients can delay critical desaturation. This has great importance in the case of a postinduction endotracheal intubation attempt or if an emergency surgical airway is needed.

Awake intubation is an option in those patients with known or high likelihood of a difficult airway. With awake intubation, the patient maintains spontaneous ventilation, which provides a longer time and increased safety to manage the airway. Possible limiting factors include an uncooperative patient or the presence of blood or other liquids in the upper airway. In this case, a rapid sequence for endotracheal intubation is required. The safety of maintaining spontaneous ventilation is lost; however, a better laryngoscopy is gained by adequate neuromuscular blockade [35]. With the knowledge and the new devices available for clinical care, it is possible to ensure safety and comfort for most patients.

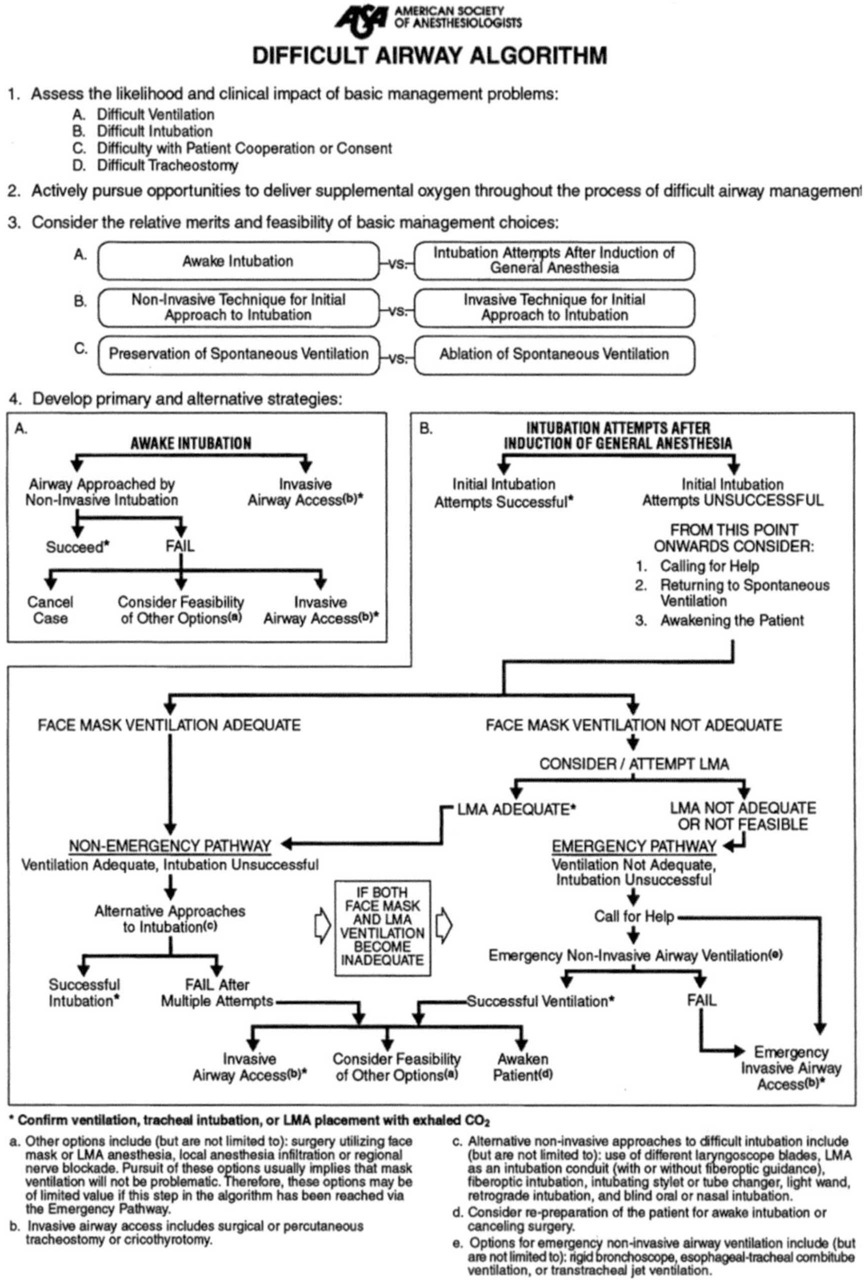

Fig. 24 Difficult-airway algorithm flowchart from the American Society of Anesthesiologists

Conclusion

Adequate airway management requires knowledge of a wide range of techniques and skills to avoid complications. Understanding of anatomy, combined with practical training, is of fundamental importance. Adequate assessment and prior reference will allow optimal choice of equipment and appropriate techniques. Whether the aim is to ensure the patency of the airway or to aid ventilation, the professional must remain calm, focused, and attentive, avoiding waste of valuable time and preventing the situation from becoming chaotic in the face of the challenge. There must always be a clear strategy, with the necessary equipment available and pretested.

Disclosure

Many devices for airway management have been developed in recent years. Omission of any such device from this chapter does not imply that it might not be useful in clinical management.

None of the authors has any conflict of interest.

References

1. Szmuk P, Ezri T, Evron S, Roth Y, Katz J. A brief history of tracheostomy and tracheal intubation, from the Bronze Age to the Space Age. Intensive Care Med. 2008;34(2):222–8.
2. Cook TM, MacDougall-Davis SR. Complications and failure of airway management. Br J Anaesth. 2012;109(S1):i68–85.
3. Bannister FB, Macbeth RG. Direct laryngoscopy and tracheal intubation. Lancet. 1944;244:651–4.
4. Burkle CM, Zepeda FA, Bacon DR, Rose SHA. historical perspective on use of the laryngoscope as a tool in anesthesiology. Anesthesiology. 2004;100(4):1003–6.
5. Gonzalez H, Minville V, Delanoue K, Mazerolles M, Concina D, Fourcade O. The importance of increased neck circumference to intubation difficulties in obese patients. Anesth Analg. 2008;106(4):1132–6.
6. Samsoon GL, Young JR. Difficult tracheal intubation: a retrospective study. Anaesthesia. 1987;42(5):487–90.
7. Langeron O, Masso E, Huraux C, Guggiari M, Bianchi A, Coriat P, Riou B. Prediction of difficult mask ventilation. Anesthesiology. 2000;92(5):1229–36.
8. Ketherpal S, Han R, Tremper KK, Shanks A, Tait AR, O'Reilly M, Ludwig TA. Incidence and predictors of difficult and impossible mask ventilation. Anesthesiology. 2006;105(5):885–91.
9. Tanoubi I, Drolet P, Donati F. Optimizing preoxygenation in adults. Can J Anaesth. 2009;56(6):449–66.
10. Weingart SD, Levitan RM. Preoxygenation and prevention of desaturation during emergency airway management. Ann Emerg Med. 2012;59(3):165–75.
11. Futier E, Constantin JM, Pelosi P, Chanques G, Massone A, Petit A, Kwiatkowski F, Bazin JE, Jaber S. Noninvasive ventilation and alveolar recruitment maneuver improve respiratory function during and after intubation of morbidly obese patients: a randomized controlled study. Anesthesiology. 2011;114(6):1354–63.
12. Adnet F, Borron SW, Dumas JL, Lapostolle F, Cupa M, Lapandry C. Study of the "sniffing position" by the magnetic resonance imaging. Anesthesiology. 2001;94(1):83–6.
13. Greenland KB, Edwards MJ, Hutton NJ, Challis VJ, Irwin MG, Sleigh JW. Changes in airway configuration with different head and neck positions using magnetic resonance imag-

ing of normal airways: a new concept with possible clinical applications. Br J Anaesth. 2010;105(5):683–90.
14. Buis ML, Maissan IM, Hoeks SE, Klimek M, Stolker RJ. Defining the learning curve for endotracheal intubation using direct laryngoscopy: a systematic review. Resuscitation. 2016;99:63–71.
15. Collins SR. Direct and Indirect Laryngoscopy: Equipment and Techniques. Respir Care. 2014;59(6):850–64.
16. Cormack RS, Lehane J. Difficult tracheal intubation in obstetrics. Anaesthesia. 1984;39(11):1105–11.
17. Knill RL. Difficult laryngoscopy made easy with a "BURP". Can J Anaesth. 1993;40(3):279–82.
18. Takahata O, Kubota M, Mamiya K, Akama Y, Nozaka T, Matsumoto H, Ogawa H. The efficacy of the "BURP" maneuver during a difficult laryngoscopy. Anesth Analg. 1997;84(2):419–21.
19. Brazil V, Grobler C, Greenslade J, Burke J. Comparison of intubation performance by junior emergency department doctors using gum elastic bougie versus stylet reinforced endotracheal tube insertion techniques. Emerg Med Australas. 2012;24(2):194–200.
20. Cook TM, Kelly FE. Time to abandon the 'vintage' laryngeal mask airway and adopt second-generation supraglottic airway devices as first choice. Br J Anaesth. 2015;115(4):497–9.
21. Ramachandran SK, Kumar AM. Supraglottic airway devices. Respir Care. 2014;59(6):920–31.
22. Henderson J. Airway management in the adult. In: Miller RD, editor. Anesthesia. 7th ed. Philadelphia: Elsevier Churchill Livingstone; 2010. p. 1573–610.
23. Bein B, Scholz J. Supraglottic airway devices. Best Pract Res Clin Anaesthesiol. 2005;19(4):581–93.
24. Van Zundert A, Brimacombe J. The LMA Supreme—a pilot study. Anaesthesia. 2008;63(2): 209–10.
25. Kleine-Brueggeney M, Greif R, Schoettker P, Savoldelli GL, Nabecker S, Theiler LG. Evaluation of six videolaryngoscopes in 720 patients with a simulated difficult airway: a multicentre randomized controlled trial. Br J Anaesth. 2016;116(5):670–9.
26. Kaplan MB, Ward D, Hagberg CA, Berci G, Hagiike M. Seeing is believing: the importance of video laryngoscopy in teaching and in managing the difficult airway. Surg Endosc. 2006;20(Suppl2):S479–83.
27. YC S, Chen CC, Lee YK, Lee JY, Lin KJ. Comparison of video laryngoscopes with direct laryngoscopy for tracheal intubation: a meta-analysis of randomised trials. Eur J Anaesthesiol. 2011;28(11):788–95.
28. Niforopoulou P, Pantazopoulos I, Demestiha T, Koudouna E, Xanthos T. Video-laryngoscopes in the adult airway management: a topical review of the literature. Acta Anaesthesiol Scand. 2010;54(9):1050–61.
29. Zaouter C, Calderon J, Hemmerling TM. Videolaryngoscopy as a new standard of care. Br J Anaesth. 2015;114(2):181–3.
30. Timanaykar RT, Anand LK, Palta S. A randomized controlled study to evaluate and compare Truview blade with Macintosh blade for laryngoscopy and intubation under general anesthesia. J Anaesthesiol Clin Pharmacol. 2011;27(2):199–204.
31. Lu Y, Jiang H, Zhu YS. Airtraq laryngoscope versus conventional Macintosh laryngoscope: a systematic review and meta-analysis. Anaesthesia. 2011;66(12):1160–7.
32. Berkow LC, Greenberg RS, Kan KH, Colantuoni E, Mark LJ, Flint PW, Corridore M, Bhatti N, Heitmiller ES. Need for emergency surgical airway reduced by a comprehensive difficult airway program. Anesth Analg. 2009;109(6):1860–9.
33. Frerk C, Mitchell VS, McNarry AF, Mendonca C, Bhagrath R, Patel A, O'Sullivan EP, Woodall NM, Ahmad I. Difficult Airway Society 2015 guidelines for management of unanticipated difficult intubation in adults. Br J Anaesth. 2015;115(6):827–48.
34. Apfelbaum JL, Hagberg CA, Caplan RA, Blitt CD, Connis RT, Nickinovich DG, Benumof JL, Berry FA, Bode RH, Cheney FW, Guildry OF, Ovassapian A. Practice guidelines for management of the difficult airway: an update report by the American Society of Anesthesiologists Task Force on Management of the Difficult Airway. Anesthesiology. 2013;118:251–70.
35. Combes X, Andriamifidy L, Dufresne E, Suen P, Sauvat S, Scherrer E, Feiss P, Marty J, Duvaldestin P. Comparison of two induction regimens using or not using muscle relaxant: impact on postoperative upper airway discomfort. Br J Anaesth. 2007;99(2):276–81.

Bronchoscopy Before and After Tracheostomy

Marcus Antônio de Mello Borba, André Leonardo de Castro Costa, Daniela Silva Santos, and Terence Pires de Farias

Introduction

Bronchoscopy, or direct examination of the respiratory tract, has been developed over time. The first person to create an instrument for endoscopic use was Hippocrates, in 400 BC. The term *endoscopy* is derived from the Greek words *endo* (meaning "in") and *scopia* (meaning "look"). But it was only on March 30, 1897, in Freiburg, Germany, that the physician Gustav Killian performed the first, still rudimentary, procedure of what was to be called *direct bronchoscopy*. Gustav Killian performed removal of a foreign body through visualization of the right main bronchus, where a solid body (bone) was identified using a Kirstein laryngoscope. Because of this, Johann Gustav Killian is considered the "father" of bronchoscopy [1].

M.A. de Mello Borba, Ph.D. (✉)
Faculty of Medicine, Department of Experimental Surgery and Surgical Specialties, Federal University of Bahia, Salvador, BA, Brazil

Department of Head and Neck Surgery, Portuguese Hospital, Salvador, BA, Brazil

Department of Head and Neck Surgery, Aristides Maltez Hospital, Salvador, BA, Brazil
e-mail: marcusmelloborba@gmail.com; marcus.borba@ufba.br

A.L. de Castro Costa
Department of Head and Neck Surgery, Portuguese Hospital, Salvador, Bahia, Brazil

Department of Head and Neck Surgery, Aristides Maltez Hospital, Salvador, Bahia, Brazil

D.S. Santos, M.D.
Department of Head and Neck Surgery, Portuguese Hospital, Salvador, BA, Brazil

T.P. de Farias, M.D., Ph.D., M.Sc., Researcher.
Department of Head and Neck Surgery, Brazilian National Cancer Institute—INCA, Rio de Janeiro, RJ, Brazil

Department of Head and Neck Surgery, Pontifical Catholic University, Rio de Janeiro, RJ, Brazil

T.P. de Farias (ed.), *Tracheostomy*, https://doi.org/10.1007/978-3-319-67867-2_21

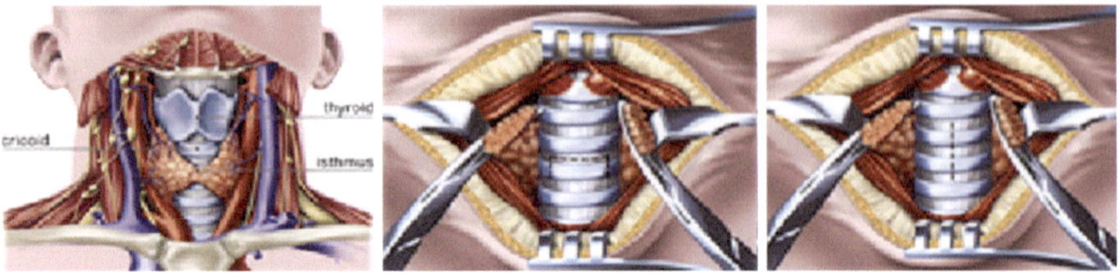

Fig. 1 Tracheal exposure in conventional tracheostomy. (Adapted from Cheung et al. [7], with permission)

Over time, new devices were developed and adapted, which facilitated direct visualization of the respiratory tract. As well, the technique has been refined and expanded. An exponent of great importance for the development of the endoscopic technique was the physician Chevalier Jackson, who was responsible for the creation of a school and abundant literature on the subject. His first book—*Tracheobronchoscopy, Esophagoscopy and Bronchoscopy*—was published in 1907 and reissued in 1914, detailing the necessary instruments, technique, and indications for the procedure [1].

Similarly, *tracheostomy*—a term of Greek origin meaning "to expose the trachea to the outside"—is a procedure known about 3500 years ago and also developed over time [2]. This exposure is maintained through the use of cannulae or through suturing of the tracheal wall to the skin, as in the case of definitive postlaryngectomy tracheostomy [3]. Currently, tracheostomy is one of the most common procedures in intensive care units (ICUs), being performed in about 20% of patients receiving mechanical ventilation, and is widely recommended in patients with prolonged orotracheal intubation [4–6].

The communication generated by the tracheostomy with the external environment reduces anatomical dead space by up to 50%, ultimately facilitating pulmonary mechanics, and is therefore strongly indicated in the ICU setting to help patients with reduced pulmonary reserve. It also reduces the discomfort of mechanical ventilation and facilitates weaning when it is no longer needed, in addition to reducing the complications generated by prolonged intubation.

The disadvantages of tracheostomy include changes in respiratory and digestive physiology, leading to tracheobronchial hypersecretion and difficulty in swallowing, which may increase the risk of airway infection and bleeding.

Conventional tracheostomy, which is the object of detailed study elsewhere in this publication, involves dissection of the pretracheal tissues and insertion of a tracheostomy tube into the trachea under direct vision, according to the representation schematically summarized in Fig. 1 [7].

In 1955, Shelden et al. described the first percutaneous tracheostomy technique [8]. Percutaneous tracheostomy emerged as an alternative, facilitating the procedure at the bedside in intensive care, and being faster and less expensive, with low risk and results similar to those obtained with the traditional technique [9]. Unlike conventional tracheostomy, the percutaneous procedure is often still performed "blindly." It consists of a technique in which the airway is punctured with passage of a guide wire, tracheal dilation, and introduction of the tracheostomy cannula, as shown in Fig. 2 [7].

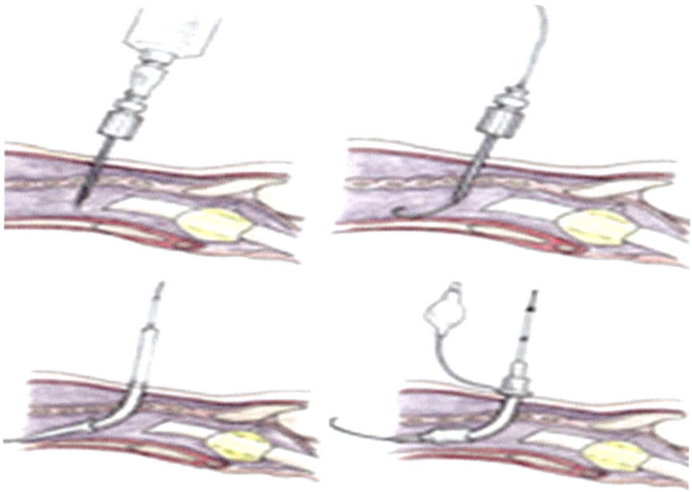

Fig. 2 Percutaneous dilation tracheostomy. (Adapted from Cheung et al. [7], with permission)

Table 1 Frequent indications for bronchoscopy

Diagnostic indication	Therapeutic indication
Chronic cough, hemoptysis, and dysphonia	Guidance during percutaneous tracheostomy
Endobronchial masses/biopsies	Hemoptysis
Respiratory infection	Cleaning of the tracheobronchial tree
Staging of lung and esophageal cancer	Foreign body
Tracheoesophageal fistula	Dilatation of stenosis
Cervical and thoracic trauma	Tracheobronchial tree prosthesis placement
Evaluation of chronic patients with tracheostomy	Drainage of pulmonary abscesses
Persistent or recurrent atelectasis	Difficult intubation and/or extubation failure
Foreign body	Bronchopleural fistula
Airway burn	Brachytherapy

General Bronchoscopy Indications

The use of bronchoscopy in the medical environment is extremely relevant and increasingly common. One proof of this is that in the USA, nearly 500,000 bronchoscopies are done each year [10].

Bronchoscopy is a fundamental technique in the study of respiratory diseases. It provides direct visualization of the upper airways and initial divisions of the tracheobronchial tree, and allows samples to be removed from the trachea, bronchi, mediastinum, and pulmonary parenchyma [11].

In a summary form, and only for didactic reasons, we can divide the indications for performing bronchoscopy into diagnostic and therapeutic indications. We can group the main indications as described in Table 1 [1].

Legislation and Competency

Bronchoscopy is a medical procedure that, despite its increasing use, still has few guidelines to ensure the minimum skills and competencies required for its accomplishment. According to the Federal Council of Medicine (CFM) in Brazil, as documented in opinion 06/2016, a Medically licensed doctor is legally authorized to practice medicine in full, assuming responsibility for their medical acts, including in the civil, criminal, and ethical spheres, even without being a specialist.

Although some believe that these procedures should be performed only by a pulmonologist, intensivist, or thoracic surgeon, it seems that the most important thing is proper training of physicians interested in performing them accurately and quickly so as not to compromise patient safety [10].

The contraindications to bronchoscopy are relative and include absence of suitably trained staff to assist the bronchoscopist during the examination and absence of consent from the patient or their caregiver [1].

Instruments

The minimum equipment required for bronchoscopy is a bronchoscope (rigid or flexible), light source, cytology brushes, biopsy forceps, aspiration equipment, syringes, specimen storage containers, supplemental oxygen, pulse oximeter, sphygmomanometer, and materials and equipment required for cardiorespiratory resuscitation (Fig. 3). Fluoroscopy and a monitor are useful accessories, although not essential, for functions such as facilitating the execution of certain transbronchial biopsies [10].

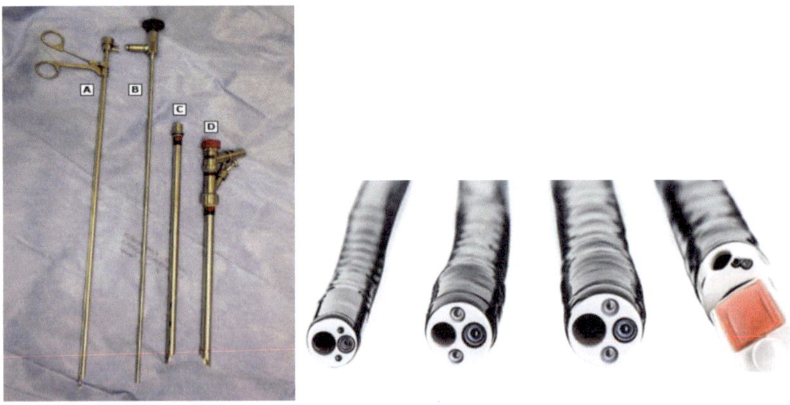

Fig. 3 Instruments for rigid and flexible bronchoscopy. *Left:* rigid biopsy forceps (A), rigid optical telescope for visualization (B), rigid bronchoscope (C), and rigid tracheoscope (D). *Right:* bronchoscopes in increasing size; an ultrathin bronchoscope is shown on the *left*, and an endobronchial ultrasound (EBUS) scope is shown on the *right*. The remaining pieces are routine bronchoscopes of two different sizes. The ultrathin and routine bronchoscopes have a light source, a camera, and a suction port, seen at the tip. (Adapted from Ernst et al. [10], with permission)

Summary of the Bronchoscopy Technique in General (Including in Tracheostomized Patients)

Among the different types of bronchoscopy, flexible bronchoscopy (FB), which was introduced in 1968 by Ikeda et al., is the most widely used technique, although there are other types, such as rigid bronchoscopy (RB) or ultrasound-guided bronchoscopy. Rigid bronchoscopy is used mainly in therapeutics (laser therapy, electrocauterization, or cryotherapy), placement of tracheobronchial stents, tumor resection, tracheobronchial stenosis dilation, and foreign body extraction, particularly in children [11].

The procedure can be performed in an endoscopy room, surgical suite, emergency room, intermediate respiratory care environment, or radiology room, or at the bedside in the ICU. The patient should be placed in a horizontal dorsal decubitus position. Fasting for at least 4 h prior to the procedure is recommended in elective situations and those requiring general anesthesia [11].

The device may be introduced nasally or orally, but the nasal route is preferred because it allows examination of the nasopharynx and is more comfortable for the patient. After topical (nose or mouth) anesthesia, tracheal anesthesia is performed either by puncture of the thin-walled cricothyroid membrane or by indirect laryngoscopy with instillation of anesthetic (lidocaine 1% or 2%). It is recalled here that the oral route of introduction requires the use of a mouth guard between the teeth, to avoid the risk of inadvertent biting and consequent damage to the device.

The procedure can be performed using local anesthesia with or without sedation, or under general anesthesia, depending on the level of complexity. Rigid bronchoscopy is usually performed under general anesthesia in the operating room, while therapeutic flexible bronchoscopy—for example, for transbronchial lung biopsy—should preferably be performed under moderate sedation with midazolam and fentanyl in a unit dedicated to bronchoscopy, due to the risk of endobronchial bleeding and pneumothorax [12].

After the anesthesia/sedation stage, the oral/nasal cavity is examined, followed by the rhino-/oropharynx and larynx, including the vocal cords in adduction and abduction. When entering the trachea, it is advanced one third of the way through, when 3–5 ml of additional anesthetic is instilled by the working channel of the device to complement the anesthesia of the tracheal carina and left main bronchus. [1, 10]. Fig. 4 shows a schematic of the positioning and the passage of the flexible apparatus.

Role of Bronchoscopy Before and After Tracheostomy

Guidance During Percutaneous Tracheostomy

As previously pointed out, there are several indications for performing bronchoscopy; some are diagnostic and others are for therapeutic purposes (Table 1). Among the therapeutic indications, one of the most common nowadays, mainly within ICUs, is for aid during percutaneous tracheostomy, which is widely discussed in the scope of this publication and is reviewed briefly in this chapter [1].

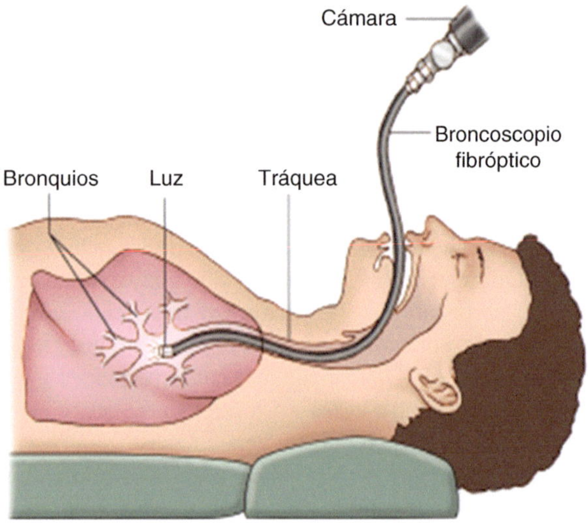

Fig. 4 Flexible bronchoscopy. *Broncoscopio fibróptico* fiberoptic bronchoscope, *Bronquios* bronchus, *Cámara* camera, *Luz* light source, *Tráquea* trachea. (Adapted from Zias et al. [12], with permission)

Percutaneous bronchoscopic tracheostomy is a safe procedure when performed by an experienced intensivist within a tertiary care institution. Flexible bronchoscopic guidance serves to visualize the anterior entry site of the needle, avoiding posterior tracheal injury and ensuring that the guide wire and dilator advance safely. Thus, there is a reduction in the risk of major complications, besides helping to manage minor complications. Figure 5 demonstrates the performance of a tracheal puncture under bronchoscopic assistance [13, 14].

Evaluation of Tracheostomized Patients in Postoperative Surgery of the Airways

Auchincloss and Wright [15], in a recently published study, emphasized the importance of bronchoscopy evaluation, among other measures, in the prevention and treatment of postoperative complications in respiratory tract surgery. In this study, bronchoscopy was performed per protocol in all patients, about 1 week after surgery.

According to the authors, direct visualization of the anastomosis is the most sensitive way to evaluate wound healing and, if necessary, initiate aggressive management of subclinical anastomotic problems. If any of the symptoms described below were present, bronchoscopy was performed prior to completion of the week as a means of preventing significant morbidity and death. Stridor, voice alterations, excessive secretions, subcutaneous emphysema, or wound infection were signs that could represent a problem requiring early bronchoscopy.

Aspiration, Collection, and Tracheobronchial Biopsies

Fibrotracheobronchoscopy may be indicated for visualization and, therefore, facilitation of aspiration of tracheobronchial secretions. In this way there is the possibility of collecting material and/or secretions for histological and laboratory tests. It is possible in cases of pneumonia-related and bronchial-source sepsis, bronchoaspiration and cleansing of the tracheobronchial tree, bronchoalveolar lavage, and lower respiratory assessments as method of airway culturing in tracheostomized patients, including children, with greater practicality, requiring less time and sedation, and thus reducing costs and facilitating a repeatition of the procedure if necessary (Figs. 6 and 7) (methods of airway culturing in tracheostomized children).

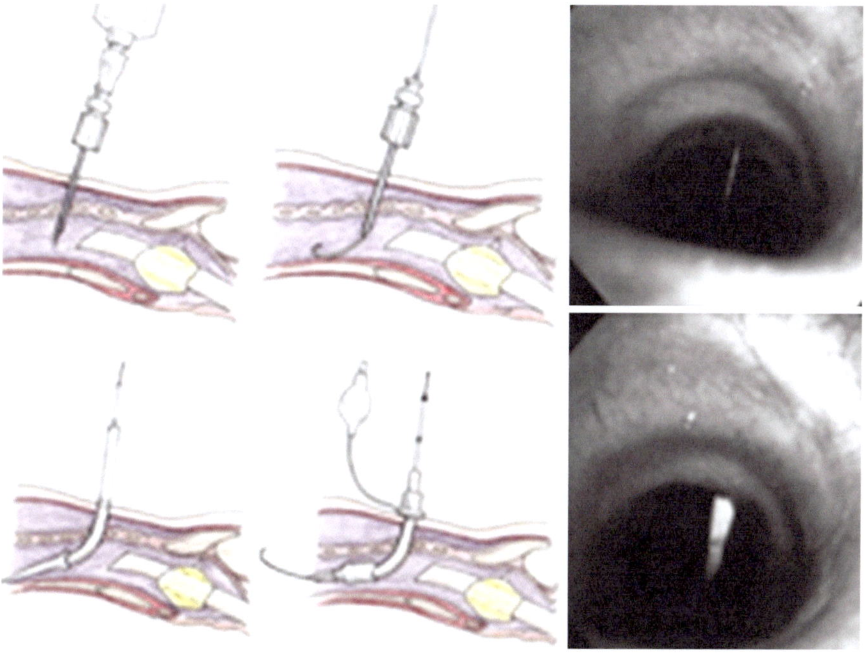

Fig. 5 Tracheal puncture under bronchoscopic aid. (Adapted from Gobatto et al., with permission) [13]

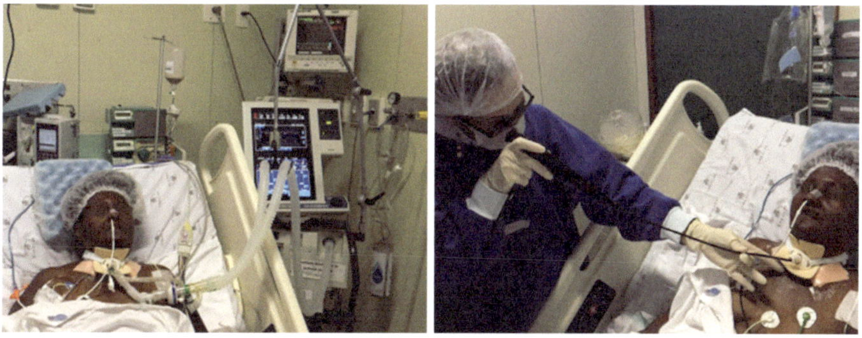

Fig. 6 Fibrotracheobronchoscopy for bronchoalveolar lavage in a critically ill patient in the intensive care unit. (Adapted from Hinerman et al. [14], with permission)

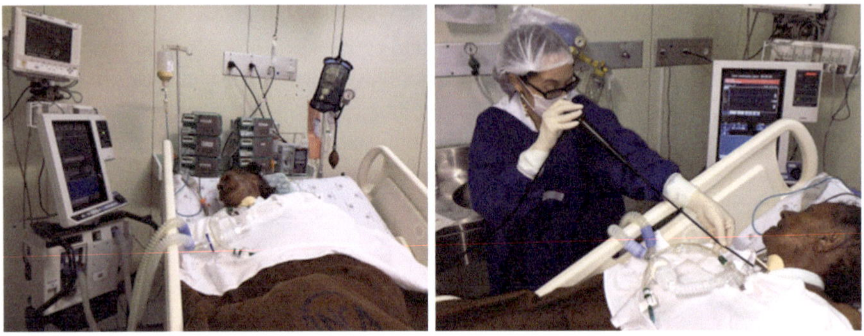

Fig. 7 Repetition of fibrotracheobronchoscopy in a critically ill patient in the intensive care unit

Table 2 Main complications of tracheostomy

Early complication	Late complication
Pneumothorax	Pneumonia
Pneumomediastinum	Tracheal and laryngotracheal stenosis[a]
Subcutaneous emphysema	Tracheoesophageal and/or tracheoinnominate fistula
Incisional bleeding	Cannula obstruction
Aspiration	Aspiration
Aphagia	Dysphagia
Cannula displacement[a]	Infection and granulomas of the stomach[a]

[a]Complication diagnosed by bronchoscopy

Evaluation of the Position and Adequacy of the Tracheostomy Cannula

Some services recommend fibrolaryngotracheobronchoscopy early after tracheostomy to evaluate, confirm, or adapt the position of the tracheostomy cannula.

Diagnosis and Treatment of Possible Complications After Tracheostomy

The main complications of tracheostomy are summarized in Table 2 [16]. In some series, the mortality attributed directly to tracheostomy is relatively low, reaching up to 6.9% [17]. Late complications can occur in up to two thirds of patients. Among these complications, the most common are granulomas at the stoma site, and the most serious are chondromalacia, laryngotracheal stenosis, and vascular or tracheoesophageal fistulas. Fibrolaryngotracheobronchoscopy (FLTB) plays a fundamental role in the diagnosis and treatment of several of these complications, and is indicated, shortly after tracheostomy and before decannulation, to diagnose acute laryngeal lesions and later complications, as indicated in Table 2 [18].

Diagnosis of Tracheoesophageal Fistula

Tracheoesophageal fistula is a rare complication of tracheostomy, with an incidence of less than 1% among all complications. Despite this, it is the third most common late complication, with high rates of morbidity and mortality. It may be the result of infectious pleuropulmonary disease but occurs mainly after trauma or iatrogenically. Its symptomatology may be nonexistent or nonspecific, with tracheal hypersecretion, vomiting, dyspnea, and cough; no isolated symptom defines the diagnosis, except for a direct view of a fistulous tract via (1) esophagoscopy and/or fibrolaryngotracheobronchoscopy; (2) radiological visualization by imaging methods; (3) surgery; or even (4) autopsy. Application of dyes such as methylene blue in the esophagus via the nasogastric probe may facilitate the diagnosis through fibrolaryngotracheobronchoscopy.

Resection of Tracheal Granulomas

In addition to biopsies of lesions at the sites included in the examination, a diagnosis can also be made by means of resection of benign fibroestenotic and inflammatory lesions, such as granulomas (Fig. 8).

Posttracheal Intubation and Posttracheostomy Stenosis

The therapeutic indications are for dilation and/or resection of laryngeal, tracheal (Fig. 9), or laryngotracheal stenosis, when associated with laryngoscopy or bronchoscopy.

Flexible diagnostic bronchoscopy is initially used to identify the type, location, and severity of the stenosis. The degree of stenosis can be estimated with an instrument that measures the diameter of the stenotic area and the diameter

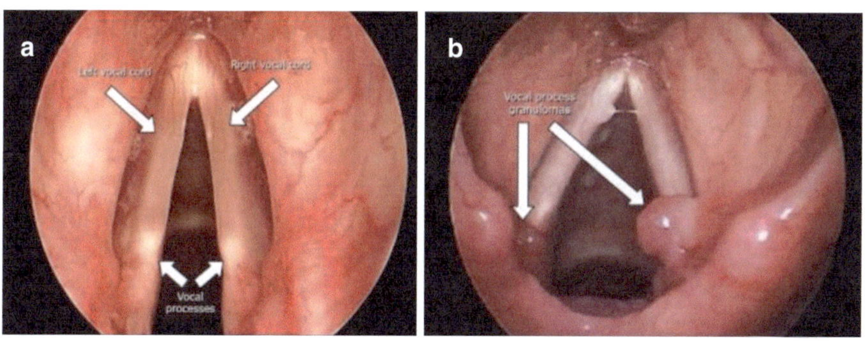

Fig. 8 Fibrolaryngotracheobronchoscopy (FLTB). (**a**) Operative view of a benign granuloma. (**b**) close view of the same granuloma

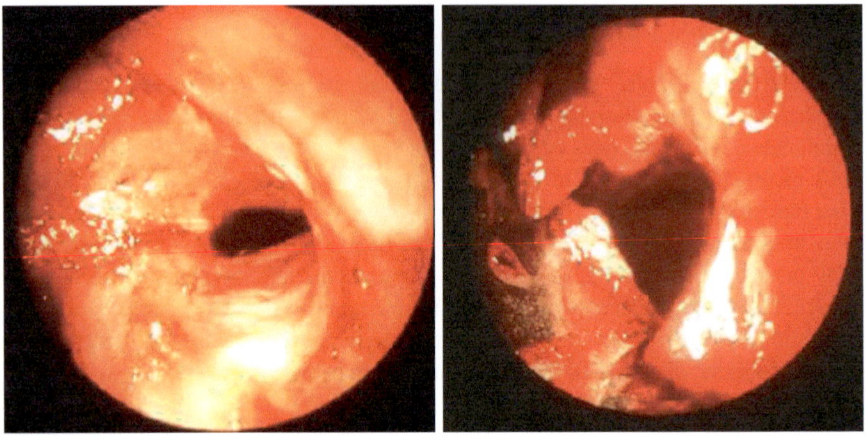

Fig. 9 *Left:* bronchoscopic view of a severe tracheal stenosis in a patient with respiratory failure. *Right:* the same patient after dilation of the stenosis with the rigid bronchoscope

of the lumen of the trachea above and below the stenotic site. In some cases, stenosis can be estimated by imaging tests including tomography with three-dimensional reconstruction and even virtual bronchoscopy. Multiple therapeutic modalities may be used, including resection of fibroestenotic tissue for mechanical debulking and dilation with rigid bronchoscopy, balloon dilatation, laser photocoagulation, stenting, or electrocoagulation with an electric or argon plasma scalpel [12].

Interventional bronchoscopy should be the first approach in the therapeutic management of these patients. It can serve as a bridge for surgical treatment and, more importantly, may be the only treatment needed in most patients [12].

An Integral Part of the Scheduled Decannulation Protocol

The decannulation process can be either accidental or programmed. Accidental decannulation should obviously be avoided, and appropriate training of patients and caregivers is extremely important. Intentional decannulation involves two techniques. The most common involves gradual and progressive reduction of the caliber of the tracheostomy cannula associated with intermittent occlusion of the tracheostomy cannula. The other method of programmed decannulation is done at a single stage (and is therefore called *single-stage decannulation*) and involves removal of the cannula after routine clinical and bronchoscopic evaluation in the absence of obstructive signs or symptoms [19].

Some intensive care, head and neck surgery, and thoracic surgery services include fibrolaryngotracheobronchoscopy or tracheobronchoscopy as a mandatory part of the protocol for decannulating patients undergoing tracheostomy. At this examination, there should be no sign of airway obstruction. If this criterion is satisfied, with absence of predictive signs of bronchopulmonary aspiration, the patient can be decannulated. Figure 10 shows part of an endoscopic evaluation for decannulation after tracheostomy. Fig. 11 shows a normal fibrolaryngotracheoscopy with no signs of obstructive lesions such as stenosis and granulomas [18, 20].

Aspiration of Foreign Bodies

In children, rigid bronchoscopy is the technique of choice for the removal of most foreign bodies. In contrast, in adults, flexible bronchoscopy is used initially for diagnostic purposes, and soon thereafter, in treatment, for removal of a foreign body. An exception is represented by asphyxiating foreign bodies, where rigid bronchoscopy should be considered the first choice [21].

Kin and collaborators (2011) reported two cases of removal of a tooth aspirated in a polytraumatized patient through fibrolaryngotracheobronchoscopy with simultaneous tracheostomy.

Bronchoscopy is the gold standard procedure for diagnosis and treatment of foreign body aspiration (Senturk and Sem, 2011). Although foreign bodies are more common in the pediatric population, a definitive tracheostoma represents a risk

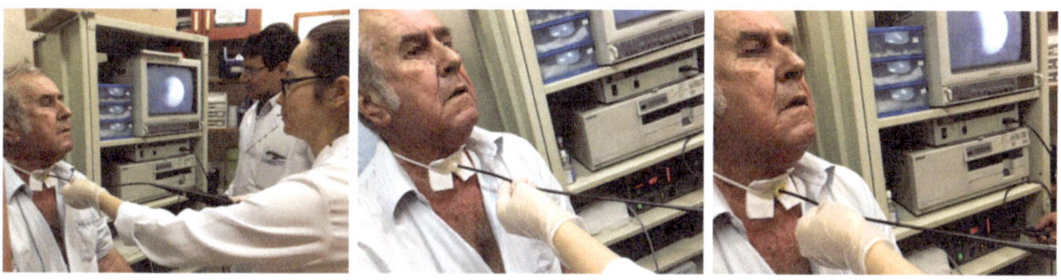

Fig. 10 Fibrotracheobronchoscopy for evaluation of decannulation

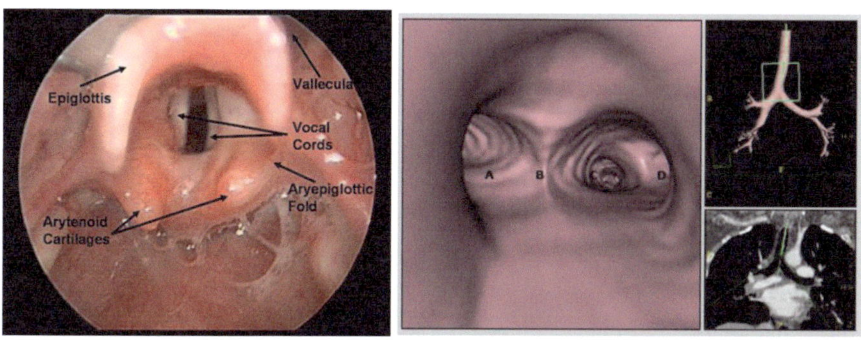

Fig. 11 *Left:* normal fibrolaryngotracheochoscopy. *Middle:* virtual fibrolaryngotracheochoscopy showing the left mainstem bronchus (A), carina (B), bronchus intermedius and segmental orifices (C), and right upper lobe bronchus (D). *Top right:* external shaded surface display (computed tomographic bronchography). *Bottom right:* coronal multiplanar reconstruction

factor for aspiration of various foreign bodies in adults, especially when there is an association with alcohol abuse. Aspiration of a tracheoesophageal vocal prosthesis is a rare occurrence, reported fewer than ten times in the literature, where the use of tracheobronchoscopy was effective for removal [21].

Diagnosis and Staging of Synchronic and Metachronous Lesions of the Distal Airways

Patients with squamous cell carcinoma of the head and neck, especially those located in the larynx, constitute a high-risk group for development of second primary tumors. The risk of developing second tumors after diagnosis and treatment of laryngeal cancer is greater than 10%. A considerable fraction of these tumors are located in the lungs and have a metachronous occurrence, causing some authors to recommend baseline bronchoscopy during the initial investigation of these laryngeal tumors and during follow-up at regular intervals [22, 23].

Tracheobronchoscopy

Bronchoscopy is a very useful tool for screening patients at high risk for lung cancer. It is important to highlight the role of bronchoscopy when performed after total laryngectomy for the treatment of laryngeal cancer. In this scenario, where there is a definitive stoma, tracheostomy is used as the initial route for the endoscopic procedure, consisting of examination via tracheobronchoscopy and requiring minimal intervention [24].

Differently from the other described situations, in which the larynx is absent, even with the presence of the tracheostomy, the bronchoscopic examination should not be abbreviated to a fibrotracheobroncoscopy, and must consist of complete endoscopic evaluation of the proximal airway starting through fibrolaryngotracheobronchoscopy.

A fibrobronchoscope or video fibrobronchoscope is used, coupled to the light source, and the nasal, oral, or stomal route can be used—the latter in patients with definitive tracheostomy. Anesthesia is performed with transcricoid infiltration of up to 5 ml of 1% lidocaine, or directly into the tracheostoma by instillation of the anesthetic for subglottic and tracheal desensitization.

Alternatives to Bronchoscopy

There are alternative imaging methods with the justification of less invasiveness than endoscopic examination of the airways. Among these methods, we can enumerate helicoidal and linear computed tomography, magnetic resonance, and, in particular, virtual bronchoscopy.

Virtual bronchoscopy (Fig. 11)—the result of advances in computer science and the development of helical tomography—uses the technique of reconstructing three-dimensional images in real time to simulate images obtained with the bronchoscope without actual introduction of an instrument into the airway [25]. In addition to noninvasiveness, the production of retrograde anatomical images of the laryngotracheobronchial and external walls of the airway is among the advantages of virtual examination.

Despite this advancement, bronchoscopy remains the examination of choice for diagnosis of severe obstructions of the airway, with the possibility of differentiating benign lesions from malignant lesions. In the near future these tests will probably play an important and complementary role in the diagnostic evaluation and planning of treatment for respiratory tract diseases, especially for laryngotracheal stenosis after tracheal intubation or posttracheostomy.

Consent for Publication Informed consent was obtained from all individual participants for whom identifying information is included in this article.

References

1. Andrade CF, Sánchez PG, Cardoso PF. Broncoscopia. Revista AMRIGS. 2005;49(3):178–82.
2. Frost E. Tracing the tracheostomy. Ann Otol Rhinol Laryngol. 1976;85:618–24.
3. Zacharias M, Zacharias E. Dicionário de Medicina Legal. São Paulo: Instituição Brasileira de Difusão Cultural Limitada. Curitiba: Editora Universitária Champagnat; 1991. p. 450–1.
4. Castella X, Gilabert J, Torner F. Laryngeal damage from intubation. Chest. 1990;98(3):776–7.
5. Esteban A, Anzueto A, Alía I, Gordo F, Apezteguía C, Pálizas F. How is mechanical ventilation employed in the intensive care unit? An international utilization review. Am J Respir Crit Care Med. 2000;161(5):1450–8.
6. Wood DE. Tracheostomy. Chest Surg Clin North Am. 1996;6:749–64.
7. Cheung NH, Napolitano LM. Tracheostomy: epidemiology, indications, timing, technique, and outcomes. Respir Care. 2014;59(6):895–915; Discussão 916-9. https://doi.org/10.4187/respcare.0297.
8. Shelden CH, Pudenz RH, Tichy FY. Percutaneous tracheotomy. JAMA. 1957;165(16):2068–70. https://doi.org/10.1001/jama.1957.02980340034009.
9. Al-Ansari MA, Hijazi MH. Clinical review: percutaneous dilatational tracheostomy. Crit Care. 2006;10:202.
10. Ernst A, Silvestri GA, Johnstone D. Interventional pulmonary procedures. Guidelines from the American College of Chest Physicians. Chest. 2003;123:1693–717.
11. Esquinas A, et al. Bronchoscopy during non-invasive mechanical ventilation: a review of techniques and procedures. Arch Bronconeumol. 2013;49(3):105–12.
12. Zias N, Chroneou A, Tabba MK, et al. Post tracheostomy and post intubation tracheal stenosis: report of 31 cases and review of the literature. BMC Pulm Med. 2008;8:18. https://doi.org/10.1186/1471-2466-8-18. PMCID: PMC2556644. http://www.portalmedico.org.br/pareceres/CFM/2016/6_2016.pdf; acesso em 06/03/16.
13. Gobatto AL, Besen BA, Tierno PF, et al. Ultrasound-guided percutaneous dilational tracheostomy versus bronchoscopy-guided percutaneous dilational tracheostomy in critically ill patients (TRACHUS): a randomized noninferiority controlled trial. Intensive Care Med. 2016;42:342–51.
14. Hinerman R, Alvarez F, Keller CA. Resultado da traqueostomia percutânea de cabeceira com orientação broncoscópica. Cuidados Intensivos Med. 2000;26:1850–6.
15. Auchincloss HG, Wright CD. Complications after tracheal resection and reconstruction: prevention and treatment. J Thorac Dis. 2016;8(Supl. 2):S160–7. https://doi.org/10.3978/j.issn.2072-1439. 2016.01.86.

16. Coelho MS, Zampier JA, Zanin SA, Silva EM, Guimarães PSF. Fístula traqueoesofágica como complicação tardia de traqueostomia. J Pneumol. 2001;27(2). Disponível em: https://doi.org/10.1590/S0102-35862001000200010.
17. Zeitoun AG, Kost KM. Tracheostomy: a retrospective review of 281 cases. J Otolaryngol. 1994;23(1):61–6.
18. Rodrigues LE. Importance of flexible bronchoscopy in decannulation of tracheostomy patients. Rev Col Bras Cir. 2015;42. https://doi.org/10.1590/0100-69912015002003.
19. Lewarski JS. Long-term care of the patient with a tracheostomy. Respir Care. 2005;50(4):534–7.
20. Coelho M d S. Influência da traqueostomia longitudinal e da traqueostomia de ressecção sobre a estenose traqueal. Tese: Doutorado Universidade Federal do Paraná; 2001. p. 155.
21. Conte SC, et al. Aspiration of tracheoesophageal prosthesis in a laryngectomized patient. Multidisciplinary Respiratory Medicine. 2012;7:25.
22. de Vries N, Snow GB. Multiple primary tumours in laryngeal cancer. J Laryngol Otol. 1986;100(8):915–8. PMID:3746107.
23. Croce A, de Vincentiis M, Primerano G, Gallo A, Rendina EA, Venuta F. Early diagnosis of pulmonary tumors in patients treated for laryngeal cancer. Acta Otorhinolaryngol Ital. 1989;9(2):139–47. Review. Italian. PMID:2669438.
24. Cetinkaya E, Veyseller B, Yildirim YS, Aksoy FJ, et al. Value of autofluorescence bronchoscopy in patients with laryngeal cancer. Laryngol Otol. 2011;125:181–7. https://doi.org/10.1017/S002221511000229X. Epub 2010 Nov 9.
25. Haponik EF, Aquino SL, Vining DJ. Virtual bronchoscopy. Clin Chest Med. 1999;20(1):201–17. Review. PMID:10205726.

What Is the Best Way to Take Care of a Patient with a Tracheostomy Tube?

Lica Arakawa-Sugueno

Introduction

Tracheostomy is a scheduled or emergency procedure to facilitate temporary or permanent breathing. Like any surgical procedure, fashioning of the tracheal stoma is associated with risk and complications.

The professional team caring for tracheostomized patients should be able to change the cannula, fix it properly to the neck, manage the hygiene of the tracheal stoma, perform an aspiration procedure, and handle the cuff. Resuscitation training and knowledge of emergency actions are necessary.

The same team will be responsible for guiding and informing caregivers and family members about breathing mechanisms in the presence of the tracheostomy, the tracheal cannula function and type, basic care, and possible complications related to tracheal breathing.

This chapter discusses the general and specific care needed to avoid possible complications related to a tracheostomy.

Tracheostomy Care

The morbidity and mortality rates in the tracheostomized pediatric population are two to three times higher than those in adults [1]. Incidents related to the cannula in children occur much more frequently, being four times more frequent in the first

L. Arakawa-Sugueno, Speech Therapist.
School of Medicine, University of São Paulo-USP, São Paulo, Brazil
e-mail: lica.sugueno@gmail.com

T.P. de Farias (ed.), *Tracheostomy*, https://doi.org/10.1007/978-3-319-67867-2_22

postoperative week and also more frequent in the immediate or early postoperative period [2].

Tracheostomy care includes learning to identify the color, consistency, odor, viscosity, and volume of secretions. Records of vital signs and patient temperature are also constant measures.

The multidisciplinary team at Great Ormond Street Hospital for Children (GOSH) in the UK makes use of an acrostic as a reminder of tracheostomy management—"TRACHE"—which represents the following: *T* = tapes, regarding the use of tapes for cannula fixation; *R* = resus, regarding knowledge of resuscitation methods; *A* = airway, allowing airflow; *C* = care, regarding care of the stoma and cannula, and neck hygiene; *H* = humidity, regarding the need for moisture to fluidify secretions; *E* = emergency, regarding the need to always have an emergency kit and training to use it [3].

T—*tape*
R—*resus*
A—*airway*
C—*care*
H—*humidity*
E—*emergency*

Cannula Fixation

Cotton tape is ideal to fix the tracheal cannula to the neck. Velcro material is more practical, but cotton is considered safer.

Both placement and replacement of fastening tapes require care.

The hands should be washed for the procedure. The professional should wear gloves and a protective mask. Gauze and saline are required for local cleaning around the stoma, with scissors to cut the tape to the required size. The patient should be placed in a suitable position (adults and older children preferably seated, and smaller children lying supine on a rolled-up towel to allow visibility of the stoma). Strong neck pressure should be avoided.

Especially when caring for children, it is recommended to have one more person present to help.

The tape should be placed only on clean and dry skin, but the procedure must be fast and efficient. Avoid tying knots before the final adjustment by making arcs in the fixing holes of the cannula itself. As a test for comfort, it should be possible to pass a finger under the tape. If it is too tight and it is difficult to move your finger comfortably, it is recommended to make an adjustment. After checking the comfort and tension adjustment of the tape, knots can be made on both sides. The procedure is detailed in Table 1.

Resuscitation Procedure

All professionals working with tracheostomized patients should undergo cardiopulmonary resuscitation training.

Table 1 Cannula fixation procedure

Action	Observation
Cut the piece of tape long enough to make two laps around the neck	Leave an extra piece of tape to fix it
Cut and remove the old tape	In conscious adults, the patient themselves can hold the cannula to prevent it from moving in the event of a cough If this is not the case, it is safer to have a second person to assist in the procedure by holding the cannula during removal of the old tape and placement of the new one
Insert the ends of the tape into the two cannula lateral holes to secure the tape	Fix one side first and, when adjusting the other side, check that there is enough space for a finger between the tape and the neck so it is not too tight, before making the knot (Fig. 1).
Placing protective gauze between the cannula and the skin flaps is an option for comfort and reduction of injury	In this case, it is suggested that the open portion of the gauze faces upward (Fig. 2)

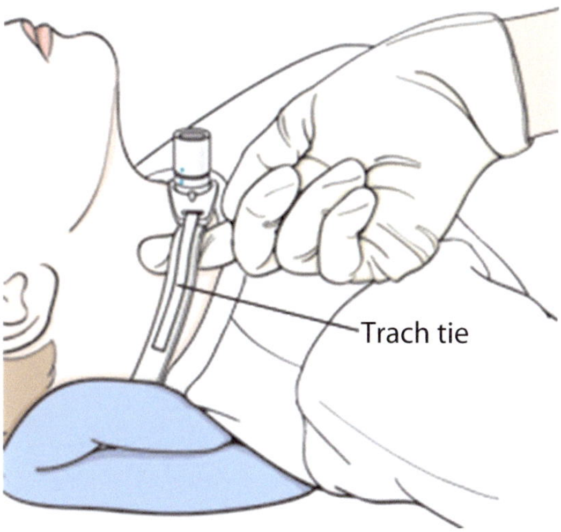

Fig. 1 Check space to a finger (https://www.fairview.org/patient-education/88997)

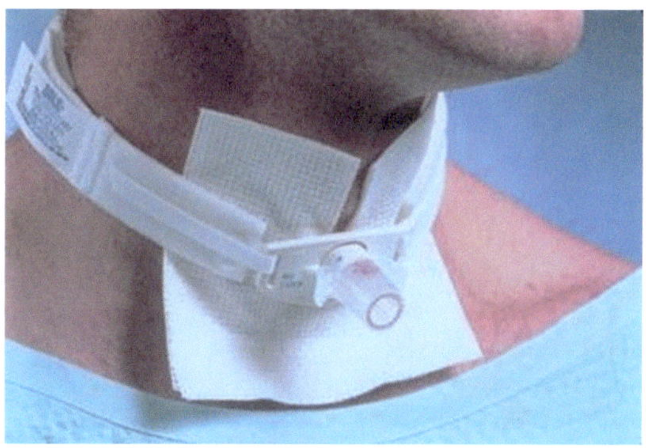

Fig. 2 Protective gauze (rehabmart.com)

Enabling air passage is the greatest emergency. After an emergency service call, the patient should be positioned with the chin up without pressure on the soft tissue of the submandibular region to allow more chance of ventilation. The presence of corneal secretions, blood crusts, or tube displacement are frequent complications and should be investigated.

If obstruction occurs, the intermediate cannula (if any) should be removed (Fig. 3). A single-tube cannula needs to be aspirated with a catheter. Solid obstructions (dry secretions) may persist. In this case, it will be necessary to remove the cannula, replacing it immediately with a new one of the same size. For this reason, the emergency exchange kit should always be available.

In some cases, the stoma may close very fast, especially in the early postoperative period. The use of the Seldinger technique is characterized by the use of the catheter tip as a guide in the tracheal orifice for placement of the tracheal cannula. It may be an indication in some cases of fast closing. There is a tracheal dilator, but there are contraindications related to this procedure [4].

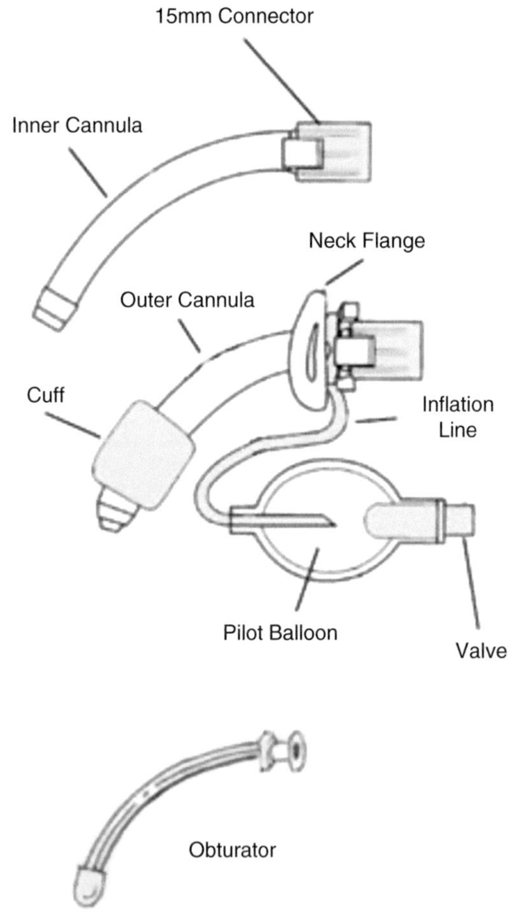

Fig. 3 Parts of cannula (http://trachs.com/parts-of-a-trach-tube/)

If ventilation has not yet been achieved, rescue breathing methods such as mouth-to-mouth or a ventilation mask should be used.

After the tube is replaced, it is necessary to monitor the patient for respiratory comfort. The patient should not be left alone. If the cannula fixation is adequate, If the cannula fixation is adequate, it is important to initiate the ventilation support conduct.

Suction

Care in the suction procedure should take into account the following aspects:

- Length of suction tube (catheter): a shorter tube may not allow adequate aspiration while a volume of secretions persists in the unreached area, whereas a longer tube may cause trauma to the tracheal wall.
- Diameter of the catheter: there is There is suggested size for safe suction pressure and to avoid discomfort [5]. A catheter size of 12 French is recommended for cannula sizes 6–9, or 10 Fr for a smaller cannula.
- Side holes smaller than the distal orifice in the catheter: this allows less adherence to the mucosa with less risk of injury.
- Valve: this allows vacuum control with digital occlusion.
- Catheter markings: these allow the insertion of the catheter to be done more accurately.
- Equipment with a variable vacuum control unit.
- Personal protective equipment: procedure gloves before sterile gloves, protective mask, goggles.
- Bottled water in a clean container.
- Equipment for waste disposal.
- Training/practice.

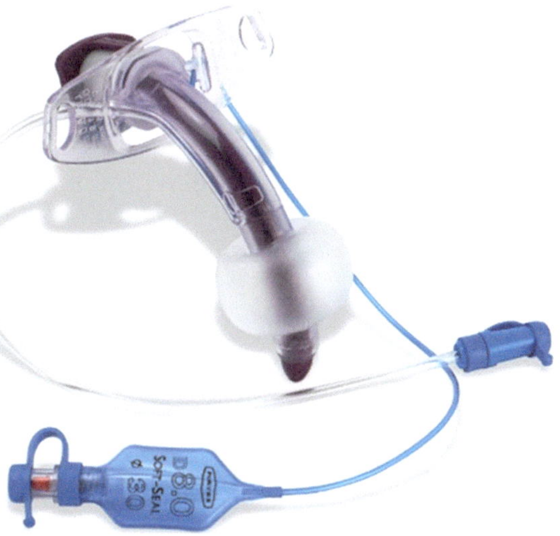

Fig. 4 Cannula with supracuff probe (Cuffed Blue Line Ultra® Suctionaid)

If the tracheal cannula is of the type containing a supracuff probe (Fig. 4), it should be aspirated directly with the suction tube before attachment of the sterile catheter.

Suction should be started only at the return of the catheter and not at the insertion. It is not necessary to rotate the catheter if there are lateral orifices. Avoid twisting the catheter to obtain a vacuum. Greater pressure is not always what is needed for suction. The aspiration should not be slow, but rather quick, and its indication and frequency will be related to the need and the degree of severity. It is recommended that each suction never exceed 15 s. This minimizes the risk of complications such as hypoxia and cardiovascular changes [6]. The catheter should be discarded if the tip is contaminated (by contact with any surface) prior to insertion.

Saline should not be used routinely before suction, but only when there is difficulty in suction of secretions because of thickened consistency or presence of obstructive dry secretion stopper.

The procedure should be documented, with a description of the quality of secretions regarding the color, consistency, odor, viscosity, volume, and presence of blood.

In young children, it is recommended that the tip of the catheter does not extend beyond the end of the tracheostomy cannula. Some children require oxygen therapy before the suction procedure, so check for this.

Mistakes in the suction procedure can lead directly or indirectly to hypoxia, distal granulation, ulcerations, cardiovascular changes, pneumothorax, atelectasis, bacterial infections and, in extreme cases, intracranial complications.

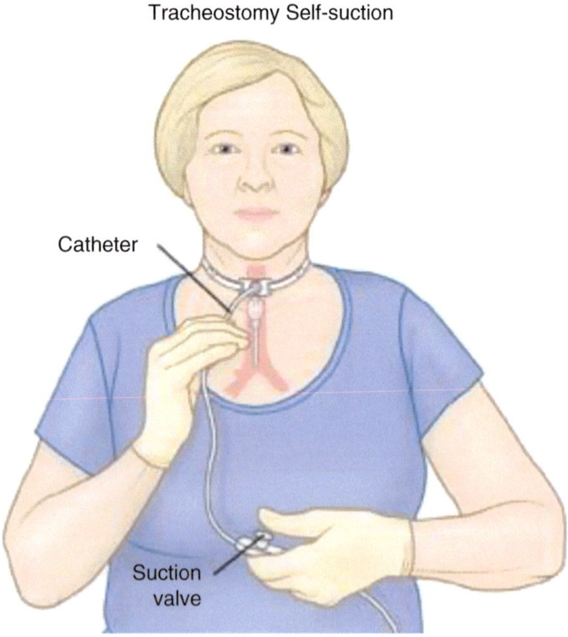

Fig. 5 Self-suction (https://www.allinahealth.org/mdex/ND0413G.HTM)

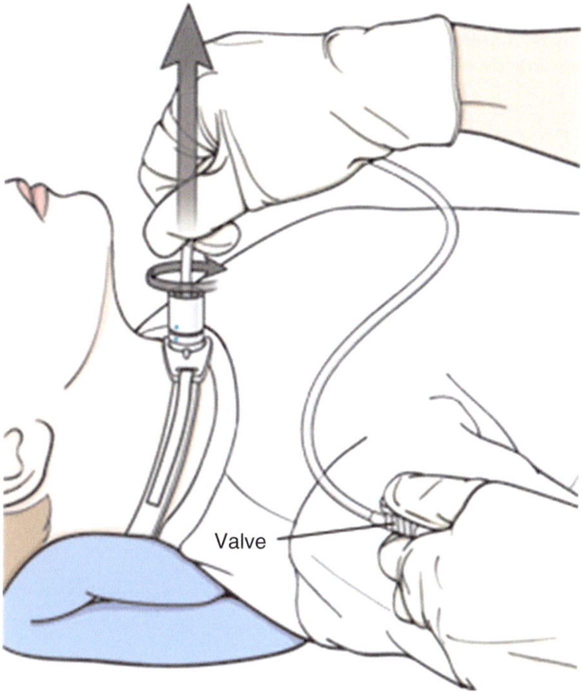

Fig. 6 Suction with catheter (https://www.mountnittany.org/articles/healthsheets/7411)

The suction procedure is as follows:

1. Immerse the catheter in a clean container with sterile water.
2. The patient should sit comfortably in front of the mirror (Fig. 5).
3. Insert the catheter 10–15 cm without occlusion of the suction valve.
4. Occlude the suction valve with a thumb to promote aspiration while withdrawing the catheter in a rotating movement (in a catheter without lateral orifices) (Fig. 6).
5. If there are more secretions, immerse the catheter in sterile water and repeat the procedure until the secretions are minimized.
6. It is not a comfortable procedure; however, it is important that the patient has time to calm down and not get too agitated.
7. Discard the catheter after use.

Care of the Cannula, Stoma, and Neck

Skin evaluation and careful daily cleaning can avoid complications such as skin trauma, epidermolysis bullosa, vascular problems, and lymphatic malformations, especially with a long-term cannula.

Cleaning of the inner cannula is done once a day or, if necessary, more often. Running water and a cleaning brush are sufficient.

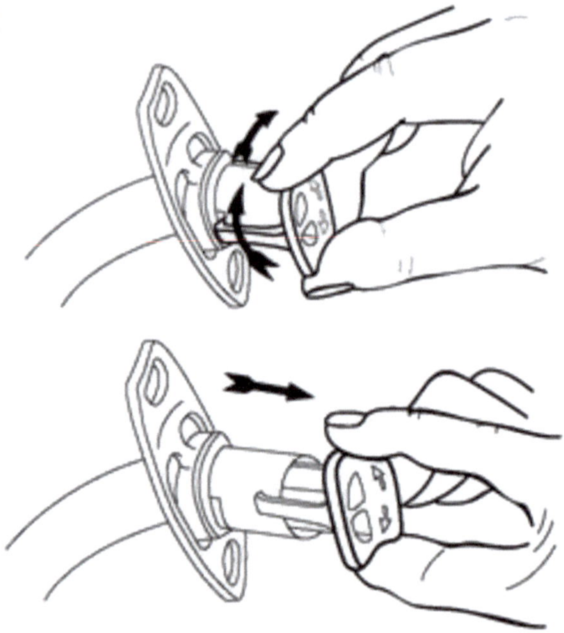

Fig. 7 Inner cannula removal (http://purecath.com/en/cpshow1.html)

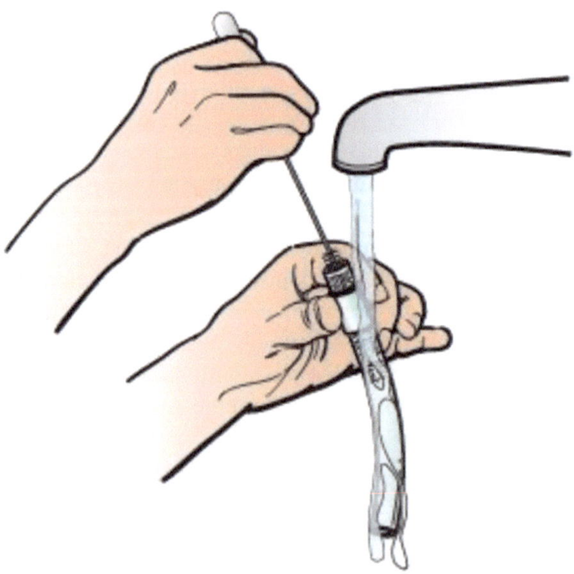

Fig. 8 Cleaning with brush under running water (https://www.mskcc.org/cancer-care/patient-education/caring-your-tracheostomy)

The procedure to clean the inner cannula is as follows:

1. With clean hands (gloves for the health professional), remove the inner cannula and wash it under running water (Fig. 7).
2. Ask the patient to cough to avoid obstructions in the external cannula, and perform a suction procedure if necessary.

3. Clean the internal cannula with a brush to release all adherence of secretions (Fig. 8).
4. Remove excess liquid from the cannula, drying it only by shaking it in the air, without using any material.
5. Replace the inner cannula.
6. Wash the hands.

The region around the cannula (peristoma) is also cleaned daily. If the frequency of accumulation of secretions is high, this procedure should be repeated as frequently as needed.

The procedure to clean the tracheal stoma (around the cannula) is as follows:

1. For the patient, it is recommended to use a mirror and a seated position.
2. Remove the old bandage.
3. Wash the hands.
4. Clean the skin and the outer cannula with clean gauze wet with sterile water.
5. Use saline if there are more viscous or dry secretions.
6. Dry with a clean towel after cleaning.
7. If necessary, use a bandage on the ends of the cannula to avoid contact lesions.
8. Document and inform medical staff if you observe edema, bleeding, irritation, or secretions with an altered color (greenish, bloody, etc.).

Humidity

Air flow directly through the trachea does not allow the humid environment (100% relative humidity) and 37 °C body temperature that the nose offers in normal breathing. For this reason, especially in the first few weeks, it is important to artificially offer warm moisture to avoid thick, sticky secretions.

Medications or combined use of oxygen therapy are individually targeted interventions to be used as needed.

A nebulizer provides humidification via a direct aerosol in the lower airway, with a mask on the tracheostomy cannula.

Intake of water orally or via a feeding tube should be indicated for systemic hydration. On average, intake of two liters of water per day is recommended.

Other humidification systems will be discussed by the multidisciplinary team on a case-by-case basis.

Emergency Kit

It is imperative that the following materials are always available in a clean and dry place to avoid contamination and to be easily accessible.

- Suction equipment
- Suction catheters or tubes—length and gauge suitable for the patient's age and physical structure

- Inhaler equipment/vaporizer with a suitable mask (size)
- Two packs of sterile gauze pads
- Saline solution
- Personal protective equipment (PPE)—goggles, gloves, face mask, and apron
- Clean receiver containing bottled water
- 2 mL syringe and ampoule of 0.9% sodium chloride for cleaning
- 10 mL syringe for cuff manipulation (in a cannula with a cuff)
- Manometer for the cuff (in a cannula with a cuff)
- Pump for waste disposal
- Reserve tracheostomy cannula (same size/make/gauge)
- Shiley cannula smaller than the size used by the patient
- Water-based lubricant
- Round-tipped scissors
- Tracheal cannula tapes
- Rolled towel or blanket to assist in positioning if the patient is a child

It is recommended that only trained individuals perform cannula replacement in the event of an accidental decannulation [7]. For this, it is important that caregivers or family members responsible for the patient also undertake training for such emergencies. If the patient is a child, it is important to have one more person to help.

After checking that the necessary materials are available, the cannula exchange procedure should be performed as follows:

1. Wash the hands and put on the personal protective equipment.
2. The patient should be positioned to facilitate the exchange. If the patient is a child, they should lie supine, with a support under their shoulders, such as a rolled-up towel. An adult patient can be seated if they are not obese.
3. Cut the fastening tapes if there is an intention to change them, or untie the knots (or remove the Velcro) if there is a need for reuse.
4. Water-based lubricant on the tip of the new cannula with a setter (or shutter) facilitates passage.
5. In the case of a cannula with a cuff, it must be completely deflated with a syringe before withdrawal. Remove the cannula by performing a curve movement, immediately insert the new cannula into the curvature, and then follow the midline. Remove the setter to allow air to pass through.
6. Before fixing, clean and dry the region around the stoma.
7. Fasten with tape and do the finger test to check that it is not tight, before tying knots or fastening the Velcro.
8. If use of an inflated cuff is indicated, reinflate it and measure for appropriate pressure with the manometer.

Pulmonary Protection

Pulmonary protection care for the tracheostomy involves use of cotton pads or disposable material made for this purpose.

As discussed earlier, specific filters of the HME (heat and moisture exchange) type are indicated on a case-by-case basis but should not be used for general care.

There is a bathing protector available, made of neoprene material, which covers the stoma during showering without limiting tracheal breathing.

A variety of products have been developed for total laryngectomies, such as silicone cannulae for a permanent hole with a risk of stenosis, specific phonation products, and a snorkel adapted for a tracheal stoma for use when diving and swimming, among others.

Complications

The most frequent complications can be resolved as long as the patient, caregiver, and/or professionals involved are attentive in identifying the problem and resolving it calmly.

Accidental Decannulation or Tube Displacement

This occurrence should be considered an emergency. It is always important to know that this risk is quite possible and, in advance, the family or caregiver must have an accessible telephone number to call in these situations. Accidental decannulation occurs in approximately 5% of the pediatric population [1].

When a tracheal cannula is out of the orifice (partially or totally), it must be reintroduced without being forced. Guidelines for placement of the cannula have been discussed previously.

Prevention is always the best course. Always direct the family or caregiver to check that the tape tension is adequate—neither too tight nor too loose. The type of tape used should also ensure comfort. Side gauzes can be used for assistance, provided they are of a quality ensuring that gauze lint is not aspirated by the patient.

In some cases, there is a need to fix the cannula with a suture to the patient's skin. Although this may bother or frighten the patient and the caregiver/family member, it may make the difference to prevent extrusion and the risk of significant respiratory discomfort.

A chest X-ray is indicated to confirm the position of the tube and rule out any complications such as pneumothorax and surgical emphysema [8].

Pneumothorax

This is a postoperative risk. Check for air passage by feeling with the hands in front of the cannula. Observation of bilateral thoracic movement should be done, along with bilateral pulmonary auscultation.

Respiratory obstructions should be reported immediately to the emergency service.

Hemorrhage

There is also a risk of hemorrhage in the early or late postoperative period. Bleeding, even in a small volume, that persists for more than 24 h should be notified to the medical staff.

The pulse oximeter will identify oxygen saturation and cardiorespiratory frequency.

Obstruction

The cannula should always be kept clean. Inspiratory noises are a sign of turbulence of air flow in contact with secretion residue. In the immediate postoperative period of 12–24 h after surgery of the stoma, it is necessary that hygiene procedures be performed constantly, in some cases as often as every 30 min.

After this period, suction with a catheter is required whenever the volume of secretions causes respiratory difficulty. Intensive care is needed in the first week because obstruction can cause serious problems.

Pulmonary Emphysema

Air leakage may occur into the surrounding tissue. Local edema may be a warning of a risk of emphysema.

Cannula fixing tapes that look tighter may suggest a risk of this type of edema. It is important that medical staff conduct an evaluation as soon as possible.

Infection

Infectious processes are usually noticed by the characteristics of the secretions. The color, consistency, odor, viscosity, and volume are clinical parameters used as indicators of infection.

Humidification

It is recommended not to use HME tracheal protectors in the first week after tracheostomy surgery.

Vaporization or inhalation is indicated for at least 1 week after surgery.

Feeding/Swallowing

There is a very negative expectation of feeding related to tracheostomized patients, especially due to studies that have revealed the relation between dysphagia and tracheostomy. It is known that many patients with dysphagia are tracheostomized. This does not mean that the cause of dysphagia is the presence of the tracheal orifice or the cannula. Tracheostomy is rarely the only cause of dysphagia. Many patients who use a cannula have dysphagia, but investigation of an association with underlying neurological or oncological disease is essential for relation of the etiology to the dysphagia. The speech therapist is a professional qualified to evaluate and treat mechanical or neurological oropharyngeal dysphagia. Joint intervention with a physiotherapist is essential in rehabilitation of a dysphagic patient with a tracheostomy. This issue is addressed in the chapter on rehabilitation of a tracheostomized patient.

Speech/Voice

The possibility of oral communication should be investigated by the team. In patients whose laryngeal anatomy is preserved, albeit with dysfunction, it is possible to produce phonation if an insufflated cuff is not being used and if the lateral column to the tracheal cannula allows airflow for vibration of laryngeal phonation structures. Indication of phonatory valves may also be an option. However, any of these possibilities requires a speech–language evaluation for safe indication, since complications may ensue. Patients undergoing total laryngeal resection have a permanent tracheostoma, but the phonatory production process involves completely different rehabilitation (an electronic larynx, tracheoesophageal prosthesis, or esophageal voice). This theme is also addressed in the rehab chapter.

If oral communication cannot be restored at this time, paper and pen or alternative forms of communication should be offered, such as a board with figures and letters. This will offer some comfort during the initial period of adaptation to the presence of the tracheal cannula.

Comments

The impact of a tracheostomy is overwhelming in various respects: aesthetic, functional, and hygienic (bathing), among many others commented on in this book. The quality of life of the tracheostomized patient depends on the care offered by the professionals and performed by caregivers and the patient themselves.

Professionals, caregivers, and family members must, first and foremost, demonstrate calm and safety to the tracheostomy patient. The best way to demonstrate these qualities is to have prior experience, knowledge, and training.

Adult patients who are conscious and have motor skill need to be guided to maintain the hygiene of the cannula and tracheal stoma, and to manage pulmonary secretions and cannula exchange. The professionals involved in the multidisciplinary team are responsible for providing such information and training.

Websites Consulted

Atos Medical. www.atosmedical.com

Care of Adult Patients with a Tracheostomy Tube (previously Tracheostomy Care Guideline). Version 11. January 2015. Nepean Blue Mountains Local Health District. http://www.aci.health.nsw.gov.au/

Inhealth. www.inhealth.com

Living with a tracheostomy—information for families. Great Ormond Street Hospital for Children NHS Trust, 2001. http://www.gosh.nhs.uk/

Patient and Family Guide, 2016. Tracheostomy Care at Home. Nova Scotia Health authority. http://www.nshealth.ca

References

1. Alladi A, Rao S, Das K, Charles AR, D'Cruz AJ. Pediatric tracheostomy: a 13-year experience. Pediatr Surg Int. 2004;20:695–8.
2. Corbett HJ, Mann KS, Mitra I, Jesudason EC, Losty PD, Clarke RW. Tracheostomy—a 10-year experience from a UK pediatric surgical center. J Pediatr Surg. 2007;42(7):1251–4.
3. National Tracheostomy Safety Project (NTSP). National Tracheostomy Safety Project paediatric emergency algorithms. http://www.tracheostomy.org.uk/Templates/NTSP-Paeds.html (2017). Accessed 9 Mar 2017.
4. Lyons MJ, Cooke J, Cochrane LA, Albert DM. Safe reliable atraumatic replacement of misplaced paediatric tracheostomy tubes. Int J Pediatr Otorhinolaryngol. 2007;71(11):1743–6.
5. Ahn Y, Hwang T. The effects of shallow versus deep endotracheal suctioning on the cytological components of respiratory aspirates in high-risk infants. Respiration. 2003;70(2):172–8.
6. Davies K, Monterosso L, Bulsara M, Ramelet AS. Clinical Indicators for the initiation of endotracheal suctioning in children: an Integrative review. Aust Crit Care. 2015;28(1):11–8.
7. Roberts FE. Consensus among physiotherapists in the United Kingdom on the use of normal saline instillation prior to endotracheal suction; a Delphi study. Physiotherapy Can. 2009;61(2):107–15.
8. Tarnoff M, Moncure M, Jones F, Ross S, Goodman M. The value of routine post tracheostomy chest radiography. Chest. 1998;113(6):1647–9.

When and How to Remove a Tracheostomy

Priscila Rodrigues Prado Prado Zagari and
Roberta Melo Calvoso Paulon

Introduction

Tracheostomy is a surgical procedure used to facilitate prolonged ventilatory support in critically ill patients, allowing early discharge from the intensive care unit (ICU) and lower mortality associated with mechanical ventilation. This procedure, previously performed only in a surgical center, is increasingly used in ICUs. Indications for tracheostomy placement include unsuccessful weaning off mechanical ventilation, neurological patients unable to protect airways, excessive secretions, and upper airway obstruction [1].

The tracheostomy tube is placed below the cricoid cartilage through the trachea, between the third and fourth tracheal rings, creating a secondary airway (larynx), allowing for a greater volume of inspired air being available for oxygenation [2]. There are several types of tubes that are classified according to the material used in their manufacture, their style, and their type [3].

The types of materials that can be used to make the tubes are plastic (PVC), which is commonly used but can cause an inflammatory reaction and formation of granuloma tissue, and cannot be resterilized; silicone, which is not porous and allows resterilization, being a synthetic material more commonly used in bioengineering due to its high degree of biocompatibility; and metal, which is present in rigid and heavy tubes, and has the drawback of transmitting heat and cold to the patient but is more hygienic than PVC tubing. Plastic and silicone tubes are generally preferred to metallic ones because of their flexibility, providing greater comfort to the patient [4].

The standard tracheostomy tube has an external tube, an inner tube, a mandrel, an anchoring cord on the neck, and a small device to occlude the tube when necessary. As for the type, they can be fenestrated or nonfenestrated, with or without

P.R.P.P. Zagari, Speech Therapist. (✉) • R.M.C. Paulon, Ph.D., M.Sc., Speech Therapist.
Hospital Sírio-Libanês, São Paulo, SP, Brazil
e-mail: cilaprado@yahoo.com.br

T.P. de Farias (ed.), *Tracheostomy*, https://doi.org/10.1007/978-3-319-67867-2_23

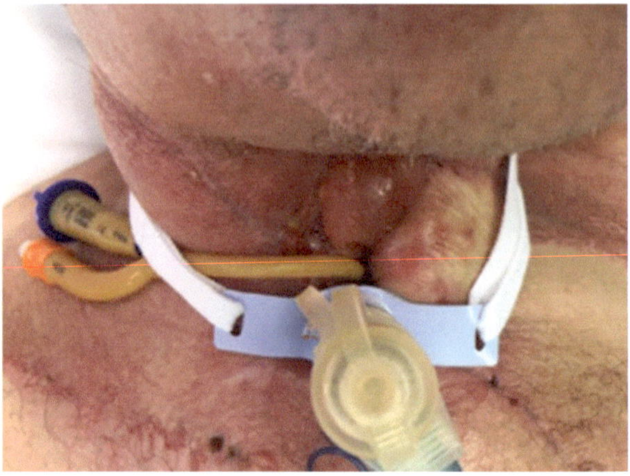

Fig. 1 Complications due to prolonged use of tracheostomy

a cuff, and with or without internal tubing. Fenestrated tubes have small holes that allow air to pass through to the vocal folds, restoring airflow normalization. The cuff is a small balloon at the distal end of the tube, which can be inflated and deflated according to need. It is indicated in two situations: in patients requiring mechanical ventilation and in patients with chronic aspiration [4].

Tracheostomy, when compared with an orotracheal tube, has some advantages, including less time for weaning off mechanical ventilation, less resistance to airflow, less dead space, less movement inside the trachea, greater patient comfort, and more efficient swallowing [5]. However, some studies report that prolonged tracheostomy favors the appearance of late complications, such as tracheal stenosis, bleeding, fistulae, infections, hemorrhages, and bronchoaspiration [6] (Figs. 1 and 2). Others report that mortality is higher in patients who are still tracheostomized when they are discharged from the ICU to the ward. Therefore, removal of the tracheal tube is a key step in the rehabilitation of the critical patient [5–7].

Decannulation

Decannulation is the process of restoring the physiological pathway of respiration with the withdrawal of the tracheostomy tube. In order to obtain successful weaning, attention should be given to the need for sedation, mechanical ventilation, acute or chronic respiratory failure, airway obstruction (due to edema, a tumor, or other causes), prior surgeries to the head and neck, vocal fold paralysis, and glottic or subglottic stenosis—in short, any problems that may impact the upper airway, preventing the restoration of adequate airflow passage.

Some other predictors of success in decannulation include patient stability, absence of secretions in amounts that may compromise the respiratory pattern, total weaning off mechanical ventilation, ability to manage saliva and other upper airway secretions in the absence of a cuff, and no signs of bronchoaspiration. The patient

Fig. 2 Complications due to prolonged use of tracheostomy

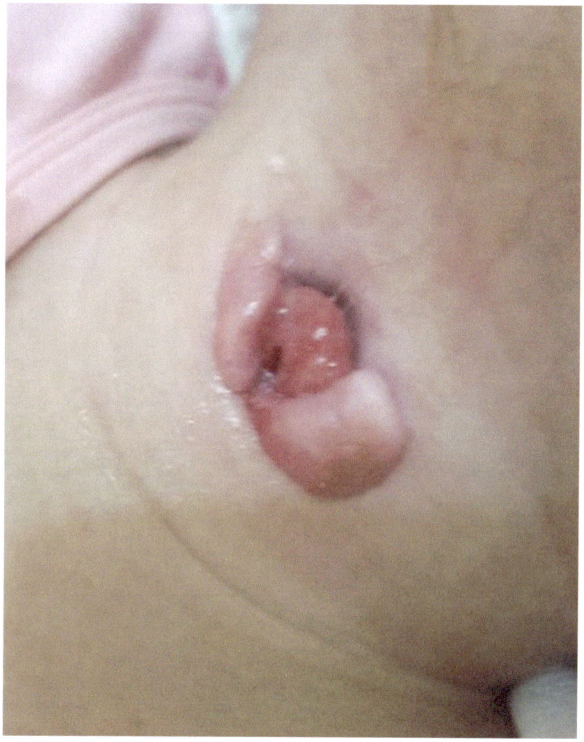

should be able to breathe through the upper airway upon withdrawal of cuff pressure and tracheostoma occlusion without any sign of obstruction, resistance, or respiratory distress (Fig. 3). The expiratory flow should also be sufficient to generate enough force for the patient to cough and speak [8]. If the patient's clinical condition is favorable, the physician authorizes the start of weaning off the tracheostomy.

It is common to follow specific rules for tracheostomy indication, but there are no rules determining the withdrawal process, since clinical conditions and therapeutic evolution are individual. Chronic diseases and lack of protocols for weaning and decannulation based on evidence make it difficult to predict the results of this process, given the particulars of each patient [9].

The decision on when to start weaning the patient off the tracheostomy is made by the team, aiming to minimize any factor that is predictive of failure [4]. Lages and Neumamm [10] propose decannulation as soon as the patient has adequate respiratory mechanics without the need for mechanical ventilation, without upper airway obstruction, with secretions controlled, and with swallowing already evaluated.

Hernández et al. [11] inferred that classification of tracheostomized patients based on the indication for tracheostomy (mechanical ventilation with prolonged weaning or inability to manage respiratory secretions, including patients with

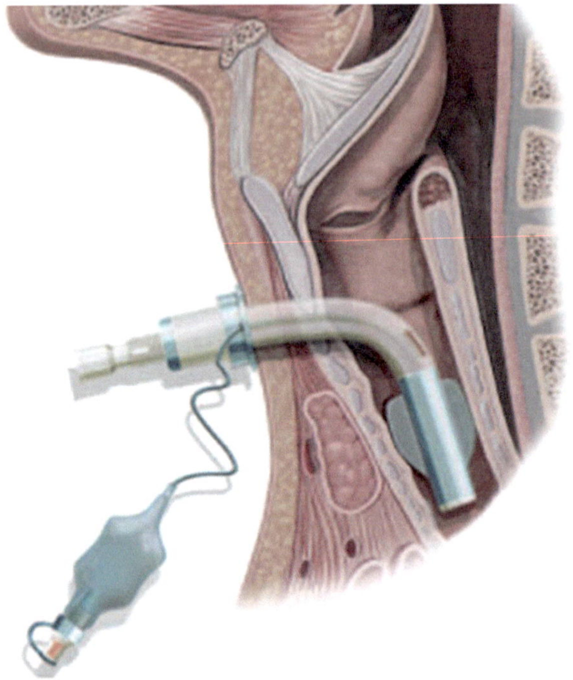

Fig. 3 Relationship between cuff tracheostomy and structures involved with swallowing and breathing functions

deterioration of the level of consciousness due to brain damage) is a fundamental step in the development of protocols for decannulation.

According to a study by Tobin and Santamaria [12], the main criteria for decannulation include the ability to tolerate a deflated cuff for 24 h, an effective cough with the ability to eliminate secretions through the mouth, intact upper airways, swallowing capacity, speech with a phonation valve or occlusion of the tracheostomy, and lack of need for oxygen support. The same criteria were observed in the study carried out by Stelfox et al. [6], which aimed to characterize contemporary practices for decannulation, through an interview applied to physicians and respiratory therapists in the USA. As a result, the four most important criteria for the decision regarding decannulation were determined as the ability to tolerate tracheostomy tube occlusion, secretions, cough effectiveness, and the patient's level of consciousness [6]. A decreased level of consciousness has been described as a factor related to oropharyngeal dysphagia, associated with aspiration and pneumonia [4].

The process of decannulation is complex and highly individual, and some studies have shown the importance of the joint action of speech–language pathology and physiotherapy in this process. The physiotherapist's responsibility is to check the tracheostomy tube and the oxygen system, discussing daily issues of tracheostomy care with the nursing team, patient, and family. The speech–language pathologist should evaluate the patient's ability to tolerate the speech valve (i.e., assess the level of consciousness, airway protection, phonation, and secretion management) and make recommendations regarding the use of the speech valve and/or strategies for communication [13].

It is important to consider six criteria for speech–language evaluation in the decannulation process: (1) the level of consciousness; (2) breathing (plastic or metallic tube, cuff inflated or deflated, and, when the cuff is inflated, whether the patient maintains a stable respiratory pattern during deflation); (3) tracheal secretion (quantity, appearance, and color); (4) phonation (presence or absence, and presence of vocal quality); (5) coughing (presence of voluntary cough, reflex, and whether it is effective or not); and (6) swallowing (assessing the level of impairment) [4].

Swallowing is evaluated by the speech–language pathologist through a blue dye test—a procedure involving use of blue dye to stain saliva (blue dye test) or food (modified blue dye test modified), to identify saliva/food aspiration in tracheostomized individuals [14]. The presence of bluish secretions in the tracheal or peritracheal region is indicative of aspiration of saliva or offered food that is stained with blue food aniline. In cases where there is aspiration of saliva or food content, this test result qualifies as positive for aspiration.

A study of 30 patients who had undergone treatment for head and neck cancer submitted the patients to a modified blue dye test and concomitantly to nasofibrolaryngoscopy of swallowing. This study demonstrated that the modified blue dye test had 95.24% sensitivity and 100% specificity to detect aspiration in patients after treatment for head and neck cancer [15].

Belafsky et al. [16] performed a modified blue dye test in 30 tracheostomized patients with a mean age of 65 years and found that the sensitivity and specificity of the test were 82% and 38%, respectively. Santana et al. [14] applied a questionnaire to speech–language pathologists who treat tracheostomized patients, and found that all interviewees used the blue dye test as a resource in clinical evaluation of swallowing to detect aspiration. Garuti et al. [17] suggest use of the test to detect the presence or absence of aspiration and propose association between episodes of desaturation and respiratory complications to aid in the decision regarding decannulation.

In order to initiate the process of decannulation in patients undergoing mechanical ventilation, it is very important to have a respiratory physiotherapist (whose objective is to reduce respiratory pressures) identify respiratory and peripheral muscle weakness and facilitate adaptation of the speech valve, considering that patients undergoing tracheostomy and prolonged mechanical ventilation suffer loss of strength and resistance of overall musculature, due to disuse [18].

According to Santana et al. [14], mechanical ventilation leads to changes in the physiology of swallowing, presenting a change in the tonicity and amplitude of the movement of the oropharyngeal structures, thus compromising laryngeal elevation and coordination of swallowing and breathing.

For Frank et al. [19], the main aspect in the treatment of swallowing in tracheostomized patients is the process of deflating the cuff and stimulating swallowing and coughing functions with the deflated cuff. However, standardized protocols for the evaluation of swallowing are still scarce in the literature. Frank at al. [19] suggest the use of a protocol created in the year 2000 at the REHAB rehabilitation center in Basel, Switzerland. In this protocol the functions of the speech therapist are to deflate the cuff during expiration and, if the patient tolerates the deflated cuff, to perform digital occlusion of the tube or to adapt the speech valve, increasing the intervals with the cuff deflated daily until the patient tolerates it for at least 20 min, performing at this time stimulation of swallowing, vocal production, cough, and secretion management.

The speech valve is a resource that can be used to contribute to decannulation [20, 21]. It can be adapted to patients who breathe spontaneously and tolerate tracheostomy occlusion, and the adaptation should always occur when the cuff is deflated. The use of this device allows air to flow into the tube during inspiration, but during expiration, air is directed to the vocal folds and upper airways, producing the voice [22] (Figs. 4 and 5).

Sutt et al. [21] stated that with the use of the unidirectional speech valve, fenestrated tubes or occlusion of the tracheostomy, the adequacy of phonation and swallowing in tracheostomized patients occurs through re-establishment of air passage through the glottis, increased subglottic pressure, and stimulation of peripheral and central nerve endings. For better tolerance of the speech valve and to reduce muscular effort, it is advisable to replace the tube of the tracheostomy with another with a size number 1–2 units smaller, reducing the expiratory resistance (although inspiratory force becomes increased) and also improving the handling of secretions, which must be expectorated by the airways naturally [20] (Fig. 6).

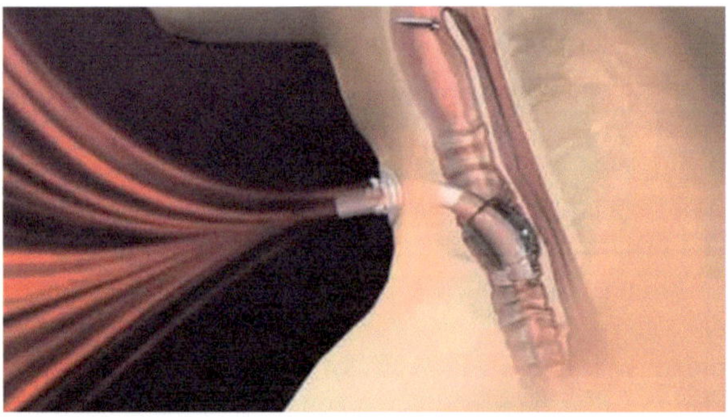

Fig. 4 Breathing via tracheostomy without phonation valve adaptation

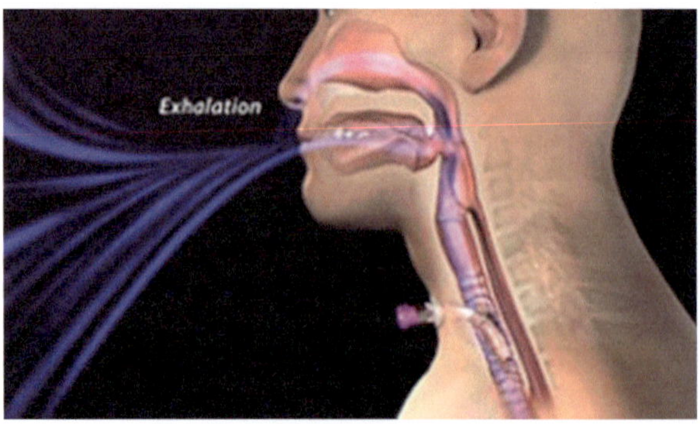

Fig. 5 Breathing via tracheostomy with phonation valve adaptation

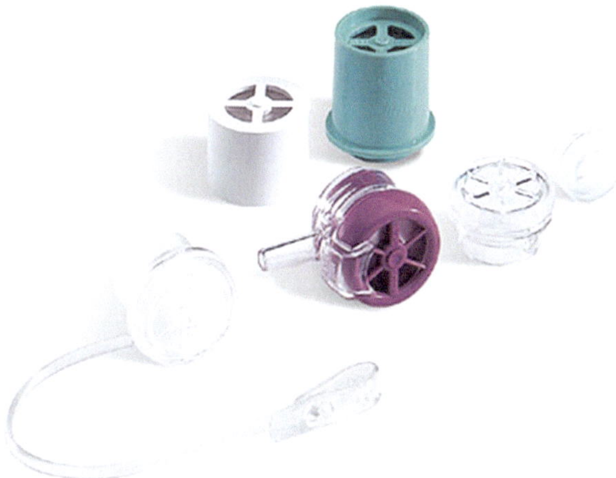

Fig. 6 Passy-Muir type valves (www.passy-muir.com)

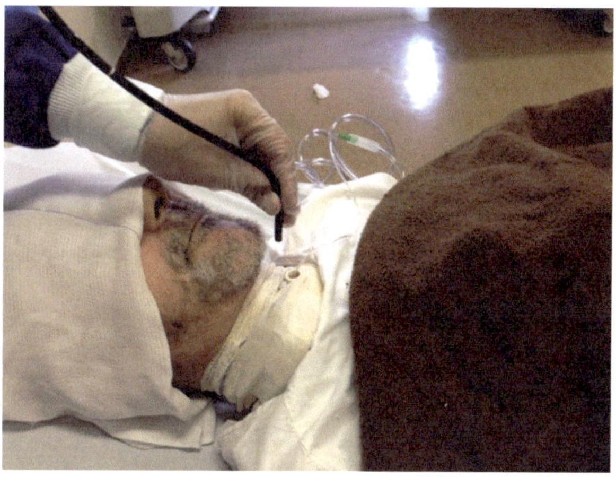

Fig. 7 Endoscopic inspection via tracheostomy

For O'Connor and White [9], endoscopic airway inspection, while not essential for decannulation, may be useful. This procedure is performed by nasoendoscopy with an optical fiber in the subglottic space. It is a safe procedure and requires only topical anesthesia (Fig. 4). In a substantial number of patients, endoscopic evaluation identifies pathologies that require otorhinolaryngological or thoracic surgery before the decannulation process (Fig. 7).

Recently, Santus et al. [22] published a systematic review that aimed to identify quantitative and semiquantitative parameters for decannulation and to elaborate a clinical score, involving phonoaudiological and physiotherapeutic evaluations. Among the quantitative parameters, the authors included measures of cough (expiratory muscle strength ≥40 cm H_2O, peak cough flow >160 L/min) and tube occlusion ≥24 h, each parameter receiving a score of 0 in the case of commitment or 20 if appropriate. The semiquantitative parameters were the level of consciousness (drowsy/alert), secretions (thick/thin), swallowing (compromised/normal), partial pressure of carbon dioxide ($PaCO_2$ <60 mmHg), airway clearance (tracheal stenosis <50% seen by bronchoscopy), age <70 years, indication for tracheostomy (other/pneumonia or airway obstruction), and comorbidities ($\geq$1 or none). Each semiquantitative parameter received a score of 0 (compromised) to 5 (adequate).

The performance of the multidisciplinary team increases the chances of faster, complication-free, and safer decannulation for the patient. There is still no validated protocol for the decannulation process, and studies are needed to define a model that may be applicable to this population.

Studies that establish criteria for weaning off tracheostomy are still scarce, implying that the decision regarding decannulation is still based on subjective evaluations, as opposed to standardized protocols. Thus, all professionals involved in the treatment of tracheostomized patients need to be alert to the following warning signs for complications: saliva or food residue in the trachea, changes in the color or appearance of secretions, fever, worsening of oxygenation, lowering of the consciousness level, and abrupt alteration of radiological images [23].

Difficulties with Decannulation

Despite the fact that it offers enormous benefits to the patient when compared with the use of an orotracheal tube, tracheostomy should be performed with an appropriate technique and properly applied care, since (although they are not frequent) complications can be fatal [24].

According to Choate et al. [25], the major cause of failure in decannulation is secretion retention. Difficulties in removal of the tube also occur in situations where there is persistence of the cause that led to the tracheostomy, displacement of the anterior tracheal wall, obstruction of the tracheal lumen, mucosal edema, intolerance of increased air resistance through the passage of air into the nostrils (common in children and the elderly), stenosis, or tracheomalacia [25].

According to Lages et al. [10], it may be difficult to eliminate the manifestation of obstructive and restrictive respiratory conditions during nighttime mechanical ventilation, due to hypoventilation or sleep apnea. These patients may benefit from noninvasive nasal ventilation with an occluded tracheostomy tube overnight until they are finally decannulated.

O'Connor and White [9] note the need to monitor patient oximetry within 24 h after decannulation. When the stoma closes, vocalization tends to return to normal, which can take between 5 and 7 days in patients with no associated comorbidities. The presence of fibrous scarring at the stomatal closure may be aesthetically embarrassing and may also contribute to dysphagia due to adherence of the skin to the trachea, making laryngeal elevation difficult. These cases can be corrected surgically.

Accidental decannulation can result in serious consequences if the tracheostomy is recent and if the patient has a difficult course. At more than 7 days after tracheostomy tube placement surgery, replacement is usually easy. If the decannulation occurs at less than 7 days, recannulation may occur improperly. Patients with a short neck or increased neck circumference are at increased risk of this occurrence [10].

Choate et al. [25] conducted a prospective and descriptive study with 981 patients, in which 823 were decannulated. Decannulation was considered unsuccessful if the tube needed replacement prior to hospital discharge. Using this criterion, there were 40 episodes of failure (4.8%). According to the authors, if recannulation had been considered as a failure criterion in the 48 h period after decannulation, the failure rate would have been 3.5%.

Another important complication found in tracheostomized patients is immobility, followed by generalized muscle weakness in subjects who remain dependent on mechanical ventilation for long periods [26, 27], and this may be a factor in failure during the decannulation procedure. Lima et al. [28] verified the influence of peripheral muscle strength on the success of decannulation in 57 patients, with 46 successes and 11 failures. Subjects who were successfully decannulated presented with significantly greater peripheral muscle strength than those in the failure group (41.11 ± 11.52 versus 28.33 ± 15.31, $p = 0.04$). In this study, strength assessment was performed using the Medical Research Council (MRC) scale.

Final Considerations

Decannulation depends on many factors, and because it is a complex process, the importance of a multidisciplinary team to make the process more effective and safe must be considered.

Speech–language pathology during the decannulation process aims to adapt swallowing, making it effective and safe, as well as acting in the protection of lower airways, working the sphincter function of the larynx and cough.

References

1. Mendes F, Ranea P, Oliveira ACT. Protocolo de desmame e decanulação de traqueostomia. Revista UNILUS Ensino e Pesquisa. 2013;10(2), ISSN (impresso): 1807-8850, ISSN (eletrônico): 2318–2083.
2. Lewis K, Liss JM, Sciortino KL. Bases fisiológicas das etiologias estruturais da disfagia e estratégias de tratamento—anatomia clínica e fisiologia do mecanismo de deglutição. São Paulo: Cengage Learning; 2009.
3. Filho EDM, Gomes GF, Furkim AM. Manual de cuidados do paciente com disfagia. São Paulo: Lovise; 2000.
4. Zanata IL, Santos RS, Hirata GC. Tracheal decannulation protocol in patients affected by traumatic brain injury. Int Arch Otorhinolaryngol. 2014;18:108–14.
5. Martinez GH, Fernandez R, Casado MS, Cuena R, Lopez-Reina P, Zamora S, Luzon E. Tracheostomy tube in place at intensive care unit discharge is associated with increased ward mortality. Respir Care. 2009;54(12):1644–52.
6. Stelfox HT, Crimi C, Berra L, Noto A, Schmidt U, Bigatello LM, Hess D. Determinants of tracheostomy decannulation: an international survey. Crit Care. 2008;12:R26.
7. Hsu CL, Chen KY, Chang CH, Jerng JS, CJ Y, Yang PC. Timing of tracheostomy as a determinant of weaning success in critically ill patients: a retrospective study. Crit Care. 2005;9:46–52.
8. Pannunzio TG. Aspiration of oral feedings in patients with tracheostomies. AACN Clin Issues. 1996;7(4):560–9.
9. O'Connor HH, White AC. Tracheostomy decannulation. Respir Care. 2010;55(8):1076–81.

10. Lages NCL, Neumamm LBA. Decanulação em traqueostomia: uma abordagem prática. 2011. Revista InterFISIO. http://interfisio.com.br/?artigo&ID=446. acesso em 18 de julho de 2013.
11. Hernández G, Ortiz R, Pedrosa A, Cuena R, Vaquero Collado C, González Arenas P, García Plaza S, Canabal Berlanga A, Fernández R. La indicación de la traqueotomía condiciona las variables predictoras del tiempo hasta la decanulación en pacientes críticos. Med Intensiva. 2012;36(8):531–9.
12. Tobin AE, Santamaria JD. An intensivist-led tracheostomy review team is associated with shorter decannulation time and length of stay: a prospective cohort study. Crit Care. 2008;12(2):R48.
13. Mestral C, Iqbal S, Fong N, LeBlanc J, Fata P, Razek T, Khwaja K. Impact of a specialized multidisciplinary tracheostomy team on tracheostomy care in critically ill patients. Can J Surg. 2011;54(3):167–72.
14. Santana L, Fernandes A, Brasileiro AG, Abreu AC. Critérios para avaliação clínica fonoaudiológica do paciente traqueostomizado no leito hospitalar e internamento domiciliar. Rev CEFAC. 2014;16(2):524–36.
15. Winklmaier U, Wüst K, Plinkert PK, Wallner F. The accuracy of the modified Evans blue dye test in detecting aspiration in head and neck cancer patients. Eur Arch Otorhinolaryngol. 2007;264(9):1059–64.
16. Belafsky PC, Blumenfeld L, LePage A, Nahrstedt K. The accuracy of the modified Evan's blue dye test in predicting aspiration. Laryngoscope. 2003;113(11):1969–72.
17. Garuti G, Reverberi C, Briganti A, Massobrio M, Lombardi F, Lusuardi M. Swallowing disorders in tracheostomised patients: a multidisciplinary/multiprofessional approach in decannulation protocols. Multidiscip Respir Med. 2014;9:36.
18. Mendes TAB, Cavalheiro LV, Arevalo RT, Sonegth R. Estudo preliminar sobre a proposta de um fluxograma de decanulação em traqueostomia com atuação interdisciplinar. Einstein. 2008;6:1–6.
19. Frank U, Mäder M, Sticher H. Dysphagic patients with tracheotomies: a multidisciplinary approach to treatment and decannulation management. Dysphagia. 2007;22:20–9.
20. Fernández-Carmona A, Penas-Maldonado L, Yuste-Osorio E, Díaz-Redondo A. Exploración y abordaje de disfagia secundaria a vía aérea artificial. Med Intensiva. 2012;36(6):423–33.
21. Sutt AL, Cornwell P, Mullany D, Kinneally T, Fraser JF. The use of tracheostomy speaking valves in mechanically ventilated patients results in improved communication and does not prolong ventilation time in cardiothoracic intensive care unit patients. J Crit Care. 2015;30(3):491–4.
22. Santus P, Gramegna A, Radovanovic D, Raccanelli R, Valenti V, Rabbiosi D, et al. A systematic review on tracheostomy decannulation: a proposal of a quantitative semiquantitative clinical score. BMC Pulm Med. 2014;14:201.
23. Garrubba M, Turner T, Grieveson C. Multidisciplinary care for tracheostomy patients: a systematic review. Crit Care. 2009;13:R177.
24. Ricz HMA, Mello-Filho FV, Contide Freitas LC, Mamede RCM. Traqueostomia. Medicina (Ribeirão Preto). 2011;44:63–9.
25. Choate K, Barbetti J, Currey J. Tracheostomy decannulation failure rate following critical illness: a prospective descriptive study. Aust Crit Care. 2009;22:8–15.
26. Chambers MA, Moylan JS, Reid MB. Physical inactivity and muscle weakness in the critically ill. Crit Care Med. 2009;37(10 Suppl):S337–46.
27. Chiang LL, Wang LY, CP W, HD W, Wu YT. Effects of physical training on functional status in patients with prolonged mechanical ventilation. Phys Ther. 2006;8(9):1271–81.
28. Lima CA, Siqueira TB, Travassos ÉF, Macedo CMG, Bezerra AL, Paiva Júnior MDS, et al. Influência da força da musculatura periférica no sucesso da decanulação. Rev Bras Ter Intensiva. 2011;23:56–61.

Rehabilitation After Tracheostomy

Priscila Rodrigues Prado Prado Zagari,
Roberta Melo Calvoso Paulon, and Luciana Paiva Farias

Introduction

Tracheostomy is a surgical procedure often performed in emergency situations in patients presenting with surgical diseases of the head and neck (re-establishment of the airways in cases of obstructive disease and protection of the airway after major surgery of the oral cavity and oropharynx, as well as in partial laryngectomy), respiratory insufficiency, hypoxia, inflammatory processes, foreign bodies in the respiratory tract, bronchial hypersecretion, congenital anomalies, neuromuscular diseases, and/or respiratory muscle fatigue (usually caused by some disease) [1, 2].

In most cases, tracheostomy is also indicated for patients with prolonged mechanical ventilation, in the management of patients with difficult weaning from a ventilatory prosthesis, or to facilitate airway hygiene, thus providing greater patient safety and comfort. This procedure is characterized as the best alternative for removal of the tracheal tube and reduction of sedation during mechanical ventilation, which may reduce the artificial ventilation time, incidence of pneumonia, and length of hospital stay [3]. For these patient profiles, tracheostomy can bring great benefits, such as a lower rate of self-extubation, the possibility of phonation and oral ingestion, improvement of oral hygiene, and easier management of the patient by the team.

On the other hand, researchers and clinicians have discussed the impact of tracheostomy on the functions of the stomatognathic system, especially regarding the

P.R.P.P. Zagari, Speech Therapist. (✉) • R.M.C. Paulon, Ph.D., M.Sc., Speech Therapist.
Hospital Sírio-Libanês, São Paulo, SP, Brazil
e-mail: cilaprado@yahoo.com.br

L.P. Farias, MSc., Speech Therapist.
Sirio Libanes Hospital, Sao Paulo, SP, Brazil

Department of Neurolinguistics, Faculty of Medicine, Hospital das Clinicas, University of Sao Paulo, Sao Paulo, SP, Brazil

Federal Speech Therapist Council, Belo Horizonte, MG, Brazil

T.P. de Farias (ed.), *Tracheostomy*, https://doi.org/10.1007/978-3-319-67867-2_24

biomechanics of swallowing and speech. Studies have shown that prolonged use of a tracheostomy tube can compromise the sensory and motor functions of the mechanisms involved in swallowing, leading to aggravation of dysphagia, which is most often caused by a basic disease (neurological, pulmonary, or oncological, among others) or in the appearance of late complications, including tracheal stenosis, bleeding, fistulas, infections, hemorrhages, and bronchoaspiration [4]. From the point of view of the biomechanics of swallowing, tracheostomy will alter the structures and physiology of the respiratory system, influencing the mechanisms of airway protection, vocal production, and the digestive system. Regarding the biomechanics of speech, there will be insufficient directing of expiratory airflow to the upper airway, thus compromising the glottic coaptation necessary for efficient phonation during oral communication. It should be noted that the occurrence and severity of these changes will depend on many variables, from the underlying disease to the appropriate choice of tube type for each patient [5, 6].

The aims of speech–language pathology assessment of the tracheostomized patient are to know the patient's clinical status, analyze the history of the swallowing disorder, and carefully evaluate the structures and functions of the stomatognathic system (focusing on respiration–phonation–swallowing) to determine the diagnosis and course of treatment to be followed. Clinical speech–language pathology assessment criteria are essential to ensure a safe approach and appropriate management of tracheostomized patients. These criteria involve multiple and complex factors that must be considered, such as cognitive–linguistic, behavioral, respiratory, phonatory, and orofacial motor aspects [7, 8].

Although the benefits of tracheostomy are explicit, there are controversies in the literature and clinical practice regarding its indication, the correct choice of tube, and also the actual complications of this procedure for swallowing, breathing, and speech functions. Likewise, there are discussions in the theoretical field and clinical practice about the impact of the inflated cuff on the biomechanics of swallowing.

The cuff is indicated for sealing the lower airway during mechanical ventilation, preventing bronchoaspiration of secretions, foods, and gastric contents [7, 9]. However, it is known that the inflated cuff causes a negative impact on the pharyngeal phase of swallowing, as it compromises the excursion of the hyolaryngeal complex and, when hyperinflated, compresses the anterior wall of the esophagus, making esophageal transit difficult and facilitating the occurrence of food reflux.

Considering these changes in the physiology of swallowing, there is a high risk that secretions, saliva, and food (in the case of oral alimentary intake) will be imprisoned in the supracuff region, with a great possibility of dripping of these residues down the sides of the trachea, thus promoting immediate or late bronchoaspiration. Therefore, even if the cuff is inflated, there is no total protection of the lower airway during an oral diet, as well as for secretions and/or gastric contents.

We have seen that the reason for indicating tracheostomy, the type of tube, and careful evaluation of the structures and functions of the stomatognathic system are important factors for the design of the therapeutic plan, although the prognosis of the rehabilitation of the patient's swallowing does not depend exclusively on the presence of tracheostomy.

Swallowing

Implications of Tracheostomy for Swallowing

Swallowing is a neuromuscular response initiated by a combination of voluntary and involuntary actions involving precise coordination mainly between the oral and pharyngeal phases of swallowing and a complex interaction between various muscles and nerves, whose function is to transport food from the oral cavity to the stomach. Efficient (physiological) swallowing results from anatomical and functional integrity of various structures and muscles (orofacial, pharyngeal, laryngeal, esophageal, and stomach), which are controlled by the central and peripheral nervous systems [7]. Didactically, it is possible to divide the swallowing process into five phases—anticipatory, preparatory, oral, pharyngeal, and esophageal—since they occur interdependently [7]:

- *Anticipatory phase:* This corresponds to the intention and the will to feed, hunger, visual and olfactory aspects, the environment, and all of the factors that can facilitate (or not) the next phase, which is the preparatory phase.
- *Preparatory phase:* This is the moment of preparation of the bolus, from the capture to the grinding to the formation of a homogeneous bolus. This phase can take different times, according to the characteristics of the bolus, such as the quantity, consistency, viscosity, and temperature of the food.
- *Oral phase:* This begins after the formation of a homogeneous bolus when it is transported from the oral cavity to the pharynx.
- *Pharyngeal phase:* This triggers the moment when the bolus, together with anteroposterior movement of the tongue, stimulates the afferent region of the oropharynx and begins sequential movements to protect the airways from the food, and for the bolus to be transported directly into the esophagus. In the physiology of the pharyngeal phase of swallowing, when the bolus reaches the oropharyngeal region, the palatine veil elevates and the larynx anteriorly elevates and closes at three levels (the vocal folds, vestibular folds, and arytenoids with the epiglottis) so that concomitantly the pharyngeal–esophageal transition relaxes and the bolus progresses from the pharynx to the esophagus.
- *Esophageal phase:* This begins after the passage of the bolus through the pharyngeal–esophageal transition, when peristaltic waves start moving the bolus to the stomach.

Changes in swallowing, when unidentified and not properly diagnosed, may have consequences for the general health of the individual, such as malnutrition, dehydration, bronchopneumonia, and even death.

This change in swallowing, called *dysphagia*, is characterized by any failure that occurs from the entrance of the food into the oral cavity until it reaches the stomach; however, it is important to consider that in the context of cognitive disorders, there is not necessarily a flaw in the biomechanics but perhaps in the anticipatory phase of swallowing, which may compromise the patient's performance in the later stages. In general, the main videofluoroscopic findings in patients with dysphagia are oral incontinence, increased oral transit time, premature oropharyngeal bolus loss, nasal reflux, food residue in the vallecula and/or pharyngeal recesses after swallowing, laryngeal penetration, tracheal aspiration, change in the opening/relaxation of the pharyngoesophageal transition, and esophageal dysmotility. The bolus can enter the airways, causing laryngeal penetration (when it reaches the level of the vocal folds) or aspiration (when the bolus exceeds the level of the vocal folds). Therefore, laryngeal penetration and/or aspiration of the bolus occur when there are sensorial, motor, pressure, and/or incoordination changes of the structures in their respective sequential functions.

The vast majority of tracheostomized patients have been previously intubated and are characterized as a population at risk for dysphagia due to various factors, such as intubation time, and their respective sequelae. Intubation time influences the severity of dysphagia, as it may damage the mucosa and the laryngeal and pharyngeal musculature, leading to sensory and motor changes that cause dysphagia manifested by premature loss of bolus and/or change of laryngeal mobility (elevation and stability) and the closing movement of the vocal folds, vestibular folds, and aryepiglottic folds for consequent protection of the airways; laryngeal penetration and/or aspiration before, during, and/or after swallowing; and food stasis in the vallecula and pharyngeal recesses, as previously described [10–13]. The size of the tube and the weight and presence of the cuff are also factors that hamper laryngeal mobility, which consequently contributes to bolus entry into the airways before, during, and/or after swallowing. The restriction of elevation of the larynx in the neck is another mechanical factor that should be considered. Some surgeries that use techniques such as horizontal incision can leverage the restriction of vertical movement of the larynx, along with the size and weight of the tube and a highly inflated cuff (Fig. 1).

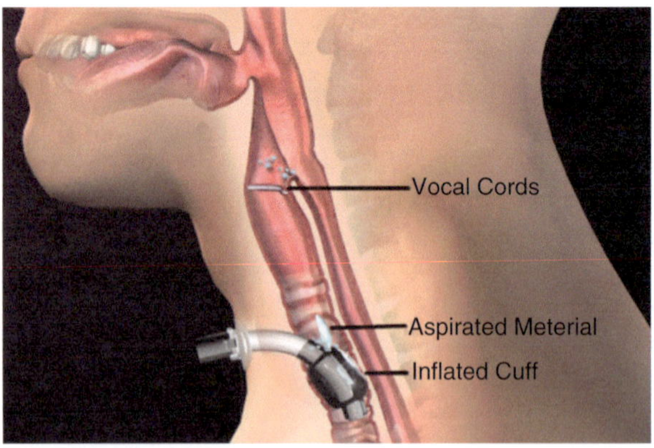

Fig. 1 Inflated cuff interfering with swallowing

With the presence of tracheostomy, there is a reduction of the pressure and quantity of airflow to the upper airway, causing the absence of a protective cough and the cleaning effect if food enters the airways or if there is stasis [7]. This protective cough can be characterized as absent or present but with weak intensity or ineffective, characterizing a worsening of the individual's swallowing status.

It should also be considered that with airflow diversion to the tracheostomy, the individual may present with changes of smell and taste, making the anticipatory phase of swallowing difficult, leading to reduced appetite and reduced laryngeal sensitivity, causing silent aspiration [14, 15].

Patients who are dependent on mechanical ventilation also present with changes in the physiology of swallowing, since the period of the respiratory pause in swallowing (the pharyngeal phase) will also be modified and the patients will have to adapt to the different phases of inspiration and expiration starting from then, which should be set with ventilator parameters [7].

Therefore, all of these factors added to the underlying disease have great repercussions for swallowing and speech [7].

Speech–Language Pathological Assessment of Swallowing in the Presence of Tracheostomy

Speech–language assessment consists of identification and differentiation of sequelae of the underlying disease and tracheostomy. It is necessary to carry out a rigorous structural and functional evaluation of the phonoarticulatory organs—taking into consideration the aspects of symmetry, sensitivity, mobility, strength, resistance, presence or absence of physiological and/or pathological reflexes, amount of orotracheal secretion, presence and general condition of dentition, oral control of saliva, and oral hygiene—and to evaluate the risks and benefits of a swallowing assessment.

In order to perform a speech–language assessment in patients with an inflated cuff, dependent (or not) on mechanical ventilation, it is necessary to discuss with the multidisciplinary team the risks and benefits of deflating the cuff to evaluate the integration of respiratory versus swallowing functions. For cases where the cuff can be deflated, a Passy-Muir valve is commonly indicated, which is a small device that, when placed in the tracheostomy tube, allows air to enter the lungs and exit through the upper airway. The air then reaches the vocal folds by normalizing the airflow [16].

In some situations, when the patient is able to have the cuff deflated, some professionals from the multidisciplinary team choose to perform stoma occlusion training, either digitally and/or with a syringe plunger, to assess swallowing that is closest to physiology. If the patient tolerates the occluded tracheostomy tube, they should be guided in relation to the phases of respiration (inspiration and expiration) and coordination for phonation and swallowing, causing a conscious restoration with this entire process.

One of the screening tests most commonly used by the speech–language pathologist to assess swallowing in tracheostomized patients is the *blue dye test* (BDT), which is an easy procedure to perform but requires adequate criteria and methodology for its use in clinical practice. This screening test consists of the dripping of four drops of food coloring on the back of the tongue of the user of the tracheostomy tube, and the procedure of tracheal aspirations should occur at intervals of 4 h over 48 h to identify the presence or absence of salivary aspiration. The small amount of dye may also be mixed with different food consistencies to screen for functional swallowing and to record whether or not there is aspiration, which is named the *modified blue dye test* (MBDT). The test is followed immediately by endotracheal aspiration and monitoring of aspiration secretion staining by the nursing/physiotherapy team during the proximate periods. The result is characterized as negative or positive, indicating absence or presence of stained tracheal secretion, respectively. Some studies show that both tests have a low sensitivity rate due to false negative or false positive results, so in order to perform such tests for screening, it is important that the speech–language pathologist be skilled in the performance of the procedure and critically analyze the results, taking into consideration possible flaws [17].

Some analyses should be considered when it is possible to evaluate the function of swallowing for different foods:

1. The consistency, quantity, and temperature of the food to be offered (remembering that it is important to discuss the clinical profile of each patient with the multidisciplinary team).
2. Observation of the frequency and effectiveness of spontaneous swallowing of saliva.
3. Staining of the food with food aniline, preferably in a blue color, to facilitate identification of the characteristics and quantity of the material aspirated in the lower airway, knowing that the presence of this colored material in the aspiration is a positive sign of aspiration of the food offered, but its absence cannot be immediately considered a negative result, since there may be a false negative result. Therefore, whenever possible, it is important to take advantage of complementary instrumental evaluations (cervical auscultation associated with pulse oximetry) to increase the reliability of the evaluation.
4. Observation of the respiratory pattern and the behavior of the patient during and after each offer of food [17].

In addition to clinical assessments, in many cases, further instrumental evaluations are required to complement the findings of clinical assessment, such as nasofibrolaryngoscopy (fiberoptic endoscopic evaluation of swallowing (FEES) and flexible endoscopic evaluation of swallowing with sensory testing (FEESST)) and/or swallowing videofluoroscopy. Through these instruments, swallowing phases can be analyzed separately and seamlessly, giving the speech–language pathologist a sum of important findings for clinical clarification and for future elaboration of compensatory or rehabilitative strategies for swallowing.

Swallowing Therapy in the Presence of Tracheostomy

The planning of therapies for dysphagia occurs after evaluation and understanding of the condition through the correlation of the patient's previous history, underlying disease, structural observation, and functionality of the phonoarticulatory organs. For tracheostomized patients, an approach prior to specific care for swallowing dysfunction is required. Therapy begins when the patient is stable from the hemodynamic point of view. If possible, orotracheal aspiration, consecutive deflation of the cuff, and respective tube occlusion to direct airflow to the upper airway are performed with the objective of physiological re-establishment of respiration, phonation, and swallowing.

In cases in which the patient does not tolerate cuff deflation, it is necessary to evaluate the reason why it is not possible to perform such a procedure and the real benefit of the introduction of the oral route with the cuff inflated, considering that the physiology will be altered by all of the variables above. If the intolerance of cuff deflation occurs due to sialorrhea and/or massive aspiration of saliva, a medical evaluation is essential for determination of complementary courses of medical and/or surgical treatment, depending on the severity of the case.

A speech valve, being unidirectional, is usually an important device for patients who do not tolerate total occlusion of the tracheostomy tube, which additionally benefits the therapeutic process and the possibility of reintroduction of the diet by the oral route to some patients who are dependent (or not) on mechanical ventilation. For these patients in particular, it is essential to discuss the ventilatory mode and parameters of the patient together with the medical and physiotherapy team, and, if possible, adjust them to favor adaptation of a speech valve and consequent training of speech and swallowing functions.

Oral Communication

Implications of Tracheostomy for Speech

Phonoarticulation involves the participation of five motor systems coordinated by the central and peripheral nervous systems: respiratory, phonatory, articulatory, resonantal, and prosodic.

In principle, the presence of the tracheostomy tube compromises respiration and phonation, leading the individual to be unable to perform phonation effectively. The impact of tracheostomy on the individual's speech can be divided into two categories: mechanical and physiological.

The mechanical impact is when the patient has a history of previous intubation, which can lead to temporary or permanent sequelae, and unilateral or bilateral sequelae, in the larynx and in vocal production.

Some sequelae of intubation include reduction of laryngeal sensitivity, fixation of cricoid and arytenoid cartilage, change of movement and/or laryngeal muscle force, and edema in the vocal folds. All of these changes may cause a greater or lesser impact on vocal physiology. These sequelae resulting from traumatic and/or prolonged intubation may still be present in the patient even after extubation and will add to the changes in vocal physiology due to the presence of the tracheostomy tube. One of the factors that alter pitch modulation is the vertical movement of the larynx during phonation. Restricted excursion of laryngeal elevation may occur due to different factors, such as the presence of the tracheostomy tube, the surgical technique adopted at the time of the surgical procedure (horizontal or vertical incision), the tube size and weight, and the cuff status (inflated or deflated) [7, 18–20] (Fig. 2).

Whenever possible, an indication for a speech valve is extremely valued in relation to the various benefits it can provide for the patient. Quite differently from what many people think, it can make it easier to wean the patient off mechanical ventilation, improve the quality of swallowing, and allow the patient to resume oral communication.

In cases of patients who are dependent (or not) on mechanical ventilation, adaptation of a speech valve may also be indicated. The main situations that contraindicate a speech valve are unconscious comatose patients (if the objective is only for speech), acute medical instability, severe obstruction of the airways, very reduced pulmonary compliance, massive aspiration of saliva, presence of thick secretion, a large tracheostomy tube size (which does not allow expired air to pass through), an adapted tube with a foam cuff, inability to deflate the cuff, or use of mechanical ventilation in a high-frequency mode or ventilation with release of airway pressure [21].

For adaptation of a valve, it is important to take a multidisciplinary approach and accomplish a preliminary evaluation that includes the cognitive state, pulmonary condition, tolerance of cuff deflation, good management of secretions, adequate swallowing of saliva, and individual appraisal of the valve choice for each case [4] (Fig. 3).

For adaptation of a speech valve in a tracheostomized patient under mechanical ventilation, the presence of a physiotherapist specializing in the respiratory area is necessary to adjust the parameters of the device according to the patient's needs and to follow these steps: observation of vital signs and need for aspiration of the upper and/or lower airways, (depending on the pulmonary condition) cuff deflation, adequacy of ventilation parameters, valve placement, and observation and monitoring of respiratory behavior [4] (Fig. 4).

The most widely used phonation valves are Passy-Muir, Shiley, Portex Montgomery, Olympic, and Kistner. However, Passy-Muir provides better vocal

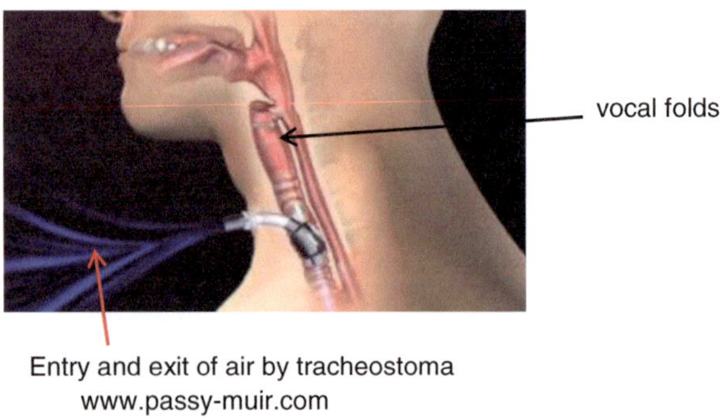

Fig. 2 Inflated cuff interfering with vocal production

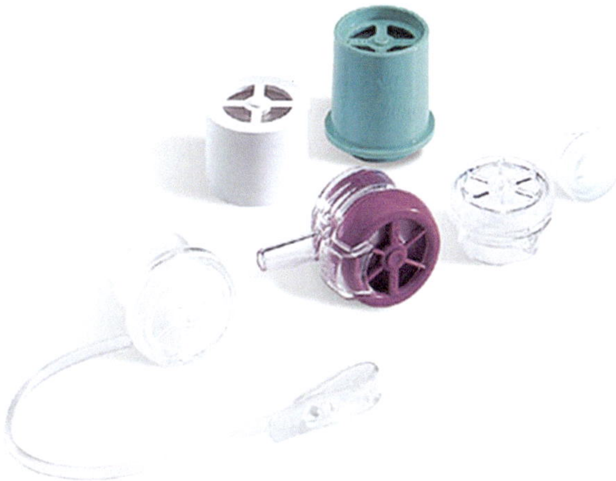

Fig. 3 Types of Passy-Muir valve

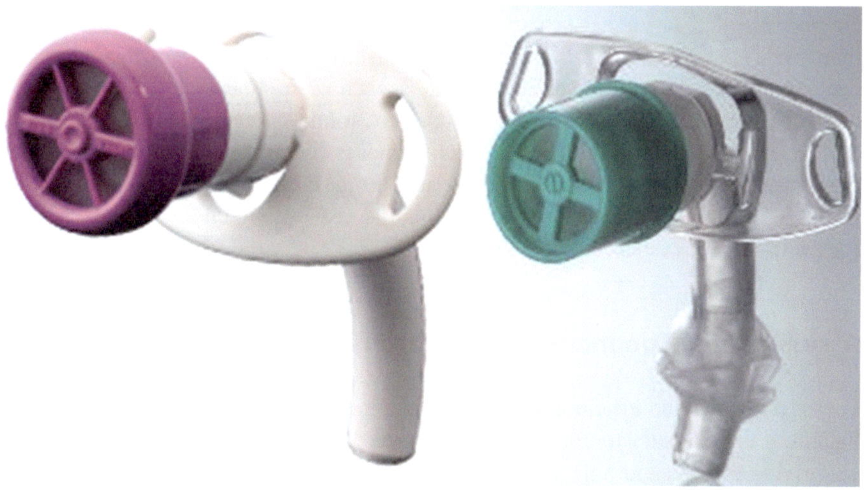

Fig. 4 Phonatory valve adapted to a plastic tracheostomy tube with or without a cuff (deflated)

quality, verified by both listeners and patients themselves, as reported in the literature. This presents the lowest rates of mechanical problems [22]. Speech valves are unidirectional, allowing air to be drawn through the tracheostomy tube during inspiration (with small inspiratory pressure), and have an automatic closure mechanism, which directs airflow into the upper airway during the expiratory phase, allowing glottic coaptation (voice).

The speech valve is a resource that can be used to contribute to decannulation [23, 24]. In patients who breathe spontaneously and tolerate tracheostomy occlusion, a speech valve may be adapted to occlude the tube orifice while the cuff is being deflated.

With the use of a unidirectional speech valve, fenestrated tubes, or occlusion of the tracheostomy, the adequacy of phonation and swallowing in tracheostomized patients occurs through the re-establishment of air passage through the glottis, increased subglottic pressure, and stimulation of peripheral and central nerve endings [25]. For better tolerance of a speech valve and to avoid muscular effort, it is advisable to replace the tube of the tracheostomy with another that has a size number 1–2 units smaller, reducing the expiratory resistance (although the inspiratory force becomes increased) and also improving the handling of secretions, which must be expectorated by the airways naturally [23].

The occlusion of the tracheostomy using a phonatory valve not only promotes more favorable swallowing but also favors the re-establishment of the patient's oral communication [7]. The benefits are related to increased ventilation and blood oxygenation, air filtration preventing infections, decreased secretions, increased olfactory sensation, and decreased vocal effort, initiating or resuming speech with longer and stronger emissions, and also as an aid to the process of weaning from the ventilator and/or tracheostomy [24].

The unidirectional speech valve is associated with a reduction in the incidence and severity of aspiration of thin liquids, likely due to re-establishment of subglottic air pressure and laryngeal sensitization [25]. However, one study identified that there was no reduction in the incidence of aspiration due to tracheostomy tube occlusion and/or the use of a unidirectional speech valve. In this study, only a small number of speech–language pathologists were found to use a speech valve as a therapeutic resource, despite the numerous benefits cited in the literature. In view of these findings, it is assumed that there are limitations to the acquisition of this resource, from bureaucratic and financial points of view, which have repercussions for the use of the resource [26].

Assessment of Communication in the Presence of Tracheostomy

For an objective and efficient assessment of the communication of a tracheostomy patient, it is necessary to consider the cause of the need for the tracheostomy. The underlying disease and pulmonary clinical conditions are critical factors for understanding patient communication [7]. It is necessary to observe and investigate the following factors: alertness; linguistic–cognitive aspects (ability to understand and express the language of the patient) in which the means of communication is more effective in the absence of a laryngeal voice; the sensory and motor integrity of the phonoarticulatory, laryngeal, and pharyngeal organs; and the respiratory rate, heart rate, and oxygen saturation in different situations (open tracheostomy and during digital occlusion).

There is a need for multidisciplinary clarification of the risks and benefits of initiating tracheostomy occlusion training for the re-establishment of laryngeal functions such as breathing, swallowing, and phonation. If tracheostomy occlusion is well accepted, it should be indicated as early as possible for the return of laryngeal functions.

In cases where the aforementioned tests are negative, the speech–language pathologist should evaluate other forms of nonlaryngeal communication and orientate those involved regarding the use of sign language, orofacial mime, writing, laryngeal vibrator adaptation, indication for tracheoesophageal prosthesis, and/or alternative supplementary communication.

Oral Communication Therapy in the Presence of Tracheostomy

Tracheoesophageal Prosthesis

The use of a tracheoesophageal prosthesis is indicated for patients undergoing total laryngectomy due to head and neck cancer. The production of a tracheoesophageal voice is the most similar to a laryngeal voice, thus it is considered the gold standard. Some studies have shown that this prosthesis favors improvement in vocal rehabilitation after total laryngectomy. It yields a good-quality and socially acceptable voice when compared with the electronic larynx, and success rates are often higher than those of the esophageal voice (being 90% better) [27].

The choice of tracheoesophageal prosthesis should be based on three factors [28]:

- The patient's ability to manipulate the tracheostoma to sanitize the prosthesis
- The cost of the prosthesis
- The presence of a low-pressure valve on the prosthesis to make phonation easier

Implantation of a tracheoesophageal prosthesis is indicated for patients who are still motivated during rehabilitation for esophageal voice communication but are unable to develop it, preventing their return to family and social life. Before pursuing this indication, it is important that the individual be evaluated in several aspects, which include considering the existence (or not) of tracheal stenosis, manual ability of the individual to maintain the prosthesis and occlusion of the tracheostoma, motivation in relation to communication, absence of mental illness, tracheostoma diameter, and understanding of the anatomy and mode of operation of the prosthesis and the possibility of acquisition. However, some institutions offer all types of rehabilitation, including prostheses, for laryngectomized patients.

Contraindications to implantation of a prosthesis are severe stenosis (narrowing) of the pharyngoesophageal segment and/or tracheostoma, and radiotherapy at doses greater than 70 Gy for 7 weeks, increasing the risk of tissue necrosis in the fistula itself and the region surrounding the tracheoesophageal fistula, and making implantation inadvisable under these conditions (Figs. 5 and 6).

Vibrating Larynx or Electronic Larynx

The laryngeal vibrator or electronic larynx is a battery-powered amplifier, which emits a continuous sound wave. This sound vibration is transmitted to the bucconasopharyngeal resonator which, together with the articulatory organs, enables the patient to communicate. The voice is limited in terms of frequency, intensity, and modulation, with metallic, strident, and monotonous qualities. It is an excellent

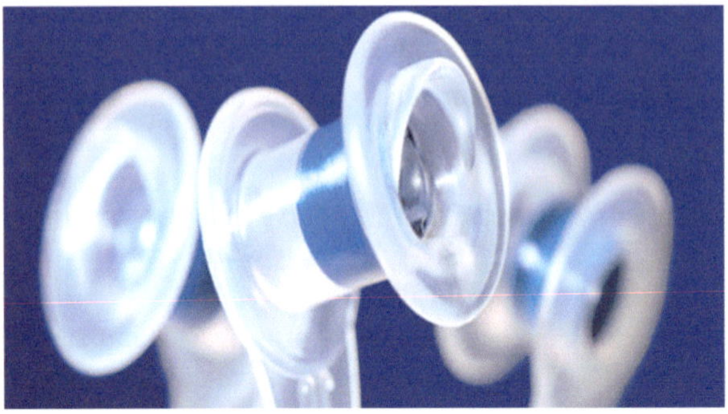

Fig. 5 Tracheoesophageal prosthesis

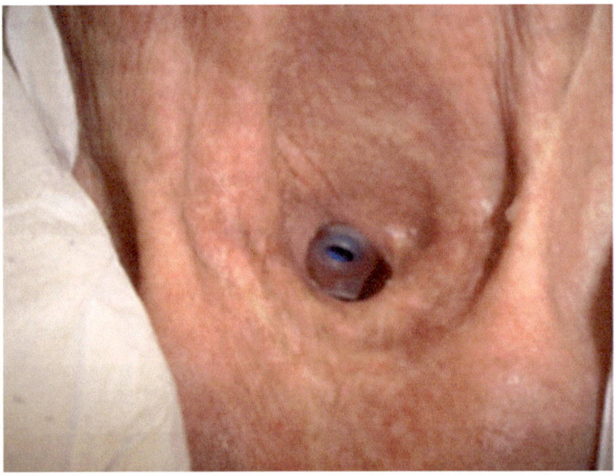

Fig. 6 Positioning the tracheoesophageal prosthesis in the stoma

alternative for immediate use, especially for voice professionals, providing postoperative emotional security, greater independence, and easy learning with minimal effort. However, it requires use of one hand, creates an electronic noise that can mask speech, requires a flexible cervical area for the propagation of sound toward the vocal tract, compromises differentiation of deep and sonorous sounds, and requires technical assistance, with high costs for maintenance and acquisition [29] (Figs. 7 and 8).

Augmentative and Alternative Communication

Not much attention has been given to work in the area of augmentative and alternative communication (AAC) with patients who use a tracheostomy tube, whether or not they are mechanically ventilated, even in the face of the "devastating" experience of losing their ability to speak.

Lack of knowledge about the assessment process, tool identification, appropriate strategies, and proper implementation of the AAC resource is still considered a significant barrier to patient care, as training and information on these resources are not available to most professionals who make up the "front line" in tracheostomy patient care. It is observed that some speech–language pathologists—although they

Fig. 7 Electronic larynx

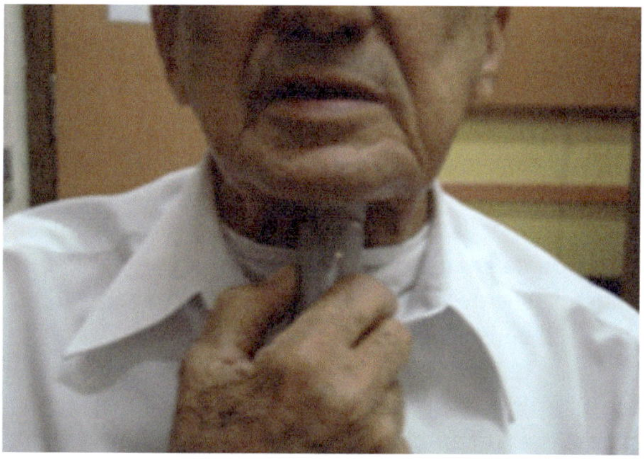

Fig. 8 Electronic larynx

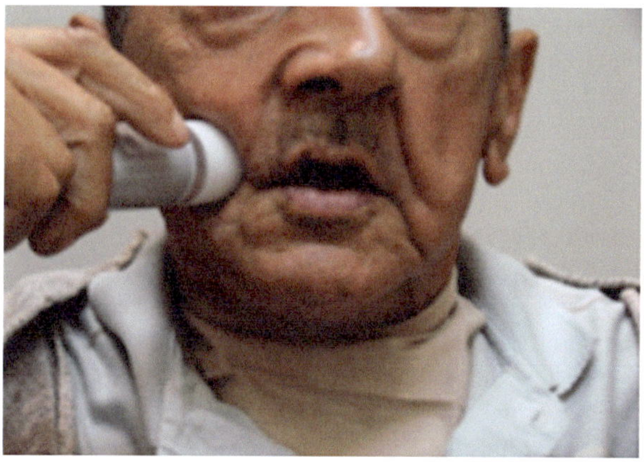

recognize the importance of working in the area of voice, speech, and language with patients deprived of oral communication—demonstrate that they are not familiar with the work of AAC in this context and are not prepared to act in situations that involve this type of work with tracheostomized patients.

In the same way that there are demands, space, and incentives for the training of speech–language pathologist specialists in the different areas of speech therapy, there is a need to rescue a generalist view based on a refined reflection on the possible speech–language interfaces in the care of the tracheostomy patient. First of all, speech–language pathology is a science with the aim to study human communication in regard to its development, improvement, disorders, and differences in relation to the aspects involved in central and peripheral auditory functions; vestibular, cognitive, oral, and written language; speech; fluency; orofacial voice functions; and swallowing [30]. Therefore, the attribution of the speech–language pathologist in this field legitimately needs to be expanded since there is a great demand from patients who are deprived of communication and are not candidates for immediate use of devices that enable the production of voice/speech.

In parallel, it is necessary to open space for clinicians and researchers in the language area to discuss the peculiarities inherent in the care of the tracheostomy patient, especially with regard to the diagnosis for which tracheostomy is indicated, types of mechanical ventilation and tracheostomy tubes, existent techniques, and devices that favor the biomechanics of voice and/or speech (digital tracheostoma occlusion, speech valve, tracheoesophageal prosthesis, electronic larynx, etc.). Prior knowledge of these practices will allow the speech–language pathologist a basis for work on augmentative and/or alternative communication with tracheostomized patients who need specific techniques and dialogue exchange strategies to take part in varied conversations in different contexts.

In the field of speech–language pathology, it is possible to say that there is a point of intersection between the specialties—dysphagia, voice, and oral language (speech)—so that certain therapeutic interventions are common to favoring different functions from the physiological point of view. We can mention the use of a speech valve, which is a device indicated to re-establish subglottic pressure in patients who use a tracheostomy tube and who are able to remain with a deflated cuff. This device is carefully indicated by speech–language pathologists who are specialists in dysphagia, since such an indication depends on the evaluation and the clinical reasoning pertinent to this field of action. In addition to providing an improvement in the biomechanics of swallowing, a speech valve allows redirection of airflow to the upper airway, favoring phonation and oral communication, when possible, for the patient [21]. Thus, it is clear that not all patients with tracheostomy tubes or even mechanical ventilation patients are candidates for the use of AAC resources, because in the first instance, the speech–language pathologist must assess the criteria for adapting a speech valve [31].

On the other hand, an AAC resource (temporary or permanent) can be indicated for individuals who use tracheostomy tubes under the conditions listed in Table 1.

Table 2 lists the clinical diagnoses of the most frequent communication disorders presented by tracheostomized patients in a private hospital in São Paulo, Brazil.

AAC is an area of interdisciplinary clinical activity that aims to attend to the important proportion of individuals with communicative needs, with the purpose of compensating (temporarily or permanently) for difficulties of individuals with

Table 1 Profiles of tracheostomized patient candidates for use of augmentative and alternative communication (AAC) resources [31–34]

Neurological disorders	Mechanical disorders	Physiological limitations
Cerebrovascular accident Dementia Cranioencephalic trauma Neuromuscular disorder Extrapyramidal disease Brain aneurysm Brain tumor Neurological syndrome Coma (minimum state of consciousness)	Spinal cord trauma Cardiac disorder Lung disease Respiratory disease Head and neck cancer	Lack of criteria for use of a speech valve, tracheoesophageal prosthesis, or electronic larynx Training and adaptation to these devices

Table 2 Characterization of communication disorders of hospitalized tracheostomized patients [31]

Neurological disorders	Mechanical disorders	Psychogenic disorders
Aphasia Oral communication disorder (right-hemisphere lesion) Cognitive–linguistic disorder	Dysarthrophonia	Cognitive–linguistic disorder
Pragmatic changes Speech apraxia Dysarthrophonia/jumbled speech	Aphonia (due to the presence of a tracheostomy tube)	Pragmatic changes

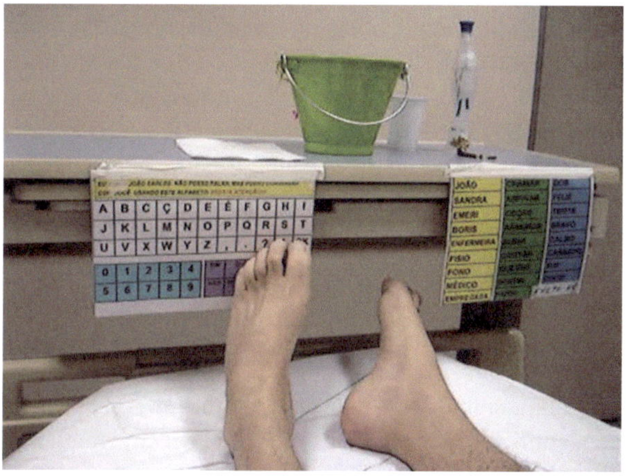

Fig. 9 Patient J.C., aged 56 years, male, diagnosed with amyotrophic lateral sclerosis, with a tracheostomy tube and dependent on mechanical ventilation, using alphabet and word plates through direct access with the right lower limb

severe speech disorders—that is, with speech, language, and writing impairments [35]. AAC is also considered one of the areas of assistive technology and comprises an integrated group of components, which include symbols, resources, techniques, and strategies used by the user for the communication process to occur. This area of knowledge of an interdisciplinary nature enables the involvement of users, family members, and many professionals such as occupational therapists, speech–language pathologists, physiotherapists, nurses, psychologists, social workers, physicians, prosthetists, engineers, architects, etc. [36] (Fig. 9).

This area of clinical practice is anchored in one of the theoretical presuppositions of language, thus it is important for the speech–language pathologist to know about these different conceptions to establish points of approximation and distance in their clinical practices.

Communication is the instrument of social interaction par excellence, which develops throughout life, through multiple relationships, and in continuous transformations, which can occur in verbal or nonverbal forms [37]. The verbal form can be transmitted by oral means (speech) or graphic means (writing), whereas the nonverbal form can be transmitted by means of paralinguistic elements (voice intonation) and/or extralinguistic elements (indicative, representative, or symbolic gestures and orofacial mime). Language can be defined as a dynamic and complex system of conventional symbols, which is used in different modalities for thought and communication, and which has integrated components: cognitive (attention, memory, perception, praxis), linguistic (phonological, morphological, syntactic, semantic), pragmatic (use of language in communication), and phonetic (in its acoustic and articulatory components) [38]. According to this conception, for the production of oral language (speech) to occur, cortical activation is necessary, besides the action of various combinations of contraction of the phonoarticulatory muscles to produce certain phonemes (speech sounds).

This theoretical assumption of language dialogues with the medical model found in the different health services, which has its recognized importance when it values the observable clinical findings and objectives, the complaint, the diagnosis, the pathology, the application of techniques, and the specific treatment, regardless of what the subject brings. To think of alternative communication in this conception is to consider a work marked by skill training, improvement of the use of the resource to guarantee greater communicative effectiveness, and development of teaching–learning strategies. This may be a path, but not the only one, as there are other aspects of the work that are inscribed in the dimensions of language functioning, such as each patient's mode of meaning (which depends on their life history), strategies to deal with situations of communication, discursive construction, and production of meaning (which is not subject to training, since it happens in the act and changes with each enunciation process) [39], as well as psychosocial and environmental factors, motivation, and social roles that determine the use of language and are fundamental in human interaction [40]. The relational model articulates these conceptions, so it proposes that the speech–language pathologist clarify the most objective questions of an organic nature, and at the same time contextualize these findings with knowledge about the interactional history of the patient [41]. From this point of view, it is not enough to collect the information by itself or to apply a certain therapeutic technique; it is also necessary to listen to the data given by the professional, whether verbal or nonverbal, and the articulation that can be established between them, aiming at not only the disease but also the subject who manifests the symptoms reported. In this model, listening to all of those involved in the process is fundamental, be they family members, caregiver(s), and/or the interdisciplinary team itself.

Partial loss or absence of oral communication of tracheostomized patients can directly impact the family, since these individuals often present with feelings of fear and insecurity and are unable to explicitly communicate their needs, doubts, and desires. Many relatives report that even when they are exhausted, they refuse to sleep because they think that if the patient calls, no one will be around to help, or because they think that the patient may feel abandoned.

Another barrier faced by the family is not knowing how to deal with the frustration of not understanding what the patient is talking about and not knowing how to use strategies that facilitate communication, which triggers wear for all of the people involved and can negatively impact the recovery of the individual [33].

In addition to the impact on the patient, the family, and the team, the patient who is unable to communicate also generates a cost increase to the paying source, since in this condition, if the patient is hospitalized, they may be hospitalized for a longer time and prone to "medical errors," often undergoing unnecessary use of sedation and medication for pain, in addition to having low adherence to treatment, due to the inability to get involved with the care team (make comments, ask questions, etc.).

Some studies show that hospitalized patients with access to communication receive less sedation, present clinical improvement, and have better satisfaction with the health plan, a shorter hospitalization time, more control and participation in the process of self-care, and better management of pain [43], noting that partial or total deprivation of communication may impact all patients, but the selection and implementation of AAC is not the same for everyone.

Among other measures adopted to improve communication, one study has shown that structured family care, in structured sessions with the participation of the interdisciplinary team, improved some aspects of client satisfaction, particularly in situations of decision making [44].

Due to the great demand of patients in this condition, it is necessary to increase the number of professionals working in the AAC area, to train and assist professionals who will offer AAC services to tracheostomized patients in situations of vulnerable communication, and to develop projects for the institution to include in its budget the acquisition of tools, in addition to the use of AAC strategies, which should be available immediately for assessment and intervention.

Proposals for Use of Augmentative and Alternative Communication for Tracheostomized Patients: Many individuals who use a tracheostomy tube with partial or total deprivation of oral communication can improve their social participation by increasing the frequency of their interactions and making decisions about their own lives when using some type of AAC resource.

In Brazil, work with AAC in tracheostomized patients is still little publicized and recognized, so it is incumbent upon each professional to identify and understand access barriers (physical, motor, cognitive, cultural, visual, and auditory) that make the participation of the patient in the recovery process unfeasible, but also to adopt intervention measures in the face of barriers to opportunities in terms of institutional policies, multidisciplinary practices, vocational training, and the use of resources in the environment.

The primary role of the speech–language pathologist is to provide the multidisciplinary team and family members with information, clarification, support, and specific indications on how best to communicate with the patient, as well as identifying and elaborating action plans against barriers to opportunities and access to the use of AAC. Thus, the professional must guarantee the right of communication of the important part of the population that needs these resources in the most complete way possible, as established by the American Speech–Language–Hearing Association (ASHA) [45], and the central focal point should be people, not resources [46, 47].

For selection of the AAC resource, it is important to consider several factors: the clinical profile; underlying disease; alert conditions; motor, perceptual and sensory conditions; presence of tracheostomy and mechanical ventilation (invasive and noninvasive); cognitive and language impairment; fatigue; prior user experience; support of communication partners; participation of a facilitator; adverse reactions to medications; educational level of patients; and environmental interference. Interventions in the AAC area vary according to the case analysis from an interdisciplinary point of view, and according to the clinical conditions presented by each patient, so that they meet the shared needs and expectations through dialogue with the candidate.

Regarding the evaluation procedures, the use of open or semistructured interviews, evaluations in functional and/or standardized situations, and protocols that investigate the linguistic–cognitive, sensory, motor skills, and communicative needs of the patient with a disorder of communication is recommended. The objectives of the evaluation are to adopt measures to eliminate communication barriers and facilitate the participation of users in dialogue situations with different speakers in different contexts, thus allowing them an active role in the recovery process, autonomy, and better professional/patient interaction, social integration, and quality of life. Permanent dialogue with the family, caregivers, and staff is fundamental and is part of the routine of the speech–language pathologist; as with communication, there can be various doubts and expectations that overlap in relation to the patient's speech recovery, e.g., will AAC solve the problem of patient communication; can AAC hinder the process of adaptation and training of voice and/or speech with other devices; will AAC prevent speech recurrence if the patient is decannulated; and will AAC minimize communication difficulties or will it leverage improvement of other skills? These questions are frequently asked at the outset by the multidisciplinary team and family members, and they deserve attention on the part of the speech–language pathologist, since all of those involved in this process must visualize that the resources are legitimate for the interactive and communicative processes; if this recognition does not exist, the procedures will not be effective, regardless of their importance and scope.

The aim of the intervention is to promote the development of communication so that people with complex communication needs can develop, reconstruct, or maintain communicative competence in their relationships, exchange information, and participate in social activities [46, 47].

In health services in general, there are simple tools and strategies available to improve patient communication, but these are generally not used (e.g., paper, pen, white board, etc.). The devices can be of low technology (e.g., use of indicative, representative, and symbolic gestures and orofacial expressions), medium technology (e.g., drawn and written graphic emissions, concrete objects, or boards with an alphabet, words, phrases, and pictograms), or high technology (e.g., vocalizers and computerized systems). The success and effectiveness of these interventions lie in the combination of nontechnological resources (linguistic, paralinguistic, and extralinguistic) associated with low-technology and/or high-technology resources, since the communicative situations vary according to the speaker, the extension and intention of the message, the environment, and the context. The indications for high-technology features for tracheostomized patients include different symbols, mode and access options (speed, paused/interruptions, and filtering), voice output options, message formulation, word prediction, storage, retrieval, and interconnectivity.

In this sense, we must consider the importance of multidisciplinary work in assistive technology, including (in addition to the speech–language pathologist) the occupational therapist and/or physiotherapist, to favor postural adequacy of the patient by providing accessibility of AAC devices and adaptation of equipment, the environment, and activities [36]. This considers that the indication for an appropriate AAC resource involves not only linguistic–cognitive criteria; articulatory competence (orofacial movement); and sensory, motor, and accessibility condition; but also a "task force" of several participants. This will ensure that:

- The communication of the individual is monitored.
- Referral for evaluation with the AAC resource is done in a timely manner.
- The indication for an AAC resource is accepted by the patient.
- Technology is acquired (purchased).
- Instructions for use are complete.
- Adaptations of the resource are made according to communication needs.

Considering the criteria of orofacial mobility (articulation) and the motor and accessibility profile, it is possible to group some patient candidates for the use of some devices and strategies in AAC:

- *Group 1: Preserved articulatory (orofacial) and manual function. Purpose:* To monitor communication and provide information on the possibilities of expanding the communicative function.
- *Group 2: Committed articulatory (orofacial) function, manual function, and global mobility preserved. Purpose:* Alphabetical supplementation, writing (portable), direct selection of low- and high-technology resources and calling devices (Figs. 10, 11, 12, 13, 14, 15, 16 and 17).
- *Group 3: Impaired articulatory (orofacial) function, preserved manual function, and mobility of other compromised structures. Purpose:* Similar to that of Group 2, except that the AAC features can be assembled and transported in a wheelchair or walker. Access to AAC and other assistive technology needs to be integrated.
- *Group 4: Articulatory (orofacial) function and manual function compromised; mobility present of some other structure of the body. Purpose:* Alternative access (pointer, eye scan, or trigger); not necessarily portable. Access to AAC and other assistive technology needs to be integrated (Figs. 18, 19, 20 and 21).
- *Group 5: All motor functions compromised. Purpose:* Indirect access (similar to that of Group 5). Access to AAC and other assistive technology needs to be integrated (Figs. 22, 23, 24, 25, 26, 27 and 28).

Patients who learn to use communication tools, such as boards with pictograms or words and simple communication devices, report improvement in satisfaction and comfort in comparison with care that lacks this support [48–50]

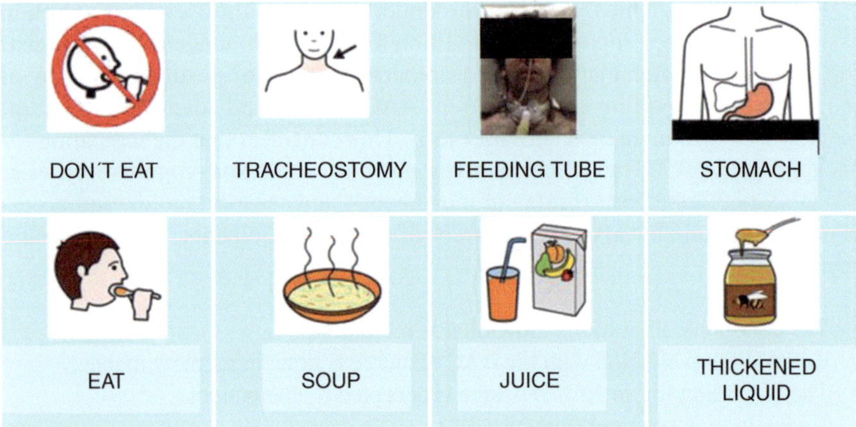

Fig. 10 Boards with pictograms or photographs aimed at self-care, basic needs, body/comfort, and personal interests

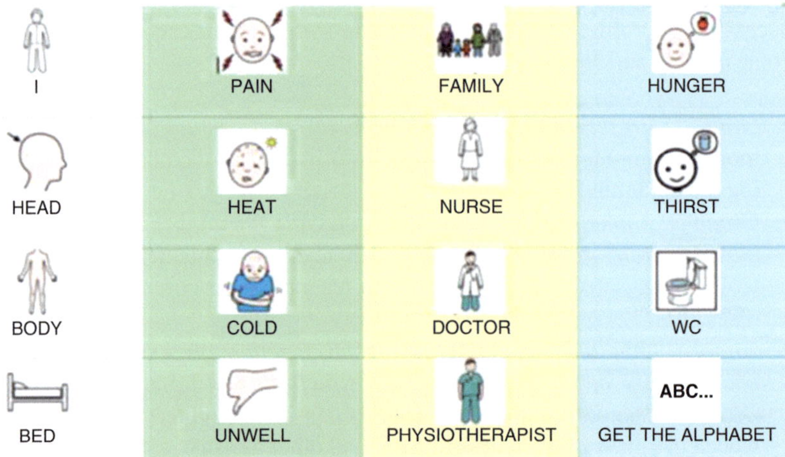

Fig. 11 Boards with pictograms or photographs aimed at self-care, basic needs, body/comfort, and personal interests

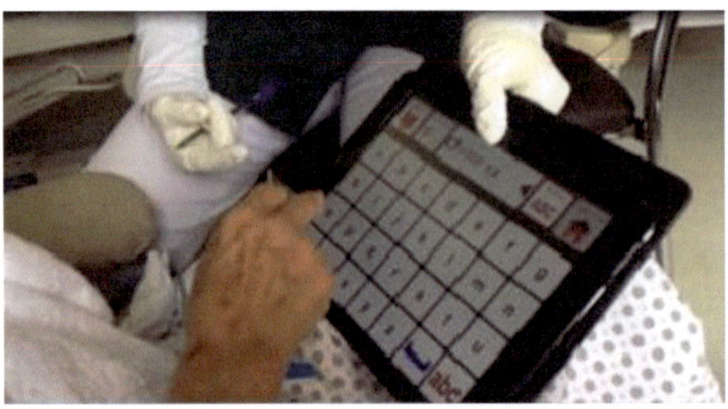

Fig. 12 SonoFlex for iPad and Android tablets (CIVIAM)

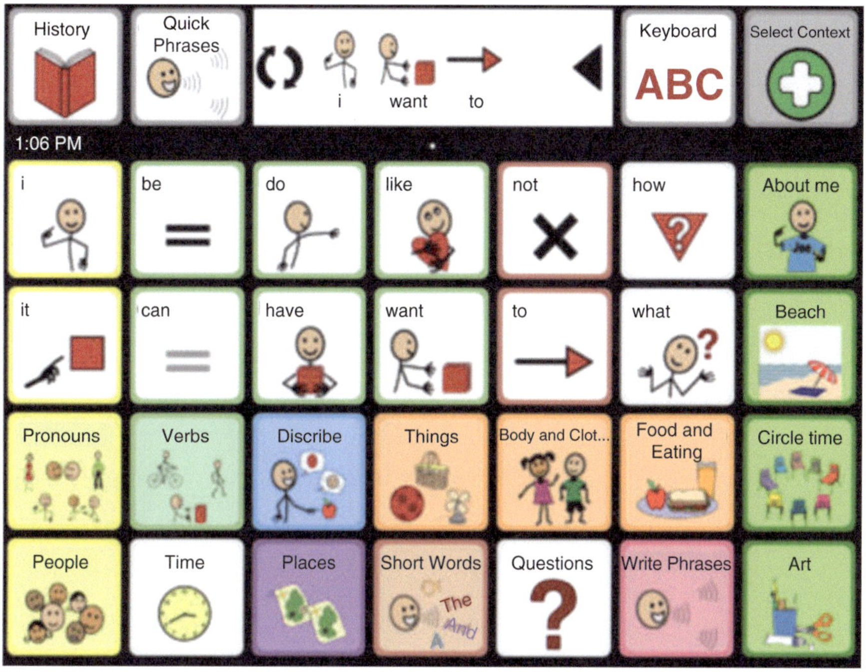

Fig. 13 SonoFlex for iPad and Android tablets (CIVIAM)

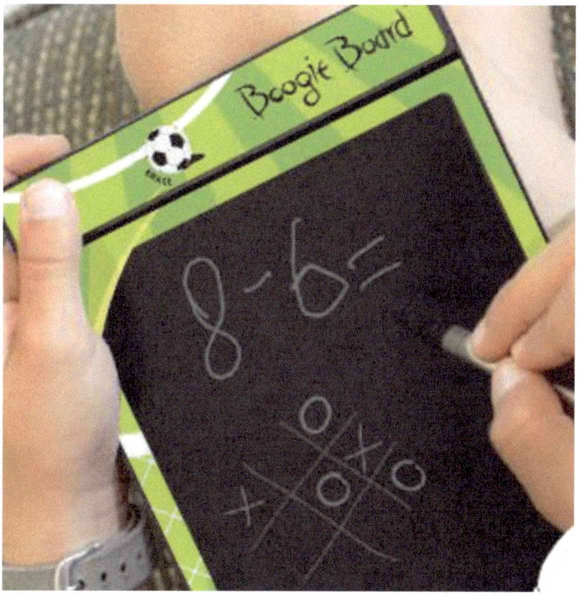

Fig. 14 Writing boards

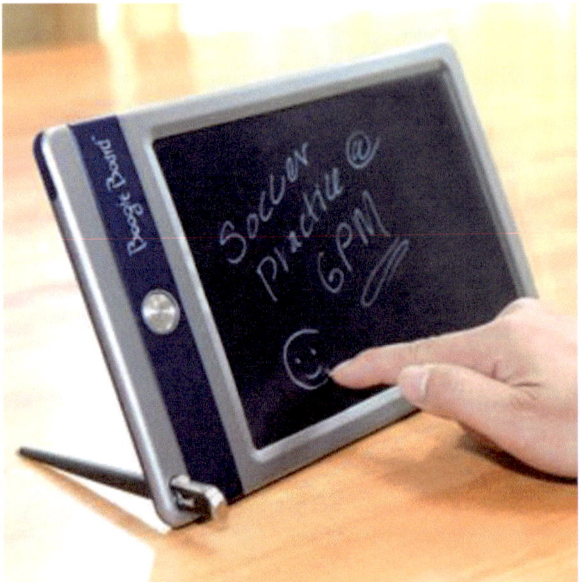
Boogie Board
Soccer practice @ 6PM

Fig. 15 Writing boards

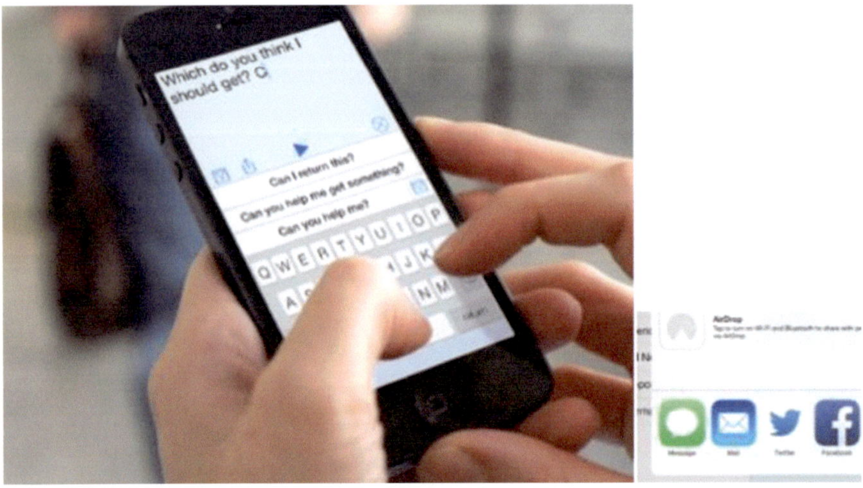
Which do you think I should get? C
Can I return this?
Can you help me get something?
Can you help me?

Fig. 16 Word predictor: *Proloquo 4 Text* (source: http://www.assistiveware.com/)

For AAC to succeed, sophisticated tools are not required. In addition to the necessary training for professionals and family members who accompany the patient in the hospital, at home, or in other places and contexts, the most important thing is to favor the patient with an "easier" form of communication, considering a simple resource for independent use by the user. More elaborate technology or techniques are indicated only for patients with learning ease.

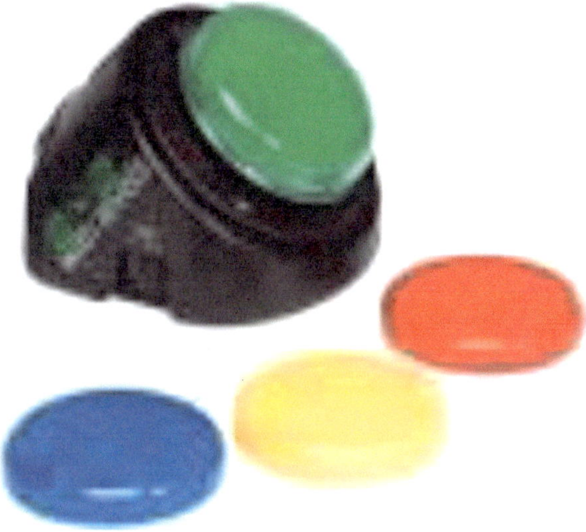

Fig. 17 Simple communicator: *Go Talk* (source: http://clik.com.br) [39]. The simple communicator can be used to call for attention, for social interactions, for participation in activities, and to establish cause and effect

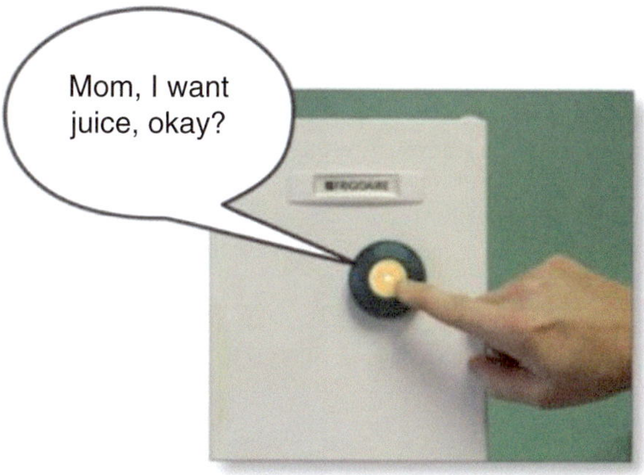

Fig. 18 Simple communicator: *Go Talk* (source: http://clik.com.br) [39]. The simple communicator can be used to call for attention, for social interactions, for participation in activities, and to establish cause and effect

Some situations that may limit work with AAC are [42]:

- Patients in the acute phase of an illness who require intensive multidisciplinary assistance for care
- High frequency of examinations, procedures, medical evaluations, and family visits
- Clinical instability of the patient
- Oscillation of the level of consciousness
- Short time frame for functional use

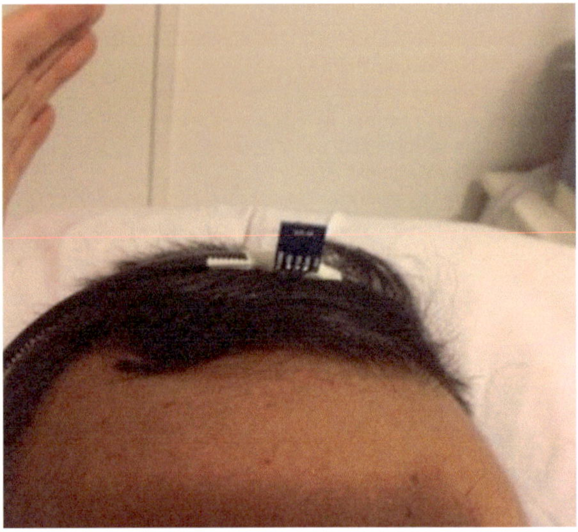

Fig. 19 Custom trigger integrated into a computerized alternative communication system. By an alphabetical auditory scan and cervical movement, the patient selects graphical images for writing on the computer

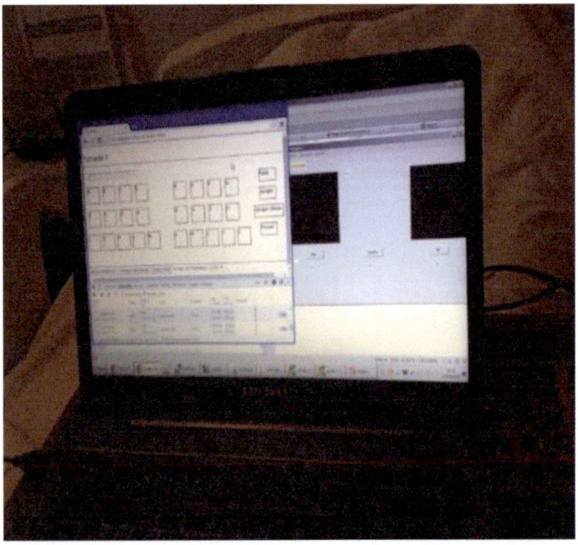

Fig. 20 Custom trigger integrated into a computerized alternative communication system. By an alphabetical auditory scan and cervical movement, the patient selects graphical images for writing on the computer

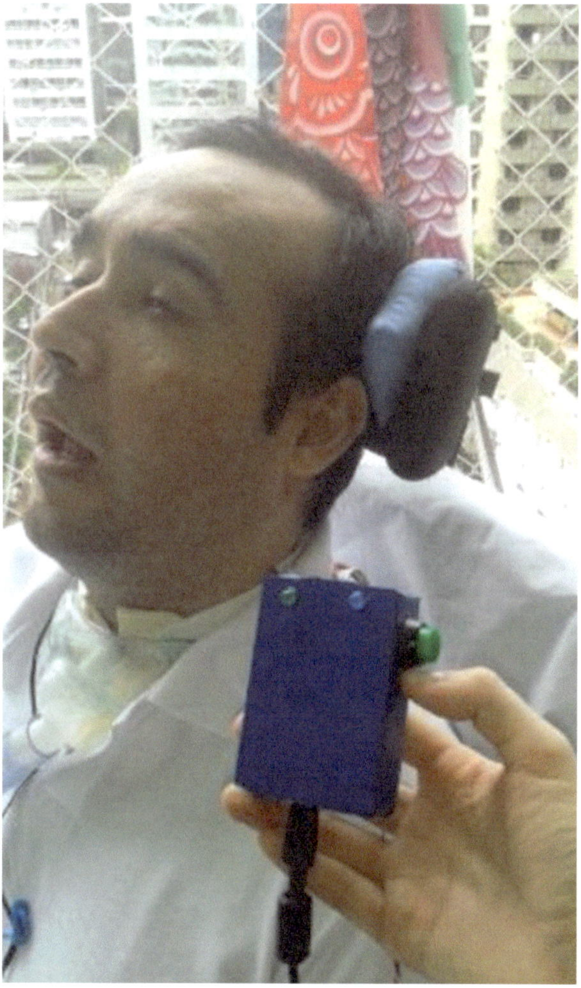

Fig. 21 Emergency call system adapted to a wheelchair, with a bell activated by a discreet cervical movement. It can be used as a trigger to be adapted to the computer

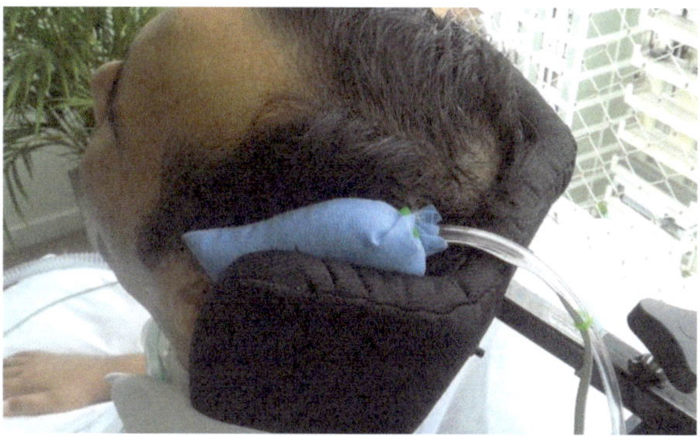

Fig. 22 Emergency call system adapted to a wheelchair, with a bell activated by a discreet cervical movement. It can be used as a trigger to be adapted to the computer

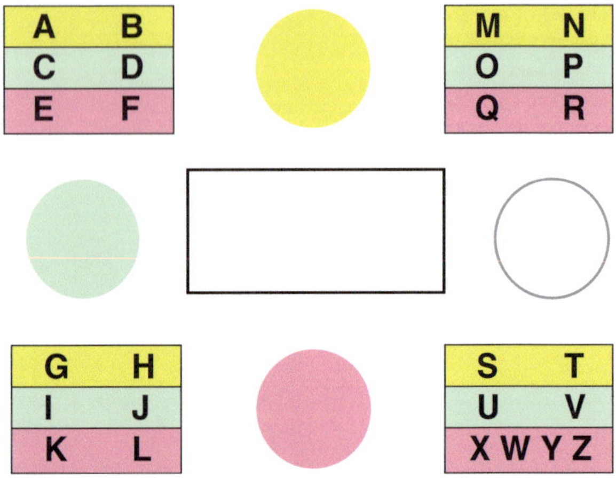

Fig. 23 *Speakbook*, developed by Patrick Joyce (source: http://www.speakbook.org/), accessed by visual scanning

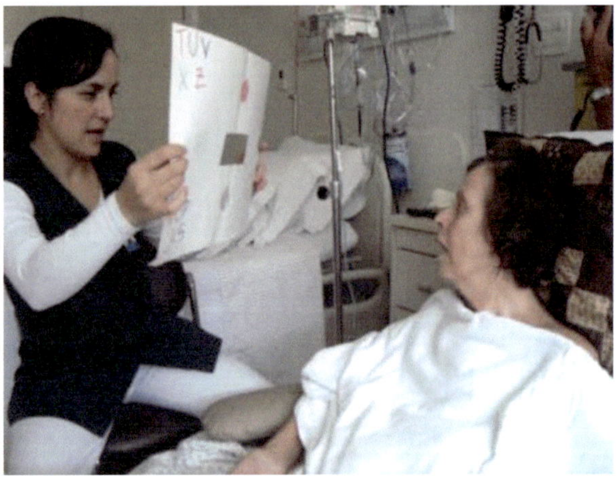

Fig. 24 *Speakbook*, developed by Patrick Joyce (source: http://www.speakbook.org/), accessed by visual scanning

Some studies have shown reasons why some patients with amyotrophic lateral sclerosis refuse to use AAC features [51]:

- Excessive concern of the patient with the evolution of the disease itself
- "Condition of immobility"
- Inappropriate recommendation of the type of communication system
- "Cultural" limitations
- Lack of guidance for family and professionals regarding the functional use of the communication system
- Associated cognitive impairment
- Expectations in communicating with the user
- User personality

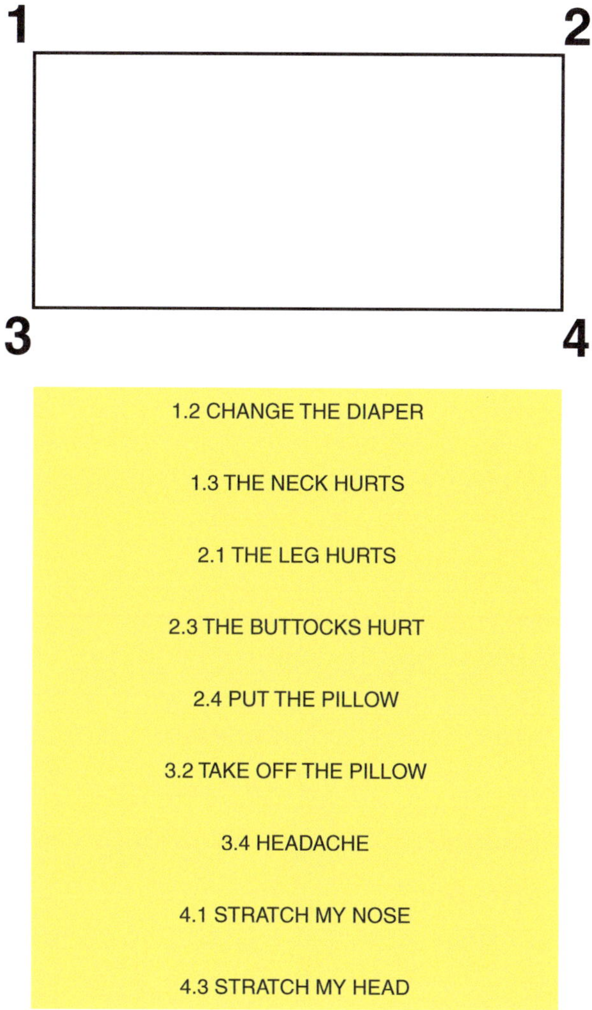

Fig. 25 Strategies for decoding by visual scanning (low technology)

Privileging the dialogue exchange between the patient and their other speakers in different places and contexts is considered a priority research topic. It is necessary that this teamwork be guided by a common assistance project, in which the professionals seek to develop an interaction action among themselves and with all of those involved in the AAC implementation proposal. For this, it is essential to develop communicative practice oriented toward mutual understanding of each other's knowledge and the interdisciplinary "exercise."

Conflict of Interest There are no commercial and/or financial interests on the part of the authors regarding the assistive devices presented in this work.

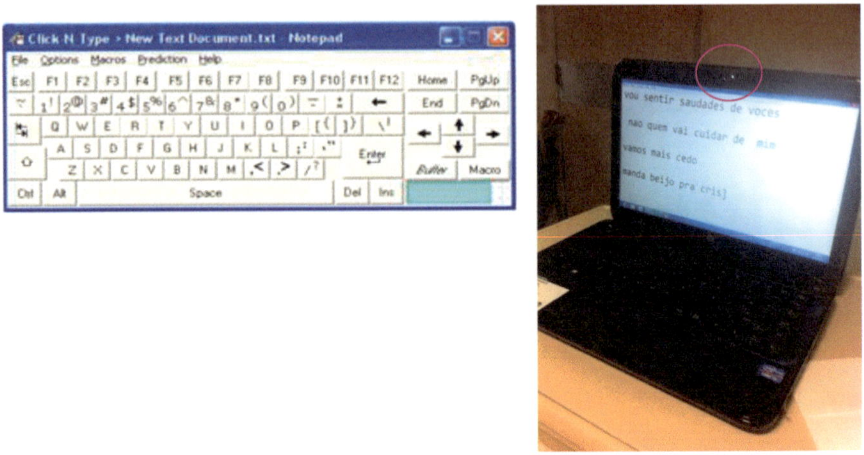

Fig. 26 *Click-N-Type* keyboard and camera mouse, used together with Windows® Notepad

ABOUT ME...

Name:	Soccer team:	Lengua:
Age:	Favorite odors:	Vocational:
Technology:	Favorite objects:	________
Favorite color:	Favorite book:	________
Music Style:	Hobby:	________
Favorite food:	School Education:	________

In spaces (____) other patient's preferences intensity can be filled.

Fig. 27 Plate fixed to the bedside of a young man diagnosed with cranioencephalic trauma, in a minimal state of consciousness in an intensive care unit, the purpose of which is to enhance the communicative intentions of the team and their relatives with the patient [39]

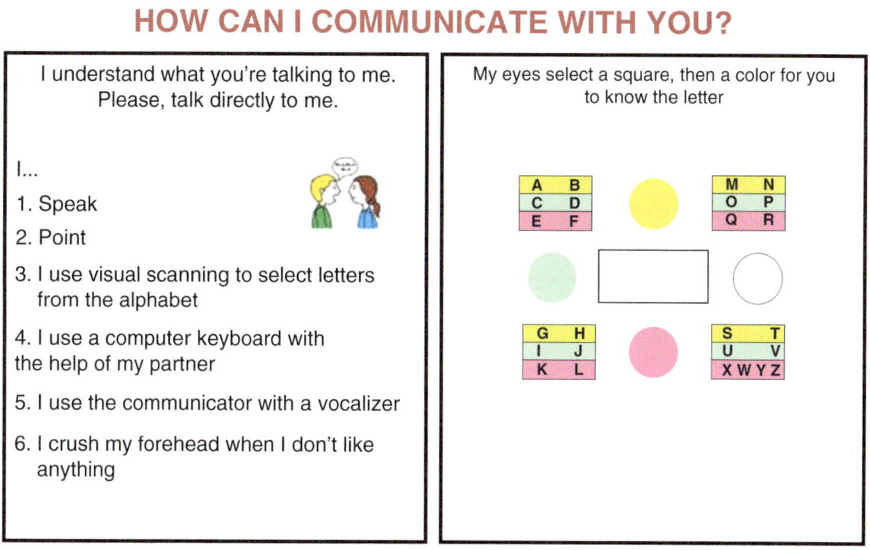

Fig. 28 Adhesive plate at the edge of the bed, used to identify the communication feature used by the patient, allowing easy access and viewing by communication partners [39]

Consent for Publication Informed consent was obtained from any individual participant for whom identifying information is included in this article.

References

1. Ferreira RB. Impacto das Traqueostomias nas Funções de Deglutição, Respiração e Fala. Trabalho de conclusão do curso de pós-graduação lato sensu em Motricidade Orofacial: Enfoque em Disfagia e Atuação em Âmbito Hospitalar pela Universidade Tuiuti do Paraná. Paraná; 2010.
2. Macedo E, Gomes GF, Furkim AM. Manual de Cuidados do Paciente com Disfagia. São Paulo: Lovise; 2000.
3. Mendes F, Ranea P, Oliveira ACT Protocolo de desmame e decanulação de traqueostomia. Revista UNILUS Ensino e Pesquisa, vol. 10, n. 20, jul./set. 2013, ISSN (impresso): 1807–8850, ISSN (eletrônico): 2318–2083.
4. Higgins DM, Maclean JC. Dysphagia in the patient with a tracheostomy: six cases of inappropriate cuff deflation or removal. Heart Lung. 1997;26(3):215–20.
5. Mendes TAB, Cavalheiro LV, Arevalo RT, Sonegth R. Estudo preliminar sobre a proposta de um fluxograma de decanulação em traqueostomia com atuação interdisciplinar. Einstein. 2008;6(1):1–6.
6. Ghion LG. Traqueostomia e válvula de fala. In: Furkim AM, Santini CS, editors. Disfagias orofaríngeas. 2nd ed. São Paulo: Pró-Fono; 2008. p. 49–54.
7. Barros APB, Portas JG, Queija DS. Implicações da traqueostomia na comunicação e na deglutição. Rev Bras Cir Cabeça Pescoço. 2009;38(3):202–7.
8. Logemann JA, Pauloski BR, Colangelo L. Light digital occlusion of the tracheostomy tube: a pilot study of effects on aspiration and biomechanics of the swallow. Head Neck. 1998;20(1):52–7.

9. Padovani AR, Andrade CRF. Perfil funcional da deglutição em unidade de terapia intensiva clínica. Einstein. 2007;5(4):358–62.
10. Almeida ST. Detecção dos sons da deglutição através da ausculta cervical. In: Jacobi JS, Levy DS, LMC S, editors. Disfagia. Rio de Janeiro: Avaliação e Tratamento, Revinter; 2003. p. 373–81.
11. Lundy DS, Casiano RR, Shatz D, Reisberg M, Xue JW. Laryngeal injuries after short- versus long-term intubation. J Voice. 1998;12(3):360–5.
12. Ellis PD, Bennett J. Laryngeal trauma after prolonged endotracheal intubation. J Laryngol Otol. 1977;91(1):69–74. 21
13. Goldsmith T. Evaluation and treatment of swallowing disorders following endotracheal intubation and traqueostomy. Int Anesthesiol Clin. 2000;38(3):219–42.
14. Shaker R, Milbrath M, Ren J, Campbell B, Toohill R, Hogan W. Deglutitive aspiration in patients with tracheostomy: effect of tracheostomy on the duration of vocal cord closure. Gastroenterology. 1995;108(5):1357–60.
15. Sasaki CT, Suzuki M, Horiuchi M, Kirchner JA. The effect of tracheostomy on the laryngeal closure reflex. Laryngoscope. 1977;87(9 Pt 1):1428–33.
16. Dikeman K, Kazandjian M. Communication and swallowing management of trachestomized and ventilator dependent adults. San Diego: Singular; 1995.
17. Sugeno LA, Pires E. Uso do teste de corante azul na avaliação da deglutição. In: Furkim AM, Rodrigues KA, editors. Disfagias nas Unidades de Terapia Intensiva, vol. 12. São Paulo: Editora Roca; 2014. p. 133–8.
18. Furkim AM, Silva RG. Programas de reabilitação em disfagia neurogênica. Frôntis Editorial: São Paulo; 1999.
19. Leder SB. Perceptual rankings of speech quality produced with one-way tracheostomy speaking valves. J Speech Hear Res. 1994;37:1308–12.
20. Fernández-Carmona A, Peñas-Maldonado L, Yuste-Osorio E, Díaz-Redondo A. Exploración y abordaje de disfagia secundaria a vía aérea artificial. Med Intensiva. 2012;36(6):423–33.
21. Rodrigues KA, Ghion G, Gonçalves MIR. Válvula de Fala Passy-Muir. In: Furkim AM, Rodrigues KA, editors. Disfagias nas Unidades de Terapia Intensiva, vol. 18. São Paulo: Editora Roca; 2014. p. 201–16.
22. Ding R, Logemann JA. Swallow physiology in patients with trach cuff inflated or deflated: a retrospective study. Head Neck. 2005;27(9):809–13.
23. Leder SB, Joe JK, Hill SE, Traube M. Effect of tracheotomy tube occlusion on upper esophageal sphincter and pharyngeal pressures in aspirating and nonaspirating patients. Dysphagia. 2001;16(2):79–82.
24. Leder SB, Ross DA, Burrell MI, Sasaki CT. Tracheotomy tube occlusion status and aspiration in early postsurgical head and neck cancer patients. Dysphagia. 1998;13(3):167–71.
25. Leder SB. Effect of a one-way tracheotomy speaking valve on the incidence of aspiration in previously aspirating patients with tracheotomy. Dysphagia. 1999;14(2):73–7.
26. Leder SB, Ross DA. Investigation of the causal relationship between tracheotomy and aspiration in the acute care setting. Laryngoscope. 2000;110(4):641–4.
27. Healton JM, Parker AJ. In vitro comparison of the Groningen high resistance, Groningen low resistance and the Provox speaking valves. J Laryngol Otol. 1994;108:321–4.
28. Lennie TA, Christiman SK, Jadack RA. Educational needs and altered eating habits following a total laryngectomy. Oncol Nurs Forum. 2001;28:667–74.
29. Lerman JW. The artificial larynx. In: Salmon SJ, Mounts KH, editors. Alaryngeal speech rehabilitation. Austin: Pro-Ed; 1991. p. 27–45.
30. Conselho Federal de Fonoaudiologia. Lei Federal 6965/81. 2004.
31. Farias LP. A comunicação vulnerável do paciente na unidade de terapia intensiva e a comunicação suplementar e alternativa. In: RYS C, Reily L, Moreira EC, editors. Comunicação Alternativa: ocupando territórios. São Carlos: Marquezine & Manzini: ABPEE; 2015. p. 171–94.
32. Hafsteindóttir TB. Patients experiences off communication during the respirator treatment period. Intensive Crit Care Nurs. 1996;12:261–71.

33. Magnus VS, Turkington L. Communication interaction in ICU: patient and staff experiences and perceptions. Intensive Crit Care Nurs. 2006;22:167–80.
34. Correia SM, Mansur LL. Abordagem da Comunicação e da Linguagem em pacientes na Unidade de Terapia Intensiva. In: Furkim AM, Rodrigues KA, editors. Disfagias nas Unidades de Terapia Intensiva, vol. 21. São Paulo: Editora Roca; 2014. p. 241–9.
35. Beukelman D, Mirenda P. Augmentative and alternative communication: management of severe communication in children and adults. Baltimore: Paul H Brookes Publishing Co; 1998.
36. Bersch, RCR, Pelosi MB. Portal para ajudas técnicas.Tecnologia Assistiva: recursos de acessibilidade ao computador. Brasília: MEC/SEESP; 2007. http://www.educadores.diaadia.pr.gov.br/arquivos/File/pdf/tecnologia_assistiva.pdf.
37. Rabadán O. Lenguaje y envejecimiento. Bases para la intervención: Barcelona; 1998.
38. American Speech–Language–Hearing Association Committee on Language. Definition of language. ASHA 1983; 25: 44.
39. Duarte EN. Linguagem e comunicação suplementar e alternativa na clínica fonoaudiológica. (Dissertação de Mestrado). São Paulo: Pontifícia Universidade Católica; 2005.
40. Mansur LL, Radanovic M. Neurolinguística—princípios para a prática clínica. Edições Inteligentes: São Paulo; 2004. p. 343.
41. Spinelli M. Distúrbios no desenvolvimento da linguagem. In: Assumpção Jr F, editor. Psiquiatria da Infância e da Adolescência. Santos: São Paulo; 1994.
42. Costello JM, Santiago R. AAC assessment and intervention in the intensive care/acute care settings: from referral through continuum of care. Lisboa: ISAAC Bienal Conference; 2014.
43. Happ MB, Roesch TK, Garrett K. Electronic voice-output communication aids for temporarily non speaking patients in a medical intensive care unit: a feasibility study. Heart Lung. 2004;33(2):92–101.
44. Jacobowski NL, Girard TD, Mulder JA, et al. Communication in critical care: family rounds in the intensive care unit. Am J Crit Care. 2010;19:421–30.
45. American Speech–Language–Hearing Association. Roles and responsibilities of speech–language pathologists with respect to augmentative and alternative communication: technical report. ASHA Supplement. 2004; 24:1–18. http://www.asha.org/policy/PS2005-00113.htm.
46. Light J, McNaughton D. Putting people first: re-thinking the role of technology in augmentative and alternative communication intervention. Augment Altern Commun. 2013;29(4):299–309.
47. Chun RYS, Romano N, Zerbeto AB, Moreira EC. Comunicação Suplementar e/ou Alternativa no Brasil: Ampliação de Territórios e Saberes Científicos e Locais. In: RYS C, Reily L, Moreira EC, editors. Comunicação Alternativa: ocupando territórios. São Carlos: Marquezine & Manzini: ABPEE; 2015. p. 17–37.
48. Patak L, Gawlinski A, Fung NI, et al. Patients' reports off health care practitioner interventions that are related to communication during mechanical ventilation. Heart Lung. 2004;33:308–21.
49. Costello JM. AAC intervention in critical care unit: the Children's Hospital Boston model. AAC. 2000;16(3):137–53.
50. Stovsky B, Rudy E, Dragonette P. Comparison of two types of communication methods used after cardiac surgery with patients with endotracheal tubes. Heart Lung. 1988;17:281–9.
51. Ball LJ, Beukelman DR, Pattee GL. Communication effectiveness of individuals.with amyotrophic lateral sclerosis. J Commun Disord. 2004;37(3):197–215.

Index

T.P. de Farias (ed.), *Tracheostomy*, https://doi.org/10.1007/978-3-319-67867-2

Q

R

S

U

V

W

MIX
Papier aus verantwortungsvollen Quellen
Paper from responsible sources
FSC® C105338

If you have any concerns about our products,
you can contact us on
ProductSafety@springernature.com

In case Publisher is established outside the EU,
the EU authorized representative is:
Springer Nature Customer Service Center GmbH
Europaplatz 3, 69115 Heidelberg, Germany

Printed by Libri Plureos GmbH
in Hamburg, Germany